Principles of
Human

Principles of Human Nutrition

Second edition

Martin Eastwood
Edinburgh, UK

Blackwell
Science

© 2003 by Blackwell Science Ltd,
a Blackwell Publishing Company

Editorial Offices:
9600 Garsington Road, Oxford, OX4 2DQ, UK
 Tel: 01865 776868
Blackwell Publishing, Inc., 350 Main Street, Malden,
MA 02148-5018, USA
 Tel: +1 781 388 8250
Iowa State Press, a Blackwell Publishing Company,
2121 State Avenue, Ames, Iowa 50014-8300, USA
 Tel: +1 515 292 0140
Blackwell Publishing Asia Pty Ltd,
550 Swanston Street, Carlton South,
Victoria 3053, Australia
 Tel: +61 (0)3 9347 0300
Blackwell Wissenschafts Verlag, Kurfürstendamm 57,
10707 Berlin, Germany
 Tel: +49 (0)30 32 79 060

First edition published 1997 by Chapman & Hall
This edition first published 2003 by
Blackwell Science Ltd

Library of Congress
Cataloging-in-Publication Data
is available

0-632-05811-0

A catalogue record for this title is available from the
British Library

Set in Times and produced by Gray Publishing,
Tunbridge Wells, Kent
Printed and bound in Great Britain by
The Bath Press, Bath

For further information on
Blackwell Publishing, visit our website:
www.blackwellpublishing.com

Contents

Acknowledgements

While the responsibility for this book is entirely mine, there are many people who have given help and encouragement: Neil Eastwood, Gill Poole, Janet Lambert, Ann de Looy, Bizan Pourkomailian, Rosalind Skinner and Jon Warner.

I am grateful to Nigel Balmforth at Blackwell for his kindness, understanding and support during the preparation of this new edition. Also his very supportive staff. Robert Gray and his staff have been so helpful during the production of this book.

*This book is dedicated to Jenny for all
the reasons she knows and without
whom it would not have been possible.*

1

Introduction and overview

This book looks at nutrition as an exciting discipline that draws on all branches of biology. Nutrition is both an art and a science: it observes, measures and tries to explain the constantly changing process of the optimal mix of chemicals necessary for the functioning of an individual at all stages of life.

This book is written at a number of levels to encompass:

- traditional nutrition (Chapters 2–6, 8–17, 39–45)
- evolving nutrition (Chapters 20, 22–26, 31–37, 46)
- complex concepts, which although not currently central will influence the future of nutrition: an awareness of these will be necessary for the next generation of nutritionists (Chapter 7, and parts of Chapters 11, 18, 19, 21, 27–30, 38).

Take what is appropriate for your requirements at different stages of your development in nutrition.

The selection, processing and manner of eating food will be strongly influenced by what is available and by the history, social stability and economy of the community. What and how a person eats is significantly affected by their family background and traditions, although travel is increasingly changing food choices. War, pestilence and famine can restrict food availability, and food may also be contaminated by pollutants from the environment.

Being able to eat optimal amounts is dependent on agriculture and the political, educational and social organisation in which the person lives. The chemical substances should be available in optimal amounts and in an attractive form for metabolism. Nutrition identifies, measures and recommends optimal dietary intakes of the nutrient chemicals in health and disease.

All living creatures require a range of dietary chemicals for metabolism, growth and activity. These chemicals are obtained from a range of sources. The digestion, absorption and metabolism of ingested nutrients are determined in each individual by many factors, including inherited constitution, gender, age, activity, growth, fecundity and lactation. A person needs an adequate energy intake as well as essential nutrients to provide for the needs and control of a genetically determined constitution (genome), which dictates protein and enzyme structure and hence metabolism. This brings nutrition to a central role in the story. The synthesis, maintenance, functioning and control of the protein complex and hence overall metabolism rely on ingested nutrients.

This book is written in the belief that the basis of nutrition lies in molecular biology, genetic make-up, biochemistry and physiology. Even the mysteries of the cooking art are dependent on physicochemical transformations of raw food into available edible food.

The book is divided into seven parts.

Parts I and II deal with food in the community. The first part deals with the historical influences that decide what food a community eats and how it is cooked. This is followed by a description of those environmental factors that can adversely affect food availability. Part II looks at the calculation of how much food a community requires and actually eats. The remaining parts deal with the individual.

Part III looks at how a person metabolises nutrients in an individual manner dictated by genetic make-up, then Part IV describes the measurement of the individual nutritional status.

Part V describes the core nutrients, essential, non-essential and non-nutrients, and Part VI their selection for eating, ingestion and subsequent digestion, absorption and metabolism. Part VII looks at special nutritional requirements in the normal condition and for some specific diseases.

At the end of each part there are key points for understanding and learning, and thinking points. Important references are listed at end of each chapter.

Some companion material relating to this book will be available on Blackwell Publishing's web pages: please look at details of the book, which can be found on the publisher's website: www.blackwellpublishing.com.

LITERATURE

The enjoyable and productive analysis of the literature is important, and there are many great books and journals. The following may be of help and interest to the reader:

- **Biological dictionary**
  Oxford Dictionary of Biochemistry and Molecular Biology (1997). Oxford University Press, Oxford.
- **Nutrition reference books**
  Sadler, M.J., Strain, J.J. and Caballero, B. (eds) (1999) *Encyclopedia of Human Nutrition*. Academic Press, San Diego, CA.
- **Biochemistry and biology reference books**
  Nelson, D.L. and Cox, M.M. (eds). (2000) *Lehninger's Principles of Biochemistry*, 3rd edn. Worth, New York.
- Lodish, H., Berk, A., Zipursky, S.L. *et al.* (eds) (2000) *Molecular Cell Biology*, 4th edn. WH Freeman, New York.
  Jones, L. and Atkins, P. (2000) *Chemistry, Molecules, Matter and Change*. WH Freeman, New York.
- **Journals**
  American Journal of Clinical Nutrition, British Journal of Medicine, British Medical Journal, Nutrition Journal, Nutrition Review, New England Journal of Medicine, Science, Annual Review of Nutrition, British Journal of Nutrition, European Journal of Clinical Nutrition, Lancet, Nature and *Proceedings of the Nutrition Society.*

- **The Internet**
  The manner in which written information is handed on is changing rapidly with the availability of the World Wide Web. The printed textbook can be seen as a primer, an introduction at varying levels of sophistication. From this sound knowledge base educated forays can be made into the Internet for retrieval of information. This book is intended to provide a good basic knowledge for such rewarding searches. It is recommended that this book is supplemented by using Medline and other searches, e.g. Google or Metacrawler. These are a starter pack and it is suggested that readers develop their own list of favourite websites which can be upgraded. The website associated with this book will be kept up to date with new references and links. Navigating around the Internet is facilitated by the use of helpful search engines. Even so, the top 11 search engines only reach 42% of the Web. The search engines can be based on the directory model placing sites into categories and subcategories. This requires human input and has the potential for error. 'Robots', 'spiders' and 'crawlers' navigate through the following links pages and return to the database with the result.

  Specialist sites dealing with a subject are more specific, e.g. PubMed and Medline. PubMed was developed by the National Library of Medicine and developed in conjunction with publishers of biomedical literature as a search tool for accessing literature citations and linking to full-text journals at websites of participating publishers.

  Medline is the National Library of Medicine's premier bibliographic database covering the fields of medicine, nursing, dentistry, veterinary medicine, the health-care system and the pre-clinical sciences. Medline contains bibliographic citations and author abstracts from more than 4000 biomedical journals published in the USA and 70 other countries. The file contains over 11 million citations dating back to the mid-1960s. However, it is important to appreciate that the citations miss the massive literature preceding the 1960s and these have to be traced by traditional library methods. Coverage is world-wide, but most records are from English-language sources or have English abstracts.

OVERVIEW

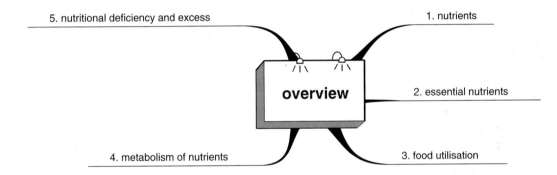

Fig. 1.1 Chapter outline.

NUTRIENTS

A definition of a nutrient is any chemical substance that can be used by an organism to sustain its metabolic activities. These metabolic activities in humans and other animals include the provision of energy, growth, renewal of tissues, reproduction and lactation.

The status of some chemicals as nutrients is assured: amino acids, carbohydrates, essential fatty acids, vitamins and trace elements. Other chemicals, such as dietary fibre and secondary plant metabolites, are part of the food but may not so readily be classified as nutrients.

ESSENTIAL NUTRIENTS

Some nutrients are essential in that these molecules cannot be synthesised within the body and can only be provided by the diet. Such essential nutrients provide for metabolic processes: vitamins, e.g. ascorbic acid, and trace elements, e.g. selenium; and for structure, e.g. proteins, essential amino acids, vitamins and trace elements.

The science of nutrition is devoted to defining requirements for essential nutrients, amino acids, essential fatty acids, vitamins and trace elements. Recommendations for daily requirements of nutrients made by expert committees are dependent on diverse factors such as growth, pregnancy and illness and are only carefully determined approximations. Implicit in the requirement for essential dietary constituents is that the human race is not independent of the environment. Thus, people are part of a food chain as recipients or producers of food.

FOOD UTILISATION

An important aspect of nutrition is the availability of dietary sources of nutrients. Causes of dietary deficiencies range from a lack of all nutrients (famine), to absence or omission of individual food items from the diet for social, economic, cultural, religious or personal reasons. Nutrients may not be absorbed from the intestine in some illnesses. A deficiency or excess of overall calorie intake or of individual nutrients may result in nutritional disorders.

Ingested food is broken down to chemicals of a molecular size that is readily absorbed and utilised by the body. The process of absorption is dictated by the nutrient needs of the body and bioavailability value.

> **Bioavailability** is a measure of the relative amount of the ingested nutrient that is absorbed from the intestinal content and reaches the systemic circulation. It is described as the rate and extent to which the nutrient is absorbed and becomes available to the body's metabolic processes.

In general, energy-providing nutrients are readily absorbed and have a high bioavailability value, whereas there are more controls on the absorption of micronutrients and their bioavailability value is lower and more variable. Some nutrients, e.g. divalent cations, calcium and magnesium, are only absorbed in an amount necessary for the needs of the body, as an excess can be toxic.

Waste products of metabolism are excreted in breath (carbon dioxide), urine [in general, water-soluble compounds of molecular weight less than 300 Daltons (Da: a unit of measure of atomic and molecular mass)] and bile (in general, fat-soluble, molecular weight more than 300 Da). The accu-

mulation of metabolic waste products has disadvantageous effects on growth, metabolism and well-being.

Nutrients contribute to bodily needs in several ways:

- provision of energy
- creation of structure
- provision of essential small molecular substances that the body cannot synthesise.

Some nutrients are sources of carbon and nitrogen, which pass into the metabolic pool to meet the body's general needs, e.g. carbohydrates, fats and amino acids. Carbohydrates and lipids are necessary fuels for metabolic activity, to a variable extent for structure and in some instances in the synthesis of hormones. The whole range of amino acids is relevant for adequate structural growth. Amino acids may also be utilised at times of nutritional deprivation as a source of energy.

METABOLISM OF NUTRIENTS

The metabolism of nutrients by enzymes is dictated by the individual's gene structure and the induction of enzymes and, in turn, by species and gender. These distinctions are complex, subtle and only partially understood (Figure 1.2).

The nutrient needs and subsequent metabolism by the individual will be influenced by growth in the young and in pregnancy, and modified by disease, drugs, alcohol and tobacco. As the person ages there are important changes in the effectiveness of the absorption and utilisation of the nutrients consumed.

It has been suggested that diet may affect behaviour. In some ancient cultures certain foods were thought to have magical qualities capable of giving special powers of strength, courage, health, happiness and well-being. It is possible that some food constituents may affect the synthesis of brain neurotransmitters and thus modify brain functions. It is therefore important to integrate dietary effects on brain chemicals into our wider understanding of human behaviour.

Until there is an understanding of such nutritional and metabolic mechanisms, confused advice

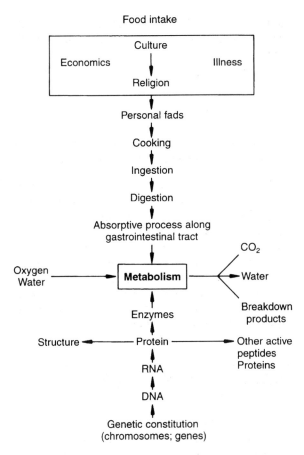

Food intake

Culture

Economics   Illness

Religion

↓

Personal fads

↓

Cooking

↓

Ingestion

↓

Digestion

↓

Absorptive process along
gastrointestinal tract

↓ CO_2

Oxygen ———   ↗
Water ———→ **Metabolism** →→ Water

↓   ↘
Enzymes   Breakdown
↑   products

Structure ←——— Protein ——→ Other active
↑   peptides
RNA   Proteins
↑
DNA
↑
Genetic constitution
(chromosomes; genes)

Fig. 1.2 Metabolism represents a relationship between food intake and the enzymes characteristic of an individual, which are dependent on genetic constitution. Also important are oxygen and water intake and the ability to excrete carbon dioxide, water and metabolic breakdown products.

may be disseminated. Pathology that is provoked by the metabolic response in even a small proportion of the population may erroneously be applied to the population as a whole.

NUTRITIONAL DEFICIENCY AND EXCESS

It is not possible to live for more than 2–3 min without oxygen. However, human life can continue without water for between 2 and 7 days, depending on the ambient temperature and the amount of exercise being taken. Survival without any food at all, but with water, may be for 60–120 days, depending on the body stores. Females and those with considerable subcutaneous fat generally survive for longer than slightly built males.

There are individual responses to nutritional deficiency and excess, although in general weight increase is associated with overall excessive eating and weight loss is associated with inadequate dietary intake. A failure to provide amino acids, fats, vitamins and trace elements leads to specific lesions which may progress to morbidity and death. There is no nutritional explanation for the apparent synthesis of essential vitamins by some individuals. When scurvy was a problem in the Royal Navy the fleet would come into land every 2 months to take on board provisions specifically to reduce the prevalence of scurvy. However, on the long sea voyages some individuals died quite quickly of scurvy, whereas others appeared to be unaffected. Similarly, the different types of beri-beri suggest individual metabolic responses to thiamin deficiency.

In general, the body copes better with an excess than with a deficiency of nutrients, with the exception of alcohol. Consequently, there is an inclination to eat somewhat more than is required. The body copes less well with an excess of dietary fatty or fat-soluble compounds than an excess of water-soluble dietary components. Fatty nutrients, e.g. lipids, are stored and, if the storage load becomes excessive, then the body is disadvantaged. Water-soluble dietary excesses may be excreted, metabolically modified or unchanged in the urine. Excess dietary protein and lipid intakes may be metabolically modified to structural or storage tissues, or possibly be excreted in bile and urine. The variable pathways whereby these processes occur will be determined by the range of variants of the same enzyme (isoenzymes) that forms the metabolic enzyme structure of the individual.

THINKING POINT

What are the criteria for classifying a dietary chemical as a nutrient?

Part I

Factors influencing the food that a community eats

- History of food
- Social, population and environmental influences on nutrition

2

History of food

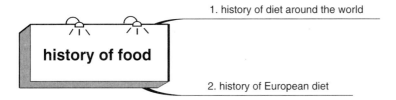

1. history of diet around the world

history of food

2. history of European diet

Fig. 2.1   Chapter outline.

Cookery books are the recordings of how food was prepared and reflect the cooking practices of the era in which they were written. Babylonian clay tablets and Ancient Egyptian scrolls contain recipes. Cookery books in English are to be found from the fourteenth century from the cooks serving Richard II. Now cookery books are major sellers, being of universal interest.

Ancient Egypt

Grain, bread and porridge have been the basis of the human diet since the beginning of nutritional history. In Egypt, bread was made as flat cakes from toasted grains of barley, wheat or millet. The meal mixed with water in a paste was either dried in the sun or baked on the flat stones of the hearth. Primitive grains required toasting before the hard outer husks could be removed. However, the Egyptians found a strain of wheat that could be threshed without being toasted, and consequently dough could be made from a raw flour. Subsequently, the Egyptians found out how to produce beer and used this knowledge in bread making to create sponginess in the dough when baked, and so leavened bread was produced.

Egyptian bread is said to have had a sour taste, suggesting they used lees of beer or a sour dough for their leaven. Sour dough is a piece of fermented dough saved from a previous baking and is used to start the fermenting process of the new dough.

In thirteenth century BC Egypt, it was usual for people to eat two meals a day, a light morning meal and a more substantial evening meal consisting of several dishes.

Ancient Greece

The Greeks made unleavened bread from coarse wheat, which they favoured over barley meal, baking their bread in hot ashes and later in bread ovens. Increasingly, they used flour which had been finely sieved to remove most of the chaff. A wide range of breads was available to both the Ancient Greeks and the Romans. For leaven, like the Egyptians, both the Greeks and the Romans used sour dough.

The Roman Empire

The earliest Romans were a rural people who ate a thick porridge of barley or beans and green vegetables with flat barley bread, hard-baked in ashes. Cheeses were made from goat's milk, meat was a rarity and fish was hardly used. Food was flavoured with garlic, parsnip, olives and olive oil. When Rome became all-powerful, the poor still ate thick grain soups of millet and coarse bread, together with a little turnip or a few beans. Raw olives, goat's cheese and figs were delicacies, and occasionally cooked pork or meatballs were available; these were produced in cook shops which were found throughout the cities. For long periods in Rome bread was given without payment.

The wealthy few had food from all over the known world: spices from India, south-east Asia and China, wheat from Egypt, ham from Gaul and wine from Greece. Ginger came from China through central Asia; cloves from Indonesia by sea to Ceylon and then on by sea and land to Alexandria.

Pepper was a very important element in Roman cooking and was brought overland from India through Egypt. A meal might consist of hors d'oeuvres: a salad of mallow leaves, lettuce, leeks, mint and fish dishes, garnished with sliced eggs, rue and tuna. The main course included a kid, meatballs and beans, together with chicken and a ham. The meal finished with a dessert of ripe apples and vintage wines. The salads were dressed with wine, oil and vinegar and liquamen, a sauce made from fermented salted anchovies. Hams were boiled with dried figs and bay leaves, and baked with honey in a pastry coating. Chickens were roasted or boiled in a variety of spiced sauces. Roman manors had their own oyster tank to ensure a fresh supply. The Roman physician Galen taught his followers that it was harmful to eat fruit with a meal.

By the second century BC cooking had become an art in Rome. The Romans ate three meals a day. Breakfast, between 8 and 10 am, consisted of bread and cheese and a glass of water. Lunch, eaten at noon with little ceremony, was usually bread with cold meat and vegetables, and fruit with a little wine. Dinner was eaten at about 8 pm in winter and 9 pm in summer. Most food was eaten with the fingers, which were rinsed occasionally, although the diners were provided with knives, toothpicks, spoons and napkins.

The requirement for grain necessitated the importation of wheat on a large scale from Egypt, Sicily and north Africa. Special docks and lighthouses were built for these grain ships. Rotary mills powered by animals were used and sophisticated ovens with systems of draughts and chimneys controlled the heat. The flour was milled into various grades, ranging from the finest white to coarse flour considered suitable only for slaves.

The Roman army stretched from the Scottish border through to Egypt and as far east as the edge of the Black Sea. The soldiers were issued with daily rations of grain or bread, meat, wine and oil, and the cost was deducted from their pay. Cheese, vegetables and salt were included in their basic rations. When the legions were on the march they carried a scythe to cut crops, a metal cooking pot, a mess tin and 3 days' emergency food of hard tack, dried cooked grain which could be eaten without further cooking, salted pork and sour wine. Meat was boiled or grilled and the soldiers were issued with spits as standard equipment. A quern to grind flour and a portable oven were carried for every ten men. During peacetime a soldier was expected to grind his own grain and bake his own bread. Soldiers supplemented their diet by hunting. In wartime troops foraged from the enemy countryside. Soldiers made their own cheeses from the milk of animals kept at the forts.

Roman army officers lived on fresh meat and imported edible snails, olives, vintage wine, pepper, fish sauce, hams and oysters. The Roman army was huge: 300 000 men in the first century AD. This required substantial organisation in supplying the garrison and moving food around the Empire. The cost of such provision of food eventually became an intolerable burden on the Roman taxation system.

Mosaic dietary laws

The Jewish diet is established under Mosaic law, which defines clean and unclean food. Blood was seen as the life-force and was forbidden, so all food animals had their blood drained as in kosher ritual slaughter. Fish that swim with their fins and had scales were accepted as clean; shellfish that have neither fins or scales but swim in water were unclean. Cows, sheep and goats, which chew the cud and have cloven hooves, were clean; the pig, which cannot live on grass, was difficult to herd and had little stamina for the nomadic way of life, was unclean. The modification to that diet depended on the dispersal of the Jewish race either to the north of Europe or along the southern shores of the Mediterranean Sea. Eastern European Jews adopted central European cooking, e.g. 'gefilte fish', poached fish cakes made with the flesh scraped from the skin and bones, and mixed with onions, seasoning and breadcrumbs bound with egg. The Jews of the Mediterranean lands used fish, fruit, nuts and vegetables.

India

Indian philosophers stressed the importance of food for the uplifting of the soul and the health of the body. They suggested that spices such as cloves and cinnamon were warming; coriander and cumin cooling. They also believed in pure and impure foods: rice and honey were considered purer than other foods.

The Indus valley was the centre of civilisation around 2000 BC, when it was invaded by Aryan invaders from Iran and Afghanistan. The economy of these Aryan warrior nomads was based on cattle. They lived primarily on meat and milk products. Barley was the staple grain, ground into flour and cakes and eaten with butter. Crushed toasted barley was mixed into a gruel with curds, clarified butter and milk. Food was eaten by hand. Thick gruels were licked off the fingers and thin ones drunk from bowls or cups made of clay. The inhabitants of the Indus valley were driven south into India. Aryans gradually adopted the use of rice, wheat and beans, and learned the use of spices, including tumeric, long peppers (pepper from vines similar to black pepper), sour oranges and sesame, but continued to use clarified butter for cooking. Rice was cooked with mung beans into a thick gruel or khicri. Raw ginger was eaten after meals to aid digestion. The juice of the soma plant was mixed with rice or curds.

The early Aryans were tribal and their society was divided into castes. The Brahmins were the highest caste, with strict rules of purity, particularly concerning food. Food could be polluted by being touched by lower caste people, as this was believed to affect its purity. To protect themselves from pollution, strict laws governing the toilet and behaviour of cooks were developed. Brahmins could only eat food prepared by other Brahmins. There were huge blood sacrifices, particularly of cattle, and until the end of the fifth century AD the meat was eaten after the sacrifice. As society developed, effigies of horses and cows made of dough were substituted and a ban on killing cattle was introduced.

Beliefs were very austere and did not allow the eating of meat, fish or eggs, and the people were consequently strict vegetarians. Other Hindus, also strict vegetarians, do not eat rank-smelling foods, and ban onions and garlic from their kitchens. There may be a separate side kitchen in which onions and garlic may be cooked for dishes not considered ritually pure.

The Buddhist diet was a compromise between the diets of the Hindus and Brahmins. Buddhists were not forbidden meat, merely not allowed to kill for food. Vegetarianism was, however, encouraged for all people. The cow was sacred and no longer killed for food or sacrifice. In the temple in modern India Hindu gods are offered vegetarian dishes.

Until the fifteenth century AD the rulers of northern India came into contact with and were influenced by Persian culture. Many of the dishes had a Persian origin, particularly the samusak pastries. Samosas made of meat, hashed and cooked with almonds, walnuts, pistachios, onions and spices, were presented. The word samusak comes from the Persian word sanbusa, a triangle, and is similar to the samosas sold as snack foods in modern times. Meals would start with sherbet and bread in the form of thin, round cakes. Roasted meat was cut into a large sheet, which was divided into six pieces, one piece being placed before each person. Round dough cakes made with ghee were stuffed with a mixture of flour, almonds, honey and sesame oil. On the top of each dough cake was a brick-shaped sweet cake made of flour, sugar and ghee. Meat was served in large porcelain bowls, and cooked with ghee, onions and green ginger. In addition, rice cooked in ghee was served with chicken.

At the end of the fifteenth century, northern India was invaded by the Mughals, who came from Uzbekistan in central Asia. Their cuisine was similar to that of the Persians, with a variety of grains, green vegetables and meats, which were oily, sweet and spicy.

China

In the China of the last millennium BC, grains were cooked whole as flour milling did not come into general use until about the first century AD. An Imperial Court banquet would include roast turtle and fresh fish, bamboo shoots and reed tips. Meanwhile, the common people lived on a diet of beans and grains flavoured with sour or bitter herbs. Salt and sour plums were the earliest seasoning used. Around the second century BC fermented salted soya beans became popular and were produced on a commercial scale. By the fifth century Chinese cooks had a choice of herbs and pickled meats for bitter flavours: honey and maltose from grains for sweet flavours, and prickly ash, mustard or ginger for hot flavours.

The Chinese knelt on mats or flat cushions to eat. The food was laid out either on the floor or on tables. Chopsticks were beginning to be widely used, but soup stews were eaten with spoons and grains were eaten with the fingers. Soup stews were very popular. For the rich there were beef soups seasoned with sour plums, pickled meat sauce and vinegar. Other soups contained venison, salted fish, bamboo shoots and rice, beef, dog or turnip. The poor had soups made of vegetables and grain without meat.

In the Imperial courts of China from AD 960 to 1280 Chinese cooking reached great heights. Seasoning was important, primarily sesame, anise, ginger, black pepper, onion, salt, cardamoms and vinegar. Other seasonings such as orange peel, soy sauce, peppermint, cinnamon and liquorice were used. Rice was brought in from Vietnam at the beginning of the eleventh century, with resulting nutritional advantage. China became one of the richest countries and as a result of trading, new foods and culinary skills were available. From India came the refining of sugar and black pepper; from Persia came coriander and pastries.

Stir-frying became a central cooking method. Woks came into common use and wheat-flour doughs and pastries were mastered. Bean curd was discovered and became increasingly popular, and noodles became generally used. Sweet sauces made from fermented flour were used to flavour stir-fry dishes. Raw meat and fish were both great delicacies, being flavours that were intense and natural. Preserved pickled meats and fish were very popular. Sparrows were pickled with fermented rice and barbecued.

As the Chinese Empire developed up to AD 1600, a very complicated system of cooking was developed by the northern Chinese aristocracy. Vinegar, fermented bean paste and soy sauces were developed. In the winter meat and fish were preserved by pickling or made into fermented sauces. Vegetables were pickled with salts. At festivals, popular foods included gruels and packets of grain wrapped in cucumber leaves. A small bear was steamed with onion, ginger, orange peel and salt after being marinated in fermented bean sauce. The fat from a boiled pig was skimmed off for separate use. Discs of boiled dough were made from wheat flour, and other doughs from a balm of white rice and wine were left to simmer by the fire. Dishes were spiced with ginger, rice wine, prickly ash pepper and fermented bean sausages, as well as the bitter bark of magnolia.

A Chinese proverb says: 'you are what you eat'. Chinese attitudes to food and health were dependent on this. The Chinese held to the humoral belief that the universe and everything in it was composed of four elements: fire, air, earth and water; and four qualities: heat, cold, moisture and dryness. Treatment for bodily disorders was based on the strength and interaction of these elements and qualities. The basic division of the Chinese beliefs was between the bright, dry, warm, male principle, Yang, and the cold, dark, moist, female principle, Yin (Yang and Yin).

The human body was a reproduction of the cosmos. To be healthy was a reflection of the general harmony among the various virtues, while illness was a sign of disharmony of heat, cold, moisture and dryness. These elements were controlled by food which also had the four qualities. Fundamental to the Chinese theories on nutrition was the idea that food and cures come from the same source. Cooling foods such as green vegetables and fruit treated fevers and rashes, while heating foods such as liver and chicken could treat debility and weakness.

In China, soup was used as a tonic to maintain health. A healthy soup proposed for the liver was made of dog meat, sour plums, Chinese leeks and hemp, while for the lungs a soup of yellow millet, chicken, peach and onion was recommended. Chicken soup was meant to be particularly good after childbirth. (It is also interesting that the Jewish general belief is that chicken soup is a universal panacea.)

A goat's heart marinated in rose water and barbecued with safflower was a prescription for tachycardia, and a goat's leg and cardamom for strength. Tisanes made from ginger were recommended for general strengthening. Chestnuts or salted bamboo shoots and sesame were served several times a day, and the women of the house frequently drank strengthening gruels. A bean gruel made with a little salt and ginger was regarded both as being good for the kidneys and as a cure for vomiting.

Buddhism came to China from India at about the time of Christ. With it came preaching against the killing of animals for food. As Buddhism progressed in China the prohibitions of meat eating were not accepted generally, except in Buddhist monasteries, which were famous for the excellence of their cuisine where the cooking followed strict Buddhist regulations. However, they also insisted on five colours: red, green, yellow, black and white; five flavours: bitter, salt, sweet, hot and sour; and five styles of cooking: raw, simmered, barbecued, fried and steamed. All were represented in a temple meal. Dishes were contrived to create the illusion of eating meat; flour and water pastes were made to resemble animal barbecues. Gluten was used for both stir-fry dishes and barbecues.

In Europe during the Dark Ages trade with the east stopped and pepper disappeared from northern Europe. By the time of the Norman conquest of England, eastern spices and pepper were once again being traded by Arabs living in Spain and sending trading ships to India, south-east Asia and China. This trade was then developed in Venice, which eventually became dominant in trading, bringing food from the east to the markets of northern Europe.

When sweet potatoes were introduced into China they were an immediate success because they grew readily in poor soils and adverse weather conditions. They were also attractive because they were sweet, in an area where sugar and sweeteners were expensive. By the beginning of the nineteenth century sweet potatoes were a staple food for half of the population of northern China. Similarly, chillies arrived in China around AD 1700 and were introduced into Schezuan yunnan cooking. Maize was added to the Chinese diet around the middle of the sixteenth century, but was never as popular as rice, and wheat flour became more popular.

Japan

Buddhism moved to Japan from China and Korea during the seventh century. When Buddhism came to Japan the emperor forbade the eating of any meat except by the sick. Within 100 years both chicken and fish were exempted from this rule. A stricter interpretation of Buddhist law came in the twelfth century with the spread of Zen Buddhism from China. The attempts to introduce a rigid vegetarian diet were only partially successful.

Until the mid-nineteenth century the Japanese were somewhat reluctant to kill four-legged animals, particularly cattle, for food. However, most modern Japanese eat beef.

Zen Buddhism developed and formalised the tea ceremony which had been present in China some 700 years previously. Zen belief in restraint, and simplicity was expressed in the tea ceremony with its strict rules of formal behaviour. These ceremonies were undertaken in the Zen temples. Only foods in season could be used. Two main styles of tea ceremony cooking developed: one at the Daaitokuji temple near Kyoto in the fourteenth century and the other at the Obakusn temple near Tokyo in the sixteenth century. At Daaitokuji the meal was prepared in individual servings. The Obakusn meal was based on Chinese vegetarian cooking and retained the Chinese practice of serving all food in large dishes in the centre of the table, from which diners could help themselves. Such a meal started with green tea and a sweet cake served according to the formal tea ceremony style, followed by a plate of cold hors d'oeuvres and a clear soup with bean curd and ginko nuts. Next came a number of different foods cooked by simmering: bean curd balls, aubergine, rolls of thin bean curd sheets, mushrooms, bamboo, lotus roots, chillies, ginko nuts and pine needles. After this arrived a steamed dish followed by a dish of braised vegetables, a deep-fried dish, a salad of chrysanthemum leaves with a walnut dressing, a vegetable stew, fruit and finally rice cooked with a little green tea. Such a feast is known as Lohan's delight, Lohan being a Buddhist saint.

Ancient Persia

The Persian Court in the sixth century AD regarded the rearing of animals and birds for the table as being very important. Wild asses were fattened with clover and barley and then cooked with yoghurt and spices. Chickens were reared on hemp, oil and olives and after being killed were hung for 2 days by the feet and then by the neck before they were cooked. Other dishes included milk-fed kids and calves and fat beef cooked in a broth of spinach, flour and vinegar. Hares and pheasants were made into ragouts. In the summer the Persians ate nut and almond pastries made with gazelle fat and fried in nut oil. Foods imported from Europe and Asia were available to the Persians. Fresh coconut was served with sugar and dates and stuffed with nuts. They also ate sweet preserves of lemons, quinces, Chinese ginger and chestnuts, and drank sweet wine.

Islam

Mohammed preached that food was a gift from God, 'So eat of what God has given you, lawful and good, and give thanks to God's favour if Him it is you serve'. Pork or any animal found dead, blood or animals killed as an offering to a pagan god, fish without scales (including shellfish), alcohol and fermented liquids were all forbidden, or halan. Carnivorous animals and birds were forbidden. Permitted foods were halal. Animals killed for food had to be slaughtered by an approved butcher who had to say 'In the name of God, God is most great', and cut the animal's throat to allow the blood to drain out. Animals who died by disease, strangulation or beating were not acceptable. This practice is still followed by modern Muslims.

The month-long fast of Ramadan is in memory of the prophet's revelations and is for the health of the soul. Fasting is a way of reaping spiritual rewards. Nothing is eaten or drunk during daylight hours in the month of Ramadan. Each evening after sunset the fast is broken with three dates and water, followed, after final sunset, by prayer and a meal. All Muslims must follow Ramadan after the age of responsibility, 12 years in girls, 15 years in boys. Exceptions are the elderly in poor health, pregnant and nursing women, menstruating women,

the sick, travellers and labourers. The meal is of an ordinary size, not extra quantity to fill the stomach after fasting. In Saudi Arabia today people eat a meal of bread, milk or sour milk, together with a braised or stewed meat dish.

The lifestyle of the Arab Califs who ruled Egypt, Iran and the eastern Mediterranean in the thirteenth century AD was influenced by the Persian traditions, including cooking. Trade with the east brought a wide range of foods to the Arab world and was of a high level of sophistication and luxury. Cleanliness was all-important, in particular the cleaning and preparation of the food and hand-washing. Meat, usually lamb, was cooked with fruit such as oranges, lemons, pomegranates, redcurrants, apples and apricots. Fresh vegetables such as carrots, onions, aubergines, spinach and leeks appeared in many meat dishes. Meat was fried in the rendered down fat from sheep's tails. Some meats were fried before boiling, and almonds and other nuts were used to make gravies. Spices such as ginger, cinnamon, pepper and caraway from China and India, as well as local spices, cumin and coriander, were used with meat dishes. Rice was a luxury and was mixed with meat into a pilau-style dish.

The New World

Many of the foods eaten in Europe, and which are regarded as Mediterranean foods, came originally from central or meso America. The early hunters in Central America lived on mammoth or barbecued bison and relied on gathering seasonally available plants. Alternative sources of protein were gophers, squirrels, rabbits and mice. These hunter–gatherers had necessarily to be nomadic.

In the warm, well-watered central valleys there was an abundance of fish and fowl. The new concept of returning seeds to the ground for harvesting was the beginning of agriculture. The avocado pear and some kind of squash were the first to be cultivated. Between 5000 and 3000 BC maize and beans were cultivated, but at that stage provided only 10% of the total diet. Even then, Mexican food was already heavily spiced with chilli.

Villages in this area date from approximately 3000 BC and a basic triad of maize, beans and squash was grown. Early maize was only the size of a strawberry plant. The diet was supplemented with fish and deer from lagoons and neighbouring forests. Cannibalism may also have been practised.

During the Olmec period of middle America from 1500 to 100 BC the basic crop was maize, which even today accounts for 90% of the inhabitants' diet. It was possible to obtain two crops of maize per year. The agriculture was based on slash and burn; that is, a patch of forest was felled during the short dry season, the wood was burnt, seeds were sown using a simple digging stick and the crops were harvested. This was repeated until the ground became arid, when it was then allowed to rejuvenate over the next 5 years. Such a system supported both the Olmec and the Mayan civilisations. It sustained only a limited number of people, however, and both civilisations collapsed when it was no longer possible to grow sufficient food to sustain the populations. In the Olmec period the growth of food was complicated by the flooding of large rivers. At this stage, the dog and the turkey had been domesticated and served as sources of food. Limitations for these civilisations were that the plough had not been invented and there were no draught animals, the beast of burden being man. The cities of meso America had a carefully planned supply and control of water, with main aqueducts carrying water to the city.

After the land had been cleared, weeds would grow very readily and the great cities that developed would disappear quite quickly after the agricultural land had been exhausted and the population moved on to new and fertile land.

By the time of the Spanish conquest, the Aztecs grew maize as the main crop, chillies as seasoning, with additional squashes and beans. The latter provided nitrogen and protein in the diet. There were no dietary dairy products and very little meat was eaten. Chia was used to make a kind of porridge. Maguey was an all-purpose plant; the spikes served as needles, the fibre was used for making cloth and the juice from the heart of the plant was used to make the alcoholic beverage 'pulque', which is still drunk in Mexico. During the Aztec period pulque was used for ritual intoxication and may have been used to sedate people waiting to be sacrificed. Central to Aztec agriculture was human sacrifice, as it was believed that the safeguarding of the crop cycle depended on such rituals. At its

most intense 50 000 people a year were sacrificed to ensure the rising of the sun and continued crops. Maize was the staple diet for the Mayans, but they ate domesticated plants such as the anone, avocado, tuayaba, passion fruits, zucchini, tomatoes, carrots, beans and sweet potatoes. The surplus of these crops was stored in underground rooms. This diet was supplemented with fish, crabs, molluscs and turtles.

The Spanish brought many of the foods grown in central America back to Spain. They were then grown in Spain and are now associated with what is called the 'Mediterranean diet'.

Other imports from the New World included nasturtiums from the West Indies, used for their flowers and leaves in salads, and potatoes, turkeys and chocolate from Central America. Potatoes also came to Europe from the mountainous parts of South America. Initially, they were a curiosity in English cooking and in mainland Europe potatoes were not eaten to any great extent. In Ireland, by the middle of the seventeenth century they were an established staple food. Turkeys were introduced into England about 1524, having been imported from Spain. They replaced swans, peacocks and bustards as festive foods, being relatively cheap, readily stuffed, roasted and baked in pies. Fruit and vegetables from Central America included sweet potatoes, peanuts, maize, chillies, tomatoes and kidney beans.

The Crusades

After the Crusades, spices and new foods were brought into northern Europe. Sugar was unknown until the eleventh century when it came to Europe, first from the Middle East and then from Spain, but by the seventeenth century, sugar plantations, run by slave labour in the Caribbean and Brazil, enabled Europe to indulge its fast growing taste for sugar. Spiced sugar comfits were nibbled in the long fasting hours of Lent as a medicinal aid.

Cooking practices began to change. Crusaders learned to cook meats in almond milk and to fry meat first without boiling. The Middle Eastern custom of cooking meat with fruit began to be adopted in European dishes. Rice grown by the Arabs in Spain was imported into French and English cooking. Another Arab custom of highly coloured dishes was also imported into London and Paris; foods were dyed green with parsley, yellow with egg yolks, and red with sandalwood, cinnamon or alkenet.

Rice, oranges, figs, dates, raisins, spinach, almonds and pomegranates were all imported. Dishes were made with rose hips, shredded almond, chicken, red wine, sugar and strong pepper and thickened with rice flour. Other recipes included eels seasoned with ginger, cinnamon, cloves, cardamoms, galingale, long peppers and saffron. Galingale is a rhizome belonging to the ginger family. Cloves, cardamoms, nutmegs, mace and rose water were all Arab ingredients which were imported after the Crusades. Blancmange, made with rice sweetened with sugar and flavoured with almonds, is a Middle Eastern dish. The Arabs, who were the mainstay of culture in the European Dark Ages, maintained much of the Greek and Indian philosophies and science. They applied these philosophies to food, whereby foods were classified and used to balance the humours in people.

In contrast, the early Christians believed that only Christ had healing powers. Illness was a punishment for wrong-doings, to be treated by fasting and prayer. However, by the time of the Crusades, some foods were seen as having medicinal properties. This all emanated from the Salerno School near Naples, founded by Benedictine monks. Knights returning from the crusades often stopped there and were cured. Even 400 years later, the English physician Andrew Boorde was influenced by the Salerno school of teaching. Foods were still regarded as hot or cold, dry or wet, according to the humoral theory. Fruits, milk products and red meat were all to be eaten with caution. Specific foods were believed to be suitable or unsuitable for different diseases and there were even different diets for different types of men. 'Sanguine men, who are hot and moist, should be careful in eating meat, but not eat fruit.' Such people had to be careful with their food or they would become fat and gross. 'Phlegmatic men are cold and moist and should not eat white meat, herbs or fruit, but only onions, garlic, pepper, ginger and hot and dry meats. Choleric men are hot and dry and should avoid hot spices and wine. Melancholic men are cold and dry and should not eat fried or salted meats and drink only light wines.'

Cannibalism

Cannibalism is a taboo subject, causing great distress when mentioned. It occasionally occurs with starving groups and is variably reported in various societies, e.g. the head-hunters of Papua New Guinea.

HISTORY OF EUROPEAN DIET

Mediaeval Europe

In late mediaeval Europe feast alternated with famine. Large trenches of hand-baked coarse bread were cut into oblongs to serve as plates. There were jugs of water and wine on side tables. Diners were provided with a broad knife and spoon, and rinsed and dried their hands after taking their place at the table for large and important meals. Most meals were taken by hand from the serving plates. Fine white bread was trimmed into finger-shaped sops and used to mop up liquid, including wine. Potage or soups were eaten with spoons from shared bowls and mopped up with sops. Meats and other foods were sliced and placed on the bread trenches. The meat slices were held with the fingers, and before being eaten, were dipped in a sauce the consistency of mustard. At the end of each course the softened trenches of bread were collected to be given to the poor. These were replaced by a soteley, which consisted of coloured scenes sculpted from marzipan made with ground almonds and sugar. These were often decorated with banners which might depict the four seasons or the Christmas story.

At large banquets there would be a boar's head with gilded tusks, a heron, a sturgeon and a pie made with cream, eggs, dates, prunes and sugar. The next course might include venison served in spice, wheat gruel, stuffed suckling pig and peacocks, skinned, roasted and served in their plumage. The third course had more roast birds, quinces in syrup, grilled pork rissoles, custard tarts and pies of dried fruit and eggs.

The essence of mediaeval cookery lay in mixture. The quantities of spices used were quite significant. For example, one fifteenth century house used five pounds (2.2 kg) of pepper, two-and-a-half pounds

(1.1 kg) of ginger, three pounds (1.4 kg) of cinnamon and one-and-a-quarter pounds (0.6 kg) each of mace and cloves in a year. Sugar was expensive and regarded in a similar fashion in cooking as a spice. Raisins, dates and saffron were introduced to northern Europe from the Middle East. Pastry and the stylish shaping of pies came from Persia, along with recipes for traditional Chinese pastries.

The diet of ordinary people was very different from the nobility at court. Such people lived on cheeses, curds, cream and oatcake. Others, more fortunate, ate two or three meals a day and enjoyed wine or beer, pork or meat, cheese, dried beans and bread, with the occasional chicken, eggs, pepper, cumin, salt, vinegar and sufficient vegetables.

Potage, a porridge-like soup thickened with cereal or bread, was popular in England. A porridge made of boiled ground wheat, moistened with milk and covered with saffron, was served with venison at the court of Richard II. The poor, when they could afford meat, made a potage of dried beans boiled in bacon stock, mashed and served with bacon.

Throughout Europe peasants lived on a similar diet of bread, cheese and pork, which was usually salted. In northern Europe peasants ate more rye or black bread than in the south. A Lenten bread was made of barley and oats. In times of shortage, bread was made of oats, peas or beans. The leaven would probably have been sour dough. The bread was heavy, hard-crusted and coarse. In England it was usually baked on a hearth, stone or in a pot buried in the fire embers. In France, peasants were forced to use bread ovens belonging to their landlords, for which they paid with a portion of bread dough. Rats and mice polluted the stored grain, weevils burrowed into the dried beans, bacon was rancid, cheese mouldy and wine sour. Bread was made from rye infected with ergot fungus, which brought with it the terrible consequences of induced abortions. There was never enough fodder through the winter to keep alive more than the few animals needed for breeding. In the autumn animals would be killed for their meat, salted or smoked, and preserved for the winter and spring. Turnips, beans and peas were dried. During times of famine the poor would only have cabbages and turnips without bread or salt.

In the Middle Ages, towns were relatively small. Within the city were private gardens and around the city walls were fields and vegetable gardens. The offal from various meats and fish was dumped anywhere, with resulting pollution of the streams.

In the Christian calendar there were 200 fast days a year, when meat, milk and eggs were all forbidden, and only fish or vegetables were allowed. There were particular privations during Lent at the end of winter, when food stocks were already low. The one meal a day allowed for the 6 weeks of Lent offered a daily diet of salted fish, stock fish or red salted herrings with mustard sauce. Fresh fish was also permissible; consequently, some monasteries had their own fish pools. The only soup allowed was dried peas boiled in water and flavoured with fried onions. More prosperous individuals could use dried fruit such as currants, figs and dates, and sweetmeats of crystallised ginger or candied violets.

Cooking techniques changed during Lent. Milk made from ground almonds replaced cow's milk for poaching and stewing. Oil was used rather than butter or lard. Sea-birds were sometimes allowed in religious houses because they were a form of water creature. Fast or fish days continued in England until after the Reformation and it was not until the mid-seventeenth century that statutory fish days were abandoned in England. The long fasts of Advent and Lent ended with Christmas and Easter. Christmas in England was celebrated not only with new wine from Gascogny, but also with certain days of feasting and entertainment. The end of Lent was celebrated with a great feast on Easter Sunday; meals on that day traditionally included a lamb or a kid in many European countries. In mediaeval times it was usual to give gifts of hardboiled eggs painted with vegetable dyes on Easter Sunday. This practice has continued to the present.

Food supply and balances were at their limits. The supply of food to the developing cities was yet to reach levels of sophistication. Many countries experienced long periods of starvation. Bread, oats and cooked vegetables were the peasants' food, with water and whey for drinking.

Sixteenth and seventeenth century Europe

By the sixteenth century came the development of printing and cookery books. During this period English merchants became extremely rich, with fortunes made from trade to India and the West Indies. There was little ability to store food, so the diet reflected seasonal availability. Some of the cookery books discussed the curative properties of specific diets. A recipe for whitening and retaining teeth recommended rose water, sage, marjoram, alum and cinnamon. Rosemary was believed to have almost miraculous powers and was used to treat colds, toothache, aching feet, bad breath, sweating, lack of appetite, gout, consumption and madness. Bed-wetting could be cured by eating fried mice.

In England in 1603 breakfasts of cold meat, cheese and egg were eaten between 6 and 7 am. Dinner, the main meal of the day, was between 11 am and 12 noon, and a light supper was taken at about 6 pm. By the late eighteenth century fashionable people in London were eating as late as 7 pm, although this was not the pattern in the country. Breakfast was a meal of cold meats and ale, eaten at about 9 or 10 am in towns, and supper had become a late-night snack. Afternoon tea was taken between breakfast and dinner, with tea and bread and butter or buttered toast. Dinner plates of pottery or pewter replaced the mediaeval trench of bread, and forks were slowly introduced. Nevertheless, monarchs such as Louis XIV of France always ate with their fingers. The dishes, both sweet and savoury, were laid out on the table in geometric patterns. The third course of fish and confection was similarly presented.

Around the periphery of London there were small, intensive market gardens, manured by excrement. Fruit and vegetables were grown for the population of the capital and were sold from barrows or in markets, e.g. Covent Garden.

In the seventeenth century increasing trade meant a new concept of food storage for the mariners. Fish could be caught, but water and fresh fruit and vegetables could not be stored, with consequences for vitamin C status until the findings of Lind were adopted. A year's store of food was taken, the basic being hard tack, a cake of wheat flour baked twice for better preservation. Venetian ships carried salt pork, wine, cheese and broad beans. Protein-calorie malnutrition was a feature of the early, long voyages. Queen Elizabeth of England's fleet consisted of swift and small ships, limited in storage and hence ill-adapted for long journeys. The food at sea was salt beef and pork,

beer, pease, cheese and butter, biscuit and salted fish. London was the only port large enough to victual a ship with these specialist foods. During the Napoleonic wars and the blockade of the French channel ports a major agricultural industry developed: the walking to London of cattle from the Scottish Highlands by drovers, and geese from East Anglia, all for the feeding of the fleet. This trade was central to the Highland economy.

In the seventeenth century increasing trade among European countries led to new diets. Trade with India and China resulted in tea being imported. A variety of beverages, such as tea, coffee and chocolate, was introduced into Europe.

The Chinese habit of drinking tea is believed to date from the time of Emperor Shen Nung (2737 BC). Japan, India and Sri Lanka have a long tradition of tea drinking. The Portuguese brought tea to Europe in the middle of the sixteenth century. The Dutch brought small quantities to France, and by the mid-seventeenth century large amounts were introduced into England by the East India Company. The first teas imported were green teas (now coming from the Zhejiang province of China). The leaves were picked, rolled and steamed to prevent further fermentation. Initially, very weak tea was made and drunk with sugar but no milk. By the end of the seventeenth century bohea or black tea (China, India and Sri Lanka), which is a stronger and less astringent tea, was available. Cream or milk was then added to the tea to counteract the acidic effects of the tannin. Oolong is a partially fermented red tea from the Fujian province of south-east China and Taiwan. Tea became popular throughout all social classes and was drunk throughout the day. Tea replaced beer as the drink for many English farm labourers.

Coffee was introduced into Europe during the seventeenth century. The coffee shrub is native to Ethiopia. By the sixteenth century coffee was drunk throughout the Muslim world. It was introduced to Europe through Venice by the beginning of the seventeenth century. The first coffee shop opened in Oxford in 1650. Many of the early coffee shops became associated with dining clubs and were important centres of political and social life.

Drinking chocolate became popular throughout Europe during the seventeenth century. Chocolate was initially imported by the Spanish from Mexico, where it had been drunk by the Mayans and

Aztecs. When first introduced into Spain it was a secret maintained by monasteries. The Spanish added sugar, cinnamon and vanilla in place of the chillies in the Aztec recipe. By the middle of the seventeenth century drinking chocolate was available throughout Europe, although it was not until the mid-eighteenth century that chocolate bars were produced.

Tea, coffee and chocolate replaced the previously widely drunk mulled wine. As they were rather bitter in flavour, sugar was taken to improve the flavour.

France was the most important European wine producer in the mediaeval era, sustaining a tradition that had existed since Roman times. Wines were exported to England from the Weine basin and from Gascogny. The new wines from Bordeaux arrived in England just in time for Christmas. Mediaeval wines were lighter than the modern ones and were at their best after about 4 months. They were stored in wooden barrels. The Parisians preferred light white wines, whereas the English liked red wines. By the end of the sixteenth century wines from the warm south were recognised as having a higher alcohol content than those grown in the north. These stronger wines could be kept for several years and would improve with keeping.

The favourite wine during the second half of the seventeenth century was champagne. Champagne wines were first developed under Henry IV of France at the beginning of the century. It was only slowly that their capacity to form a sparkling wine was appreciated, largely under the guidance of Dom Perignon from the Abbey of Hautvillers near Rheims. Champagne was the most popular wine at the court of Charles II in London.

Claret was imported in barrels from Bordeaux, usually drunk warmed with spices as mulled wine. Younger wines were more expensive than older wines because wines kept in barrels tended to deteriorate after a year or two. Maturing of wine in bottles later became more common and with this development the concept of wine improving with age.

By the mid-seventeenth century the great tradition of French cooking had begun. This was a cuisine based on a series of techniques: basic preparation, bouillon and roux, the use of bouquet garni, egg whites for clearing consommé, and stuffings made with mushrooms and other vegetables. Pieces of meat and mutton were slowly cooked. Eighteenth century French and subsequent cooking preferred the infusion of carefully selected flavours. The previous menus containing multiflavoured sauces and exotic game birds were thus replaced.

From the seventeenth century, with the increasing availability of sugar, puddings were slowly established as a regular feature of a meal and served with other savoury dishes in the second course. There was a wide range of fruit pies, fool's cream, syllabubs and fritters. The English pudding was transformed by the introduction of the boiling cloth. Before this innovation boiled puddings, both the sweet and spicy versions of sausage and savoury puddings, were cooked in animal intestines. These had to be fresh, so boiled puddings could only be made during the seasonal autumn slaughter of livestock for the winter. However, once boiled puddings were cooked wrapped in cloth, they could be enjoyed at any time of the year. Quaking or shaking puddings of cream, breadcrumbs, sugar and eggs flavoured with spices were cooked in well-floured bags in simmering water. Apple puddings of apple, sugar and butter were wrapped in pastry skin and boiled in a cloth. The boiled sweet pudding became the national dish, consisting of flour, suet, milk and eggs, and was usually boiled in the same utensil as the meat of the day, the square of bacon, cabbage or other green vegetables in one net, the potatoes in another and the roly poly in a cloth. Roly poly pudding with dried fruit was served as a first course, with a similar purpose to the Yorkshire pudding, to reduce the appetite for the more expensive later courses. Plum puddings with dried fruit developed during the seventeenth and eighteenth centuries, with fruit, sugar and spices such as cinnamon, nutmeg, ginger, cloves and maize.

Eighteenth and nineteenth century Europe

Butcher's meat required specialised killing and cutting, which often took place in remote towns, whereas rabbits, chickens and pigs were killed locally. During the Industrial Revolution in Britain, workers crowded into the rapidly growing towns to operate the new machines. Women worked in factories and were also responsible for the preparation and cooking of family meals, without the training they had previously received from their totally domesticated and now distant mothers. There was a resulting decline in nutrition.

In the eighteenth and nineteenth centuries rural life was very much dominated by the availability of seasonal fresh fruits and game from the rural activities of fishing and hunting. Fishing towns supplied cod, lobster, sole, skate and whiting. Fresh vegetables were grown in the garden, with strawberries and raspberries in June, and peaches, nectarines, plums and pears in September. Asparagus and cucumber were also grown.

The farmworkers had a very simple diet. There was bacon from the family pig, kept in a sty at the back of the cottage, eaten with fresh vegetables, bread and home-made lard flavoured with rosemary. However, many of the farmworkers came close to starvation, particularly during times of poor harvest. They lived on potatoes, and in Scotland on oatmeal, milk and sometimes fresh herrings. Potatoes were increasingly popular as they were easy to cook and provided the essence of a hot meal. They also had the advantage of lasting for three-quarters of the year. Fresh meat was a luxury, eaten only on Sundays. A pot roast was made by placing the meat with a little lard or other fat in a covered iron saucepan kept over the fire. In the north, oatmeal and tea were provided for workers. Rural workers in the south did not necessarily have gardens provided and lived almost exclusively on bread, with little salt, bacon or cheese.

The introduction of the potato into rural Ireland and Scotland gave a readily grown nutritious crop. By the nineteenth century the potato was a staple of the diet in both town and country. When the fungus *Phytopthora infestans* infected potatoes in Ireland, the resultant destruction of the crop resulted in widespread famine for poor Irish populations living on a marginal diet. The infection was increased during a period of high humidity which occurred during 1845–1847. The Irish famine ensued (1845–1852) and one million survivors of the potato famine emigrated. Later, potatoes resistant to the blight were developed in Scotland and the USA.

The development of restaurants followed the French Revolution when chefs, who had lost their aristocratic employers, opened restaurants, resulting in a more general, intense and continuing inter-

est in recipes and food. There was a defining of cooking styles, with precise cooking instructions for the preparation of purées, essences, sauces and garnishes, with a perfect balance between well-chosen flavours. This led to an almost total domination by French cooking of food in Europe. It has been suggested that, by the mid-nineteenth century, the urban British middle-class, unlike the French, had lost contact with their own country origins and consequently an understanding of the origins of their foods. The British cooking pattern was plain, leaving foods to taste of themselves, whereas the French haute cuisine depended on the cook adding to their flavour.

The introduction of spices into Britain came from exposure to India. The recipe for Worcester sauce was brought back from India and curries were introduced through the East India Company. The first recipes for mulligatawny soup, using curry powder, appeared at the beginning of the nineteenth century. Such soups were thickened with barley, bread or split peas. The British community living in India combined Indian and British foods, one such being the development and increasing popularity in the eighteenth century of chutneys made with tamarinds, mangoes, limes and aubergines. which were previously unknown in Britain at that time, although known in southern Europe.

In the industrial areas there was considerable starvation. During the 1840s the diet of the majority was stodgy and monotonous, and for many, deficient in both quantity and nutriment. Badly housed parents lost many of their children and those who survived were undernourished, rachitic and sometimes deformed. Meat was often eaten only two or three times a week, with the main or even sole food source being bread and potatoes.

At the beginning of the nineteenth century the British soldier's daily ration was one pound of bread (450 g) and a quarter of a pound (110 g) of meat. In the army barracks there were two coppers for each company, one for meat and the other for vegetables, so the food could only be boiled. There were no canteens. There were two meals, one at 7.30 am and the other at 12.30 pm. On overseas service soldiers were provided with salt pork, salt beef or dried biscuits.

There were considerable problems of storage during this period, with resulting mass adulteration and upgrading of food. Bakers bleached inferior grades of flour with alum to make bread appear white. Flour was diluted with ground peas and beans, beer was adulterated with acids, milk was thickened with arrowroot, the skins of Gloucester cheese were coloured with red lead, and old port crusting was imitated by lining the bottle with a layer of super-tartrate of potash. Hedgerow clippings were used to adulterate tea; leaves of blackthorn, ash and elder were boiled, dried and coloured on copper plates. Ground coffee was diluted with chicory and toasted corn. Flour was mixed with chalk, pipe clay, powdered flints and potato flour. Second-hand tea leaves were sold by servants to merchants. The tea leaves were then mixed with gum and dried with black lead before being sold as fresh tea leaves. It was only in the 1870s that parliament legislated against food adulteration.

The introduction of the railways enabled food to be carried rapidly around the country. By the end of the eighteenth century, fresh salmon in ice could be brought from Scotland to London, initially by road and later by the railway. In the 1860s and 1870s the development of the railway system into the mid-west of the United States and the cattle lands of South America opened up new fertile sources of food. The railway and rapid ship movements meant that grain and cattle could be brought from North America and South America to the industrial areas of Europe. Later came the introduction of reaping machines and self-binders, requiring fewer workers, which increased the cheap production of wheat and other crops.

Canned meats and vegetables were used by the Royal Navy in the Napoleonic wars, but preservation through canning was only partially successful. By the late nineteenth century canned Californian pineapples and peaches were available in Britain.

The long period of urban malnutrition became apparent during the Boer war, when nearly 40% of the British volunteers had to be rejected because of being physically impaired by inadequate diet. The result of this and other findings, such as the Rowntree Report on poverty, resulted in parliamentary Acts providing free school meals for children of poor families and pensions for the elderly. By the middle of the nineteenth century, advances in the knowledge of nutrition enabled adequate nutritional provision to be made for developing schoolchildren.

Despite this knowledge, was the failure of one of the most famous expeditions of all times, Scott's attempt to be the first man to reach the South Pole. Not only was he beaten by Amundsen, but he and his party died on the way back through cold and poor nutrition. One of the early expeditions to climb Everest used hampers from Fortnum and Masons as the food supply.

Twentieth century Europe

The diet of the British working classes at the beginning of the twentieth century was dominated by bread, sugar, lard, cheese, bacon and condensed milk. Meat was brought chilled from Argentina or frozen from New Zealand.

In Europe, factories were attracting workers from the land, so that as the available agricultural production was reduced the diet was augmented by overseas food. Novel methods were found to preserve foods on long journeys. Cattle in Argentina were slaughtered solely for their skins for leather. Later, the development of a meat concentrate, e.g. Bovril, made the proteins available for use by distant populations. The introduction of refrigerated ships enabled meat to be carried over long distances in prime condition.

Later in the twentieth century, food could be carried by refrigerated lorries, so that lettuces, strawberries and melons could be brought in good condition from France to Britain. Successful canning was another important development. Canned salmon and canned peaches became the traditional Sunday tea for many people during the Second World War.

The long working hours in factories resulted in eating problems, because the traditional time for the working man's main meal was the middle of the day. Good employers provided canteens where workers could eat at that time. At the Cadbury's works canteen a meal of roast beef and two vegetables was available at midday. For the majority of workers, canteens were not available until the 1940s. Often food was taken to work to be eaten at midday. This might be a pie, a basin of meat and vegetable stew or cold sandwiches, and tea. Coal miners would take a bottle of cold tea and a tin of sandwiches. There were no set meal breaks and they ate as they worked. Other workers relied on stalls in market places close to the factory. When possible, men returned to their homes for their midday meal. However, changes in working patterns altered eating patterns throughout the world. At the same time, the women, who were either working or having virtually annual pregnancies throughout their childbearing years, were not even given these facilities.

War makes great demands on a population's nutrition. The First and Second World Wars made great demands on both the civilian and military personnel. Civilians often experience famine during wars. One of the greatest nutrition experiments ever was food rationing in Great Britain during the Second World War, under the charge of J.C. Drummond. Many of the poor ate better than previously during this period, with an equitable sharing of food. The supply of food to armies moving over distances provides a constant problem for their generals. When Ghengis Khan entered Europe there were nearly half a million cavalry horses, which caused considerable feeding problems. The members of the Chinese Communist Army carried rice with them on the long march. In contrast, a British regiment facing an enemy charge opened their ammunition boxes to find that they had been provisioned with biscuits.

Concentration camps for civilians and prisoner of war camps resulted in controlled starvation beyond comprehension.

History of eating patterns in Scotland

An example of the development of eating patterns in an industrial society can be found in Scotland. In 1949, Kitchin and Passmore described three distinct eras of nutrition in the general Scottish population. The first era was that of a self-supporting agricultural community. The diet was in the Viking tradition, which included rye, wholemeal bread, oat and barley porridge; fish (especially herring); boiled meat and broths of sheep, lamb, goat, ox, calf and pig; cheese, butter and cream; beer and mead, and among the wealthy, wine. The most common vegetables were cabbage and onions; apples, berries and hazelnuts were also popular.

The second era was the age of the Industrial Revolution. As industry expanded and the population increased, so food requirements exceeded home food production, necessitating the import of food from overseas. Significant differences in health appeared between the urban and rural populations, in part because of the better quality of the country people's diet. During the nineteenth century, 10% of the population were too poor to buy sufficient food for themselves. Such malnutrition, in addition to bad sanitation, inadequate overcrowded housing, insufficient land for farming, and a host of acute and chronic infectious diseases, led to rickets, poor stature, and high maternal and infant mortality.

A study in 1903 by Patton, Dunlop and Inglis of the diet of the labouring classes in Edinburgh identified a large proportion of poorly developed and undersized children and adults. Two groups were studied: families with assured and adequate incomes, and the poor, who were unable to buy the necessities of life, either because of inadequate income or because of employment that was only casual. Some families living in poor housing on small, irregular wages refused to take part in the study. The range of expenditure on food varied from 2.5 to 9.5 pence per man per day. The daily nutrient intake per man varied from 1100 to 4800 kilocalories (kcal). The wife and children of the poor families lived on tea, bread and potatoes, the tradition being that the man ate butcher's meat daily. The larder was replenished with small quantities of food bought each day. Alcohol was a great problem, affecting work records and hence income. In contrast, the families of workmen receiving regular wages ate meals consisting of bread, potatoes, oatmeal, eggs, beef, mutton, ham, butter, herrings, cod, sugar, rice and barley. Fresh vegetables were confined to potatoes, cabbage and peas.

In Edinburgh before the First World War, over 12% of the milk contained tubercle bacilli. The consequence was that the bovine, milk-borne form of tuberculosis occurred in 32.4% of tuberculosis patients aged under 5 years, 29% aged 5–16 years and 2.9% of adults.

The third era was that of state planning. During and after the Second World War, the government was obliged to control and provide an adequate food supply for the whole population, so that malnutrition could, despite the obstacles to the importation of food, be avoided as far as possible. This was the golden age of the nutritionist. Good nutritional practice, school meals and works canteens were available to the entire population. The consequences were striking. During the period 1941–1945, boys 13 years old in Glasgow grew to be on average three-quarters of an inch (2 cm) taller and 3 pounds (1.4 kg) heavier than those in the same age group in 1935–1939, and $3^{1}/_{2}$ inches (9 cm) and $12^{1}/_{2}$ pounds (5.7 kg) heavier than those of 1910–1914.

Since then, a fourth era has emerged, the era of the supermarket and a free market. Increasing overall prosperity, more efficient home farming practices and ready availability of food from all over the world mean that many have the choice of a wide range of foods from an efficient wholesale and retail system. The constraints now are personal and communal preferences, and financial limitations. There have been considerable increases in height, weight and lifespan. The population now has new and unprecedented opportunities for inappropriate or excessive indulgences; in general, however, the human race copes better with nutritional excesses than with insufficiency.

An important consequence of the advent of this fourth era is that Scotland's nutrition is dominated by a common range of choice on supermarket counters, selected by a few supermarket purchasing managers. The modern consumer is presented with an unprecedented range of 20 000 lines in major stores. The pattern of restaurant eating has changed, with Indian and Chinese restaurants having a prime place in contemporary eating. Chicken tikka masala is now Britain's most popular meal.

A development in the provision of food in Europe is the long distances that food may travel to ensure that the supermarkets have a broad range of edible fresh items for the shelves. This 'globalisation' has undoubted advantages, but is not without its hazards:

- **Zoonosis**: this is the spread of diseases over long distances as a consequence of travel. This includes AIDS, Lassa fever and Ebola, and animal diseases such as bovine spongiform encephalopathy (BSE), foot and mouth disease, and salmonella.
- **Transport**: a manufactured food may contain ingredients from several countries which have travelled a total of some 1000 km to meet together.
- **Cash crops**: poverty-stricken countries may grow crops such as tobacco, oranges and opium, which are exported, neglecting the local population's food needs.
- **Inefficiency**: for every calorie of carrot flown from South Africa to the UK, 66 calories of fuel are consumed.
- **Regional issues**: supermarket buying managers may spend only defined periods in any one section, and not make contacts and contracts with local producers.

A new element has entered the delivery of food. Farming practice has changed, with the number of types of any one plant or animal being very much reduced, but the range of plants and animal sources of food greatly increased. There is a growing group of people who do not believe that mass farming, with its heavy use of pesticides and herbicides, is healthy. From this has developed a significant support for organic farming. Similarly, for various reasons, distaste for the way in which animals are farmed or even the killing of animals for food has led to a group who are vegetarian, the definition of which varies in degree of strictness. The supporters of both organic farming and vegetarian practices have had significant effects on the food industry.

Despite diligence in ensuring that our food is clean and wholesome, there are widespread concerns about chemical additives ('E numbers'), bacterial and viral infections, pesticide residues, and the perils of excessive intake of proteins or saturated fatty acids. Food, long recognised as a vector of infectious disease, is now seen to have a role in the aetiology of non-infectious disease such as coronary heart disease, maturity-onset diabetes and obesity.

Quality of life is important. Well-being and protection from stress are not inappropriate ambitions. The French have a reverence for food that has nothing to do with their concern for longevity. They are fortunate in being blessed with both exciting food and longevity. A rigidly controlled diet may not result in longer life, it may only seem longer. The value of survival and quality of life will vary with circumstances and may be judged only by the individual or possibly the community. Mencius (Chinese, second century BC) supported the principle of equilibrium in agriculture and the food production industry between the past, the present and those who come after, based on an understanding of balance and the right time and the right way to do things. This has governed the Chinese approach to food until the present day.

KEY POINTS

1. The intention of this chapter is to show how throughout history, communities have developed a dietary structure that made the most of local resources.
2. The cooking of this food depended on the population, the manner in which society developed and contact with other populations.
3. Religion and social structure have been important determinants of diet.
4. Diets changed once travel and migration became the norm and populations became aware of other modes of life and cooking.
5. The industrialisation of agriculture and food delivery systems, e.g. supermarkets, has profoundly changed nutrition in the developed world.
6. Nutrition throughout much of the world has become more interdependent.

THINKING POINTS

1. How does your diet now differ from that of your parents and grandparents at your age?
2. Trace the sources of the food that you ate at your last three meals. Where did the various items originate?
3. How does the transport of food over the globe affect the energy used its production?

NEED TO UNDERSTAND

The food we eat is not prescribed by recommendations from statutory bodies, but by choices provided by contact with other communities, commerce, economics and what is enjoyed.

FURTHER READING

Aslet, C. (2002) Clocking up food miles. *FT Weekend*, 23/24 February, I.

Burnett, J. (1989) *Plenty and Want – A History of Food in England from 1815 to the Present Day*. Routledge, London.

Davies, N. (1982) *The Ancient Kingdoms of Mexico*. Penguin Press, London.

Fieldhouse, P. (1986) *Food and Nutrition, Custom and Culture*. Chapman & Hall, London.

Kiple, K.F. and Ornelas, K.C. (2000) *Cambridge World History of Food*, Cambridge University Press, Cambridge.

Kitchin, A.H. and Passmore, R. (1949) *The Scotsman's Food: An Historical Introduction to Modern Food Administration*. E & S Livingstone, Edinburgh.

Leeming, M. (1991) *The History of Food*. BBC Books, London.

Patton, N.D., Dunlop, J.C. and Inglis, E.A. (1903) *Study of the Diet of the Labouring Classes in Edinburgh*. Otto Schulze, Edinburgh.

Tannahill, R. (1995) *Food in History*. Three Rivers Press, New York.

Tansey, G. (1995) *Food System Guide*. Earthscan Publications, London.

WEBSITES

www.gti.net/mocolib1/kid/food.html   The food timetable

www.horizon.nmsu.edu/garden/history/welcome.html Where food originated

3

Social, population and environmental influences on nutrition

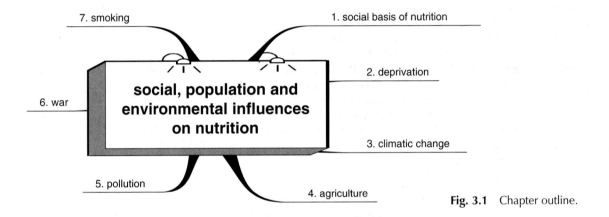

7. smoking

1. social basis of nutrition

social, population and environmental influences on nutrition

2. deprivation

6. war

3. climatic change

5. pollution

4. agriculture

Fig. 3.1 Chapter outline.

SOCIAL BASIS OF NUTRITION

The essence of a good society is that every member, regardless of gender, race or ethnic origin, should have access to a rewarding life (J.K. Galbraith). This includes access to a sufficiency of clean and nutritious food. Harmful factors in the social, population and environment are those that deprive populations of food through insufficient production or importation. Such situations arise from over-population relative to food supply from whatever cause: poverty, corruption, disease, bureaucratic sloth and war. The social and political consequences of famine continue for generations.

Malnutrition and poor water and sanitation contribute to 23% of the risk factors to the global disease pattern. The frequency of natural disasters has been increasing during the twentieth century. These lead to a breakdown in social services, failure to distribute food and hence poor nutrition (Table 3.1).

The reliable provision of food requires an organised society. The epidemiologist Rose has written, 'the primary determinants of disease are mainly economic and social, and therefore its remedy are mainly economic and social'. A society that is disorganised through war, epidemics of infections or natural disaster is less able to produce or deliver food than a well-structured stable society with a sufficiency of healthy workers. It is important that food is grown that is appropriate for the particular population's social, cultural and religious beliefs. The influences on nutrition include:

- food availability and intake
- sufficient but not excessive suitable nutrients and chemicals, which will vary with age, gender, growth and health of the population
- the provision and availability of a sufficiency of clean water

Table 3.1 One-thousand years of natural disasters and death tolls

Date	Country	Disaster	Deaths
1042	Syria	Earthquake	50 000
1281	Netherlands	Storm surge	80 000
1362	Germany	Storm surge	100 000
1622	China, Anxiang	Earthquake	50 000
1668	China	Earthquake	50 000
1693	Italy, Catania	Earthquake	60 000
1780	West Indies	Hurricane	24 000
1755	Portugal	Earthquakes	30 000
1883	Indonesia	Eruption of Krakatoa	36 000
1908	Italy, Messina	Earthquake	86 000
1915	Italy, Avezzano	Earthquake	32 000
1920	China, Gansu	Earthquake	235 000
1923	Japan, Tokyo	Earthquake	143 000
1931	China, Yangtzekiang	Flood	140 000
1935	North India, Quetta	Earthquake	35 000
1939	Turkey, Erzincan	Earthquake	33 000
1942	North-east India	Cyclone	61 000
1954	China, Dongting area	Flood	40 000
1970	Bangladesh, Chittagong, Khulna	Cyclone	300 000
1970	Peru, Chimbote	Earthquake, landslide	67 000
1976	Guatemala, Guatemala City	Earthquake	22 000
1976	China, Tangshan	Earthquake	290 000
1985	Colombia	Eruption of Mt Nevado del Ruiz	25 000
1988	Armenia, Spitak	Earthquake	25 000

- a nutrient intake that meets the requirements and constraints set by the individual's genetic constitution
- a ready disposal of breakdown products of metabolism, urine and faeces
- food that is tasty and meets with the cultural, social and religious requirements of the population.

The world's population will increase by between 2.5 and 3.5 billion by the year 2025. There are even projections that the world population will be greater than 8 billion in the year 2025, that is, it will have grown four-fold in a century. There are, however, signs that population growth is declining in many countries, e.g. China and possibly India and Indonesia. Exceptions are within Africa and the Middle East (Table 3.2). To provide adequate contraception for the world's fertile female population would cost US$ 9 billion annually, the amount the world spends on arms every 56 h. The world's population has risen by 40% during the past 20 years and food production has risen by 50%, although Africa is an exception to this. Food production will

have to rise by 75% over the next 30 years to feed 9 billion people. An indication of global priorities in spending is given in Table 3.3.

Much of our modern thinking on population comes from the essay by Thomas Malthus (1766–1834), an Englishman who pioneered economic theory. He held that the power of populations to increase is infinitely greater than the power in the Earth to produce subsistence for man. Population, when unchecked, increases in a geometric progression. Thus, the human population, irrespective of size, would double every 25 years.

If $P(t)$ is the population size during the period t, and r is the population growth rate over unit time, then the Malthus population model is:

$$P(t + 1) = (1 + r)P(t)$$

Subsistence increases only in an arithmetical ratio. The effects of subsistence and population must be kept equal. Whenever a gain occurs in food production over population growth, a higher rate of population increase is stimulated; however, if the population grows too much more rapidly than food

Table 3.2 Population characteristics: some differences between the poorest and richest countries

	Poorest countries	Richest countries
Population	Increasing	Static
Age distribution	Young	Elderly
Diseases	Infections:	Non-infectious:
	AIDS	coronary heart disease
	tuberculosis	cancer
	hunger	
Food	Insufficient	Too much
Water	Insufficient, contaminated	Plentiful, clean
Housing	Rural and urban slums	Comfortable
Agriculture	Marginal, removing trees	Intensive:
		pesticides
		herbicides
Fuel	Timber, loss of forests	Fossil fuels
		Air pollution
Pollution	People	By-products of industry, transport, packaging

Table 3.3 World's priorities: annual expenditure

	Spending (US$ billion)
Basic education for all	6
Cosmetics in USA	8
Water and sanitation for all	9
Ice cream in Europe	11
Reproductive health for women	12
Perfumes in Europe and USA	12
Basic health and nutrition	13
Pet foods in Europe and USA	17
Business entertainment in Japan	35
Cigarettes in Europe	50
Alcoholic drinks in Europe	105
Military spending world-wide	780

Source: UN *Human Development Report* (1999).

production then the growth is affected by famine, disease and war. Malthus also advocated the advisability of reducing the birth rate of the poor. This was in contrast to a British Prime Minister of the period, who proposed that the poor relief should give special consideration of large families as, 'those who enriched their country with a number of children, have a claim upon its assistance for their support'.

There is, for whatever reason, an inverse relationship between life expectancy and total fertility rates in populations. Five billion people world-wide can now expect to live to more than 60 years. The global average lifespan has increased from 48 to 66 years since 1982 and will reach 73 in 2025.

Malthus did not anticipate the technological advances that have altered agriculture and industry in general, but it should be remembered that we are only 200–300 years into the Industrial Revolution.

While the world population grew from 1.49 billion in 1890 to 2.5 billion in 1950 and to 5.32 billion in 1990, energy consumption grew from 1 terawatt (tera is 10^9) in 1890 to 3.3 terawatts in 1950 to 13.7 terawatts in 1990. Energy consumption grows as the population grows and as poor people become richer. Each individual in the developing world uses 0.28 kilowatts (kW), a year, while those in the developed world use 3.2 kilowatts and those in the USA use 9 kW. If the poor of the world were to increase their use to a modest amount of energy, say 2.3 kW a year, this could mean a seven-fold increase in world energy consumption. This, combined with a doubling of their numbers by 2050, could mean a 14-fold increase in energy consumption. At the present rate of consumption there is sufficient oil and gas to last for 50 years. Energy costs in industrialised countries are low, but energy is wasted. Energy costs in the developing world are steadily rising; cheap biomass fuels, e.g. wood, dung and crop wastes, are insufficient for needs. Over 2 billion people suffer from acute scarcity of fuel wood and lack other energy supplies. Deforestation and the growing use of tree, crop and dried

Table 3.4 Influences on global carbon availability

Source	Amount (tonnes)
Fossil fuels	5 billion
Plant respiration	50 million
Deforestation	2 billion
Biological and chemical absorption	50 billion
Plant photosynthesis	100 billion
Biological and chemical absorption to ocean	104 billion

Note: There is some disagreement in the English language on how to name large numbers; the British and the American systems vary: 10^9, UK thousand million, US billion; 10^{12}, UK billion, US trillion; 10^{15}, UK thousand billion, US quadrillion; 10^{18}, UK trillion, US quintillion. A googol is 10^{100}. The US system will be used in this book.

dung for fuel removes these vital soil replenishers. These changes in energy requirements and utilisation could have serious effects on global carbon availability (Table 3.4).

A definition of health should include the concept of sustainability or the ability of the ecosystem to support life in quantity and quality. The converse of sustainability is entrapment. Entrapment leads to dependence on outside aid, forced migration, starvation or civil war.

The human population is almost at the point where more live in cities than in the countryside. In 1950 only one city, New York, had more than 10 million inhabitants. Now there are 20, of which 16 are in the developing world. These mega-cities, e.g. Bangkok, Manila , São Paulo and Mexico City, have great problems in feeding, watering, removing waste products, and traffic. These problems have been faced and met by all developing cities through the ages. Many of the new mega-cities are in vulnerable sites on flood plains, with low-lying coastal areas and poorly constructed buildings. Successful cities, e.g. London, are comprised of suburbs or villages which coalesce into a city.

It has been noted that there is an intensification of thunderstorms over heated cities.

It is predicted that by the year 2030 the level of the sea will have risen by 18 cm owing to global warming (climate change). Global warming causes the drying of wells in some regions and an increase in rain, flooding and water levels elsewhere. Drought leads to less easily available fuel, fewer raw materials for industry, less fodder for livestock and even a decrease in availability of medicinal plants. An increase in time spent on collecting fuel and water may result in fewer livestock

and less manure for fuel or fertiliser. Money would be spent on fossil fuel and farm yields would be affected. The prospect overall is of lower incomes, and poorer nutrition and health.

Environmental damage is in itself serious, and nutritionists must be aware of the potential human nutritional consequences of this damage.

DEPRIVATION

Material deprivation is strongly linked with many common diseases and this effect is found in all societies throughout the world. Poverty means poor health and performance, wherever one lives. The definition and measurement of deprivation is important because of the relationship between deprivation, poor nutrition and ill health. One measurement scale of deprivation in Britain is the Jarman underprivileged area 8 (UPA 8) score. The variables include unemployment, overcrowding, no car, low owner occupation, social class, poor skills, pensioners living alone, single parent, lack of amenities, ethnic status, children under 5 and having moved within 1 year. Unemployment is an important single element in the definition of deprivation. Hospital admissions correlate highly with all measures of deprivation.

Gandhi described poverty as the worst form of violence. Some differences in population characteristics between the poorest and richest countries are shown in Table 3.2. Table 3.5 gives the number of deaths in developed and developing countries for 1990. Non-communicable diseases account for 77% of global mortality.

Table 3.5 Numbers of deaths (thousands) from disease in 1990 in developed and developing countries

Disease	Developed countries	Developing countries
Infections and parasites	163	9166
Respiratory infections	389	3992
Maternal and perinatal deaths	85	2812
Nutritional deficiencies	30	604
Cardiovascular disorders	5245	9082
Malignant neoplasms	2413	3611
Diabetes mellitus	176	396
Injuries	834	4251

Source: *British Medical Journal* (1997) **314**, 1367.

Poverty exists where there is a lack of resources, including:

- money and material possessions
- emotional and psychological support
- environmental protection
- education
- shelter and housing.

These factors all significantly affect health and well-being. Income inequality goes hand in hand with underinvestment in human resources. Poverty may be relative or absolute; absolute poverty is when a life-threatening state exists. Poverty should be measured by life expectation, literacy and infant mortality rate. Poverty may change with age, employment status, disability and changing local conditions. The number of people in the world experiencing real poverty is 1 billion, one-fifth of the total population. This group has 1.5% of gross national product and 1% of world trade. Poverty is the principal cause of 12 million deaths a year in children under 5 years of age, 4 million from acute respiratory tract infections and a further 3 million from diarrhoea and dysentery. Malnutrition is an underlying cause of 30% of child death, affects growth in 230 million children and is associated with severe wasting in 50 million others. Tuberculosis, malaria and maternal mortality increase in poverty-stricken areas. In 1997, 0.5 million children under the age of 15 years were infected with the human immunodeficiency virus (HIV).

The economist Amartya Sen has questioned whether inadequate food production and availability are of themselves sufficient to explain the onset of famine. Famines can occur despite reasonable food production. Starvation occurs because a substantial proportion of the population loses the means of obtaining food. Such a loss may occur from unemployment, a fall in the purchasing power of wages, or a shift in the exchange rate between goods and services sold and food bought. Climatic disasters can cause famine, as can food hoarding. Food is never shared equally by all people on the basis of total availability. Particularly vulnerable are people who depend on seasonal work and may starve between periods of employment.

CLIMATIC CHANGE

The cosmic influences on climate are due to insulation, the amount of sunlight hitting the top of the atmosphere and hence energy passing through to the Earth's surface. Local weather, a current transient state, becomes warmer, and air flow from the equator to the poles increases, causing more thunderstorms, hurricanes and monsoons until the energy runs out near the poles. The primary cause of seasonal and annual variations in the weather is the tilt of the Earth's axis. Over long periods there are minor periodic variations in the shape, orientation and tilt of the planets in relation to each other, causing repetitive changes in the climate. For example, the Earth orbits the sun in an elliptical path, influencing the distance of the Earth from the sun, and hence the weather.

El Niño

This is a major influence on global climate, due to the warming of the surface water of the Pacific. The tropical Pacific Ocean is characterised by warm surface water in the west (29–30°C) and much cooler temperatures in the east (22–24°C). The western water area is associated with intense rain and atmospheric heating. The cooler surface water of the eastern Pacific is in equilibrium with the western warmer surface water. Every 3–7 years this state of equilibrium breaks down and the ocean surface is warm throughout the Pacific. This may last for a year and is the El Niño event. The result is a disruption of weather in the higher latitudes. Following this there is a cooling phase in the tropical Pacific, La Niña. Although El Niño is local, the effect is global, with droughts in Australia and Indonesia, weakened summer monsoon rainfall over south Asia, catastrophic flooding along the Pacific coast of South America, and disappearance of fish stocks. Where the impact is felt, flooding, forest fires, loss of housing and loss of crops may occur – grain is destroyed and fisheries are ruined. Water-borne diseases (hepatitis, dysentery, typhoid and cholera) associated with El Niño have a cyclical pattern.

AGRICULTURE

Depletion of the productivity of land

An estimate of 200 kg of grain per person per year is needed for survival. The productivity of land is increasing, but climatic changes and availability of water are important factors in such increases. Some 25 billion tonnes of topsoil are lost annually from the world's crop lands. As a result, the world's area of deserts is increasing.

Deforestation

Over 11 million hectares of tropical forest are felled each year, leading to soil erosion, with resulting floods and development of desert. Subsequent flood-control measures can impede migration of fish and fishing practices. Other losses of trees result from the migration of destructive insects to new areas, e.g. Dutch elm disease, chestnut blight and gypsy moth.

Availability of soil micronutrients

Oil pollution or a change in soil pH alters the bioavailability of micronutrients to plants and thereby adversely affects the food chain.

Use of chemical fertilisers

Considerable progress has been made in agriculture with the 'green revolution' crops. High-yielding staple crops provide a consistent and predictable calorie intake in a wide number of countries. However, the fertilisers used to maintain the plants are quality sources of nitrogen, but do not necessarily contain the rich array of micronutrients, e.g. sulfur, manganese, zinc and copper, provided by the traditional manures.

The trace element content of the soil declines and this is reflected in plant growth. There is now a serious possibility that a new nutritional bottleneck is developing wherein the constraint to growth is not macronutrients, but micronutrients such as zinc.

The reduction of crop-rotation practices and other modern agricultural techniques may result in zinc deficiency in soil and hence in plants. Goitre has also been attributed to the use of fertilisers that impair the bioavailability of iodine.

POLLUTION

Large stretches of water, rivers, lakes and seas contain dangerous heavy metals and chemicals in concentrations high enough to kill fish and endanger human life. Despite legal restrictions, factories and sewerage works dump dangerous substances, e.g. mercury, cadmium, insecticides, herbicides and chemicals such as chloroform, into the sea, lakes and rivers. Some contamination also comes from old dumps and old mine workings. The food chain is adversely affected by this pollution.

Air pollution hastens the death of up to 25 000 vulnerable people a year in the UK alone.

WAR

There have been more than 150 wars in the world since 1945, mostly internal and mostly in the developing world. There has been a six-fold increase in the number of refugees since 1970, some 1% of the world's population, from Rwanda, Afghanistan and the Balkans. They often live in camps, families are destroyed and dispersed, and they suffer untold horrors. Famines, polluted wells and inadequate water supplies become the norm. Women are assaulted and raped, and even may have to kill their babies and eat them under cruel conditions. Infant mortality increases, with measles and other infections killing hungry populations. Children are recruited into armies to become killers. AIDS is rampant with rape and the loss of safe patterns of sexual conduct. Such local wars destroy social and cultural norms and the range of traditions, values and understanding that these carry. Health workers are attacked. The long-term consequence of war is the destruction of society, exacerbated by danger from land mines in strategic places, e.g. around hospitals.

SMOKING

There is considerable overlap between tobacco smoking and conditions in which bad nutrition is believed to play an aetiological role. This is considered again later.

KEY POINTS

1. This chapter gives an overview of factors affecting nutrition in the community.
2. The provision of food in amounts that allow choice and for babies to grow and to reach their potential as adults assumes a predictable structure to society.
3. This chapter looks at social and environmental factors that upset such order and have considerable consequences on nutrition in the community.

THINKING POINTS

1. What are the conditions that make for poverty, malnutrition and famine?

2. How do these occur in the developing world and in the developed world?
3. How can this happen where you live? Does it happen where you live?
4. How can adequate usage of land and a good environment coexist?

NEED TO UNDERSTAND

1. Nutrition is a global interest.
2. Each region will be fed according to the local climatic, social, economic and political climate.

FURTHER READING

Brunner, E. (1997) Stress and the biology of inequality. *British Medical Journal*, **314**, 1187–91.

Calman, K.C. (1997) Equity, poverty and health for all. *British Medical Journal*, **314**, 1472–6.

Campbell, D.A., Radford, J.M.C. and Burton, P. (1991) Unemployment rates: an alternative to the Jarman index. *British Medical Journal*, **303**, 750–5.

Galbraith, J.K. (1996) *The Good Society. The Humane Agenda*. Sinclair Stevenson, London.

Godlee, E. (1991) Strategy for a healthy environment. *British Medical Journal*, **303**, 836–8.

Gopalan, C. (1999) The changing epidemiology of malnutrition in a developing society – the effects of unforseen factors. *Bulletin of the Nutrition Foundation of India*, **20**, 1–6.

Hall, P. (1998) *Cities in Civilization*. Weidenfeld & Nicolson, London.

Leather, S. (1996) *The Making of Modern Malnutrition*. Caroline Walker Trust, London.

Lowrey, S. (1991) Housing. *British Medical Journal*, **303**, 838–40.

Marmont, M.G. (1998) Improvement of social environment to improve health. *Lancet*, **351**, 57–60.

Pena, M., Bacallao (2002) Malnutrition and poverty. *Annual Review of Nutrition*, **22**, 241–253.

Rose, G. (1992) *The Strategy of Preventive Medicine*. Oxford University Press, Oxford.

Summerfield, D. (1997) The social, cultural and political dimensions of contemporary war. *Medicine, Conflict and Survival*, **13**, 3–25.

United Nations Children's Fund (UNICEF). *Progress of Nations*. Annual Report, New York.

United Nations Development Programme (1999) *Human Development Report*, New York.

Weaver, L.T. and Beckerleg, S. (1993) Is health a sustainable state? A village study in The Gambia. *Lancet*, **341**, 1327–8.

World Bank (1997) *Sector Strategy: Health, Nutrition and Population*. World Bank Group, Washington, DC.

World Health Organisation Report (1998) *Life in the 21st Century – A Vision for All*. WHO, Geneva.

World Health Organisation Report (1999) *Making a Difference*. WHO, Geneva.

Medicine, Conflict and Survival is a journal devoted to this topic.

WEBSITES

www.alertnet.org   Up-to-date information on current natural disasters

www.unicef.org   UNICEF

www.twnside.org.sg   Third World network

www.undp.org   UN development programme

www.globalforumhealth.org   The Global Forum for Health Research

Part II

Calculating how much food a community eats

- The food chain
- Nutritional requirements
- Nutritional epidemiology

4

The food chain

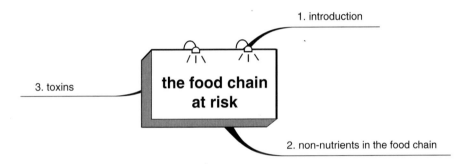

Fig. 4.1 Section outline.

INTRODUCTION

This section focuses on the adverse side of the food chain rather than the overall food chain. A complex web of events occurs before food is eaten by humans. A food web gives a more accurate picture than the more familiar food chain, as most organisms eat from a diversity of food sources. The food chain is the process whereby nitrogen and carbon are synthesised to nutrients, simple and complex, by microorganisms, sea plankton and plants. These are eaten by ruminants, vegetarian animals and fish, which are in turn eaten by omnivores and carnivores, including humans.

The amount of carbon in the atmosphere relative to that in the earth and ocean is important. The balance between net primary use for the synthesis of organic substances of carbon and subsequent decomposition is affected by a number of factors.

Climate affects the accumulation of carbon and nitrogen in the earth and water. The store of carbon in earth and water [some 2000 gigatonnes (Gt)] is three times that in the atmosphere (700 Gt). Water, particularly in the oceans, contains dissolved carbon dioxide. Oceans circulate massive currents of water and hence transport large amounts of heat, fresh water and nutrients around the world. As discussed in Chapter 3, they are also regulators of climate and nutrition. Sea ice is a crucial boundary between the ocean and the atmosphere, which varies from ocean to ocean and even between the landlocked Arctic and the sea surrounding Antarctica. The thickness of the ice cap varies with the seasons, but overall the ice cap is reducing in thickness. As the ice thaws, the salt it contains sinks and affects the circulation of water in the oceans, with further effects on climate and marine fixation of carbon and nitrogen. A warm climate increases carbon loss from the earth and decomposition.

Industry is an important source of carbon dioxide emissions.

Photosynthesis, the decay of organic substances and circulating carbon dioxide have long-term effects on the climate and carbon cycle. Photosynthesis by terrestrial vegetation accounts for half of the carbon that annually cycles between the Earth and the atmosphere. Forestry and farming practices make an important contribution to the overall distribution of carbon, to offset some of the carbon released by burning fossil fuels. The northern peat lands decay very slowly and remove carbon dioxide from the atmosphere more rapidly than it is released, and consequently contain 20–30% of the Earth's carbon stock, which is 60% of the atmospheric carbon pool. Cool conditions and poor air penetration of the soil reduce the decomposition of soil organic matter. Respiration by roots contributes a significant amount of carbon dioxide emission from the ground. Deep ploughing releases carbon from the soil.

Influences on growth

Factors affecting carbon fixation:
- light
- water
- nutrients:
  - phosphorus
  - nitrogen
  - iron and other trace elements

Nitrogen availability is also a factor in plant growth. Nitrogen fixing is mainly a function of soil microbes, and therefore the quantity of these microbes is significant. Carbon and nitrogen are utilised by ruminants, vegetarian animals and fish which, in turn, may be eaten by insects, birds, animals, fish and crustaceans. All of these, according to the prevailing local culture, may be eaten by humans. In a predator food chain a plant-eating animal is eaten by a carnivore. In a parasitic food chain a small organism consumes part of a host and may in turn may be infected by a smaller organism. In a saprophytic food chain microorganisms live on dead organic matter.

Food chains in water are known as pelagic food chains. In coastal waters the food chain is regulated by nutrient concentration, which determines the population of phytoplankton, the source of food for fish, squid and marine mammals. Plankton (5–100 µm in size) are responsible, along with a microbial food web, for most of the primary production in the sea. Plankton absorb some 5000 billion tonnes of carbon from the atmosphere each year.

The discharge of organic material by rivers into the seas and oceans is a significant source of oceanic dissolved organic carbon.

Energy is lost as it is transferred on eating, so chains are usually not more than four or five stages long. Steps may be omitted, e.g. by eating eggs rather than chickens. By shortening the food chain, energy is conserved.

Economics, religion and social advancement determine what is eaten and the manner and form in which it is eaten. An important element in the choice of what is eaten by humans is the attractiveness of the food or prepared dish. This may depend on the expected appearance, smell, taste, colour, shape, texture, flavour and consistency.

The human food chain may be disrupted by various factors:

- climatic change
- changes in soil fertility and composition
- loss of species through extinction
- pests or bacteria
- pollution of water
- drought
- war and social disruption
- incompetent food transport systems
- poor farming and fishing equipment or practices
- destruction of forests, woods and hedges
- absence of healthy labour
- disincentives to efficient farming and fishing
- over farming and fishing
- genetically modified plants and animals
- poverty
- ignorance
- illness
- cultural and religious non-acceptance of products.

NON-NUTRIENTS IN THE FOOD CHAIN

Infective agents

The most common contaminants of food products

Table 4.1 Transmissible spongiform encephalopathies

	Affected species	Source
Kuru	Human	Human
New variant Creutzfeldt–Jakob disease (nvCJD)	Human	Beef
Gerstmann–Straussler–Scheinker disease	Human	Unknown
Fatal familial insomnia	Human	Unknown
Bovine spongiform encephalopathy (BSE)	Cattle	?Maternal
Scrapie	Sheep, goats	?Maternal
Chronic wasting disease of mule deer and elk		?Maternal
Transmissible encephalopathy of mink		?Maternal

are microbes or fungi arising from improper sanitation, inadequate refrigeration during storage or insufficient cooking. Five sources of bacteria can cause food-borne illness:

- faecal matter or urine of infected humans or animals
- nasal and throat discharges of sick individuals or asymptomatic carriers
- infections on body surfaces of food handlers
- infected soil, mud, surface water and dust
- seawater, marine materials and marine life.

Some foods are contaminated by antibiotics and antiseptic agents.

Cannibalism, prions, animal feeds and disease

A form of cannibalism occurs in farming when farm animals are fed with food containing tissue products from the same animal species. The result can be very harmful, in that toxic substances and infections that are present in the species are retained within that food chain. The more the animals eat from that closed recycled system, the more concentrated is the toxicity in the species. This is known as bioconcentration. This is becoming apparent with the transmissible spongiform encephalopathies (TSEs) or prion diseases (Table 4.1). Here it is believed that brain and nervous tissue infected by prions can enter the food chain. Conditions caused by eating tissue infected by the infectious protein include kuru, where human brains are eaten by humans, bovine spongiform encephalopathy (BSE), where cattle tissue was fed to cattle, and new variant Creutzfeldt–Jakob disease (nvCJD), where infected cattle nerve tissue is eaten by humans. There is still some doubt about the prion causation of these conditions, and viruses, trace element deficiency or eating from a spectrum of foods may contribute.

The fatal conditions listed in Table 4.1 are of infectious, inherited or sporadic origin. These diseases cause behavioural changes, alterations of sensation, changes in mental state and ataxia. The typical pathology is non-inflammatory vacuolation or spongiosis in brain cells and occasionally amyloid deposition in the brain and spinal cord. The incubation periods are long and death comes after a drawn-out, progressive illness.

Chemicals

These include antibiotics, pesticides, metals, industrial chemicals and fertilisers.

Distinguishing between toxicity and hazard

Toxicity is the ability of a toxin to produce a harmful effect.
Hazard is the capacity of the chemical to produce toxicity under the circumstances of exposure.

Plants are the primary food source as they convert solar energy to food. Plants also absorb inorganic chemicals, whether they be nutrients or toxicants from the aqueous phase of the soil. Through ingestion and digestion of plants by animals, such chemicals can be transferred from one organism to another. Decaying organic matter, whether animal or plant, returns to the soil as inorganic chemicals in solution, which may be removed

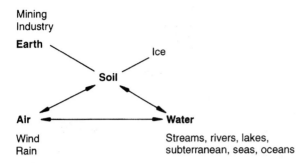

Fig. 4.2   Physical vectors of water-soluble chemicals through soil, water and air.

once again by the action of microorganisms. Rainwater dissolves soil matter and may carry these soluble chemicals from the land to the sea through streams and rivers. The chemicals may return to the terrestrial system through precipitation into stream and river sediments (Figure 4.2). Two-thirds of the world's population lives within 80 km of the sea and much of the pollution from the land runs into the sea.

The chain may be distorted or contaminated by pollutants, chemicals or infection. Mining, smelting, coal mining and coal utilisation, dredging of waterways, chemical manufacturing systems, sewage sludge, fertilisation, irrigation and traffic patterns may alter these natural cycles. These utilities, situated in localised areas, may be traced as sources of pollution entering the human food chain. Radioactive waste products are permitted to be discharged into the sea.

Nitrates are a toxin both in food and as widely used in agriculture. Nitrates are used as additives in preserving cured meats and are naturally present in celery, beetroot and lettuce, accumulating from nitrogenous fertilisers and also occurring in drinking water following leaching from farms. Microbial nitrate-reducing activity occurs in the mouth, where oral bacteria reduce nitrate recirculated in the saliva to nitrite. If the nitrate content of the water drunk by babies is increased, then nitrate reduction and subsequent absorption of nitrites can result in methaemoglobin formation. This reduces the oxygen-carrying capacity of the blood, leading to tiredness and reduced activity. N-Nitrosation occurs at low pH in the stomach from salivary nitrate, with nitrosamine formation and the potential for carcinogenic change. Most

nitrosamines are metabolised in tissues, but N-nitrosoproline, a stable nitrosated amine, is excreted in urine and indicates N-nitrosamine formation. High dietary fat reduces N-nitrosoproline excretion. There is also an endogenous non-microbial synthesis system for nitrate, which is derived from dietary protein and can be a significant source of nitrates.

Synthetic residues in animal carcasses

Such residues may arise as pollutants in the environment from veterinary prescription of drugs, the ingestion of feed or water contaminated by pesticides.

The most common types of drugs used in animal production are:

* **Antimicrobial drugs**: to control and prevent diseases and promote growth. Such antimicrobial drugs are used in the treatment of mastitis, enteritis, and pneumonia and to eradicate parasites. Feeding supplements of low levels of the antibiotics chlortetracycline and oxytetracycline improves growth rates and feed efficiency. This increases the rate of weight gain, hence reducing the time to achieve a required weight. The selective antibiotic monensin affects the rumen microbes but not the metabolism of the animal, and improves daily weight gain by approximately 16%.
* **Parasiticides and pesticides**: to control helminths, e.g. roundworms, tapeworms, liver flukes, coccidia, insects (flies, lice, mange, mites, grubs, etc.) and other parasites.
* **Hormones**: to stimulate growth, encourage the development of lean meat, increase feed efficiency, or prevent or terminate pregnancy in female cattle. Anabolic implants are growth stimulants and vary in use with the type, age and sex of the animal. Calves implanted during nursing show an average enhanced increase in daily weight gain of 9%. Cattle implanted from weaning to finishing average a 15% increase in daily weight gain. Finishing cattle average an 11% increase in daily weight gain. Melengestrol acetate, a synthetic progesterone which is a contraceptive for heifers, improves average weight gain by 11% and the feed conversion efficiency by 11%.

- **Feed additives, vitamins and minerals**: such products leak into the food chain as a result of incorrect dosage or route of administration, species and site of administration. Lack of information about a drug's turnover time, resulting in the sale of treated animals without allowing sufficient withdrawal time, premature slaughter of treated animals, contamination of feed milling equipment and bins, or exposure to water containing antibiotics used to flush alleys and waste bins may also result in additives used in animal production appearing inappropriately in food.

The enteric absorption of ingested drugs varies with the dose level, the drug formulation and the addition of an adjuvant (a compound added to lengthen the period of release). Human exposure is reduced as the animals may metabolise, excrete and dilute these compounds. Some metabolites may have a different toxicity to that of the parent compounds, and such toxicity may vary from species to species.

Industrial contaminants

The release of crude oil hydrocarbons into the sea or soil is an important contaminant.

Large power stations which are sited at the sea shore use massive amounts of water for cooling. Fish and other marine life are drawn in with the water and killed.

Phthalate esters are widely used in industry and their annual production is of the order of millions of kilograms. These spread to the environment as pesticide carriers and insect repellents. They are also used as plasticiser additives and slowly leach over a prolonged period from the plastic product into the environment. They are relatively modest in their toxicity, although they may leach from plastic bags to stored blood. Milk, cheese, lard and other fatty substances can extract phthalate plasticisers from plastic tubing used in processing and from polyvinyl chloride (PVC)-based plastic containers and film. Concentrations are generally low, in single figures per million, although the concentration is increased in fatty foods (Figures 4.3 and 4.4). The levels resulting in acute toxicity are likely to be of 50–1000 mg/kg body weight, or may reach even higher levels. The long-term effects are not known.

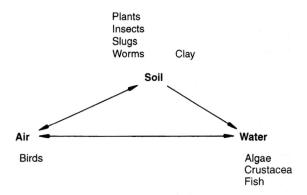

Fig. 4.3 Physical vectors of fat-soluble chemicals may be present in clays, but tend to be concentrated in the lipids of plants, birds and animals.

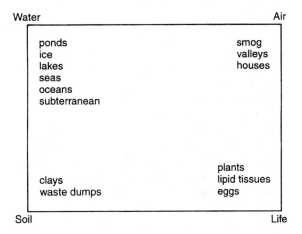

Fig. 4.4 Concentrations of chemicals in static and mobile phases: water, air, soil and life.

There is widespread distribution of these chemicals in the marine and freshwater systems. This, combined with the high lipid solubility of these compounds, raises the problem of food-chain accumulation in fish, seafood and water fowl. These chemicals are difficult to identify using standard chemical analytical methodology.

Some of the most toxic chemicals, dioxins and polychlorinated biphenyls (PCBs), are transferred by evaporation from soils, waste dumps and polluted lakes to be trapped in the ice of the Arctic. The chemicals then pass into the food chain, to be eaten by whales, seals, polar bears and Inuits (Eskimos).

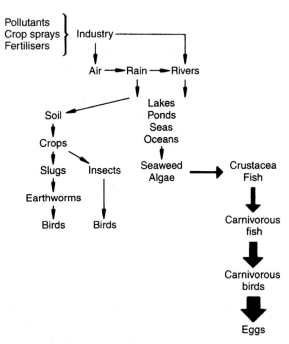

Fig. 4.5 Food-chain effect and biomagnification factor. The biomagnification factor is a sequence of concentration within organisms compared with the immediate soil or water environment in which the organisms live. The biomagnification, for example of DDT, may be of the order of 10^3 to 10^6 between algae and fish-eating birds, and between the soil and birds that eat earthworms. At all of these stages other creatures can eat intermediate stages in the chain and so concentrate chemicals in their own tissues.

Agricultural contaminants

DDT (dichlorodiphenyltrichloroethane) is no longer used in many agricultural systems because of its toxicity but, despite this, it remains in the environment. The phenomenon of *biomagnification* shows that concentrations of such chemicals can increase by 1000 to 1 000 000 times as they pass to the top of the food chain, causing serious deformities or even death (Figure 4.5). Phytoplankton may have a DDT concentration of 0.0025 ppm, which compares with lake trout at 4.83 ppm. Zooplankton may have a DDT concentration of 0.123 ppm and herring gull eggs 124 ppm. As phytoplankton collect nutrients for plant growth they also accumulate non-polar contaminants which may be in the water in very low concentrations.

The development and introduction of genetically modified (GM) crops is a major development in agriculture. They are heralded on one side as a significant development in a robust farming and ecological environment, meeting the needs of the undernourished, but cause grave concern to others concerned at the potential for such crops to alter the balance of the vulnerable environment around farms.

TOXINS

Plant toxins

Plants may serve as poisons; for example, hemlock, a member of the parsley family, has long been known as a deadly poison. Most chemicals that are natural poisons in plants are known as 'secondary' products, produced by the plant only to form part of its defence mechanism against herbivores and pathogens. Plants also produce certain 'primary' products, such as amino acids, amines and organic acids, e.g. oxalic acid, which may enter the human food chain and cause poisoning. Humans have, through trial and error, learned to avoid certain poisonous plants as foods. Some plant poisons are minimised in their toxicity by cooking.

A system within cells (p-glycoproteins), found especially in the mucosa of the gastrointestinal tract (oesophagus, stomach and colon), protects against toxic substances in plants, bacteria and fungi by pumping toxic substances from the cell. Drugs commonly used in cancer chemotherapy, against which resistance develops, have a common origin in that they are all products of plants, fungi and bacteria. Resistance appears to be related to the amount of p-glycoprotein 170 in the tumour cell. The multidrug resistance-1 gene associated with p-glycoprotein 170 is amplified in patients receiving drugs of plant or bacterial origin. This may explain why cancer in the oesophagus, stomach and colon is so resistant to chemotherapy.

Proteinaceous substances, lectins, are found throughout plants, in seeds, bulbs, bark and leaves, acting as protection against unwanted predators. They are resistant to proteolysis and bind strongly to the brush border of the small intestinal epithelium, resulting in increased growth of the small intestine. Bacterial colonisation of the small intestine can then occur. Lectins bind to specific sugars of the epithelial membrane, glycoconjugates.

Toxicants are grouped together by chemical classification, e.g. alkaloids, cyanogenic glycosides and amino acids, or by their effect, e.g. carcinogens and oestrogens.

Alkaloids
Alkaloids, of which there are possibly 6000, contain nitrogen as part of a heterocyclic ring structure and are often bitter to taste. They are present in about 25% of all plant species. Alkaloids are an important cause of liver, lung and heart damage, neurological disorders and birth defects in livestock, to which alkaloids present a much greater risk than they do to humans, because of the plants and therefore toxins consumed as food. Some, including solarium alkaloids and pyrrolizidine alkaloids, can pass into the human food chain.

- **Solanum alkaloids**: the solanum alkaloids include sugar-based alkaloids (glycoalkaloids) found in potatoes, apples, egg plants, roots and leaves of tomatoes and sugar beet roots. These alkaloids have anticholinesterase properties. The poisoning effects include influenza-like symptoms, headache, nausea, fatigue, vomiting, abdominal pain and diarrhoea. The alkaloid concentration in healthy potatoes is in the order of 2–13 mg solanine/100 g fresh weight, predominantly in the potato skin. The level of solanine is increased in parts of the potato that turn green after exposure to light, resulting in a dangerous concentration of 80–100 mg/100 g fresh weight (20 mg/100 g is the generally accepted upper limit of safety for solanine). Cooking the potato does not reduce solanine concentrations, as the solanine is stable at increased temperature.
- **Pyrrolizidine alkaloids**: some 3% of the flowering plants in the world, about 6000 species, contain pyrrolizidine alkaloids (senecio alkaloids) with about 250 different chemical structures. Pyrrolizidine alkaloid poisoning generally presents as hepatic disease, with chronic liver failure and periportal fibrosis resulting in cirrhosis and veno-occlusive disease as the central veins of the liver are blocked by connective tissue. Pyrrolizidine poisoning usually occurs from contact with weeds contaminating food crops,

including wheat or corn, harvested with the grain. The problem may be compounded by plants of Senecio and Crotalaria being used as folk medicine. They may also be taken in the form of herbal teas, e.g. gordolobo yerba. Flower stalks of *Petasites japonicus*, which are used as a cough medicine in Japan, also contain the pyrrolizidine alkaloid petasitenine.

Aconites, the dried root stalks of plants in the Aconitium family, are used as herbal medicines to treat rheumatism, neuralgia and cardiac complaints.

Cyanogenic glycosides
These are synthesised by plants and contain sugar molecules and α-hydroxynitriles (cyanohydrins). When these are degraded by plant enzymes, nitrile groups are eliminated as hydrogen cyanide, which is toxic: 50–60 mg is an average fatal dose in humans. Cyanogenic glycosides have been detected in 110 plant families and over 2000 plant species. These include the plants identified in Table 4.2.

Cyanogenic glycoside poisoning is most seen in populations eating lima beans and cassava, although the concentration in lima varies markedly from the American white bean to the Puerto Rican small black. In cassava, however, cooking removes or destroys cyanogenic glycoside and the enzymes that cause the liberation of hydrogen cyanide. Linseeds, traditionally used as laxatives, are cyanogenic; toxic effects are unknown at traditional levels of intake, but altered processing and increased intake can lead to toxicity. The cyanide content varies from batch to batch (4–12 mmol/kg) and contains the cyanogenic glucoside as cassava. Poisoning from

Table 4.2 Hydrogen cyanide (HCN) levels liberated from food crops containing cyanogenic glycosides

Food	HCN yield (mg/100 g)
Bitter almond seed	290
Peach seed	160
Cassava leaves	104
Apricot seed	60
Lima bean	
Puerto Rico small black	400
American white	10

cyanogenic glycosides can also occur from the ingestion of bitter almonds and cherry seeds, and drinking tea made from peach leaves.

Amino acids and amines
There are more than 200 *amino acids*, but only 25–30 are universally incorporated into proteins or occur as intermediates in metabolism. Some uncommon amino acids interfere with metabolism and consequently are toxic. Seeds of the lathyrus species, including chickling vetch, flat-podded vetch and Spanish vetchling, contain lathyrogens, toxic amino acids that cause lathyrism. Lathyrism is characterised by muscular weakness and paralysis of the lower limbs and may be fatal. It is particularly prevalent in times of famine when there is reduced choice in food.

Another uncommon plant amino acid that is extremely poisonous is 3-methylenecyclopropyl-propionic acid (hypoglycin A). This is found in the fruit of the tropical tree *Blighia sapida*. This plant is poisonous when the fruit is unripe or when the inadequately cooked fruit is eaten. The consequences are severe vomiting, coma, acute hypoglycaemia and death within 12 h. The toxicity is due to interference with the oxidation of fatty acids and, as a result, undernourished individuals are particularly vulnerable.

Excess ingestion of the selenium-containing amino acids, selenomethionine and selenocystine, results in dermatitis, fatigue, dizziness and hair loss. Such amino acid poisoning results from the consumption of the nuts from the monkey nut tree, *Lecythis olloria*, found in Central and South America.

Amines include serotonin, noradrenaline, tyramine, tryptamine and dopamine. These are very active pharmacologically, are potent vasoconstrictors, and are found in bananas, plantains, pineapples, avocados, tomatoes and plums. While levels of these amines normally eaten are readily detoxified, excessive consumption of these plants may prove to be poisonous. Patients receiving the monoamine oxidase inhibitor group of antidepressants, who must avoid amine-rich diets, are particularly vulnerable.

Glucosinolates
These are produced by the brassica plant family, including cabbage, kale, Brussels sprouts, cauliflower, broccoli, turnips, garden cress, water cress, radishes and horseradish, rape seed, and brown, black and white mustard. There are more than 70 different glucosinolates, of which most of the crucifer plants contain several. Glucosinolates are responsible for the pungent flavours of horseradish and mustard, and the characteristic flavour of turnip, cabbage and other related plants. They have been shown to interfere with thyroid function in experimental animals. Toxic effects arise from metabolic products formed from the action of thioglucosidase enzymes, which break the glucosinolates into glucose, organic nitriles, isothiocyanates and thiocyanate ions. These latter two substances modify thyroid function. However, effects on the thyroid gland are only noticed at very high ingestion rates of raw plants, e.g. 500 g of raw cabbage daily for 2 weeks.

Carcinogens

- **Safrole** is a carcinogen found in several oils, including oil of sassafras, camphor and nutmeg. Safrole has been found in 53 plant species and in ten plant families, and has been shown to produce liver cancer when sufficient is added to a rat diet. Safrole represents 75% of the weight of oil of sassafras, which was formerly used as a flavouring agent in root beer. Black pepper contains small amounts of safrole and larger amounts of piprine, which has been shown to be carcinogenic to mice.
- **Furanocoumarins** are carcinogenic chemicals produced by celery, parsley and parsnip. The concentration in these plants is low, but may increase in diseased plants. The most common furanocoumarins are psoralen, bergapten (5-methoxypsoralen) and zanthotoxin (8-methoxypsoralen). Cycasin is found in cycads, which are important sources of starch for tropical and subtropical populations. Such compounds can produce liver, kidney, intestinal and lung cancers in rats.
- **Pyrrolizidine alkaloids** have caused cancer in rodents, and human cancers have been reported from the use of herbal remedies containing these alkaloids.
- **Stevioside** is a very sweet glycoside from *Stevia rebaudiana*. Steviol is the aglycone resulting from bacterial hydrolysis, and has potential for carcinogenesis.

- **Cycasin** is a glycoside present in the nuts of *Cycas circinalis*. This is harmless as the glycone, but the α-glycone methylazoxymethanol is carcinogenic. The β-glucosidase which splits off the carcinogenic α-glycone is present in tissues and in colonic bacteria.
- **Oestrogens**: at least 50 plants are known to contain chemicals that have oestrogenic activity, including carrots, soya beans, wheat, rice, oats, barley, potatoes, apples, cherries, plums and wheatgerm. Oestrogens are also present in vegetable oils such as cotton seed, sunflower, corn, linseed, olive and coconut oils. The oestrogenic activity rests in isoflavones, coumestans or resorcyclic acid lactones. It is doubtful whether physiological effects would be elicited in humans by normal consumption of foods containing these weakly oestrogenic chemicals.

  Human female natural urinary oestrogens and excreted oral contraceptives can feminise male fish when sewage effluent is discharged to a river.
- **Hormone disrupters** are chemicals that affect human or animal health by interfering with normal hormonal processes. They are mediated by hormone receptors and may have an effect at low dosages. However, the response is variable and the differences in response may be due to genetic variation. Bisphenyl A, a chemical in plastics and glues, functions as a relatively potent oestrogen in some circumstances.
- **Mutagens**: the cooking and processing of meat and fish at high temperatures results in heterocyclic amines with mutagenic and carcinogenic potential as judged by the Ames' test.

Miscellaneous toxins

- **Beans**: the broad bean, or lava bean, can produce acute haemolytic anaemia (favism), which is prevalent in Mediterranean countries, China and Bulgaria. The disease is characterised by nausea, dyspnoea, fever and chills, and occurs 5–24 h after broad-bean ingestion. Individuals who are susceptible to favism are deficient in glucose 6-phosphate dehydrogenase, which also results in resistance to malaria.
- **Castor Beans**: contain ricin, a mixture of lectins, two of which ricin D (RCL_{III}) and RCL_{IV} are the most toxic substances known. These lectins are resistant to proteolytic enzyme

hydrolysis. One gram of seed yields 1 mg toxin. A seed contains 250 µg which is lethal.
- **Lentils**: red lentils (*Lensculinaris*) are pulses which produce modest crops. Similar pulses from *Vicia sativa* are sometimes substituted in the diet of some populations. Cultivars of *V. sativa* may contain two neurotoxins, L-β-cyanoalanine and γ-L-glutamyl derivatives, at a concentration of approximately 0.1%, a level capable of being toxic to animals. Most, if not all, of the neurotoxins are lost if the seeds are soaked, and soaking and cooking water is discarded. *Vicia sativa* also contains pyrilidine glucoside. *Vicia sativa* and *V. faba* can also cause favism.
- **Myristicin**: this is a potent hallucinogenic chemical produced by dill, celery, parsley, parsnip, mint and nutmeg. It is said that as little as 500 mg of raw nutmeg may produce psychoactive symptoms, while 5–15 mg of powdered nutmeg may result in euphoria, hallucinations and a dream-like feeling, followed by abdominal pain, depression and stupor.
- **Oxalates**: these may be produced endogenously by the metabolism of ascorbic acid or the amino acid glycine, which is also derived from the families Polygonaceae, Chenopodiacea, Portulacaceae and Fidoidaceae. Spinach contains 0.3–1.2%, rhubarb 0.2–1.3%, beet leaves 0.3–0.9%, tea 0.3–2% and cocoa 0.5–0.9%. The leaves of rhubarb are particularly rich in oxalic acid.
- **Gossypol**: this is the yellow colouring of cotton, *Gossypium*. It is found in the pigment glands of the leaves, stems, roots and seeds, and may form 20–30% of the weight of the gland. When ingested, the results are depressed appetite and loss of body weight, cardiac irregularity and circulatory failure or pulmonary oedema. A major source of gossypol in the diet is cotton seed oil, which may be found in salad oil, margarine and shortening. Gossypol has also been used in China with a 99% effectiveness as a male anti-fertility agent.
- **Diterpenoids**: the honey from wild rhododendrons (*Rhododendron luteum* and *Rhododendron ponticum*) may be poisonous owing to the nectar containing toxic diterpenoids (grayanotoxins).

Microbial toxins

Microbial toxins are poisonous metabolites produced by bacteria, filamentous fungi, mushrooms

Table 4.3 Relative potency of toxins

Toxin	Lethal dose to mice (μg/kg body weight)
Bacterial toxins	0.00003–1
Animal venoms	10–100
Algal toxins	10–1000
Mushroom toxins	> 1000
Mycotoxins	1000–10 000

and algae. Bacterial fungi grow commonly in food, competing for nutrients with animals and humans, as mushrooms and algae are themselves a form of food supply. Bacteria and fungi may proliferate within a food as it is stored or may proliferate on entering the gastrointestinal tract.

Bacterial toxins
Most illnesses caused by pathogenic microorganisms result from proliferation of pathogenic microorganisms in the host, usually in the gastrointestinal tract. In other cases, poisoning arises from the ingestion of toxins. Food-borne diseases usually cause gastrointestinal disturbance. Toxins produced by bacteria have different modes of action and have individual toxic characteristics (Table 4.3).

Some toxins produce the same type of cellular disorder and therefore the toxin is named after the specific action. Toxins that cause enteric disorders, e.g. cholera, salmonellosis and *Escherichia coli*, are called **enterotoxins**. Others, such as tetanus and botulinum, are **neurotoxins**. Bacterial toxins are usually either endotoxins or exotoxins. Endotoxins are released upon the disintegration or death of bacterial cells in the body. These produce specific toxic effects either in specific tissues or affecting the whole body. They are toxic when there is massive bacterial infection in the body and their effects may be due to an overreaction of the host immune system. Exotoxins are special proteins excreted by toxigenic bacteria in various foods, are generally extremely poisonous and may be fatal, e.g. botulism, cholera and gastroenteritis.

Food is only the final link in a chain of infections and as a suitable medium may determine the degree to which a product is infected. For example, cholera-causing organisms do not thrive in acid foods. Botulism is caused by food contaminated by

strains of *Clostridium botulinum*. This highly lethal organism is the most poisonous known to humans.

Mycotoxins are highly poisonous compounds, of low molecular weight, produced by moulds or fungi which are contaminants of fruit and agricultural products. If mould growth occurs on any food there is the possibility of mycotoxin production, which may persist long after the mould has disappeared. A large number of commonly consumed foods therefore may potentially contain mycotoxins. These include wheat, flour, bread, corn meal and popcorn, which may contain aflatoxin, ochratoxin, serigmatocystin, patulin, penicillic acid, deoxynivalenol or zearalenone. Peanuts and pecans may contain aflatoxins, ochratoxin, patulin and strigmatocystin. Apples and apple products may contain patulin. Cereal grains are a good substrate for toxin production, whereas seeds that are high in protein, soya beans, peanuts and cotton seeds, support certain toxins but not others.

The growth of microorganisms in food will be influenced by moisture content, relative humidity, temperature, food composition, presence of competing microorganisms and fungal strain. The critical moisture content varies with the commodity. Storage fungi are primarily aspergilli and some penicillins. Variations in the moisture content of stored materials in different areas throughout storage bins (hot spots) allow fungal growth and toxic development. Other materials in the commodity, e.g. zinc, can also affect fungal growth and toxin production, e.g. aflatoxin and soya beans.

Significant food-borne mycotoxins include aflatoxins, ochratoxin A, citrinin, patulin, penicillic acid, zearalenone, trichothecenes and alternaria toxins.

- **Aflatoxins** are produced by some strains of *Aspergillus flavus* and *A. parasiticus*. There are six main aflatoxins: B_1, B_2, G_1, G_2, M_1, and M_2. Aflatoxin B is a principal member of the aflatoxin family. Aflatoxin M is a metabolite of B_1, found in the milk of dairy cattle that have ingested mouldy feed, and readily produces cancer of the liver. It is stable in raw milk and processed milk products, and is unaffected by pasteurisation or processing into cheese or yoghurt. The widespread use of milk and milk products by children makes this toxin of importance. Foods commonly contaminated with aflatoxins include peanuts, peanut oil, corn and beans. Aflatoxin B can kill poultry and domestic animals. Aflatoxins are potent liver toxins and carcinogenic in animals but, it appears from studies in the USA of otherwise fit people, not in humans. Other studies have shown that aflatoxin contamination of food correlates with the incidence of liver cancer in high-risk areas, such as south-east Asia and tropical Africa, where malnourishment and viral hepatitis are endemic. The mortality rate from liver cancer among individuals infected with hepatitis B and who are antibody positive is ten times higher than in individuals who are antibody negative when eating small amounts of these infected materials. It has been suggested that 50% of liver cancer cases in Shanghai are related to aflatoxin exposure.

- **Ochratoxins** are produced by *Aspergillus ochraceus* and other *Aspergillus* species. They can contaminate corn, pork, barley, wheat, oats, peanuts, green coffee and beans. Ochratoxin A, which frequently occurs in wheat and barley, can cause kidney damage in rats, dogs and pigs, and may cause kidney disease in humans. Only 2–7% of the ochratoxin A in barley is transmitted to beer during processing. Over 80% of ochratoxin A is destroyed on roasting of coffee and variable losses of ochratoxin A occur when baking with toxin-contaminated flour.
- **Citrinin** is a yellow compound produced by *Penicillium* and *Aspergiculla* species, and is a contaminant of yellow peanut kernels from damaged pods. It may be strongly nephrotoxic, although in general is less toxic than ochratoxin A.
- **Patulin** is toxic to bacteria, mammalian cell cultures, higher plants and animals. Patulin, produced by a dozen *Penicillium* and *Aspergiculla* species, is a principal cause of apple rot and a common pathogen on many fruits and vegetables. It is a contaminant of fruit juices worldwide, particularly apple juice. It is unstable in the presence of sulfhydryl compounds and sulfur dioxide. When fruit juices are left to ferment, more than 99% of the patulin is destroyed.
- **Zearalenone** is an oestrogenic compound that causes vulvovaginitis and oestrogenic responses in pigs. It is produced by *Fusarium* species and is found in moist corn in autumn and winter. It is not very toxic and has not been implicated in human disease.

Mushroom toxins

There are thousands of mushroom species; in the USA there may be more than 5000. There are many species with very similar appearance and yet quite different tissues and cellular structure. Edible or poisonous species may differ quite radically in different environmental growth conditions. The poisonous *Amanita muscaria* comes in three colours, dark red, yellowish orange and white. These vary in intensity with age or exposure to sun and rain. The orange-capped toxic variety can be confused with the edible Acesarea. A characteristic feature of a species' appearance may be changed by mechanical damage, which may lead to errors in identity. There are many individual responses to the toxins, which have resulted in conflicting reports regarding edibility in the literature. Responses vary with the number of mushrooms eaten, the preparation, length of cooking, age and the health of the individual, as well as the amount of toxin present in the mushroom. There is no simple test for the toxicity of fungi.

Types of mushroom poisoning
These include cytotoxic, haemotoxic, neurotoxic, hallucinogenic, gastrointestinal, disulfiram-like activity and carcinogenic.

- **Cytotoxic**: the most important toxins in this group are amatoxins and phallotoxins. Amatoxins are 10–20 times more toxic than phallotoxins and there is no known antidote. Phallotoxins are hepatotoxic, whereas amatoxins are both strongly hepatotoxic and nephrotoxic. Fungi containing amanitin include the species *Amanita galerina* and *A. conocybee*. Among the most poisonous of mushrooms is *Amanita phalloides*: this has a large cap which is greenish brown in colour; the smell is of raw potato; the taste, reported by survivors, is said to be quite good. *Amanita galerina* are small brown to buff mushrooms with moist, sticky caps, found on logs buried deep in moss, and are equal in toxicity to *A. phalloides*.
- **Haemotoxic**: the Ear mushroom causes inhibition of blood clotting when eaten in sufficient amounts.
- **Neurotoxic**: *Amanita muscarina* and *A. pantherina* are important examples of neurotoxic mushrooms, which cause increased salivation,

lacrymation, sweating and severe gastrointestinal disturbances.

- **Hallucinogenic**: two mushrooms, *Psilocybe* and *Panaeolus*, may cause euphoria and excitement as well as muscle incoordination and weakness of arms and legs. Panic reactions may follow psychedelic visions of intense, bright-coloured patterns, and are associated with an inability to distinguish between fantasy and reality.
- **Gastrointestinal toxic**: these cause abdominal cramps, intense abdominal pain, nausea, vomiting and diarrhoea, which may be incapacitating and may even cause death in children. *Amanita agaricus* includes the widely available mushrooms sold in supermarkets, as well as a number of phenol-smelling yellow stainers. These mushrooms are variably edible or toxic, suggesting the existence of local mildly toxic forms.
- **Disulfiram-like**: these induce hypersensitivity to ethanol and when eaten with alcohol can cause severe flushing of the face, palpitations, tachycardia, nausea and vomiting. Disulfiram may be offered to alcoholics as an external deterrent to drinking.
- **Carcinogenic**: laboratory assays have identified carcinogenic and mutagenic properties in mushrooms. These include the false morel gyromitrin and two common types, the common commercial supermarket mushroom *Agaricus bisporus* and the Japanese forest mushroom *Cortinellus shiitake*. The toxins responsible are unstable to heat.

KEY POINTS

1. In the food chain, nitrogen and carbon are converted to complex and essential nutrients by microorganisms, sea plankton and plants. There is a complex chain of events, which progresses from the inorganic chemicals in the soil to plants, which are ingested and digested by animals.
2. Food additives and preservatives are substances, either synthetic or natural, which are normally not regarded as food, but added in small amounts influence the desirability of food or preserve food. Additives are also used for enrichment and fortification of nutrients.

3. Food-borne microbes or fungi are other non-nutrients in the human food chain. Antibiotics, pesticides, metals and fertilisers can enter the food chain and hence human food.
4. Industrial contaminants may leach out into the soil and be taken up by plants and enter the human food cycle.
5. Many plants, plant leaves, stalks and roots contain poisonous chemicals, which may protect the plant from being eaten.
6. Toxins can be produced by bacteria, fungi, mushrooms and algae, and are important causes of food-borne illness.

THINKING POINTS

1. How does the length of the food chain for any chosen item in the diet affect its potential for remaining uncontaminated?
2. How can food chains be enriched from the nutritional point of view?
3. How can the food can be protected?

NEED TO UNDERSTAND

1. The food chain is essential for nutrition for all creatures.
2. It generates complex compounds that are necessary for life.
3. The food chain is dependent on its size and length, and freedom from contamination.

FURTHER READING

British Medical Bulletin (2000), **56** (1).

Copley, J. (2000) Climate change. The great ice mystery. *Nature*, **408**, 634–6.

D'Mello, J.P.F., Duffus, C.M. and Duffus, J.H. (1991) *Toxic Substances in Crop Plants*. Royal Society of Chemistry, Cambridge.

European Parliament and Council Directive No. 95/2/EC (1995) Food additives other than colours and sweeteners. *Official Journal of the European Communities*, L61/1.

Kump, L.R. (2000) What drives climate. *Nature*, **408**, 651–2.

Post, D.M., Pace, M.L. and Hairston, N.G. (2000) Ecosystem size determines food-chain length in lakes. *Nature*, **406**, 1047–9.

Winter, C.K., Seiber, J.N. and Muckton, C.F. (eds) (1990) *Chemicals in the Human Food Chain*. Van Nostrand Reinhold, New York.

WEBSITES

The European Union, World Health Organisation, UK and other national websites will give details of the contaminants of the food chain.

DOMESTIC WATER

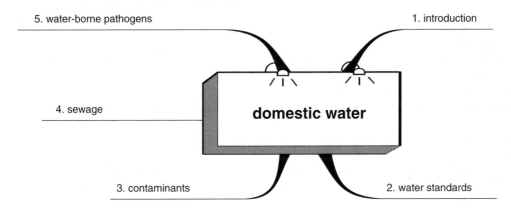

Fig. 4.6 Section outline.

INTRODUCTION

Water occurs in most foods and as free fluid. Some two-thirds of rainwater returns to the atmosphere by evaporation, so it is a renewable commodity.

In organised societies, domestic drinking water, free from bacteria and other pollutants, is made available through a piped water system. Waste products such as sewage should be removed from the domestic scene by pipes and disposed of in a manner that is safe for the population and the environment. Traditional lead pipes are a hazard and may leach lead into water, and therefore there is a vigorous policy to remove domestic lead piping.

World-wide, one thousand million people do not have access to safe water, that is safe from coliform bacteria, cholera, typhoid fever, viral diarrhoeal diseases, infectious hepatitis, poliomyelitis and parasites, e.g. ascariasis, dracunculiasis, nematodes, trachoma and hookworms. Some 1.8 thousand million people do not have adequate sanitary facilities. Water shortage is a global health problem.

The diversion of rivers by dams upstream, e.g. River Sajar in Syria, has profound effects on the populations downstream. In some developing countries women spend 5 h a day collecting water.

WATER STANDARDS

Legislation for water standards varies in the different parts of the UK, but it places a duty on water companies to supply water that is wholesome at the time of supply. This is defined by reference to standards and other requirements of the water supply (water quality). Regulations within the European Community incorporate the relevant requirements of EC Drinking Water Directives (80/778/EEC) and World Health Organisation guidelines.

In assessing the adequacy of water treatment, inspectors assess the:

- disinfection of water supplies
- provision of water-treatment facilities
- use of chemicals, products and materials of construction
- action and studies that have been undertaken to reduce lead (plumbosolvency) and parasites
- colour, turbidity, odour and taste, and the nitrate, aluminium, iron, manganese and polycyclic aromatic hydrocarbons (PAH) content of water.

There must also be sampling programmes for the microbiological quality of the water leaving the treatment works, with analysis for pesticides, protozoa (*Cryptosporidium* and *Giardia*) and bacteria, particularly faecal coliforms. Analyses are made for a wide range of pesticides, atrazine, simazine, chlortoluron, dichlorprop, dichlorvos, isoproturon, ioxynil, methyl chlorphenoxybutyric acid (MCPB), necoprop, propyzimide, 2,4-dichlorophenoxyacetic acid (2,4-D), fenpropimorph, tetrachloromethane, phosphorus, antimony, arsenic and selenium.

The disinfection of the water supply, from bacteria but not protozoa, necessarily involves the reaction of the disinfectant with organic contaminants. These are known as disinfection by-products. Chlorine is very widely used as a disinfectant in England and Wales, and this produces chlorination by-products including trihalomethanes (THM) such as chloroform. There is no strong evidence that these are harmful. Chlorine may react with organic substances in water to produce potentially carcinogenic substances. The risk from such compounds is 10^4–10^6 less than that of contracting waterborne infections. In tropical countries, leaving water for drinking in a plastic bottle, in the sun, for several hours, can disinfect water for drinking.

Most water distribution mains are constructed of cast or ductile iron. Before 1970 in Britain these were given an internal anticorrosion coating of coal tar pitch, which may contain up to 50% of PAH. This PAH may leach into the water supply in solution or in suspension, although surveys show that

Table 4.4 Permitted quantities of substances in domestic water the point of supply

Substance	Standard maximum acceptable concentration ($\mu g/L$)
Polycyclic aromatic hydrocarbons (PAH)	
(Six specific PAH)	0.2
Benzo 3–4 pyrene	0.01 (annual average)
Pesticides	
Individual substances	0.1
Total pesticides	0.5
Aluminium	200
Lead	2530
Nitrates	50 mg as NO_3
Fluoride	1.5 mg
Trihalomethanes (THM)	100 (average over 3 months)

PAH is not present in the majority of samples taken. The medical consequences of ingestion of PAH are not known.

The regulations set standards for permitted quantities of many substances. Those for PAH, pesticides, aluminium, lead, nitrates and THM are shown in Table 4.4. The main source of nitrate in groundwater is leaching from agricultural farmland. The concentration of nitrate varies across England, being higher in eastern lowland rivers (24 mg/l) than in western (13 mg/l) and other rivers (5 mg/l) (data for 1994).

CONTAMINANTS

Cryptosporidium is a protozoan parasite which causes diarrhoea in humans. Blue–green algae occur naturally in all inland waters and their concentration can alter rapidly in response to various climatic factors and the availability of essential nutrients. Sometimes these blue–green algae may release toxins, and when the algae are blooming extra precautions have to be taken to eradicate the algae. Monitoring is insensitive.

Giardia is another protozoan pathogen that may occasionally contaminate drinking water. It is desirable that these protozoa are totally absent from domestic water.

Viruses are important causes of ill-defined outbreaks of sickness and diarrhoea, and usually enter the water cycle through faecal contamination. Techniques for monitoring viruses in water supplies are complex and expensive, and there is no present provision for their identification in domestic water supplies.

Fresh water that is contaminated from industrial and domestic effluent and agricultural fertiliser run-off is at risk of allowing the growth of blooms or scums of toxic cyanobacteria. Microbiological contamination of the water supply, occurring through after-growth within the distribution system, is very difficult to eradicate.

Private water supplies may be drawn from lakes, streams, rivers, wells or boreholes in remote areas, and legislation requires regular testing of this water as there may be local microbiological and chemical problems.

SEWAGE

Effective sewerage is essential for a healthy domestic environment, the sewage being processed by secondary treatment systems even in coastal areas. It is no longer acceptable in Europe and many other parts of the world to allow sewage to be flushed untreated into the sea or lake, which has dire consequences to the marine population and bathing safety.

WATER-BORNE PATHOGENS

Cyanobacteria

Cyanobacteria are found world-wide and were described as long ago as the twelfth century, when dogs died after ingesting neurotoxins from benthic attached to the sediment cyanobacteria. Cyanobacteria are members of the genera *Microcystis*, *Anabaena*, *Aphanizomenon* and *Oscillatoria*. They contain lipopolysaccharide endotoxins or potent agpatotoxins (microcystins) and neurotoxins, e.g. anatoxins and saxitoxins. Few epidemiological studies have assessed the dangers to human health from freshwater cyanobacteria, although exposure to the cyanobacterial blooms has led to skin reactions, conjunctivitis, rhinitis, vomiting, diarrhoea and atypical pneumonia. Cyanobacteria can form blue–green, milky blue, green, reddish or dark brown blooms and scums on ponds and lakes.

Some algal toxins can cause serious liver, skin and central nervous system problems.

Saxitoxin

Most seafoods are safe and unlikely to cause illness, although in regions where reef fish live there is the danger of ciguatera, paralytic shellfish poisoning and neurotoxic shellfish poisoning. The food industry takes elaborate precautions to eliminate such contamination. However, many holiday makers may be endangered by harvesting molluscs and fishing without being aware of pollution in the water.

Saxitoxin is associated with paralytic shellfish poisoning which results from the ingestion of molluscs (mussels, clams, oysters, scallops) contaminated with the neurotoxins of the dinoflagellates *Gonyaolax catenella*. Dinoflagellates are unicellular algae-like organisms which grow in water and may fluoresce and light the sea at night. They also produce red tides or blooms, so that the colour of the water may change to yellow, red, brown or green, depending on the nature of the pigments present. The amount of poison in shellfish depends on the number of dinoflagellates in the water and the amount of water filtered by the shellfish. The molluscs are unaffected by the toxin which is, however, readily released when the mollusc is eaten. The dinoflagellate synthesises saxitoxin, which is highly neurotoxic to humans in a dose of 0.5–0.9 mg. It acts by preventing sodium ions from passing through the membranes of nerve cells and prevents neurotransmission. Saxitoxin is stable to heating and alterations in pH. Symptoms begin rapidly after eating shellfish, appearing as numbness in the lips, tongue and fingertips. This is followed by numbness in the legs, arms and neck, accompanied by general muscular incoordination. Respiratory paralysis occurs within 2–12 h.

Ciguatoxin

Ciguatera is food poisoning following the eating of contaminated fish, that have concentrated the poison while eating dinoflagellates, e.g. *Gambierdiscus toxicus*. Herbivorous fish eat algae on rocks, and accumulate toxins in their tissues. Although the dinoflagellate poison is 40 000 times more toxic than cyanide, the fish are not affected. Over 400 fish species may harbour ciguatoxin. The fish that are affected are those that swim at the bottom of the water near reefs, are found between 35°N and 35°S latitudes, and include barracuda, snapper, red snapper, jack, amber jack, grouper, chinamen fish, parrot fish, surgeon fish, moray eel, sea bass and shark. Toxic species vary from area to area. The symptoms of ciguatera include nausea, numbness and itching, aching jaws and teeth, and reversal of hot and cold sensations. The fish responsible for ciguatera vary in degree of toxicity, which may alter over a period of one to several years. There are no physical or chemical tests for the presence of ciguatoxin, only its post-ingestion effects.

Brevetoxin

Brevetoxin is a marine biotoxin from the dinoflagellate *Gymnodinium breve*, a blue–green alga abundant in the Gulf of Mexico. This causes red tides which kill many fish and infect bivalve molluscs. The growth of these dinoflagellates varies with salinity, wind and water temperature, with maximum growth occurring at between 17.5 and 18°C. Two heat-stable neurotoxins have been isolated from *G. Breve*. The symptoms are those of neurotoxic fish poisoning, but paralysis has not been reported.

Aplysiatoxin

An algal toxin that causes 'swimmer's itch' has been isolated from the widely distributed blue–green alga *Lyngbya majuscula*. This dermatitis is uncommon because the algal toxin readily decomposes when exposed to strong sunlight, although its ingestion may contribute to the risk of developing cancer.

Pfiesteria piscicida, a dinoflagellate found in the estuaries of North Carolina and Maryland in the USA, produces a toxin that may kill masses of fish. Humans may be affected, not from the affected fish, but by contact with water containing the toxin. Symptoms include developing nausea, respiratory problems and profound but slowly reversible memory loss. Exposure to lower concentrations of *P. piscicida* toxin may result in chronic ill health.

KEY POINTS

1. Most countries oblige water companies to supply water which is wholesome. Wholesomeness is defined by reference standards which include the freedom of the water from bacterial contamination, and the presence of chemicals, products and materials only at concentrations that do not present health risks. It is also demanded that the water looks and smells clean.
2. Contamination may be from faecal material, pesticides and fertilisers, and also from the piping which carries the water, e.g. the pipe coating, soldering materials or lead.
3. Protozoa and algae may be present in reservoirs, lakes and other sources of water. Such contamination is a hazard to recreational users such as wind surfers.

THINKING POINTS

1. Does the water in your locality come from a reservoir, river or lake?
2. What is its composition?
3. What are the possible sources of contamination?

NEED TO UNDERSTAND

1. Water is essential for life and cleanliness.
2. In a concentrated community clean water has to be achieved rather than taken for granted.
3. An understanding of water-borne diseases is necessary to ensure clean water.
4. Similarly, effective sanitation is mandatory for health.

WEBSITES

www.who.dk   World Health Organisation Europe
www.environment.defra.gov.uk   Quality of water, UK, Department of the Environment

5

Nutritional requirements

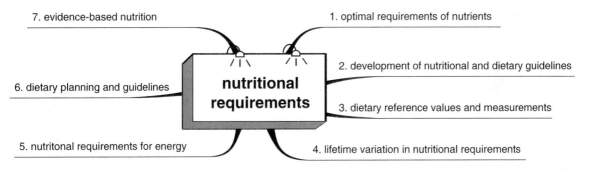

7. evidence-based nutrition

1. optimal requirements of nutrients

6. dietary planning and guidelines

nutritional requirements

2. development of nutritional and dietary guidelines

3. dietary reference values and measurements

5. nutritonal requirements for energy

4. lifetime variation in nutritional requirements

Fig. 5.1 Chapter outline.

OPTIMAL REQUIREMENTS OF NUTRIENTS

Individual nutritional requirements are determined by age, gender, environment, and genetic and isoenzyme constitution. The amount of intake for energy must be sufficient for childhood growth and adult work, leisure activities, pregnancy and lactation. The needs for a growing child who is physically active and laying down a wide range of tissue types, including neural, brain, muscle, enzyme systems, liver tissue, bone and connective tissue, are in contrast to those of the mature, exercising young adult in the physical prime of life. The pregnant or lactating woman's needs will be of a different qualitative and quantitative nature. The teenage mother who is growing as well as sustaining a growing infant has added needs. As the person ages the body requires much more care and maintenance as all activities reduce in intensity. The energy requirements of the elderly fall, but the nutrient requirement remains. The requirement for nutrients, i.e.

essential constituents of the diet, may remain unchanged during these phases of life.

> The concepts of an energy-dense and a nutrient-dense diet are important.

Requirements are also altered by stress, illness, smoking and trauma, and the extent to which these needs are met depend on the financial status of the person and the community. Adequate nutrition cannot be assumed, just because there are no obvious clinical features of deficiency disease. Indeed, some degree of malnutrition has been identified in a significant proportion of the hospital populations of affluent countries.

Optimal dietary requirements are those dietary intakes of nutrients that are most likely to ensure that the individual will attain optimum potential nutritional status for:

- successful development *in utero*
- growth
- learning potential

- quality of life
- body function
- successful pregnancies
- adequate milk production for a baby's needs
- expectation of a long and healthy life
- freedom from infection
- resistance to disease and response to diseases.

Appropriate nutrition requires that all nutrients, carbohydrates, lipids, proteins, minerals, vitamins and water are taken in adequate amounts and in the correct proportions. This is essential for normal organ development and function, reproduction, repair of body tissues, and combating stress and disease. Many nutrients require the presence of other nutrients if they are to fulfil their activity within the body.

Each nutrient is required at a certain level. The amount recommended will always exceed the precise needs because of the inefficiency of biological processes:

- **basal requirement**: that which is required to protect against clinical impairment of function due to insufficient intake
- **storage requirement** allows the body to maintain body tissue reserves. The reserve provides a supply of nutrient that can be mobilised without detectable impairment of function.
- the level required to **maximise health** and improve quality of life
- the level to required to **avoid chronic disease**.

Nutritional requirements meet:

- **fixed energy expenditure**, i.e. basal metabolic requirements, e.g. breathing, cardiac output, intestinal peristalsis
- **variable energy expenditure**, i.e. growth, movement (exercise, eating and drinking , exercise and work) on heat production, digestion, breathing, cardiac output , renal function, nervous system during active periods; also pregnancy and lactation

The variable energy output of the child and young mother is enormous, and therefore the ratio of fixed to variable energy expenditure is high. In contrast, the energy expenditure of the elderly person is much smaller and consequently the fixed to variable energy expenditure ratio is small.

Nutritionists must make recommendations based on scientifically generated facts giving guidelines for groups and individuals in the community. The definition of dietary requirements is very exacting. The important question is: requirements for what? An example of the complexity facing scientific committees is giving recommendations for the daily requirements for folic acid (200 µg/day). There are two groups in which, the recommended intake at 400 µg/day, is double, the recommended intake for the population. One group is women contemplating pregnancy and who wish to minimise the risks of neural tube defects in the baby. Another group of adults needs to reduce the plasma homocysteine concentration to reduce the risk of coronary heart disease. An intake of 400 µg/day of folic acid is only achievable through fortified foods or supplementation in tablet form, and is not possible by eating unfortified foods alone.

The fulfilment of nutritional needs is dependent on agricultural economic effectiveness, particularly in developing countries. The recognition of this basic premise has been essential for the survival of every major civilisation. The development of farming as an industry means that the whole process of food production, which is central to the health of a community, requires supervision by agencies independent of but reporting to parliament or government. Examples are the Food Standards Agency (FSA) in the UK, Agence Française de Sécurité Sanitaire des Aliments in France, and the Food and Drug Administration (FDA) in the USA.

DEVELOPMENT OF NUTRITIONAL AND DIETARY GUIDELINES

Every parent endeavours to advise their children on what to eat. Throughout history, there has been literature offering dietary advice, e.g. in the Old Testament and the Koran there are important standards for clean food policies. W.O. Atwater was the first director of the Office of Experimental Stations in the US Department of Agriculture. In 1894, he published a table of food composition and dietary standards for the US population. Atwater's dietary standards were intended to indicate the average needs of humans for total calories, protein, fat and carbohydrate. Minerals and vitamins had yet to be identified. At the beginning of the twentieth century Caroline Hunt further classified food into five groups: milk and meat, cereals, vegetables and fruit, fats and fatty foods, sugars and sugary foods. The amounts of foods were written as guides for the average family household units in familiar terms.

The recession and poverty of the 1930s changed the way in which these guides were required. Until then, ignorance was regarded as the basis of inadequate nutrition. With the recession poverty became an important factor, and cost-effective guidance became necessary. The food planners recognised that cereal foods, potatoes and dry beans supply energy and nutrients in a cheap form. Hazel Stiebeling, the writer of these new guides, drew attention to the importance of a balance between 'nutrient-dense, protective foods', e.g. calcium, vegetables and fruit, and 'high-energy and protein foods'.

The first recommended daily requirements or allowances/amounts (RDAs) were defined in the USA in 1941, and listed specific recommendations for calories and protein, iron, calcium, vitamins A and D, thiamin, riboflavin, niacin and ascorbic acid. It was essential to reinforce these with health education. In 1943 the 'basic seven' food guide was issued. Scientific RDAs were translated into ordinary foods, a format useful for the population at large. The foods that were to be eaten on a regular basis were green and yellow vegetables, oranges, tomatoes and grapefruit, potatoes and other vegetables, fruits, milk and milk products, meat, poultry, fish, eggs, dried peas and beans, bread, flour and cereals, butter and fortified margarine.

This guide also used exchanges, so that if fruit was scarce then vegetables could be an alternative. These recommendations were expanded in 1946 into a National Food Guide with recommended servings. By 1958 a simpler system was devised, with four basic food groups and a daily minimum of two helpings from four food groups: milk and milk products, meat, fish, poultry, eggs, dry beans and nuts, and four servings each of fruit and vegetables and grain products. This was a basic diet with the expectation that other foods would be eaten.

In Britain in 1940, Robert McCance and Elsie Widdowson published the Food Composition Tables, the first tables showing the chemical composition of food. They became a framework in the dietary treatment of disease and in any quantitative

study of human nutrition. These tables included composition data for raw and cooked food, complete with the sources and description of the foods and recipes used in calculating the composition of the cooked dishes of the foods analysed. These tables revolutionised nutritional practice in Britain, not least in planning food rationing during the Second World War when Britain was dependent on home-grown food.

Rationing in Britain during the Second World War was a triumph for applied nutrition. A precedent had been established in Britain during the First World War, when German submarine warfare had severely restricted the importation of food and rationing was necessary. Food was scarce, but no allowances were made for the needs of the elderly and children. In January 1918 sugar and butcher's meat were rationed, to ensure rather than to restrict supplies. During the 1930s, McCance and Widdowson had tested restricted but nutritionally complete diets under experimental conditions in normal day-to-day life. These diets met the nutritional standards of the time. In 1936, Boyd-Orr in Aberdeen published a report of a dietary survey, *Food, Health and Income*, which showed that half of the surveyed British population could not afford a diet supplying the basic nutrients, and 10% of the population was undernourished. When the war began it soon became apparent that imported foods such as tea and sugar would be in short supply. Equal shares for all were established in 1939 with the introduction of ration books. Rationing, which also included clothing, continued until 1954. This dietary regime proved to be healthy and practical, and particularly when supplemented by vegetables grown in the garden and allotments. (The government leased ground taken from parks and wasteground.) The diets of babies, children and pregnant mothers were supplemented by additional rations. Infant mortality fell during the war, helped by higher employment and perhaps a greater social awareness in the national effort.

The success of these programmes was such that by the 1970s a new approach was needed for the affluent countries, where advances in agriculture were yielding a sufficiency and variety of food. Instead of the primary concern being whether the population was eating adequately and avoiding nutritional deficiencies, it became necessary to tackle the epidemics of diseases associated with

Food rations (weekly except where otherwise stated) for one person in Britain in 1942

- Bacon and ham   100 g
- Meat   Up to 6p worth (e.g. a pork chop and four sausages)
- Sugar   225 g
- Butter, margarine or lard   225 g
- Tea   50 g
- Cheese   50 g
- Milk   1800 ml
- Sweets   350 g every 4 weeks
- Jam   450 g every 2 months

The British guidelines, *Balance of Good Health*, is a food selection guide that helps people to understand and enjoy healthy eating. The guide is in a pictorial format showing a plate with the proportion and type of foods needed for a balanced diet.

The five food groups are:

- Bread, cereals and potatoes   Eat lots
- Fruit and vegetables   Eat lots
- Milk and dairy foods   Eat moderate amounts and low-fat versions where possible
- Meat, fish and alternatives   Eat moderate amounts and low-fat versions where possible
- Foods containing fat and/or sugar Eat sparingly

It is recommended that the health benefits of eating fruit and vegetables be formulated into advice to eat 400 g of fruit and vegetables a day (varieties not specified), which translates into five portions a day.

incorrect balances in nutrient intake, excess energy, sugar and saturated fat, insufficient polyunsaturated fats and dietary fibre.

In 1977, *Dietary Goals for the USA* was prepared by a US Senate Select Committee. Quantitative goals were laid down for the dietary content of protein, carbohydrate, fat, fatty acids, cholesterol, sugars and sodium. RDAs were issued separately. These recommendations aroused controversy.

There continues to be a public demand for authoritative, consistent and achievable food guides. In 1990 the United States Department of Agriculture published seven principal statements intended to help the citizens of the USA to minimise the risk of chronic diseases in which diet was believed to have a causative role. The Swedish recommendations are similarly simplified into a helpful diagram, a pyramid giving the foods and the proportions of such foods in daily servings. This suggested a moderate diet, which was sufficient to meet nutritional needs and provided variety.

The US FDA recommends:

- **level 1**: bread, cereal, rice and pasta, 6–11 servings
- **level 2**: vegetable group, 3–5 servings; fruit group, 2–4 servings
- **level 3**: milk, yoghurt and cheese group, 2–3 servings; meat, poultry, fish, dry beans, eggs and nut group, 2–3 servings
- **level 4**: fats, oils and sugars to be used sparingly.

The diet should be reduced in salt, fat and saturated fat, and alcohol intake should be moderate. The guide recommended a substantial intake of vegetables, fruit and grain products.

DIETARY REFERENCE VALUES AND MEASUREMENTS

Current recommendations for a nutrient look at the needs of healthy, normal individuals and populations and regards the body as a biochemical machine. The nutrients listed meet the basic needs of human nutrition: protein, energy, vitamin A and carotene, vitamin D, vitamin E, vitamin K, thiamin, riboflavin, niacin, vitamin B_6, pantothenic acid, biotin, vitamin B_{12}, folate, vitamin C, calcium, iron, zinc, selenium, magnesium and iodine.

Recommended nutritional or dietary allowances or intakes define the differing nutritional needs, established by physiological and metabolic studies, for defined population groups, e.g. babies, toddlers, and pregnant and lactating women, in a healthy

Table 5.1 References terms relating to energy and nutrient intake

AI	Adequate intake: if the scientific evidence is insufficient to establish a requirement, then a figure for AI is obtained from the best available information
Basal requirement	The dietary requirement of a nutrient to prevent any clinically demonstrable impairment of function (defined by FAO/WHO)
DRI (USA, Canada, 2000)	Daily reference intakes: a collective name referring to four nutrient-based reference values, EAR, RDA, AI and UL
DRV (UK, 1991)	Dietary reference value; a term used to cover LRNI, EAR, RNI and safe intake
DV (USA)	Daily values: single figures created by the US FDA. A term used in USA nutrition labelling for a reference intake level. Two types of reference intake are defined, RDI (reference dietary intake) for minerals and vitamins, and DRV (daily reference value) for certain other nutrients)
EAR	Estimated average requirement for a group of people for energy, protein, vitamins or minerals.
LRNI	Lower reference nutrient intake for protein, vitamins or minerals. An amount of the nutrient that is enough for only a few people in a group who have low needs
Normative storage requirements	The dietary requirement of a nutrient to maintain a reserve in body tissues
RDA (USA,1941)	Recommended daily allowances: the level of intake of essential nutrients considered to meet the functional needs of practically all healthy persons. Statistically, this intake would prevent deficiency disorders in 97% of the population. The term was devised to allow modification with changing knowledge and was not intended to imply a minimum or an optimal requirement. Superseded by dietary values
RDA (UK, 1979)	Recommended daily amount: the average amount of a nutrient that should be provided in a group of people if the needs of practically all members of the group were to be met. These are averages for the group, not amounts that individuals must eat. Superseded by RNI in the UK, but European RDAs are used in food labelling
RDI (UK, 1969)	Recommended daily intake of nutrients. The recommendation applies to food as actually eaten
RNI (UK, 1991)	Reference nutrient intake for protein, vitamins or minerals. An amount of the nutrient that is enough or more than enough for about 97% in a group. If the average intake of a group is the RNI, then the risk of a deficiency in the group is extremely small. The value is equivalent to RDA or RDI
Reference values for nutrient intake (German-speaking countries, 2000)	Nutrient intakes which meet the demands of 97.5% of a population group, and for evaluation of the nutrient supply of the population
Safe intake	Indicates intake or range of intakes of a nutrient for which there is not enough information to estimate RNI, EAR or LRNI. It is an amount that is enough for almost everyone, but not so large as to cause undesirable effects. An upper limit of safe intake is not, however, implied by this recommendation
UL (USA)	Tolerable upper limit: the highest amount of nutrient intake unlikely to pose any risk of adverse health effects to almost all individuals in the general population
USRDA (USA, 1968)	Recommended daily allowances: a selection of the highest values for 20 nutrients from the RDAs and used as standards for labelling

For each dietary recommendation, consideration is given to:

- function
- metabolism
- dietary intake patterns
- requirement levels for different categories of people
- toxicity
- basal requirements
- safe intake levels and intakes
- tolerable upper intake levels
- variations between individuals within a population

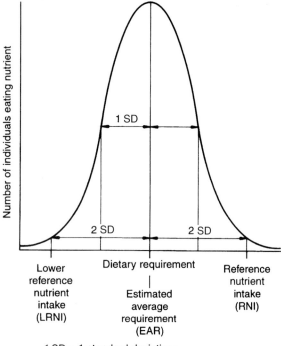

1 SD = 1 standard deviation;
68.3% of observations lie within 1 SD
2 SD = 2 standard deviations;
95.45% of observations lie within 2 SD

Fig. 5.2 Estimated average requirements (EAR), lower reference nutrient intake (LRNI) and reference nutrient intake (RNI). LRNI and RNI are two standard deviations below and above the EAR, respectively.

population. Nutritional and dietary guidelines also define intakes of individual categories of food.

It is important to distinguish requirement (for individuals) from recommendation (for populations). There is a movement towards a nutritive rather than a preventive approach. A person may meet a requirement for a specific nutrient but eat less than the recommendation for the entire population.

A requirement for a nutrient is the amount that an individual must consume to avoid deficiency as defined by clinical, physiological and biochemical criteria, and varies from individual to individual.

Various terms are used by different national authorities to prescribe or recommend values for food energy and nutrient intakes (Table 5.1). The terms reflect evolving views about guidance and prescribing recommendations for a population that is becoming more educated. The terms are gradually becoming less prescriptive and indicate best practice rather than absolute values. The original RDA values in the USA were written primarily to indicate nutrient intakes that would prevent clinical deficiency. The new approach is to maximise health and improve quality of life, including the avoidance of chronic disease, and to suggest guidelines for groups and individuals.

No single value defines the requirements of each nutrient for the whole range of people who make up a population. The notional mean requirement is the estimated average requirement (EAR) (Figure 5.2).

Dietary reference value (DRV) is a term used to cover LRNI, EAR, RNI and safe intake, introduced in 1991 by COMA (the UK Committee on Medical Aspects of Food and Nutrition Policy). When no DRV has been defined for a nutrient, a 'safe level' is useful for evaluating diets and for defining and reversing unsatisfactory low intake.

The UK DRVs are estimates of reference values and have moved away from the more prescriptive recommendations for intakes (e.g. RNI or RDA), although the values are similar. They are standards by which nutrients in the food eaten by different sections of the community can be defined. However, it is difficult to establish DRV with great confidence for every nutrient. There are different DRVs according to age and gender and during pregnancy. For most nutrients no increment for pregnancy is necessary in the mature Western mother; however, the growing teenage mother or marginally sustained mother does have extra and very real needs to increase dietary intake. DRVs have been set only for infants fed with artificial feed as it is assumed that human breast milk will automatically provide all of the baby's requirements.

Expert committees in many countries have used similar principles to establish their own values, e.g. daily reference value (USA and Canada), reference values for nutrient intake (German-speaking countries) and dietary reference intakes (The Netherlands).

Every year the British National Food Survey examines the diets of the population by region and family size and income. In addition, the National Diet and Nutrition Survey has a rolling programme examining the diets of individuals within certain population groups. In this way shortcomings in the diet can be identified.

When planning diets for groups in institutions, e.g. old people's homes, prisons and the armed forces, it is important that the overall diet meets the DRVs. In planning food supplies, international agencies use reference values to plan long-term aid for developing regions and to calculate food supplies for famine relief. There are different RDAs for most countries, reflecting their respective diets.

The USA has adopted dietary reference intakes, as part of the move from avoidance of deficiency to maximising health and improving quality of life. This again is a collective term, to include estimated average requirements, recommended dietary allowance, adequate intake and tolerable upper intake level. Thresholds differ among different members of the general population and will depend on genomic constitution, age, possibly gender and the overall diet.

Many countries rely on the Food and Agriculture Organisation (FAO) and the World Health Organisation (WHO) to establish and disseminate dietary allowances. Others use their reports as the basis of their standards. The public health and clinical significance of too little and too much intake must be revised every 10–15 years as knowledge expands, and this information is specific to each country.

LIFETIME VARIATION IN NUTRITIONAL REQUIREMENTS

The requirement for a nutrient varies from one person to another, and may alter with the composition and nature of the diet as a whole. There is no absolute requirement for fat, sugars or starches, although there are for essential fatty acids, vitamins and minerals. Estimates of requirements may be made from:

- the intake of a nutrient by individuals or by groups which is associated with the absence of any signs of deficiency disease
- the intake of a nutrient to maintain a given circulating concentration or degree of enzyme saturation or tissue concentration
- the intake of a nutrient needed to maintain balance, noting that the period over which such balance needs to be measured differs for different nutrients and between individuals
- the intake of a nutrient needed to cure clinical signs of deficiency
- the intake of a nutrient associated with an appropriate biological marker of functional nutritional adequacy.

Different groups have different nutritional needs:

- **Infants**: the baby's nutritional needs are adequately provided for by its mother's milk until 4 months. WHO recommends exclusive breast feeding for about six months. Iron and iodine provided in breast milk may be inadequate but do not require supplementation. Thereafter, the increasing nutritional demands of growth require the introduction of weaning to solid food.
- **Children 1–3 years**: essential nutrients and the great energy expenditure and growth needs of the toddler must be provided by the diet.
- **Children 4–10 years**: energy and protein, vitamin and mineral intake must meet the demands of activity and growth.
- **Children 11–18 years**: energy and protein needs continue to increase, particularly for boys, who require increased intakes of vitamins and minerals. In girls, once menstruation begins there are increased requirements for iron.
- **Adults 19–50 years**: growth is completed and the frenetic activity of youth is over. Energy

requirements are reduced, but the requirements for protein and most vitamins and minerals remain the same.

- **Pregnant women**: the most important requirement is for folic acid supplementation before and in early pregnancy. There is increased requirement for some but not all nutrients to provide for the energy needs associated with the growing foetus.
- **Lactating women**: the energy demands of milk production are reflected in increased dietary requirements of protein, minerals and vitamins if maternal good health is to be maintained.
- **Adults 50+ years**: the elderly are less energetic and protein requirement is less in men, although maintained in women. After the menopause the requirement for iron is the same in women and men. Vitamin and mineral demands are unchanged, except for increased vitamin D needs after the age of 65 years.

NUTRITIONAL REQUIREMENTS FOR ENERGY

The energy requirement of an individual is the energy intake of food that will support energy expenditure requirements in a person who requires economically and socially desirable physical activity consistent with body size, composition and long-term good health.

Energy is not a nutrient but is released from the carbohydrates, fat, protein and alcohol in food, and is therefore a composite term. Energy requirements are very individual and variable, and depend on metabolic processes, physiological functions, muscle activity, heat production, growth and synthesis of new tissue. It is needed for immediate use or, in industrial terms, just-in-time energy.

There are few methods available to measure energy status, although a constant weight or a body mass index (BMI) of 20–25 is a reasonable guide. The energy requirements in healthy people could be defined as the food energy needed to maintain a predetermined BMI and physical activity. In endurance athletes the glycogen content of muscle gives a clue to stamina.

Involuntary energy expenditure consists of different components:

- resting metabolism: the energy costs of the normal metabolic processes of the body
- adaptive involuntary energy expenditure to cope with cold conditions
- energy associated with absorbing and metabolising food

The Harris–Benedict equation is used to measure basal energy expenditure (BEE). It is important that the equation is used as originally designed in 1919. The temptation is to round off the long decimal places, which introduces errors of between 7 and 55%, depending on the particular figures rounded off.

For men,

$$BEE = 66.4730 + (13.7516 \times \text{weight in kg}) + (5.0033 \times \text{height in cm}) - (6.7750 \times \text{age in years})$$

For women,

$$BEE = 655.0955 + (9.5634 \times \text{weight in kg}) + (1.8496 \times \text{height in cm}) - (4.6756 \times \text{age in years})$$

Total caloric requirements = BEE × the sum of the stress and activity factors

> The **metabolic energy** content of a foodstuff is a measure of the proportion of the ingested food that appears to be available for metabolism in the body. Only after absorption does the nutrient attain full value, with the exception of proteins.

Dietary energy is the EAR for different age and gender groups. EAR for energy reflects estimates based on total energy expenditure (TEE). TEE is calculated by multiplying the basal metabolic rate (BMR) by physical activity level (PAL):

$$TEE = BMR \times PAL$$

The BMR is the rate at which the body uses energy when the body is at complete rest. Values depend on age, gender and body weight. For a 65 kg man BMR is approximately 7.56 MJ/day. For a 55 kg woman, BMR is about 5.98 MJ/day.

The PAL is the ratio of overall daily energy expenditure to BMR. A PAL of 1.9 would reflect a very active work pattern. The physical activity level of 1.4 is a minimum of activity at work and leisure. A physical activity level of 1.5 should be used for individuals aged 60 years. Old people have low levels of energy expenditure and dietary intake, with a consequent risk of nutritional deficiency.

In the 1985 report of the FAO/WHO/UNO Expert Consultation Committee, the maintenance energy needs were calculated as $1.4 \times BMR$ for both men and women, while the other components were expressed as a function of BMR. The average daily requirements of an elderly person might be approximately 1.55 to $1.75 \times BMR$.

Energy intake in excess of these requirements is stored as fat until needed. Thus, energy intake should meet just-in-time requirements.

DIETARY PLANNING AND GUIDELINES

No matter how carefully dietary guidelines are constructed, it is necessary to ensure that the population understands the thinking behind the scientific recommendations, and that the recommendations can be translated into recipes for delicious food and pleasurable meals.

Many agencies, at the local, national and EU level, along with the FAO and WHO, have made great efforts to define nutrient recommendations for their populations. The task of the FAO and WHO is particularly demanding because of the range of communities served, from the poverty-stricken in frozen, temperate and tropical countries, to the affluent and well-fed.

Dietary guidelines are also written by government agencies and associations interested in preventing and coping with specific diseases, e.g. heart disease or cancer. They aim to provide a diet that may, in their opinion, minimise the chance of acquiring such a disease.

Recommendations vary from country to country, but the general theme is as follows.

- Enjoy your food.
- Eat a nutritionally adequate diet drawn from a variety of foods.
- Reduce the consumption of fat, especially saturated fat (total fat should supply 30–35% of daily calories):
  - 8–10% of total calories from saturated fatty acids
  - up to 10% of total calories from polyunsaturated fatty acids

- up to 15% of total calories from monounsaturated fatty acids.
- Achieve and maintain an appropriate body weigh.
- Increase the consumption of complex carbohydrates and dietary fibre.
- Reduce the intake of sodium (< 6 g/day).
- Consume alcohol in moderation (not more than 2 drinks/day). Children and pregnant women should abstain.
- Carbohydrates should provide 55–60% of the daily energy intake, a high proportion of which should be fruit, vegetables and wholewheat products. (This figure is for meat and fish eaters, and will be quite different for vegetarians.)

EVIDENCE-BASED NUTRITION

The health professions are moving towards evidence-based practice. The evidence base used in clinical decision making is supported by statistical methods that are sound and readily interpreted. Within the science of nutrition and dietetics, current thinking does not always fulfil these criteria. The statistical principles that have clinical and population consequences are different from laboratory experiments. The use of confidence limits, clinical significance curves and risk–benefit contours improves the evidence of statistical reporting and decreases the chance of results being misinterpreted.

KEY POINTS

1. Adequate nutrition requires that all nutrients, carbohydrates, lipids, proteins, minerals, vitamins and water are consumed in sufficient amounts for normal organ development and function, reproduction, repair of body tissues, and combating stress and disease. The nutrient energy intake should be appropriate for sustained activity and effective physical work.
2. Dietary reference values for food energy and nutrients include BMR (basal metabolic rate), PAL (physical activity level) and PAR (physical activity ratio). Terms relating to energy and

nutrient intakes include and have included the RDI (recommended daily intake) and RDA (recommended daily amounts) of food energy and nutrients, EAR (estimated average requirement) for a group of people, LRNI (lower reference nutrient intake) and RNI (reference nutrient intake) for protein, vitamins and minerals, safe intake and DRV (dietary reference value).
3. Dietary guidelines translate these values into practical statements, for real-life nutrition. Recommended nutrient and dietary allowances indicate the requirements of individual nutrients for defined population groups, e.g. babies, toddlers, and pregnant and lactating women. Nutritional and dietary guidelines recommend intakes of food, milk, meat and vegetables, etc.
4. The energy requirement of an individual is the level of energy uptake for food that will balance energy expenditure when the individual has a body size and composition and level of physical activity consistent with long-term good health, and allow for economically necessary and socially desirable physical activity. In women who are pregnant or lactating, the energy requirement includes the deposition of tissue or the secretion of milk at rates consistent with good health.

THINKING POINTS

1. The construction of recommendations for the intake of nutrients is a very important task for nutritionists.
2. Central to these recommendations is the science upon which the recommendations are based. How robust is the scientific background to these recommendations?
3. Also of importance are the eating habits of the populations that are to receive the recommendations.
4. What are the practicalities of food guidelines for a nutritionist?

NEED TO UNDERSTAND

1. The science of nutrition has practical objectives.
2. The guidelines must try to meet the goals and aspirations of the community being served.

3. Each generation of the community must feel well fed, and the nutritionist must also feel that that community is sufficiently fed for its needs and to allow best growth and maintenance of function.

FURTHER READING

Anon. (2001) Clinical effectiveness, clinical guidelines and clinical standards 'from history to the future', Proceedings of the Royal College of Physicians of Edinburgh, **31** (Suppl. 9), 1–76.

Ashwell, M. (ed.) (1993) *McCance and Widdowson, A Scientific Partnership of 60 Years: 1933 to 1993*. British Nutrition Foundation, London.

Baranowski, T., Cullen, K.W. and Baranowski, J. (1999) Psychosocial correlates of dietary intake: advancing dietary intervention. *Annual Review of Nutrition*, **19**, 17–40.

Beaton, G.H. (1986) Towards harmonisation of dietary, biochemical and clinical assessments: The meanings of nutritional status and requirements. *Nutrition Reviews*, **44**, 349–58.

British Nutrition Foundation (1989) *Recommended Daily Amounts: What Are They and How Should They be Used*. Briefing Paper 19. British Nutrition Foundation, London.

British Nutrition Foundation Task Force (1992) *Unsaturated Fatty Acids: Nutritional and Physiological Significance*. Chapman and Hall, London.

Department of Health (1991) *Report on Health and Social Subjects*, No. 41, *Dietary Reference Values for Food Energy and Nutrients for the United Kingdom*. Report of the Panel on Dietary Reference Values of the Committee on Medical Aspects of Food Policy. HMSO, London, pp. 2–3.

Dewey, K.G. (1997) Energy and protein requirements during lactation. *Annual Review of Nutrition*, **17**, 19–36.

Food and Agriculture Organisation/World Health Organisation/United Nations (1985) *Energy and Protein Requirements*. Technical Report Series No. 724. WHO, Geneva.

Food and Agriculture Organization/World Health Organisation (1994) *Fats and Oils in Human Nutrition*. FAO, Rome.

Food and Agriculture Organisation/World Health Organisation (1998) *Carbohydrates in Human Nutrition*. FAO, Rome.

Grundy, S.M. (1998) The optimal ratio of fat-to-carbohydrate in the diet. *Annual Review of Nutrition*, **19**, 325–41.

Harris, J.A. and Benedict, F.G. (1919) *A Biometric Study of Basal Metabolism in Man*. Publication No. 279, Carnegie Institute of Washington, Washington, DC.

Hexted, D.M. (1975) Dietary standards. *Journal of the American Dietetic Association*, **66**, 13–21.

Liu, J.-Z. and Guthrie, H.A. (1994) Nutrient labelling, a tool for nutritional education. *Nutrition Today*, **17**, 16–21.

Mertz, W. (2000) Three decades of dietary recommendations. *Nutrition Reviews*, **58**, 324–31.

Potter, J., Langhorne, P. and Roberts, M. (1998) Routine protein energy supplementation in adults: systematic review. *British Medical Journal*, **317**, 495–501.

Reeds, P.J. (1990) Amino acid needs and protein storing patterns. *Proceedings of the Nutrition Society*, **49**, 489–97.

Scottish Intercollegiate Guidelines Network (1999), SIGN guidelines, Publication No. 39. SIGN, Edinburgh.

See, E.-S. and Florentino, R. (1997) Recommended dietary allowances in the SouthEast Asian region: scientific basis and future direction. *Nutrition Reviews*, **56**, S1–59.

Shakespeare, T.P., Gebski, V.J., Veness, M.J., and Simens, J. (2001) Improving interpretation of clinical studies by use of confidence level, clinical significance curves and risk–benefit contours. *Lancet*, **357**, 1349–53.

Waterlow, J.C. (1995) Whole body protein turnover in humans, past, present and in the future. *Annual Review of Nutrition*, **15**, 57–92.

van Way III, C.W. (1992) Variability of the Harris–Benedict equation in recently published textbooks. *Journal of Parenteral and Enteral Nutrition*, **16**, 566–8.

Welsh, S., Davis, C. and Shaw, A. (1992) A brief history of food guides in the United States. *Nutrition Today*, **27**, 6–11.

Williams, C. (1995) Healthy eating: clarifying advice about fruit and vegetables. *British Medical Journal*, **310**, 1433–5.

Williams, C., Wiseman, M. and Buttriss, J. (1999) Food-based dietary guidelines – a staged approach. *British Journal of Nutrition*, **81** (Suppl. 2).

Workshop on protein and amino acid requirements and recommendations. (2001) *Proceedings of the Nutrition Society*, **60**, 3–14.

World Health Organisation/Food and Agriculture Organisation/IAEA (1996) *Trace Elements in Human Nutrition and Health*. WHO, Geneva.

World Health Organisation/Food and Agriculture Organisation (1996) *Preparation and Use of Food-based Dietary Guidelines*. WHO, Geneva.

WEBSITES

www.who.int/nut   Establishing human nutrient requirements for world-wide application and technical reports

www.nal.usda.gov/fnic   Dietary guidelines around the world

http://health.gov   US dietary guidelines

www.americanheart.org   Dietary guidelines for healthy American adults

www.fao.org   Food and Agriculture Organisation of the United Nations

www.foodstandards.gov.uk   Food Standards Agency of the United Kingdom

www.nas.edu   US National Academy of Science, DRI updates and information

www.nutrition.org.uk   British Nutrition Foundation

http://ificinfo.health.org   US Department of Agriculture, Food Safety and Inspection Services

www.saspen.com   South African Journal of Clinical Nutrition

6

Nutritional epidemiology

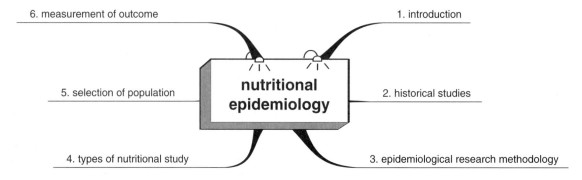

Fig. 6.1 Chapter outline.

INTRODUCTION

Epidemiology is the study of the relationship between possible determining causes and the distribution of the frequency of diseases in human populations. Epidemiological research has been one of the mainstays of our understanding of nutrition. There are three objectives for epidemiology:

* to describe the distribution and extent of disease problems in human populations
* to elucidate the aetiology of diseases
* to provide the information necessary to manage and plan services for the prevention, control and treatment of disease.

What is being studied must be carefully defined, and the interpretation of the results of the study must be within the framework of the original definition.

Nutritional epidemiology, in addition to the study of the nutritional determinants of disease, measures nutritional status in relation to environment and dietary intake. Most clinical measurements of nutritional status are used to identify deficiencies in overall intake or the intake of individual nutrients.

HISTORICAL STUDIES

The great nutritional studies of the nineteenth and early part of the twentieth century led to the discovery of dietary deficiencies in the form of beri-beri, goitre, pellagra, rickets, scurvy and xerophthalmia. These spectacular discoveries led to the concept of single dietary factors in the aetiology of disease. There is an understandable desire to identify simple and singular causes of contemporary diseases. However, it is now apparent that the system is complex, with groups vulnerable to multiple other predisposing factors in addition to nutritional factors, e.g. infection, activity levels and individual genetic variation. Furthermore, only a proportion of individuals who are at risk develop the particular nutritional problems under study.

Reaching rapid conclusions on the basis of epidemiological associations all too frequently mars the reputation of nutrition as a science, and delays identification of processes. Many recorded associations may not be causative of the condition; instead, they are markers for the net effect of many variables that influence morbidity and mortality (*post hoc*, non *ergo propter* hoc: after this, not therefore on account of this, the tendency to confuse sequence with consequences).

EPIDEMIOLOGICAL RESEARCH METHODOLOGY

A systematic approach to epidemiological research involves:

- Identifying the area of study.
- Reviewing the literature on the topic. A thorough read of a comprehensive review by an acknowledged expert and discussion with trusted colleagues is often sufficient. The detailed reading is best devoted to methodology and statistical support.
- Developing a specific study question.
- Writing a research protocol.
- Consultation with a statistician. Intelligent and understanding professional statistical advice is essential. It is mandatory that this advice be taken before the trial rather than as an after-thought or in response to the comments of the editor of a journal.
- Ethic's committee approval. The completed study protocol must be reviewed by an ethics committee. This committee must be expert but also include independent members.
- Completing the research described by the protocol.
- Analysis of the data with emphasis on (i) problems with the protocol, and (ii) statistics.
- Correct interpretation of the results, examining the relationship between exposure and outcome.

Discussions with the statistician and the ethics committee should be regarded as some of the most rewarding parts of the whole study.

The best epidemiological studies include large numbers of variables carefully and independently measured. Examples of such studies are the Framingham Study, the British Cancer Register, the British Doctors Smoking Study and the US Nurses Study.

Variables that are easy to identify but are complicated in interpretation are: smoking, gender, alcohol intake. social class, coffee consumption, and racial and national differences.

Epidemiological studies can be seen as being experimental or observational. In experimental investigations a particular set of conditions is established for subjects by the investigator. In observational studies the investigator observes and measures but has no control over the actions of the subjects.

Examples of experimental studies are community trials and clinical or field trials. Community trials use populations whose disease status is unknown but most of whom will be healthy (therapeutic trials), or studies of subjects who are known to be free from the disease at the time of the study (prevention studies). Clinical or field trials work with subjects who already have a disease. In both instances, the general design is to divide the population randomly into a treatment or exposure group and a control group, and to compare the effect of a treatment regime to a control regimen given at the same time under the same conditions. This design enables the effects of the treatment to be established. It is important that there is perfect randomisation between the control and the treatment groups. Both populations should be studied for an equivalent and biologically relevant length of time. The observer and the subject should be blind to the treatment regime, but it is important that there is constant contact, warmth and support with the subjects during the study, and when relevant the observer should watch and test whether there is compliance to the regime in question. Subjects often get bored and secretly alter the protocol.

TYPES OF NUTRITIONAL STUDY

Sources of information for nutritional studies include:

- survey of sickness

- sickness absence statistics
- notification of diseases
- general practitioner statistics
- hospital out-patient statistics
- hospital in-patient statistics (public or private)
- mortality statistics
- post-mortem statistics.

Each source has its own value and sphere of usefulness.

Ecological studies

An ecological study involves the observational study of groups who may be followed and measurements made over a certain period or at a determined time or place (country, province or city), or who have similar sociodemographic features.

Cohort studies

Cohort studies are similar to field trials, with the exception that exposure is not randomly assigned by the investigator. Here, individuals who are exposed are compared with those who are not exposed. Cohort studies accurately measure the exposure by which the outcome is not influenced. Smoking habits or exposure to a toxin or alcohol are examples. There is less chance of bias in the information as these studies provide a measure of risk. However, these studies are expensive and time consuming.

Case–control studies

The case–control study design is used to study the effects of exposure or risk (e.g. behaviour patterns and physiological measurements) on outcome. More precise outcomes can be achieved with case–control studies than with cohort studies.

Individuals with a problem, condition or disease (subjects) are compared with those who do not suffer from, or do not yet manifest the problem, condition or disease (controls). Factors thought to be involved in the condition are measured in both groups and thus the risk factor can be calculated. The definition of the population from which cases and controls are taken, and the interval from the time of exposure or removal from exposure, are significant in evaluating the results. In case–control

studies a range of exposure levels must be included, allowing a gradient of risk to be established.

Case–control studies are not expensive; they can be completed quickly and multiple risk factors can be examined at the same time. They are particularly appropriate for rare diseases. Inaccuracies may, however, arise in that the data are obtained retrospectively, exposure may not be accurately identified or the disease may influence exposure.

Cross-sectional studies

Such studies measure exposure and disease state at the same time.

The study of genes and environmental factors in complex circumstances is a new challenge to the epidemiologist.

Twin studies

The usual method involves monozygotic (identical) and dizygotic (non-identical) twins, and measurements are taken appropriate for the condition under study. Differences between the two groups gives clues to the contribution of inherited and environmental factors. Co-twin studies are made on monozygotic twins only, one of whom has the condition under study. Environmental causes can thus be followed, e.g. smoking or alcohol intake. Biometrical genetic methods allow measurements of risk factors, metabolites, behaviour, physical and psychological characteristics, especially if the twins are brought up in separate circumstances.

SELECTION OF POPULATION

It is difficult to define a normal population for research purposes. Any population will represent a wide range of gene pools. In selecting a population it is important to pose the question and then to decide what useful information can be obtained from that population. The information must be readily available and able to be defined in terms of age, gender, race and living conditions. Quality of life is an important variable. Studies in comfortable, middle-class populations may be welcomed and undertaken quite differently from individuals struggling to cope with their lot in life. Any study must be easily tolerated by the subjects, whether this be a descriptive exercise or modifying lifestyles as in clinical trials. Overall, the more fun the study the more likely it is to achieve compliance and hence to be be accurate.

Sampling

Sampling is required to obtain manageable numbers of individuals who are truly representative of the population to be studied. A system of random sampling is used.

- **Simple random sampling** is where the individuals are numbered sequentially and then the randomly numbered individuals are included in the study.
- **Systematic sampling** is a variation of simple random sampling.
- **Stratified sampling** is where measurements are made in each sampling unit, which may differ in magnitude from one subgroup to another, e.g. weight, body size, age or gender.
- **Cluster sampling** is where there are small units that may be sampled, e.g. households.
- **Multistage sampling** combines the different forms of sampling, working from larger to progressively smaller sampling frames.

The concept of 'intention to treat' must be used; that is, everyone who is recruited into a trial should be included in the results. Those who fail to complete a trial (non-responders) are a different group from those who do complete the trial (responders), and excluding non-responders may make the sample unrepresentative of the required target population. Those who remain in the study may not be representative of those of the population as a whole. It is important to describe the non-responders and to define whether or not they are representative of the population as a whole.

Epidemiological definitions

Validity: in order for a study to be valid the findings must be representative and reproducible; this is *external* validity. An alternative interpretation of validity identifies whether the measure utilised actually measures outcome; this is *internal* validity.

Sensitivity measures the proportion of truly affected subjects who are appropriately classified.

Specificity measures the proportion of truly unexposed individuals who have been correctly classified.

Repeatability, precision reliability or **reproducibility** is the consistency with which exposure is measured; similar results must be obtained if the experiment or analysis is repeated. **Confidence intervals**: 95%, 99% or greater confidence limits must be established.

Bias is any trend in the collection, analysis, interpretation, publication or review of data that leads to a conclusion which is systematically different from the truth. Bias can include selection bias, information bias, recall bias and interviewer bias.

Confounding factors are variables other than those being studied that may influence the outcome. For a variable to be a confounder it must be associated with but not causally dependent on the exposure of interest. Where possible, confounders can be controlled for in selection of subjects by randomisation, restriction or matching. *Randomisation* is where subjects are allocated to different treatment exposures to ensure that any differences that are identified do not occur by chance. In contrast, *restriction* is achieved by including only those subjects in whom the variable under study is the same. *Matching* ensures that potentially confounding factors are identically distributed in each group in the study, e.g. gender is a confounder and therefore it is necessary to study men and women separately. Other confounders are age, pregnancy, lactation, growth, activity, both physical and emotional, and stress, and these should be equivalent in both groups.

A combination of conditions may be required for a disease or condition to occur. Where time is an important prerequisite for the development of a condition, the time and duration of exposure must be identified. This is known as the *induction period*. The *latent period* is the time between the induction of the disease and the clinical manifestation that permits diagnosis. It is helpful to the theory if there is dissociation between exposure and outcome across a range of dose–response relationships.

Properties required for measurements

Validity: does the measurement measure what is intended?

Appropriateness and **acceptability**: is the measurement suitable for the study?

Reliability: are the measurements reliable?

Sensitivity: is the measure sensitive in the context of the study?

Interpretability: are the results useful for the interpretation of the study?

Data recording and interpretation

Data sheets with clear and easy places to record results and visual cues make for easy information recording.

Check lists minimise forgetting.

Illegible handwriting can be a problem.

Data sheets should always be completed when the recording is made. Memory and scraps of paper are a hazard to research.

Avoid subjective results if possible, or use visual analogue scales.

Use computers wherever possible, but always have a back-up system.

Measurements and error

Errors can arise from inadequately designed data sheets. The more care that is devoted to the data sheets, always in discussion with the statistician, the better the outcome. The manner in which the data sheet is constructed may alter the ease and manner of analysis.

The measurements that are made should be meaningful and readily achieved. It is important to discuss the methods with the people who will run the trial on a day-to-day basis and, where possible, the subjects. Babies and children are a special group and here the full co-operation of the parents is essential. Parents may, however, become over-involved, to the detriment of the results. Training is important to make the trial run smoothly and to make the accuracy of the measurements reliable.

Data collection

Questionnaires are a frequently used tool in epidemiological studies. Such questionnaires should be validated, either by the team or by well-authenticated previous studies. It is important that the questionnaire is valid for and understandable by the community being studied.

Interviews may be structured, semi-structured or unstructured. It is important that they can be translated into recordable data.

It is important to measure the variation between the same measurements in an individual. When measurements are being made, whether on the subjects, e.g. height or weight, or chemical measurements, e.g. haemoglobin or blood urea, several repeat measurements should always be made. This enables the within-subject standard deviation to be calculated.

MEASUREMENT OF OUTCOME

Having determined that an outcome can be measured with sufficient validity, sensitivity and specificity, it is important to evaluate: (i) the role of chance; and (ii) hypothesis testing.

This requires a testing of the null hypothesis, which is the state in which there is no relationship between exposure and outcome. An alternative hypothesis is that a low level of association is present. The null hypothesis for a statistical test is to establish a hypothesis for two or more groups and to test the limits in which this theory might be correct. The tests of significance between groups are expressed as a p-value, e.g. $p < 0.05$, i.e. the chance of the two groups being the same is as little as 5%.

Bradford Hill suggested nine points that may suggest causality:

- strength of association
- consistency
- specificity
- relationship in time
- biological gradient
- biological plausibility
- coherence of evidence

Statistical methods and probability

Frequentist theory

This is the commonly used system of statistics, providing techniques for collecting, analysing and testing whether the experimental data support the hypothesis or not. The data are calculated as a frequency distribution, the most common being the Gaussian normal distribution, describing the sampled population within defined limits. The methodology usually records the results as mean, median or mode, and dispersion usually as standard deviation.

Bayesian theory

This theory begins with the observation and then asks how certain we are that the statement is true. Bayesian results might say the chance that A is different to B is $p = 0.999$, and no chance of their being the same is 0. The figures are a ratio of the value of the reality to the value of the assumption. This is a flexible subjective theory adjusting to new evidence, used where there is a lack of complete information. Probabilities are estimated with some assumptions and therefore are conditional.

It is debatable whether these criteria have been met for the place of dietary fibre in the aetiology of the diseases that have been allegedly associated with fibre deficiency. The principal reason for the persistence of the assumed value of dietary fibre is that the possible health-promoting properties makes good sense, rather than that the case has been made by good science. This is the difference between the frequentist statistical confidence limits and Bayesian probability theory.

- experimental evidence
- analogy.

He set out the conditions that had to be met before it could be concluded that an association observed, in a case-controlled study, could be interpreted as indicating cause and effect. There should be:

- no bias in the selection of subjects and controls, in the way that subjects and controls report their histories or in the way that interviewers record data
- an appropriate time interval between exposure to the suspected agent and the development of the disease
- no other distinction between the affected subjects and their controls that could account for the observed association, or any common factor that could lead both to the specific exposure and to the to development of the disease.

Outcome measurements are of three types:

- the observation of the event, e.g. the first clinical sign of a disease (incidence)
- the recording of the presence or absence of disease at a particular time (prevalence), the accuracy of which may be influenced by migration or death from whatever cause
- the measurement of level of disease on a metric scale, which may similarly be subject to inaccuracies.

Nutritional epidemiological studies frequently study dietary intakes, which represent a continuum of exposure. There may be a dose–response relationship between intake and the consequent disease or condition. Recording dietary intake requires much skill and often gives a qualitative rather than a quantitative result.

Proper estimates of exposure and consequent relationship require:

- the probability distribution and measurement errors
- the distribution of true exposure and confounders in the population studied.

It may well be that both distributions are multivariate. Therefore, the variability of each component in the measurements has to be examined, as well as their interrelationship. This requires multivariate analysis.

Meta-analysis in epidemiology

Many small trials give inconsistent results. The accumulation of such small studies could be important in identifying the cause, the treatment or the risk of the condition studied. Meta-analysis is a precise statistical tool in which the results of all the relevant trials that have been undertaken can be analysed together. It is important that patients are included on an 'intention to treat' basis. All outcomes can be recorded in the same way, and all trials and all patients can be included, irrespective of their inclusion in published results. It is not clear, however, whether epidemiologists can use meta-analysis to identify hazards to health.

Epidemiological data for nutrition may not be categorised as readily as clinical trial data. Consequently, there is a subjective judgement entering into the decision to include or not to include a particular study or item within a study. All substantial studies should be considered for inclusion, whether or not they have been published, to avoid the effect of publication bias. This is most likely to occur in a situation where there is a discouragement or a reluctance to publish results that fail to show any positive effects. Consequently, in conducting a meta-analysis it is important to include unpublished studies where the cases and controls have been properly selected. A weakness of meta-analysis is the criteria for exclusion of studies. Do the results of such excluded studies differ materially from the chosen studies? If so, in what way? Any differences should be reflected in the overall conclusions.

KEY POINTS

1. Epidemiology is a study of the relationship between possible determining factors and the distribution of the frequency of disease in human populations. Nutritional epidemiology requires the measurement of nutritional status in relation to environment and dietary intake.
2. The great epidemiological studies led to the discovery of beri-beri, goitre, pellagra, rickets, scurvy and xerophthalmia.
3. The science of epidemiology demands a precise identification of the area of study, a specific study questionnaire, a research protocol, and effective analysis and interpretation of the resulting data.
4. Epidemiological studies can be experimental or observational. In experimental investigations a particular set of conditions is established for subjects by the investigator. In observational studies, the investigator observes and measures, but has no control over the actions of the subjects. Studies may be community trials, clinical or field trials.

5. Sampling is required to obtain a manageable number of individuals who are truly representative of the population to be studied. A system of random sampling is used.
6. An outcome must be measured with appropriate validity, sensitivity and specificity. It is also important to evaluate the role of chance and to test a hypothesis. Bradford Hill identified nine points that indicate causality between exposure and outcome.
7. Meta-analysis is a precise statistical tool in which the results of all relevant trials, even those that are small and may have given inconsistent results, can be analysed together.

THINKING POINTS

1. This is a very important chapter, as so much of our knowledge of nutrition comes from epidemiology.
2. The great studies have identified disordered nutrition consequent upon deficiency of one or more nutrient. The use of epidemiology for conditions arising in the presence of abundant food gives results that are less easy to interpret, where the gene–nutrition interaction is a complicating factor.
3. Statistics are the bedrock of epidemiology.
4. Design a study that looks at a deficiency condition, and another that looks at an excess intake. Identify the parts of the study where errors could occur and how you would protect the study from such errors.

NEED TO UNDERSTAND

1. The different types of epidemiological studies.
2. The strengths and weakness of this approach to nutrition in the community.
3. The importance of accuracy of the measurements, compliance of the subjects and good statistics.

FURTHER READING

Berry, D.A. (1996) *Statistics, A Bayesian Perspective.* Duxbury Press, California.

Bland, J.M. and Altman, D.G. (1996) Measurement error and correlation coefficients. *British Medical Journal*, **313**, 41–2.

Britten, N. (1995) Qualitative interviews in medical research. *British Medical Journal*, **311**, 251–3.

Clayton, D. and McKeigue, P.M. (2001) Epidemiological methods for studying genes and environmental factors in complex diseases. *Lancet*, **358**, 1356–60.

Doll, R. (1994) The use of meta-analysis in epidemiology. Diet and cancer of the breast and colon. *Nutrition Reviews*, **52**, 233–7.

Editorial (1990) Volunteering for research. *Lancet*, **340**, 823–4.

Edwards, S.J.L., Braunholz, D.A., Lilford, R.J. and Stevens, A.J. (1999) Ethical issues in the design and conduct of cluster controlled trials. *British Medical Journal*, **318**, 1407–9.

Egger, M. and Davey-Smith, G. (1997) Meta-analysis, potentials and promise. *British Medical Journal*, **315**, 1371–4.

Hawkes, C.H. (1997) Twin studies in medicine – what do they tell us? *Quarterly Journal of Medicine*, **90**, 311–21.

Higginson, I.J. and Carr, A.J. (2001) Measuring quality of life. Using quality of life measures in the clinical setting. *British Medical Journal*, **322**, 1297–300.

Horgan, G.W. (2001) Statistical analysis of nutritional studies. *British Journal of Nutrition*, **86**, 141–4.

Margetts, B.M. and Nelson, M. (1997) *Design Concepts in Nutritional Epidemiology*, 2nd edn. Oxford Medical Publications. Oxford University Press, Oxford.

Marr, J.W. (1971) Individual dietary survey: purposes and methods. *World Review of Nutrition and Dietetics*, **13**, 105–64.

Neiderhiser, J.M. (2001) Understanding the roles of genome and environment: methods in genetic epidemiology. *British Journal of Psychiatry*, **178** (Suppl. 40), s12–17.

Wright, P., Jansen, C. and Wyatt, J.C. (1998) How to limit clinical errors in interpretation of data. *Lancet*, **352**, 1539–43.

Part III

Factors influencing how an individual metabolises nutrients

- Genetics

7

Genetics

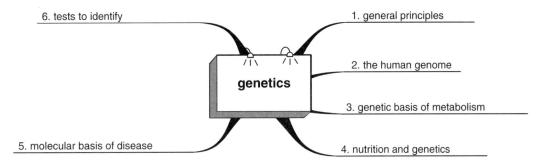

Fig. 7.1 Chapter outline.

GENERAL PRINCIPLES

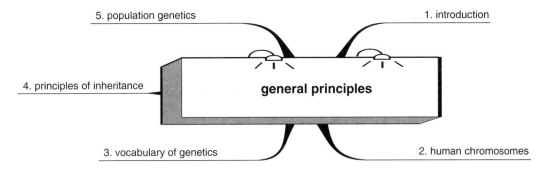

Fig. 7.2 Section outline.

INTRODUCTION

For a student of nutrition this is probably one of the hardest sections of this book and may provoke the question, 'why should I who am interested in nutrition and food concern myself with this subject?' Genetics is likely to be the key to the future of nutrition. There has been a steady progression in our understanding of food and what diets should be eaten by different groups of the population through science, and from these advances has come the discipline of nutrition. The realisation of the importance of the basic nutrients, amino acids, fatty acids and carbohydrates, then the vitamins and trace elements, enabled food guides to be written for populations and special groups, babies, children, pregnant and lactating women, for sportsmen and women, the elderly and the ill. These recommendations regard these groups as homogeneous. How-

ever, common sense, fortified by molecular biology, shows that even these subgroups are not uniform. Each of us is unique in many ways, including our metabolic response to our dietary intake.

Human genetics is the science that looks at the inherited variations in humans, a study of the mechanisms of evolution, and the process of change in gene frequency. Medical genetics is the application

Human chromosomes

Humans have 22 pairs of autosomal chromosomes (*autosomes* in the *diploid*, i.e. paired state), and the sexes are differentiated at this level by the additional pair of *sex chromosomes*, of which the female has a pair of X chromosomes and the male has XY chromosomes. During cell division there is paired exchange between closely associated *chromatids*. A chromatid is one of the two similar strands of a duplicated chromosome. The *centromere* is a compact region on a chromosome where sister chromatids join. The regions on either side of the centromere are called arms and are of unequal lengths, *long* and *short arms*.

A chiasma (Figure 7.3) is the site where chromatids are broken at corresponding points and which join in a cross-over manner, producing new chromatids. This process is called breakage and reunion, and leads to recombination. *Translocation* occurs when part of one chromosome breaks and becomes attached to a different chromosome. Translocations can be balanced, with no loss of chromosome material, or unbalanced, with loss of chromosome material. The balanced form usually has no phenotypic consequences, whereas the unbalanced may have profound effects, e.g. Down's syndrome. *Recombination* is the process by which DNA is exchanged between pairs of equivalent chromosomes during egg and sperm formation. In this process the chromosomes of the parent and offspring become different. *Deletion* is when a segment of a chromosome is missing as the result of two breaks and the loss of the intervening piece. *Inversion* occurs where there are two breaks in the chromosome with rotation of the intervening segment: *paracentric inversion* if on the same side of the centromere and *pericentric inversion* if on the opposite side.

Each pair of chromosomes is numbered, from 1 to 22, and there are also the sex chromosomes. Loss or gain in chromosomes is shown by + or −, after the chromosome number and arm designation, e.g.

5p, where p or q indicates the short or long arm, respectively. Translocation is indicated by t and inversion by inv, with the chromosome involved in the first bracket and the breakpoint in the second. The locus on the chromosome is identified by staining bands on the chromosome using cytological staining techniques, e.g. normal chromosome 9 normal band 22.

inv(9)(q22q34) means break and paracentric inversion in a single chromosomal arm, i.e. long arm q of chromosome 9 between region 2 band 2 and region 3 band 4. The segment of chromosome in between is reversed (inverted).

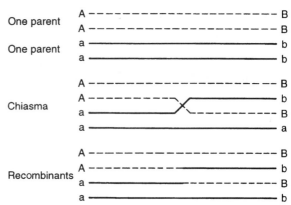

Fig. 7.3 Chiasma formation. The two identical chromosomes from one parent are shown by a broken line, the others are shown by an unbroken line. These join to form a bivalent in the meiosis. Crossing over occurs between two of the chromosomes; both are broken at the same site and the opposite ends are joined. The result is two recombinant chromosomes. The possibility of a chiasma between two points on a chromosome is proportional to the distance separating the two points. Thus, as the distance between two points increases so does the probability of a cross-over. The closer genes are to one another, the tighter they are linked and the less likely they are to be split.

of these principles to health. Medicine is passing through a revolution in how diseases are diagnosed, classified and treated as a result of the advances in genetics. Equally, nutrition is significantly the science of health, the study of how food fortifies and sustains the normal individual. Many genetic differences relate to rare conditions. The challenges are the explanation of the causes of common conditions that are secondary to disease-causing mutations, and the relationship between the genetic make-up of individuals and populations and the environment and diet of the individual.

Every individual has a specific potential for survival and reproduction that is dictated in part by genetically determined characteristics which influence metabolism, fecundity, birth, growth and death.

VOCABULARY OF GENETICS

The vocabulary of molecular biology is specialised but necessary to gain an understanding of the subject. Therefore, vocabularies are given; even these are technical and therefore it is recommended that they are referred to when reading the text.

PRINCIPLES OF INHERITANCE

Mendel clarified the process of inheritance through his studies on peas. In the mating process, paired genes from each parent separate (segregate) into single units, which pass to the next generation as individuals, independently of each other, and are never present together in the next generation. This is *Mendel's first law* (Figure 7.4). The *second law* is that pairs of genes pass to the next generation as though they were independent of one another. Mendel showed that when the newly paired genes from the parent generation are either both *dominant* or both *recessive* the offspring will be *homozygous* for that gene. If there is a mix of dominant and recessive genes the resulting individual is *heterozygous*. Homozygous is when there are two identical genes at a single site or locus of a chromosome; heterozygous is when these two genes are different. A dominant gene determines a characteristic regardless of whether or not it is in a homozygous or heterozygous pairing. The recessive gene

Inheritance

Mendel's laws

1. Each body cell has paired chromosomes. Genes are duplicated, e.g.

AA		Aa	or	aa
Homozygous	'	Heterozygous		Homozygous

2. Each ovum or sperm (gamete) has one chromosome; the genes are single

A   A   A   a   a   a

When the ovum is fertilised, then the result may be

	Homozygous		*Homozygous*	
Parents	AA	AA	aa	aa
Offspring	AA	AA	aa	aa
Parents	One parent AA One parent Aa		Parents both Aa	
Offspring	AA	AA	AA	Aa
	Aa	Aa	Aa	aa

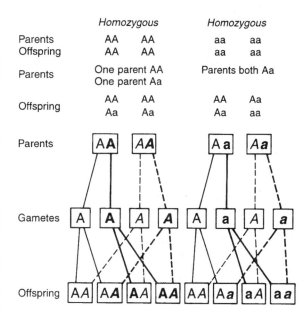

Fig. 7.4 Mendel's first law states that genes are units which segregate. Members of the same pair of genes are never present in the same fertilised ovum (gamete), but always separate and pass to different gametes. Mendel's second law states that genes separate independently. Members of different pairs of genes move to gametes independently of each other.

in the heterozygous situation does not express itself in the resultant individual. This means that in the next generation, when the paired genes are reshuffled, there will be offspring who are homozygous, and others who will be heterozygous for the dominant and recessive genes. The two parents each contribute half to the total heritage of the offspring, each grandparent contributes a quarter and each great-grandparent an eighth. The appearance of that contribution will depend on whether it is dominant or recessive. However, such characteristics do not appear equally in all offspring. A characteristic or *phenotype* from one parent may be dominant over the other parent's recessive phenotypic contribution. Phenotypes conceal a great variety of recessive genotypes which may become apparent in subsequent generations.

All genes can be pleiotrophic, dominant in one aspect of their expression and recessive in another. A favoured gene will increase in frequency and expression and a favourable characteristic will eventually become dominant. However, when circumstances change that gene may become disadvantageous and lose that dominance. Major genes have defined functions that determine specific characteristics, as distinct from *polygenes*, which are a group of genes functioning together, each of which has a small but additive effect on the phenotype. Major genes function at a single locus and may function in different allelomorphic states.

Alleles may be:

- completely dominant
- incompletely or partially dominant; the phenotype of the heterozygote is intermediate between that of the two homozygotes
- codominant and contribute equally to the phenotype.

According to Mendel's second law, in the second generation alleles assort independently so that equal numbers of each of the four types of gamete are produced. Two general types of offspring are produced:

- two parental types
- a recombinant type where the dominant of one parent and the recessive of the other parent are combined.

After conception, when two sets of chromosomes pair, the pairs of alleles determine the characteristics of the developing individual. Some inherited characteristics are probably dependent on several alleles; that is, there is a cumulative influence of several genes. Genes close together on a chromosome tend to remain close to each other during cell division (gamete production).

KEY POINTS

1. Inheritance of a genetic characteristic is determined by laws described by Mendel. Mendel's first law states that genes from each parent are in pairs which separate into single units, are passed to the next generation independently of each other, and are never present together in the next generation. The second law is that pairs of genes pass to the next generation as though they were independent of one another.
2. The two parents contribute directly to the total inheritance of the offspring and they, in turn, are affected by their own parents.

THINKING POINT

Make a list of characteristics, dominant and recessive, that may also be influenced by nutrition.

POPULATION GENETICS

The average population consists of individuals of all ages: babies, children, teenagers, some people choosing mates, some reproducing, some on the move, some growing old and some dying. The size and activity of the breeding population is important to the development of a population. The effective breeding population size may be determined by social prohibitions or an unequal sex ratio, e.g. when large numbers of men are killed during war. Social prohibitions occur when only a proportion of the population breeds, for racial, economic, social class, religious or geographical reasons, e.g. some of the population living remote from the rest, those in mixed religious cultures and celibate clergy. Some of the population of breeding age may opt not to have children. This is particularly important if that group are female. Many women now have the choice of whether or not to have children.

In a population, in each individual each genotype lasts for a generation and is unique, never to occur again. The genes, however, endure and are redistributed as alleles in each mating event. If there is inbreeding in a population then the genetic

Population genetics vocabulary

A *species* consists of a set of individuals who can actually or potentially interbreed and may adapt, but are reproductively separate from other species.

A *population* is an interbreeding group of individuals.

The phenotypic variation of a characteristic in a population usually takes the form of a *unimodal frequency distribution*, which can be described as a mean and variance.

A *heterozygote* is an individual with different alleles at a corresponding locus and a *homozygote* has the same alleles at corresponding loci on the same chromosome. As fitness to survive in an environment increases, so genetic variability is reduced; that is, inbreeding results in fewer *heterozygotic* and more *homozygotic* individuals.

There are systematic effects in which the size and direction of change are determined, including:

- *immigration* into and *migration* from a population; the effect will be dependent on the relative sizes of the immigrant and total populations

- *evolution*: a process of change in a population or species over the course of successive generations

- *unique mutations* which may provide novel forms essential for evolution.

A *microevolution* describes a change in a population either to fit into a new environment or over time to meet the challenges of a changing environment. If a population is large and there are no migrations or selective mutations, mating is random and the gene pool is large, the population will develop a genetic equilibrium after one or two generations. If a situation occurs in the environment so that a rare allele is favoured, that allele increases in frequency slowly, at a 5% increment, until equilibrium is achieved.

Homology of common ancestry, has two subclasses: parology is the relationship between genes that have originated by gene duplication, and orthology refers to genes of similar function, occurring in different species.

Mutations or changes in genotype may take place when new characteristics are needed to survive. Any mutation must be consistent with the viability of the organism if it is not to be a *lethal mutation*.

A *nonsense mutation* in a gene is one that prevents the protein specific to the gene from being synthesised. Other mutations, called *suppressers*, may allow the nonsense mutation to be overcome so that the protein can be synthesised. Spontaneous mutations occur at a rate of between 1 in 10^5 to 1 in 10^7 per locus per generation.

uniformity increases. The more a population inbreeds the more homogeneous that population becomes and the gene pool is concentrated. This may be beneficial or harmful depending on the phenotype. Polymorphism is a common phenomenon and makes people different, while sharing the same overall genome structure.

Different alleles coexist in a population, creating genetic polymorphism, the occurrence together in the same locality of two or more forms of a gene. Polymorphism is said to be transient if one gene is in the process of replacing another. It is stable if the gene frequency is at, or moving towards, a stable equilibrium. A good example in nature is melanism in the peppered moth, where the coal-black mutant becomes dominant to the usual pale speckled moth. The black pigmentation helps the moth to survive in the dirty environment of industrial areas.

An example of an evolutionary response to an environmental threat is the response in Africa and the Mediterranean countries to the threat of malaria. Mutations that cause changes in the chemistry of haemoglobin have increased the resistance to malaria, but the resistance system leads to sickle cell disease and thalassaemia.

There are numerous variants of haemoglobin in humans. Most are rare, but haemoglobin S, C and E are common in some parts of the world, dependent upon three alleles on the same locus. Sickle cell disease is an example of stable polymorphism. The sickle cell condition is caused by haemoglobin S. The abnormal forms differ from normal haemoglobin in the amino acid sequence of the haemoglobin and can be distinguished by electrophoresis. These abnormal forms are disadvantageous because they are less effective in carrying oxygen than haemoglobin A. Under conditions of low oxygen tension the red blood cells of the homozygote crenate, that is the smooth surface becomes notched. These distorted cells are inefficient in carrying oxygen and also block blood

Haemoglobin

Adult human haemoglobin is a tetramer. It comprises two α- and two β-polypeptide chains, each with an attachment site for haem, a ring molecule that binds oxygen. Important changes in the shape of the whole protein occur when oxygen and other small molecules are bound. Sickle cell anaemia, a disease of abnormally shaped red blood cells at low oxygen concentration, is caused by a change in one of the amino acids (position 6) of the 146 in the β-chain, through a single base alteration in one codon of the β-chain gene. This is not the only mutation that can occur in the haemoglobin gene: several hundred mutant haemoglobins have been identified. The consequences of each mutation on the functions of the globin chains (particularly oxygen binding and dissociation) vary, depending on the effect on their interactions in the tetramer.

vessels. The lifespan of the SS homozygote red cell is shortened to 20% of the average for other red cells. However, those heterozygous individuals who are a mix of haemoglobin A and S, i.e. haemoglobin AS type, have shown greater resistance to malaria caused by *Plasmodium falciparum*. The number of live babies born to AS women is greater than to AA women because of a reduced abortion rate in AS women.

The enzyme UDP-glucuronyl transferase catalyses the addition of glucuronic acid to bilirubin. Hereditary deficiency of this enzyme causes Crigler–Najjar syndrome type 1, a severe disease with jaundice and kernicterus, which is usually fatal in infancy. Crigler–Najjar syndrome type 2 is associated with severe deficiency of the same enzyme activity, but the jaundice is less severe and kernicterus can be prevented. Gilbert's syndrome is also associated with deficiency of UDP-glucuronyl transferase, but it is a benign, common condition usually diagnosed incidentally. Cystic fibrosis is associated with various mutations in the cystic fibrosis transmembrane conductance regulator gene, the most common being a deletion of phenylalanine at position 508. Individuals heterozygous for this change have reduced susceptibility to typhoid fever.

Selection is a complicated process in a popula-tion and depends on differential survival at any stage of the developmental cycle. Selection process-es in populations involve either elimination by loss for whatever reason or failure to breed. Gradually, there are changes in the polymorphism as beneficial traits aid survival and population increases. The newly formed fertilised egg (zygote) develops into a baby, an infant and then an adult. Each stage is vulnerable to the influence of environmental factors on the phenotype for survival. Nutrition is a key influence in this process.

J.B.S. Haldane used birth weights to look for indications of selection in human survival. Those babies with an optimal birth weight between 3.4 and 3.9 kg had a survival rate of 98.5%. The majority of those who died weighed significantly more or less than the optimal, demonstrating a selection process at the beginning of life.

Changes in gene frequency result in the elimination of unfit types under intense selection. It is possible for the population to be severely reduced until a favoured dominant phenotype becomes abundant. A large number of individuals may be lost as a result of genetic inadequacy. Haldane argued that because of the cost of evolution very few characters may be selected at one time unless they are controlled by the same genes. The rate of evolution is limited by the cost of the change. Deleterious mutations in the human population may act on the foetus before birth. The zygote may not be implanted or an embryo may be aborted at an early stage. Once a selective force eliminates a fraction of the potential population, the next selective force acts on the individuals that remain, until selection has been completed. The mode of evolution is an elementary process of change in gene frequency. Evolution is an immensely complicated process and takes place by the differential contribution of different individuals in a species to the succeeding generation.

These effects are clearly seen in humans. Skin pigmentation is an obvious genetic trait. P-glyco-protein expression linked to C3435T polymorphism in intestinal epithelial cells is more frequent in Africans than in Caucasians. P-glycoprotein is part of a defence mechanism against ingested toxic substances. There are distinct genetic attributes to be found in isolated populations, e.g. the Aborigines of Australia and the population of Iceland. Such populations are in contrast to the active pooling of gene type taking place through migration to the USA, Canada, Australia and New Zealand.

In Europe a series of epidemics over the centuries has been selective in producing subsequent populations resistant to that epidemic. The genetic makeup of a person is tested whenever that person meets a new environment or condition. There is an association between susceptibility to various infections, including malaria, tuberculosis, human immunodeficiency virus (HIV) and hepatitis B, and the major histocompatibility complex (MHC) on chromosome 6. Certain alleles of MHC complexes promote survival. In the Middle Ages in Europe the plague was rampant; in the nineteenth century, tuberculosis was common – this disease is associated with some candidate genes HLA-DR (human leucocyte antigen presentation), NRAMP1 (the divalent cation transporter gene) and VDR (the vitamin D receptor gene), and in the twentieth century and today, coronary artery disease and cancer are the main killer diseases with associated candidate genes (see Chapter 47).

The present Western generation has a wide dietary choice, clean food, good sanitation, attractive accommodation and relative freedom from lethal infectious diseases. The population is, however, exposed to an abundance of food, tobacco smoking, industrial pollution, viral and prion infections, and sedentary occupations. The population that survives a particular epidemic may be at a genetic advantage, but those genetic characteristics that enable survival in one stress situation may create a subsequently more vulnerable population in another stress situation. A constitution which in the heterozygous state is protective may be dangerous in the homozygous form, as discussed for sickle cell anaemia, thalassaemia and cystic fibrosis. The controversy remains as to whether a condition or state of development is dictated by nature or nurture, although nurture certainly presents challenges to nature.

KEY POINTS

1. Human genetics is a science that looks at the inherited variations in humans, the study of the mechanism of evolution and the process of change in gene frequency.

2. Evolution occurs when there is a change in a population either to fit into a new environment or over time to meet the challenges of a changing environment. Mutations or changes in genotype take place all the time in individuals. These mutations may or may not increase in the population, depending on whether new characteristics are favourable to survival.

3. A species consists of a set of individuals who may interbreed. Evolution is a process of adjustment by the selection of existing genetic populations. Mutations may influence the viability of the organism and population. Immigration and movement within the population may affect the genetic pool.

4. The genetic makeup of an individual or a population will be a significant factor in the ability to cope with the stresses imposed by the environment.

5. Inheritance is encoded in genes. Genes can be dominant or recessive. An allele is one of several forms of a gene occupying the same position or locus on a chromosome.

6. Humans have 22 pairs of autosomal chromosomes and one pair of sex chromosomes (X and Y), making a total of 23 pairs. The chromosome contains the genes and divides during cell division. Recombination is the process whereby DNA is exchanged between pairs of equivalent chromosomes during egg and sperm formation; the chromosomes of the offspring become different from those of the parents.

THINKING POINT

How is the genetic pool in a town, district or country that you know changing through immigration or emigration?

FURTHER READING

Brock, D.J.H. (1993) *Molecular Genetics for the Clinician*. Cambridge University Press, Cambridge.

Connor, M. and Ferguson-Smith, M. (1997) *Essential Medical Genetics*, 5th edn. Blackwell Scientific Publications, Oxford.

Emery, A.E.H. and Rimoin, D.L. (1997) *Principles and Practice of Medical Genetics*, 3rd edn. Churchill Livingstone, Edinburgh.

Horwitz, M. (2000) *Basic Concepts in Medical Genetics*. McGraw-Hill, New York.

Kwiatkowski, D. (2000) Science medicine and the future. Susceptibility to infection. *British Medical Journal*, **321**, 1061–4.

Schaeffeler, E., Eichelbaum, M., Brinkmann, U. *et al.* (2001) Frequency of expression of C3435T polymorphism of MDR1 genes in African people. *Lancet*, **358**, 363–84.

Theissen, G. (2002) Secret life of genes. *Nature*, **415**, 741.

Tudge, C. (2001) *In Mendel's Footnotes: An Introduction to the Science and Technology of Genes and Genetics from the 19th Century to the 22nd*. Jonathan Cape, London.

THE HUMAN GENOME

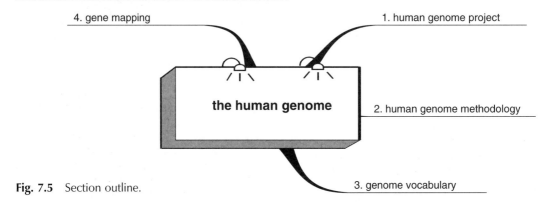

Fig. 7.5　Section outline.

The genome vocabulary

A *gene* is the store of genetic information held in the form of *deoxyribonucleic acid* (DNA). The *genome* is the complete DNA sequence of an organism. The gene-rich regions of a genome are called the *euchromatin*. The gene-poor regions of a genome which contain simple sequence repeats are called the *heterochromatin*. *Proteome* is the complete set of proteins encoded by the genome. Genes are found on *chromosomes*, structures that are composed of DNA and associated proteins, e.g. histones. The gene, which may exist in several forms, is encoded for and determines the synthesis of proteins and hence the functioning of the cells, organs and organism. *Autosomes* are all of the chromosomes except for the *sex chromosomes*. A normal somatic cell is *diploid*, that is, it has two sets of paired chromosomes. A gene can exist in more than one format on the same point or locus on a chromosome, called an *allele* or *allelomorph*. Different alleles of the same gene are called *multiple alleles*. *Gene frequency* in the population is the frequency of one kind of allele in the population.

Genes that are present in two distinct organisms or species are said to be *conserved*. Such *conservation* requires similarity at the DNA, RNA or amino acid sequence in the encoded protein. Changes in the gene's DNA are called *mutations*. The total genetic constitution of an organism is called the *genotype*, and this can also refer to the particular pair of alleles that an individual has at a given region of the genome. The *haplotype* is a particular combination of alleles or sequence variations that are close together, and hence likely to be inherited together on the same chromosome. The function and physical appearance of an individual is called the *phenotype*.

Polymorphism is a region of the genome that varies between individual members of a population, and is present in a significant number of individuals in the population. *Epistasis* occurs when one gene eliminates the phenotypic effect or the expression of another gene at another locus. A gene is said to have a high *penetrance* if it has a high frequency of expression in individuals who are carriers of that gene. A gene is said to be *pleiotrophic* if it is responsible for multiple, distinct, apparently unrelated phenotypic effects.

HUMAN GENOME PROJECT

The recent description of the human genome is the result of a monumental project organised by the publicly financed international Human Genome Project (HGP) and the commercial firm Celera Genomics. A virtually complete list of human genes and their encoded proteins has been constructed, and a compendium has thus been produced of information on inheritance, akin to the Periodic Table of elements.

HUMAN GENOME METHODOLOGY

The HGP used a *clone-by-clone* approach. Entire genomes are chopped into fragments, several hundred thousand base pairs long, by partial digestion with site-specific restriction endonucleases. These large DNA segments are inserted into bacterial artificial chromosomes (BAC), then placed into bacteria, which amplify the segments as they grew. Large amounts of clones are thus generated for analysis.

Next, each BAC is positioned on the genome's chromosomes by looking for distinctive marker sequences, sequence tagged sites (STS), the location of which has already been defined. In this way a high-resolution map of the genome is created. Clones of the BAC are shattered into small fragments by a procedure called shotgunning. Each fragment is sequenced and exposed to computer algorithms that recognise matching sequences from overlapping fragments and, from this, the complete sequence.

The Celera approach is quicker and uses existing algorithms to reassemble DNA fragments created by the shotgun technique. These fragments can then be applied to known cloned random fragments taken from the genome. Fragments are first assembled by algorithms into larger scaffolds and their positions calculated using STS.

The whole project is dependent on gene sequencing techniques developed by Fred Sanger, and analysis is further facilitated by automation of these techniques and suitable computer programs.

The accurate location on the chromosome of

Human genome vocabulary

- **Bacterial artificial chromosome (BAC):** a chromosome-like structure, constructed by genetic engineering, that carries genomic DNA to be cloned.
- **Cloning:** the process of generating sufficient copies of a particular piece of DNA to allow it to be sequenced or studied in some other way.
- **Expressed sequence tag (EST):** a short piece of DNA sequence corresponding to a fragment of a complementary DNA made from a cell's messenger RNA, and used to hunt for genes.
- **Restriction endonuclease:** an enzyme that cleaves DNA at every position where a particular short sequence occurs. Each restriction endonuclease is specific for a particular short sequence.
- **RNA polymerase II:** an enzyme that synthesises messenger RNA and some specialised RNAs. This enzyme is central to gene expression. The enzyme is a huge enzyme with 12 subunits, and must recognise thousands of promoters.
- **Shotgunning:** DNA is randomly broken into fragments of approximately the average size of genes. The fragments are cloned in suitable vectors to create a genome library.

many genes has been made possible through alignment of messenger RNA (mRNA) with sequences already known from other genome studies. Genes may also be found by looking for paralogues (family members derived by gene duplication). An alternative method is to recognise the position of identified genes in the genome, previously calculated from the relationship of that particular region with the development of a disorder. A further source of gene discovery is through mapped STS.

The maps resulting from the work of the two projects were published in *Nature* and *Science* in February 2001.

Two maps have been produced: a whole genome clone-based physical map, which provides a scaffolding upon which the sequence can be assembled, and a cytogenetic map, which plots the landmarks across the genome and places the physical map onto the underlying chromosomal positions.

The already completed sequence of the genome of model organisms has proved important in interpreting the human genome results. These existing genome descriptions include the yeast *Saccharomyces cerevisiae*, 6000 genes, the nematode worm *Caenorhabditis elegans*, 18 000 genes, the fruitfly *Drosophila melanogaster*, 13 000 genes, and the mustard weed *Arabidopsis thaliana*, 26 000 genes.

The human genome is 30 times larger than the nematode worm and the fruitfly genomes, and 250 times larger than the yeast genome.

The draft sequences for the human genome are 90% complete for the euchromatic area of the genome (weak staining and gene-rich areas). The genome is estimated to be 3.2 gigabases (Gb), 2.95 Gb of which is euchromatic. The distribution of genes, transposable elements, GC content, CpG islands and transposable elements varies throughout the genome. There are 497 transfer RNAs (tRNAs), making the human tRNA content less than that of the worm but more than the fly. The genome has regions with a relatively high content of GC bases. In the regions where the genome is rich in GC bases the gene density is greater and the average intron size lower. The number of protein-encoding genes lies between 26 000 and 31 000; the correct figure is probably 31 000. Of these, some 740 genes are non-protein-coding RNAs involved in cellular function. All of these figures are significantly lower than previously estimated. There is a discrepancy from the previous estimate of 100 000 genes, and more genes may yet emerge. Alternatively, the figure may be accurate and the overestimate may have been attributable to the indirect methods previously used for gene identification.

A major implication of the genome projects is that all human beings are 99.9% similar in their DNA complement. The size of the genome means that the genetic code varies in some 1.5–3 million places. There is a base difference every 1000–2000 bases, not necessarily at a consistent point in the genome. The spontaneous mutation rate for DNA is estimated at 0.5% each million years. More than 90% of the human genes exist as varying numbers of alleles. Not all of these changes manifest themselves, whereas others are lethal or incapacitating. The majority lead to obvious differences in the physical appearance of the person, although some attributes, such as height and weight, may be the result of the interplay between several genes and the environment (e.g. mutation).

Some beneficial gene alleles may only prove to be important on challenge, e.g. *CCR5* gene and resistance to HIV-infection. This HIV-resistant allele is present in 10% of some European populations and absent in African people. The disadvantageous alleles are discussed in the section on the genetic basis of disease.

Gene vocabulary

5′–3′ Terminology: in the polynucleotide chain, the 5′ position of one pentose ring is joined through a phosphate ring to the 3′ position of the next pentose ring, creating a backbone of 5′–3′ linkages. The nucleic acids are written and described from the free 5′ end on the left towards the 3′ end on the right.

Anti-sense: complementary in sequence to all or part of the messenger RNA or some specific RNA transcript of a gene.

DNA satellites: tandem repeats of short base sequences that show considerable variation in the number of repeats and are scattered throughout the genome. These microsatellites vary in their length in health and disease, and are characteristic for each individual. This property has been used in a system of DNA identification, known as DNA fingerprinting or genetic profiling, which is used in criminal and paternity investigations.

Exon: genes are transcribed as continuous sequences but a segment, the exon, of the mRNA molecules contains information that codes for protein.

GC content (guanine, cytosine content) and **CpG islands**: CpG islands are short, methylated regions of the chromosome, where these two bases are linked in the same strand rather than paired between strands as in the double helix. (p stands for phosphate.) Their GC content is enriched by over 50% in the guanines and cytosines in a nucleic acid sequence. These regions overlap promotor sequences in all housekeeping functions and many tissue-specific genes in vertebrates. GC-rich and GC-poor regions have different biological properties, e.g. gene density.

The cytosine base is sensitive to methylation, which is important in gene regulation. Once methylated there is an increased possibility of mutation occurring.

Gene naming: a gene is a DNA segment that contributes to phenotype or function. In the absence of demonstrable function, a gene may be characterised by sequence, transcription or homology. The naming of genes is confusing as different disciplines name genes by different systems, so that some genes have multiple names and unrelated genes may have a common name. Genes are named by virtue of having:

- a clearly defined phenotype, inherited as a monogenic Mendelian trait
- a region of no known function but associated with linkage or association with a known marker to a trait
- a non-functional copy of a gene, a pseudogene
- a cloned segment of DNA with structural, functional and expression data to be seen as a gene
- a gene structure encoded by the anti-sense strand of a known gene
- a transcribed but untranslated gene
- a cellular phenotype from which the existence of a gene may be inferred.

Gene symbols are no longer than six characters, begin with a letter, and are underlined or written in italics if the name gives genotypic information. When gene products of similar function are encoded by different genes the corresponding loci are given numbers, e.g. ADH1, ADH2, ADH3 are three alcohol dehydrogenase loci, or single letters, e.g. LDHA, LDHB, LDHC for lactate dehydrogenase loci. Homologous genes should have the same gene nomenclature. The same gene found in different species should have the same name.

Intron: a largely meaningless sequence that break up the protein coding sequences (exons) of genes.

Messenger RNA (mRNA): a messenger RNA template is fashioned (transcribed) from the protein-encoded sequence of the gene in the DNA; the RNA is processed, including splicing, to be a template for protein synthesis.

Paralogues: gene family members derived by gene duplication.

Promotor: a DNA sequence found 5′ to a gene that indicates the site for initiation of transcription. It may also influence the amount of mRNA produced.

Sequence tagged site (STS): short, single-copy DNA sequences that identify a mapping landmark on the genome. These are of known and singular sequence; they bind to yeast artificial chromosomes (YACs) and are hence identified.

Single nucleotide polymorphism (SNP): a DNA sequence is a linear combination of four nucleotides. The sequences of two combinations of four nucleotides in the same position are usually the same. When one nucleotide is different from the identically placed nucleotide in the other sequence, this sequence is an SNP. Polymorphism is caused by the change of a single nucleotide. Most genetic sequence variations between individual humans are believed to be due to SNPs. The tracking of the migration of peoples, molecular anthropology, relies on studies of SNP.

Splicing: this shows how introns, the non-protein-coding pieces of transcribed RNAs, are removed. Exons, the protein-coding portions, can also be removed. The protein that is produced depends on which exon is removed, so that different proteins can be made from the same gene or RNA. These different proteins are called either splice variants or spliced.

TATA box: this specifies the position where transcription is initiated.

Transcription: the synthesis of either RNA on a template of DNA or DNA on a template of RNA. RNA is an intermediary in the transfer of information encoded on DNA to produce the amino acid sequence of individual proteins. An arrangement of exons alternating with introns is a transcriptional unit.

Translation: the process wherein mRNA builds proteins. The m RNA enables transfer RNA (tRNA), each molecule of which carries a single amino acid to build a protein with a specific sequence of amino acids and hence a specific structure.

Transposable elements or transposon: specific mobile DNA elements that can be transferred as a unit from one replicon (a structural gene that controls the initiation and replication of DNA) to another.

KEY POINTS

1. Molecular biologists have almost completed a linkage map of the human genome. The number of protein-encoding genes is probably 31 000; of these some 740 genes are non-protein-coding RNAs involved in cellular function. Different proteins can be made from the same gene or RNA. These different proteins are called splice or spliced variants.
2. A DNA sequence is a linear combination of four nucleotides. The sequences of two combinations of four nucleotides in the same position are usually the same. When one nucleotide is different from the identically placed nucleotide in the other sequence, this sequence is a single nucleotide polymorphism (SNP). Polymorphism is caused by the change in a single nucleotide position. Most genetic sequence variations between individual humans are believed to be due to SNPs.

THINKING POINTS

1. Make sure that you are familiar with the vocabulary in this section and other sections.
2. Explore the various websites including those of the human genome.
3. The human genome is not hugely different to that of other species. What are the possible relevant species differences?

FURTHER READING

Dennis, C. (ed.) (2003) The double helix. 50 years. *Nature*, **421**, 398–453.

International Human Genome Sequencing Consortium (2001) Initial sequencing and analysis of the human genome. *Nature*, **409**, 860–921.

O'Brien, S.J. and Dean, M. (1997) In search of Aids-resistant genes. *Scientific American*, September, 43–51.

Pearson, H. (2001) Biology's name game. *Nature*, **411**, 631–2.

Smith, H.O., Yandell, M. and Evans, C.A. (2001) The sequence of the human genome. *Science*, **291**, 1304–1351.

WEBSITES

www.nature.com

www.nature.nature.com/genomics   Human and mouse genome

www.bioscience.org

www.bioscience.org/vitalink   Guidelines for human gene nomenclature

http://ca.expasy.org/   Expert protein analysis system

http://genome.cse.ucsc.edu   Genome bioinformation site

www.ensembl.org/IPI   Genome Browser and International Protein Index

www.ebi.ac.uk   European Bioinformatics Institute

www.ncbi.nlm.nih.gov/Omim/searchomim.html   Online Mendelian Inheritance in Man; contains information about human disease and genes

http://genome-www.stanford.edu   Saccharomyces Genome Database

www.celeradiscoverysystem.com   Celera Discovery system

GENOME METHODOLOGY

Isolating individual genes from the genome

Genes are small and occupy only a small part of a genome. A typical mammalian genome comprises 10^9 base pairs (bp). A gene of 10 000 bp is only 0.0001% of the total nuclear DNA.

Specific probes are used to identify particular gene sequences. Usually, mRNA that encodes a particular protein is used as the probe. A radioactive labelled probe of RNA or DNA whose hybridisation with a gene is assayed by autoradiography may be used. Another technique only requires knowledge of a small sequence of the protein; in this method short oligonucleotides are synthesised which correspond to this protein. A variety of oligonucleotides can be synthesised corresponding to possible alternative codons, especially of the third base. The triplet code can be used to trace the oligonucleotide sequences. Using this oligonucleotide synthetic technique a single strand of DNA or genome DNA can be produced.

GENE MAPPING

To isolate genes where no protein product is known it is necessary to map the identified genetic locus. Physical methods map the loci in cytogenetic terms. The nomenclature of chromosome regions is based on the bands and sub-bands of suitably stained chromosomes demonstrated by cytogeneticists. For example, Xp21 means sub-band 1 of band 2 of the short arm (p = short arm; q = long arm) for the X chromosome. Linkage methods give genetic distances in centiMorgans (cM).

Physical methods of gene mapping

In situ *hybridisation*
This is a direct method wherein a cloned DNA fragment is hybridised to a range of chromosomes in the metaphase stage of cell division. This phase of chromosome division accumulates within cells during growth after the introduction of a mitotic inhibitor such as colchicine.

The accumulated cells are fixed and spread on a slide. The chromosomes are treated with trypsin and stained with Giemsa, and the resulting dark and light bands of individual chromosomes can be identified.

Chromosomes are denatured on a slide to leave DNA single stranded but the chromosome morphology intact. The slide is then exposed to a labelled single-stranded DNA probe which hybridises to any matching sequence on the denatured chromosome. The results are analysed by examining a large number of cells and logging the chromosomal location of each silver grain in the emulsion. A histogram of grain count plotted against chromosomal position will show a strong peak at the site where the sequences match.

Somatic cell hybrids
This is a widely used technique. If mouse and human cells are fused by treatment with polyethylene glycol the resulting mixtures are unstable and tend to shed the human chromosomes in a more or less random way. Eventually, stable cell lines containing small sets of mouse chromosomes plus a few human chromosomes remain.

Once a collection of well-characterised hybrids has been prepared, the presence of other human gene products can be compared with specific, partially explored human chromosomes. If the original human cell contains a translocated or double-deleted chromosome then the hybrids can map a DNA fragment relative to the translocation break point.

However, most chromosomal abnormalities in both familial and sporadic neoplasia affect many genes and many systems. Sometimes a specific disease is associated with a small chromosomal abnormality, e.g. Prader–Willi syndrome and retinoblastoma. When chromosomes are involved in translocations or inversions, the break point may disrupt a gene and move it into a situation where its expression is inappropriate. Many tumour types are associated with specific chromosome break points.

Gene mapping linkage analysis
- **Linkage studies**: two genetic loci are linked if they segregate together in pedigrees by more than random chance. Loci are linked because they are close to each other on the same chromosome. The aim is to identify and count recombinants in suitable crosses. In a family with an autosomal dominant disease, the pedigree may have a distinct restriction length polymorphism type. Human linkage studies rely on finding exceptional families that are 'informative' to study. The problem with humans is that families are small and 'informative' families are often difficult to find, so information has to be combined from several families. In addition, sometimes the putative father is not the biological father.
- **Analysis of linkage studies**: the analysis of a linkage study requires the writing of a table showing the 'lod scores' for a disease and the identification of a marker at a range of recombination values.
- **Multilocus linkage analysis**: a set of families with an identified disease type is studied for a series of markers or evidence of a candidate region of a chromosome. Lod scores can be calculated for each marker. Standard lod score analysis cannot combine data for more than two loci. It is important to place the gene closest to a framework of known markers so that the closest flanking markers can be used as 'handles' when attempting to

Lod scores

For any linkage study data the lod score is the ratio of the probability that the loci are linked to the probability that the data could have arisen from unlinked loci. Such scores are usually calculated for recombination fractions 0.0, 0.05, 0.10 to 0.50 (independent assortment). A lod of zero means that the assumption of linkage or no linkage is equally valid. A positive lod score favours linkage and a negative lod score is evidence against linkage at the given recombination fraction. The thresholds of significance are 3 and –2. This means the odds must be 1000:1 in favour of linkage before evidence is accepted. A lod score of 3.0 means that the overall probability of linkage is 95%. A plot of lod score against recombination fraction takes several forms.

clone the gene. Computer programs can then identify the unknown locus, e.g. a known disease and a fixed framework of chromosomal marker loci, and from these it is possible to calculate the overall likelihood of these being connected in an aetiological relationship. Here, instead of a lod score there is a location score. Location score analysis is a very powerful tool and becomes more informative as the gene locations become identified.

- **Sib-pair analysis**: this is a simplified form of linkage analysis used for mapping recessive characters. If one parent has marker alleles ab and the other parent cd, then there is a 1 in 4 chance that two children will have the same types. However, if two children have the same recessive conditions, they will, of necessity, inherit the same alleles of markers, close to the gene responsible for the disease. Sib-pair analysis studies affected sibs and looks for markers that are shared more frequently than 1 in 4. This is the method by which the cystic fibrosis locus was mapped to chromosome 7.
- **Tracking disease genes using linked markers**: the prerequisite for such an exercise is a Mendelian disease with a known map location and one or two linked markers in restriction fragmentation length polymorphism (RFLP, see below). Such an analysis requires family studies. It does not require any knowledge of the molecular pathology and therefore is applicable to diseases where the gene has not yet been isolated and to heterogeneous mutation diseases. This method requires:
  - that a marker is found closely linked to the disease locus and for which the person at risk of transmitting the disease is heterozygous
  - study of other members of the family to calculate which of the marker alleles is on the chromosome carrying the disease allele
  - use of the marker to discover whether the pathological chromosome or its normal homologue was passed on to the person requiring the diagnosis.

GENETIC BASIS OF METABOLISM

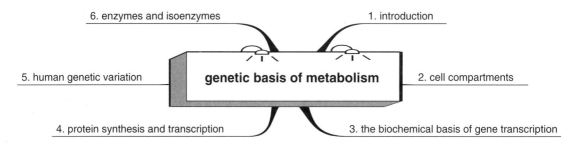

Fig. 7.6 Section outline.

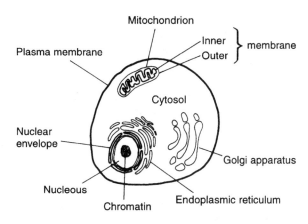

Fig. 7.7 The cell consists of a number of compartments, each separated from the cytosol by a membrane.

INTRODUCTION

The cell, the 'triumph of evolution', is the basic unit of living organisms. The cell is divided into different structures and functions forming physical and biochemical compartments (Figure 7.7). Chemicals move between compartments by specific transport mechanisms. Cells interact with their environment through chemical signals at the external surface, transduction of these signals within the cell, and secretion of synthetic products from the cell.

CELL COMPARTMENTS

The cell compartments include the nucleus, cytosol, mitochondria, endoplasmic reticulum (ER), Golgi apparatus, lysosomes and peroxisomes (Table 7.1).

Nucleus

The nucleus contains the genes encoded for the synthesis of proteins. The DNA is complexed with protein and forms exceptionally long continuous strands the chromosomes, and in humans each diploid human cell contains 23 pairs of chromosomes. The nucleus is surrounded by a double membrane, the layers of which contain pores necessary for the transfer of material to the cytosol.

All of the DNA in the nucleus is replicated when cells divide. Exact copies of each chromosome are distributed between the two daughter cells of each division. Transcription is another form of DNA copying. Small sections of the genome are selectively copied and each segmental copy (transcript) is formed of ribonucleic acid (RNA), not DNA.

Cytosol

The interior of the cell (cytoplasm) has an aqueous phase (the cytosol) in which many of the enzymes catalysing metabolic reactions function. Some enzymes, however, are membrane bound in the various organelles found within the cytoplasm.

Mitochondria

These are self-replicating organelles consisting of elongated cylinders (diameter 0.5–1.0 μm). Mitochondria may move within the cell and change shape according to the cell in which they are stationed. There are about 1000 mitochondria in each cell involved in tissue respiration. The organelles are surrounded by a double lipid membrane, the inner membrane being convoluted into cristae, which this creates two separate compartments, the matrix and the intermembrane space. Many

Table 7.1 The compartments of the cell

Compartment	Boundary	Cell volume (%)	Function
Nucleus	Nuclear envelope	5	Gene transcription
Cytosol	Plasma membrane	55	Protein synthesis
Mitochondria	Mitochondrial envelope	25	Energy production
Endoplasmic reticulum	Folded membrane	10	Protein modification
Golgi apparatus	Membrane stacks	5	Protein sorting
Lysosome	Closed membrane	< 1	Protein degradation
Peroxisome	Closed membrane	< 1	Oxidation reactions

Distribution of enzymes within a mitochondrion

Matrix: enzymes for the oxidation of pyruvate, fatty acids, tricarboxylic acid cycle, DNA and the associated genetic apparatus.
Inner mitochondrial membrane: ATP synthetase, respiratory chain enzymes and transport proteins.
Intermembrane space: kinases.
Outer membrane: cytochrome b_5, fatty acid elongation processing, monoamine oxidase, transferases.

enzymes are bound to the mitochondrial membranes, and function in transport and oxidative metabolism to produce energy that is stored in adenosine triphosphate (ATP).

All mitochondrial DNA (mtDNA) is inherited from the mother, since the portion of the male sperm that enters the female ovum has no mitochondria. There is a well-supported theory that mitochondria are descended from aerobic bacteria that invaded and then coexisted in early cells.

Endoplasmic reticulum

Membrane sheets of rough (with associated ribosomes) and smooth endoplasmic reticulum are named after their electron micrographic appearance. They form tubular channels called cisternae.

Rough endoplasmic reticulum: the attached ribosomes are the site of translation of mRNA to synthesise proteins, which are either retained in the cysternae or the lysosomes or exported from the cells. Glycoproteins are glycosylated within the cisternae.

Smooth endosplasmic reticulum: receives proteins synthesised in the rough ER, proteins being transferred from the cell for export to the Golgi apparatus, and proteins returning to the rough ER. This is also the site of phosphorylation of lysosomal proteins, lipid synthesis, and detoxification of lipid-soluble drugs and chemicals.

Ribosomes

These organelles are the site of protein synthesis, are 200 Å in diameter, and form a large complex made of several ribosomal RNA (rRNA) molecules and more than 50 proteins organised into a large subunit and a small subunit. The two subunits both contain rRNA and protein, and are classified on the basis of centrifugation characteristics as 40S and 60S. (S indicates centrifugation properties in Svedberg units, after Svedberg, the designer of the centrifuge system.)

The complex structure associates with a set of proteins to move physically along an mRNA molecule to catalyse the synthesis of amino acids into protein chains. Ribosomes also bind tRNAs, which are involved in protein synthesis.

The rRNA is encoded by genes in the nucleus. The sequence of the rRNA genes is highly conserved within species, and when differences are found between rRNA genes this information can be used as a basis for taxonomic classification and for estimating how close different species are in the evolutionary process.

Golgi apparatus

This is a stack of membrane cisternae, often found close to the nucleus, and involved in the sorting of protein from the ER for subsequent transport both within and outside the cell. The Golgi apparatus is also involved in the modification of core oligosaccharides of glycoproteins, sorting proteins for transport to defined locations and the synthesis of glycosaminoglycans.

THE BIOCHEMICAL BASIS OF GENE TRANSCRIPTION

The inheritance of living creatures is carried through the gene, DNA and RNA.

The strands of DNA are polymers of deoxyribonucleotides; and RNA of ribonucleotides. Each unit is composed of the sugar deoxyribose (DNA) or ribose (RNA), covalently linked to a triphosphate ester of a nitrogenous base. The bases are adenine and guanine (purines), and cytosine and thymine (DNA) or uracil (RNA) (pyrimidines) (Figure 7.8). The corresponding DNA nucleoside monophosphate 2′-deoxy forms are deoxyadenosine monophosphate (dAMP), deoxyguanosine monophosphate (dGMP), deoxycytidine monophos-

Extracting DNA from cells

It is simple to extract and purify the DNA from human leucocytes. Blood is collected, and the leucocytes are centrifuged into a band between the red blood cells and the plasma. Detergents are applied to disrupt external and internal cell membranes, and proteins, including those bound to DNA, can be removed by precipitation with solvents such as phenol. DNA can be precipitated by the addition of ethanol, and then resuspended in buffer. The DNA can be digested into fragments by the application of specific restriction endonucleases. These enzymes, mainly derived from bacteria, cleave DNA at particular sequences of bases. The fact that the size of the resulting fragments is variable from one individual to another implies that the cleavage sites are differently arranged between individuals, and thus that their DNA sequences are not identical.

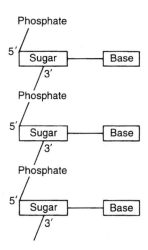

Fig. 7.9 Nucleic acid structure. The 5′ phosphate end is at the top and the 3′ hydroxyl group is at the bottom of the molecule.

phate (dCMP) and deoxythymidine monophosphate (dTMP). For RNA the ribonucleotides are adenosine monophosphate (AMP), guanosine monophosphate (GMP), cytidine monophosphate (CMP) and uradine triphosphate (UMP).

The polymer consists of phosphodiester bonds linking the 3′ carbon of one deoxyribose ring to the 5′ carbon of the next (Figure 7.9).The polymer is helical in shape, with the base moieties protruding into the centre of the helix. Two single helices of DNA interact to form a duplex strand, the double helix (Figure 7.10). The size and shape of the bases in each helix determine the ability of the two strands to interact. Because of the constraints of the helical backbone and the space within the centre of the helix, the strands will only associate if adenine and guanine on one strand lie opposite and pair with thymine and cytosine on the other. Each of the associating strands is complementary to the other, the sequence of one strand determining the sequence of the other. The base pairs, the interacting purine–pyrimidine bases on opposite strands, are non-covalently linked by hydrogen bonding (Figure 7.11).This complementation is the basis for the replication of DNA and the transcription of RNA.

Although every cell in the body has the same genetic material, the expression of this information varies from organ to organ and during different stages of life. Genes are turned off and on through

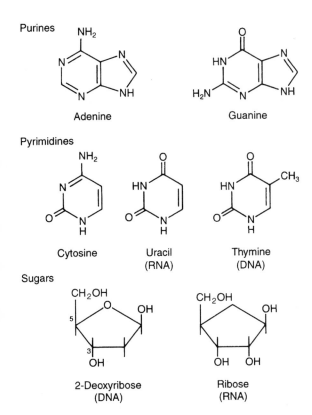

Fig. 7.8 Purines, pyrimidines and sugars present in the nucleotides of DNA and RNA.

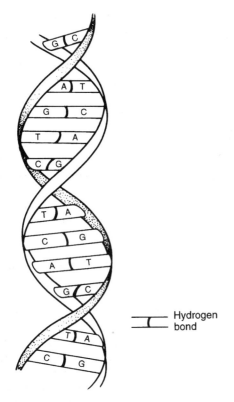

Fig. 7.10 Structure of DNA. The two bands are the sugar–phosphate backbones of the two strands which run in opposite directions. The four nucleotide bases, C, A, T and G, are linked by hydrogen bonds.

epigenetic mechanisms, an example of which is DNA methylation. The double helix has further structure and constraints imposed upon it. DNA molecules are made more compact by the coiling of the double helix around proteins, particularly histone proteins H2A, H2B, H3 and H4, to form nucleosomes. The histones (molecular weight 11–21 kDa) are rich in lysine and arginine. The flexible tails of the histones protrude from the globular DNA-wrapped nucleosomes. Histones may be acetylated, methylated, phosphorylated or ATP ribosylated; the addition or removal of these alters the charge and shape of the histone, which has important consequences for the regulation of DNA transcription. Some gene-silencing activities require the removal of acetyl groups from histones and the methylation of DNA, or the methylation and demethylation of both DNA and histones. Two proteins, SUV39H1 and heterochromatin protein 1, mark, methylate and bind to histone tails. Eventually, long tracts of bases and the gene are inactivated. Another consequence of the extensive acetylation of histone is to loosen the chromatin and to allow DNA repair systems to gain access to the genome and to seek out mutations that require repair.

The double helix DNA is further tightly folded in the nucleus in a super-coiled formation. This folding and unfolding is controlled by the enzymes

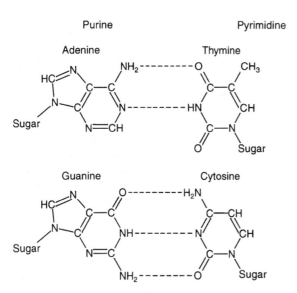

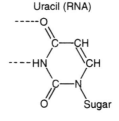

Fig. 7.11 Base pairings in DNA. Purines always face pyrimidines as complementary A–T (adenosine and thymine) and G–C (guanine and cytosine) base pairings.

topoisomerase I and II. This tightly coiled, double-helical state makes the base sequences inside the helix inaccessible for transcription. During cell division, each DNA strand divides to produce two new DNA molecules formed from an old and a new DNA strand. A new strand of DNA is synthesised in the 5′ to 3′ direction, with the 3′ end extending. One DNA duplex strand acts as a template for a complementary second strand by the polymerisation of dATP, dGTP, dCTP and dTTP.

The functions of the cell depend significantly upon proteins. Cell function, growth, differentiation and metabolism depend on the synthesis of specific proteins acting at critical times in a concerted manner in the life cycle of the cell. The proteins SUV39H1 and heterochromatin protein 1 are involved in the regulation of specific cell-cycle genes and the progression of cells through the G_1 and S-phases. The overall process is very tightly controlled, in part by methylation and removal of acetyl group histones.

The human gene system can be separated into two functions: the underlying system of cellular function which is common to all creatures, and those functions specifically required by a complex, mobile, aware human vertebrate.

Human gene and protein systems can be separated into two functions:	
• General cellular function	Intracellular and intercellular signalling
	Development
	Apoptosis
	Control of gene transcription
• Specific vertebrate systems	Neuronal complexity
	Blood clotting
	Acquired immune response

The transfer of information encoded on DNA into proteins requires the production of a single-strand RNA molecule. Gene expression progresses from the initial transcription of a gene to the translation of mRNA in the cytoplasm. In the nucleus, the sequence of transcription, pre-mRNA splicing and 3′ end formation begins with the recognition of either DNA or RNA of a multiprotein complex, which provides a scaffold on which transcription, splicing and 3′ end formation takes place.

Only 1.1–1.4% of the DNA sequence encodes protein, which is 5% of the 28% of the total genome that can be transcribed into mRNA. The protein-coding sections of the genomes are found in the exons, which are separated by non-coding sequences called introns. Most of the increase in size of genes in humans compared with other species is due to extended introns. Half of the overall DNA consists of various repeated sequences which have no known function and are a feature of the large vertebrate genome. This repetitive DNA is regarded by some biologists as junk. Whatever their function they give considerable information about biological processes and their evolution. It is now possible to establish ancestral linkages or family trees for the various components of these genome repeat regions. Within the neutral non-protein-encoded regions are regulatory regions that encode instructions for regulating gene expression. These instructions are deciphered by protein transcription factors, which recognise and enhance transcription through the recognition of DNA motifs. These switch genes on and off in specific spatial and temporal patterns during development. Many evolutionarily important changes are buried within these neutral regions or have no consequence functionally.

The discovery of a gene does not necessarily mean that this gene encodes a protein; the sequence may be a non-expressed pseudogene. Two apparently related genes may be expressed under differing circumstances, e.g. at different sites in cells or at differing stages in development or maturity. Therefore, the cellular position and control mechanisms on the gene, and hence the mode of expression, become very important.

Disordered gene transcription, or the synthesis of non-functional proteins owing to DNA mutations, can have disastrous consequences for the organism. Figure 7.12 summarises the control of gene transcription. Cells have many methods for DNA repair, but these are not discussed in this book. This might become an important topic if nutrients were shown to assist the protective processes involved when DNA is damaged.

Transcription is a highly regulated process, during polymerase binding, transcription initiation, and the elongation and termination stages, with each stage requiring specific regulatory proteins. Gene transcription begins with a transient unwinding

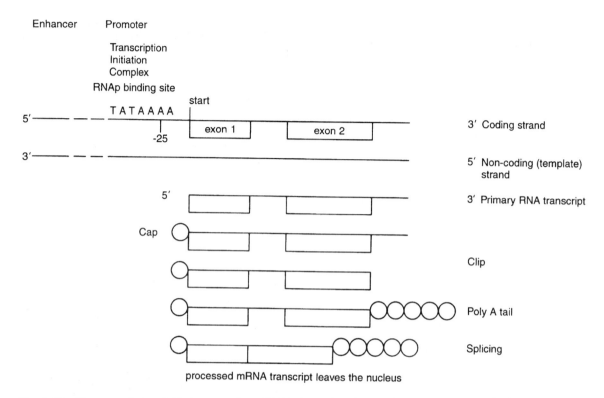

Fig. 7.12   The transcription–initiation complex of DNA-dependent RNA polymerise (RNAp) and other transcription factors assembles and binds to the coding DNA strand. The region of the binding site for this complex is called the promoter region. There are a number of conserved sequences in the promoter region, among them the 'TATA box', centred at 25 bases upstream from the transcription start site. Other regulatory sequences, 'enhancers', may be found at sites distant (and either upstream or downstream) from the start site. The primary RNA transcript is modified before leaving the nucleus. A nucleotide cap is added at the 5' end. The sequences downstream of the last exon are clipped off and a poly-adenosine tail is added. Finally, the sequences between exons are spliced out.

of the DNA coil and separation of the strands of duplex DNA in the region of the transcribed gene. One strand of the DNA acts as a template for the synthesis of single-strand RNA. The actual process of transcription requires an RNA polymerase binding to a DNA promoter sequence, which indicates the site of initiation of transcription, the amount of RNA produced and tissue specificity. TATA boxes are an example of a promotor. There are three RNA polymerases, the most important of which is RNA polymerase II, which is involved in the synthesis of mRNA and some specialised RNAs.

During transcription, protein-coding genes are transcribed by RNA polymerase II, which requires other proteins, including general or basic tran-

scription factors and transcriptional activators. The binding of proteins to sequences close to the promoter regulates gene expression, by activation or repression. These proteins assemble on the promoter to form a pre-initiation complex, which is initiated by interaction with the TATA box. Transcriptional activity is strongly stimulated by promoter-specific activators, which are sequence-specific DNA binding proteins, e.g. Cys_2/His zinc finger proteins. Specific sequences signal the completion or termination of the RNA synthesis and elongation. The RNA and DNA soon peel off and separate after replication has been completed. The newly synthesised RNA molecule is a primary transcript, the direct and total copy or transcript of the information encoded in the gene, and includes all of the introns and exons in the DNA. The primary transcript RNA has to be modified. Introns are removed, depending on the particular protein being encoded by the mRNA. The essential coding sequences, the exons, are joined to produce the specific sequence required to encode a protein. This means that the same RNA can be used to synthesise different proteins, a process called alternative splicing. The spliceosome and several other RNA enzymes require metal ions, e.g. magnesium, as essential cofactors. Pre-mRNA splicing takes place in the spliceosome, where four small nuclear ribonuclear proteins (snRNP) and other proteins interact with the pre-mRNA. A modified 5′ cap of 7-methylguanosine is added at the 5′ end. mRNAs have a 3′ poly(A) tail added after endonucleotic cleavage of the pre-mRNA. This addition of poly(A) is directed by a polyadenylation sequence just upstream from the polyadenylation site. The amount of mRNA available for translation regulates the stability and turnover of the mRNA and hence intracellular concentration. This mRNA may be translated into protein, or sequestrated in an untranslated form or degraded.

Humans have more examples of alternative splicing and complex regulatory networks than other species. This suggests that in humans there are many ways in which exons join together to create a particular functioning mRNA for translation into a protein. This process of splicing allows one gene to produce several mRNAs synthesising an extended range of proteins encoded by that gene, which requires complex regulation of the gene. By altering the pattern of introns, the genetic diversity of the genome is increased without increasing the number of genes. This flexibility becomes of particular importance in specific developmental stages and different cell types. The calcitonin gene is capable of producing calcitonin or calcitonin-gene related peptide. These nascent RNAs then associate with several nuclear proteins. This RNA–protein complex synthesised in the nucleus must be transferred to the cell cytoplasm, where protein synthesis takes place. The nuclear membrane pore complex allows fully processed mature mRNA to move out and proteins synthesised on the ribosomes to move into the nucleus. mRNA contains linear encoding for a protein and also information giving an ability to pair with rRNA, and access to the inside of ribosomes.

PROTEIN SYNTHESIS AND TRANSCRIPTION

The proteome is the sum total of all the proteins in the body. The complexity of the proteome increases from the single-celled yeast to the multicellular invertebrates, vertebrates and humans.

The human genome has at least 1300 protein families which are common to other species, animals, worms, insects and plants. These protein family groups are the conserved core proteins found throughout biology and are responsible for the basic housekeeping functions of the cell, metabolism, DNA replication and repair, and translation. Many are anabolic enzymes responsible for the respiratory chain and nucleotide synthesis. There are few catabolic enzymes in these groups. Humans have many proteins involved in cytoskeleton structure, defence and immunity, and transcription and translation. Many human proteins function in more than one capacity. Families of human proteins present in increased numbers compared with other species, e.g. worms and flies, include the families of immunoglobulins (Ig); developmental proteins, e.g. fibroblast growth factors and transforming growth factor, and intermediate filament proteins. The vertebrate olfactory receptor genes are another large gene family with some 1000 genes and pseudogenes, reflecting the importance of the sense of smell to vertebrates. Following the success of the HGP, the next phase, the study of the proteins encoded by the genes described in the HGP, to be led by the Human Proteome Organisation (HUPO), is still in its preparatory phase. The project will have three key areas of development: protein expression, protein function and a database.

Translation

Translation is the process of mRNA-controlled protein synthesis.

Three different types of RNA are involved in protein synthesis or translation.

- **Messenger RNA (mRNA)** carries the encoded message from DNA as a strand of three-base codons. These codons (triple base sequences)

Functional categories of proteins in humans

(In order of frequency in the body)

- Metabolism
- Transcription/translation
- Intracellular signalling
- Cell–cell communication
- Transport
- Defence and immunity
- Protein folding and degradation
- Cytoskeletal/structure
- DNA replication and modification
- Multifunctional proteins
- Cellular processes

Source: www.geneontology.org

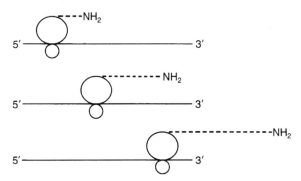

Elongating polypeptide chain

Fig. 7.13 The 40S (smaller) ribosomal subunit binds to the 5′ nucleotide cap of the mRNA. The ribosome then moves along the mRNA molecule scanning for a start codon (sequence AUG, coding for methionine). Several functional proteins (initiation factors and elongation factors) regulate the translocation of the ribosome along the mRNA molecule and the addition of amino acids (carried by transfer RNA molecules) to the polypeptide chain.

either specifically read to record either an amino acid in the resultant protein, or signal the start or end of the amino acid sequencing message (start or stop codon). After leaving the nucleus, mRNA enters the cytoplasm and becomes available to act as a template for the synthesis of protein.

- **Transfer RNA (tRNA)** is the carrier system by which amino acids are bound and transferred to the extending end of the protein being synthesised according to the dictates of the mRNA. The specificity of the system occurs because of the recognition of each codon by a tRNA, specific for each amino acid. The attachment between the two is catalysed by a specific aminoacyl-tRNA synthetase. The mRNA and tRNA function as bivalent adaptors; the tRNA contains a three-base sequence which pairs with its complementary codon in the mRNA, the anticodon.
- **Ribosomal RNA (rRNA)** is associated with a set of proteins to form ribosomes. This complex moves along an mRNA molecule to catalyse protein synthesis. The complex also binds tRNA and other molecules necessary for protein synthesis (Figure 7.13).

These three RNA types and the associated proteins in the ribosome allow 20 different amino acids in varying sequences and amounts to be the template for the synthesis of specific proteins.

The genetic code is shown in Figure 7.14. The sequence of three consecutive bases (a codon) in the RNA molecule encodes an amino acid in the

elongating polypeptide chain. After leaving the nucleus, mRNA enters the cytoplasm and forms a template for protein synthesis. The sequence of bases in the RNA, triple-base sequence or codon, is translated into a linear sequence of amino acids which forms the structural units of protein. To act as a template for protein synthesis, the mRNA must first bind to specific sites on the ribosome (Figure 7.13). This specificity relies on the recognition of each codon for each amino acid by a separate (tRNA). This allows a specific amino acid to bind to an attachment site at one end of the molecule, and recognise the codon for the amino acid by means of an anticodon triplet of bases at the other end. The process of protein biosynthesis is summarised in Figure 7.15.

It was anticipated that there would be 1310 tRNAs, but the HGP found only 497. The methodology used in the original calculation may be a reason for this discrepancy. The anticodon is a trinucleotide triplet which pairs with a specific codon on the mRNA. The code system used by the tRNA represents 20 amino acids. If three nucleotides are used for each code phrase for an amino acid then 64 codons would be required; that is, for four RNA nucleotides and four DNA nucleotides, the combinations possible are $4^3 = 64$. Some 64 codons can be decoded, but in practice 61 different anticodons

UUU	Phe	UCU	Ser	UAU	Tyr	UGU	Cys
UUC	Phe	UCC	Ser	UAC	Tyr	UGC	Cys
UUA	Leu	UCA	Ser	UAA	TERM	UGA	TERM
UUG	Leu	UCG	Ser	UAG	TERM	UGG	Trp
CUU	Leu	CCU	Pro	CAU	His	CGU	Arg
CUC	Leu	CCC	Pro	CAC	His	CGC	Arg
CUA	Leu	CCA	Pro	CAA	Gln	CGA	Arg
CUG	Leu	CCG	Pro	CAG	Gln	CGG	Arg
AUU	Ile	ACU	Thr	AAU	Asn	AGU	Ser
AUC	Ile	ACC	Thr	AAC	Asn	AGC	Ser
AUA	Ile	ACA	Thr	AAA	Lys	AGA	Arg
AUG	Met	ACG	Thr	AAG	Lys	AGG	Arg
GUU	Val	GCU	Ala	GAU	Asp	GGU	Gly
GUC	Val	GCC	Ala	GAC	Asp	GGC	Gly
GUA	Val	GCA	Ala	GAA	Glu	GGA	Gly
GUG	Val	GCG	Ala	GAG	Glu	GGG	Gly

All of the triplet codons have meaning: 61 of the codons represent amino acids. All of the amino acids except tryptophan and methionine have more than one codon. Three codons cause termination (TERM). The order of bases in a codon is written in the same way from 5′ to 3′.

Ala	Alanine	Gln	Glutamine	Leu	Leucine	Ser	Serine
Arg	Arginine	Glu	Glutamic	Lys	Lysine	Thr	Threonine
Asn	Asparagine	Gly	Glycine	Met	Methionine	Trp	Tryptophan
Asp	Aspartic	His	Histidine	Phe	Phenylalanine	Tyr	Tyrosine
Cys	Cysteine	Ile	Isoleucine	Pro	Proline	Val	Valine

Fig. 7.14 The genetic code. The codons are shown in the messenger RNA format.

are present, as only some 40 or more tRNA molecules interact with the 61 possible sense codons of mRNA. This is because of the phenomenon of the wobble rules. That is, in the process of translation during protein synthesis, the tRNA coding is not precise in the third base after the defining initial pair of G-C and A-U pairings in the mRNA. In the codon's third (wobble) position, U and C are generally decoded by a single tRNA species, whereas A and G are decoded by two separate tRNA species. The codons UAA, UGA and UAG are terminator signals for the carboxyl terminal of the protein being synthesised.

In the synthesis of protein from mRNA:

1. A specific first codon, the initiation codon UAG, indicates the beginning of the reading frame, which then runs through the codons for the consecutive amino acids for the protein being synthesised until a termination codon is reached (UAA, UAG or UGA) and the synthesis of that protein is complete.
2. There is activation of amino acids in the cytosol. Each of the 20 amino acids is covalently attached to its specific tRNA, which utilises aminoacyl-tRNA synthetase.
3. The initiation complex comprises a triad. The mRNA encoding the protein being synthesised binds to the smaller ribosomal subunit and the initiating aminoacyl-tRNA, then the larger ribosomal subunit binds. The codon of the initiating aminoacyl-tRNA base pairs with the starter codon on the mRNA. This signals the beginning of protein synthesis, a process controlled by initiation factor proteins.
4. Elongation is dictated by the codon sequence of the mRNA, the corresponding tRNA bringing the appropriate amino acid for protein synthesis.
5. Termination and release occur when a termination codon indicates that the process is finished. Release factor proteins enable the new protein to be released.
6. The new protein folds into its tertiary formation. To achieve this, amino acids are removed from

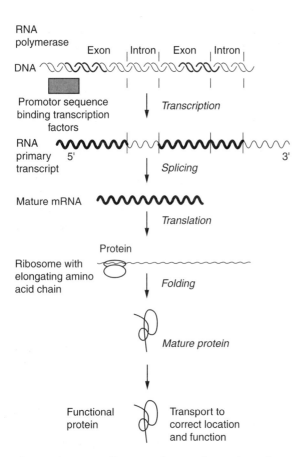

RNA
polymerase
Exon ┊ Intron┊ Exon ┊ Intron┊
DNA

Promotor sequence
binding transcription
factors

Transcription

RNA
primary　5'
transcript

3'

Splicing

Mature mRNA

Translation

Protein

Ribosome with
elongating amino
acid chain

Folding

Mature protein

Functional
protein

Transport to
correct location
and function

Fig. 7.15 An overall picture of protein biosynthesis, from gene to functional protein. Transcription of DNA occurs by a complex with RNA polymerase activity and is regulated by transcription factor proteins. The mRNA encoded by the DNA is initially created as primary transcript RNA and then spliced out as mature RNA after rearrangement of introns and exons. The mRNA is then translated on ribosomes to produce protein, which then folds and is modified to become the mature protein for transportation to the cellular location for functioning.

the amino acid terminus and methyl, acetyl, phosphoryl, carboxyl and other groups may be conjugated to the protein. This determines the charges along the protein and hence its shape.
7. Proteins that fail to fold properly or to form the correct quaternary structure are retained in the ER and are eventually degraded in the proteasomes. This is an ER quality-control system.

Proteins are the most tightly packed of any form of organic matter. This provides a rigid core upon which the arrangement of functional groups can take place, e.g. catalytic side-chains for enzymes. The basic protein folds are predetermined by the physical properties of the protein chain. The protein folds are formed from a chain of some 80–200 amino acids, producing a number of natural forms, with definite rules for the construction of each. The total number of permissible folds is somewhere between 500 and 1000. The folds are very robust and fixed, and like a steel coil will revert to a constant shape after being straightened.

Protein sorting or trafficking

All cellular proteins are synthesised on the rough ER. The 10 000 or more proteins in any one cell are directed to the site of use; otherwise, if misplaced, they are ineffective and could be a hindrance. The directing of proteins to their site of optimal activity is called protein sorting or trafficking.

Some are secreted from the cell, others are selectively distributed to various organelles and others remain within the cytosol. The mechanisms regulating protein sorting depend on a short sequence of amino acids, the signal sequence, which is specific to the protein and its eventual location. Proteins intended for the ER have the signal sequence attached to the protein amino terminus. Once the newly synthesised protein is in the lumen of the ER the signal sequence is removed.

Precursor proteins transported from the cytosol to the mitochondria have amino terminal signal sequences attached and are accompanied by cytosolic chaperone proteins. These new precursor proteins are held in an unfolded, incomplete form by chaperones, cytosolic Hsc70 and mitochondrial-import stimulation factor. The passage of the protein through the mitochondrial membrane is facilitated by proteins and selective membrane receptors, using a channel dependent on ATP or GTP hydrolysis, or a transmembrane electrochemical potential difference. The signal sequence is then removed, and the intact protein folds and settles in its directed site and to its appointed task.

Those proteins synthesised in mitochondrial ribosomes and needed locally are added directly to the appropriate compartment.

The majority of proteins are transported by the secretory pathway for proteins that are directed by a specific signal to the ER. Synthesis is completed by ribosomes on the rough ER and some proteins remain to function there. The majority move in vesicles onto the Golgi apparatus, fold into their mature form, and are then sorted and dispatched onwards or remain locally. During this process oligosaccharide side-chains are added to some proteins. Some soluble proteins (digestive enzymes, hormones and neurotransmitters) are held in vesicles to be released by suitable stimuli, in the process of regulated secretion. Other proteins are held in transport vesicles to be released by continuous secretion, in the process of exocytosis.

Most proteins undergo further transformations, forming the mature protein before secretion.

Protein synthesis → Rough ER lumen → Golgi cysternae → Secretory vesicles → Regulated
→ Exocytosed

Other proteins are synthesised on cytosolic ribosomes and are thereafter directed by signalling sequences to their destination. Within the cell, small vesicles transport proteins from one organelle to another. The protein coat of the vesicles determines where the protein is deposited.

Cells can also transport proteins from outside the cell into their cytoplasm using clathrin-coated pits and vesicles on the membrane surface, in the process of endocytosis. A specific receptor on the cell surface may bind the extracellular macromolecule, the ligand, forming a transport vesicle, within the cell of the receptor–ligand complex. Low-density lipoproteins (LDL), transferrin and insulin are good examples of such a transport system. The ligands dissociate from the receptor and return to the surface.

During cell division the nucleus is emptied when the membrane is divided. The released proteins have to be moved back into the nucleus in a recycling process using proteins, importin α and β, and a GTPase called Ran.

HUMAN GENETIC VARIATION

Within any species, populations and families, there are biological variables. Differences in our genomes account for some of these differences. The amino acid sequence of each protein is determined primarily by the codon and subsequent splicing. The function of each cell protein, including enzymes, is determined by this amino acid sequence and the folding of the mature protein, which may include enzymatic substitution of some of the amino acid residues after translation. The activity and amount of all proteins are controlled principally by the regulation of gene transcription.

In the uterus the genes of the evolving foetus are derived from the mother and father. The environment is created by the mother. Which of these competing genes at each locus of the chromosome is active or not is decided by methylation or demethylation of the maternal or paternal equivalent gene, an imprinting gene.

Haemoglobin illustrates how a single point mutation within an exon can have significant effects on the function of an expressed protein. Haemoglobin is the oxygen-carrying protein of the blood. Transport of oxygen to tissue cells is a fundamental requirement for metabolism. The transport of water and fuel (food) is subsidiary only in the sense that cell death occurs more rapidly from deficiency of oxygen than from deficiency of water or fuel. Haemoglobin is an abundant protein; it was among the first to be studied and is one of the best characterised of human proteins.

Similar mutations occur in the genes encoding other proteins. Many severe diseases are caused by alterations or premature termination of the

---

Coated vesicle transport routes

Clathrin vesicles → Plasma membrane and Golgi → Endosomes.
COP I vesicles → Golgi cisternae → Rough ER
COP II vesicles → Rough ER → Golgi
The coated vesicles also contain adapter proteins, e.g. clathrin and AP1 and AP2.

amino acid sequence of enzymes involved in metabolic pathways, leading to loss of catalytic function, e.g. phenylketonuria, galactosaemia and the 'storage diseases'.

Thus, genetically based seemingly minor alterations in the DNA and subsequent synthesis and sequence of one protein may give rise to variably severe consequences. It is highly likely that such mechanisms underlie the differences between individuals in the way in which some nutrients are handled.

The uniqueness of the DNA sequences of individuals is shown by RFLP or 'genetic fingerprinting', a technique with forensic applications.

ENZYMES AND ISOENZYMES

An important feature of enzymes, and indeed of many other functional proteins, are the domains, regions of the protein created by the local amino acids chain sequence and subsequent folding into stable globular units fashioning specific functions. In enzymes these are catalytic domains, and in membrane proteins, transmembrane domains. There may be more than one domain in an enzyme for that enzyme's function.

The complexity of proteins and the number and combinations of domains increase with evolution. Nevertheless, more than 90% of protein domains in humans are also present in other species from other kingdoms.

Adaptation to a changing environment is of paramount importance to all organisms. One such environmental change is the availability and type of nutrients and their subsequent processing by the metabolic system. Such an adaptation will depend on a responsive regulatory system, which includes enzymatic activity and transport systems. The spectrum and activity of the enzymes and transport systems synthesised by the genome of the individual are unique to that person. Hence, the metabolic response in normal, abundant and deficient dietary intakes will be dictated by the enzyme types and transport systems, and their cellular distribution and activity. Such differences in enzymatic activity and response result from the isoenzymes or enzymes. An individual metabolic pathway consists of a sequence of enzymatically catalysed reactions,

---

Interindividual differences in enzyme profile

An example is the enzymatic difference between Caucasians and Mongol races in the type and activity of the enzyme glyceraldehyde dehydrogenase. A deficiency or reduced enzyme activity as in Mongol races, results in accumulation of blood glyceraldehyde following the ingestion of alcohol, with resultant flushing.

Another enzymatic difference between individuals is the slow and fast acetylation of certain drugs. Acetylation of fat-soluble chemicals is a liver enzymatic activity which facilitates the biliary excretion of water-insoluble xenobiotic endproducts. Caffeine is eliminated in the urine after hepatic acetylation and hence becomes more soluble in water. Wakefulness after drinking coffee in the later part of the day may result from caffeine accumulation in the body due to slow clearance secondary to slow acetylator activity.

---

with different rates of activity according to the body's enzymes or isoenzyme profile. An isoenzyme, sometimes called an isozyme, is a member of a group of enzymes that are structurally similar and catalyse the same reaction, but with differing rates of activity. These isoenzymes may differ by only one amino acid or by different aggregation of subunits of polypeptides.

Before the discovery of isoenzymes, differences in metabolic activity between tissues, and to a lesser extent between individuals, were believed to be due to variations in the amounts of enzyme and substrate available, cell permeability, compartmentalisation and hormone effects. These are important, but equally important are the qualitative aspects of tissue enzymology.

Regulation of enzymatic activity

Enzymes are, fundamentally, *catalysts* of biochemical reactions. Their activity can be regulated by three mechanisms.

Enzyme molecule synthesis and degradation
In general, enzyme synthesis is constant, a zero-order reaction. Degradation is a first-order reaction, i.e. the degradation rate is a percentage of the

One enzyme initiates a major metabolic change

For example, a hormonal trigger for glycogen degradation activates adenylcyclase at the cellular membrane. Cyclic adenosine monophosphate (AMP) is synthesised from ATP and stimulates kinase, which catalyses the activation of phosphorylase kinase. Phosphorylase kinase catalyses the phosphorylation of phosphorylase *b* to the active *a* form. The active enzyme then acts on glycogen to form glucose-1-phosphate, which leads to the formation of glucose.

available enzyme pool. A steady state exists when synthesis and degradation rates are equal. Changes in the steady state result in changes in enzyme activity, which are dependent on the half-life of the enzyme.

Conversion from an inactive to an active form
This is a rapid mechanism, e.g. by phosphorylation or dephosphorylation. Glycogen synthetase and pyruvic dehydrogenase are active in the dephosphorylated form, whereas phosphorylase, an enzyme involved in glycogen breakdown, is active only when phosphorylated. A single enzyme may be responsible for the initiation of a major metabolic change.

Some enzymes, especially proteases, are synthesised as the inactive 'pro-' forms or *zymogens*, e.g. trypsinogen, chymotrypsinogen and pepsinogen, which are converted, when required, to the active form by very specific proteolytic cleavage at a peptide bond. In the lumen of the duodenum trypsinogen is cleaved by enterokinase, a small intestinal brush-border enzyme. Trypsin, in turn, activates the other pancreatic zymogens. Similar chain reactions occur in blood coagulation, fibrinolysis, hormone action and the complement system.

Changes in concentration of metabolic intermediates
Changes in concentrations of substrates, cofactors, activators and inhibitors provide the fine and immediate control of enzyme activity. Enzyme activity is related to substrate and cofactor concentration, according to the Michaelis–Menten equation:

$$V = \frac{V_m \times [S]}{K_m + [S]}$$

where V is the velocity of the reaction, V_m is the maximal velocity, K_m is the Michaelis constant, i.e. the concentration of substrate at which the velocity is half V_m, and $[S]$ is the concentration of substrate or cofactor. The Michaelis constant indicates the physiological concentration at which the enzyme will function. This identifies the possibility of catalytic effectiveness at a tissue substrate concentration.

An alternative enzymatic relationship between velocity and substrate concentration is sigmoidal in type. This occurs as a result of a co-operative binding of substrate to enzymes formed of multiple subunits. The first molecule attaches to a subunit and causes a change in the shape of the subunit, which in turn facilitates the binding of substrate to a second subunit, and so on. The best known example of this allosteric interaction is the binding of oxygen by the subunits of haemoglobin. Activation and inhibition of enzyme activity are important. Activation may originate in the cell or be mediated from an extraneous source which activates a receptor. An inhibitor may compete with a substrate for the binding site. Alternatively, the inhibitor or activator may be attached at another site and elicit allosteric interactions either to reduce or to augment enzyme activity. The effector may also alter the rate of release of product from the enzyme, thereby altering the K_m of the reaction.

Allosteric describes a protein, or more specifically an enzyme, with more than one distinct receptor site. The active site binds the substrate, while the allosteric site is separate from the active site and is affected by the same or another metabolite. The protein–allosteric effector complex reversibly alters the molecular structure of the protein and for an allosteric enzyme alters the shape of the protein and the properties of the active site (the allosteric effect). An allosteric enzyme is to be found at a branch point in a metabolic pathway. A *ligand* is any atom, ion or molecule that binds specifically to a larger one, in this case an enzyme. The ligand is chemically altered by the enzymatic reaction, and the enzyme changes shape to allow these reactions to take place at several sites on the enzyme.

Isoenzymes and metabolic reversibility

Table 7.2 highlights metabolically significant variables for which isoenzymes have been implicated.

Rate-limiting enzyme and step

This is the slowest step in a reaction sequence, the step that is catalysed by the enzyme with the slowest rate constant. The system is most readily saturated at such a step.

Table 7.2 Metabolic variables and the implicated isoenzymes

Variable	Isoenzyme
K_m	Hexokinase Pyruvate kinase Glutaminase Creatine kinase
Substrate and cofactor	Aldolase Alcohol dehydrogenase Isocitrate dehydrogenase
Allosteric properties	Hexokinase Pyruvate kinase Aspartate kinase Glutaminase Fructose bisphosphatase
Subcellular localisation	Isocitrate dehydrogenase Adenylate kinase
Dietary and hormonal control	Hexokinase Tyrosine aminotransferase Pyruvate kinase Arginase

The separation of metabolic pathways by physical compartmentalisation is an essential component of metabolism. Isoenzymes are separated into different cellular compartments. Metabolism is a series of discrete unidirectional chemical reactions catalysed by polyisoenzyme complexes. The same reaction may occur in different directions in different compartments of a cell, or in two different cells within the same organism. Each will be catalysed by a different isoenzyme, with different K_m values, and at least one will require the input of energy from a different reaction or the efficient removal of the products of the thermodynamically unfavourable reaction.

Of the ten enzymes involved in the sequential metabolism of glucose to pyruvate, nine have iso-

Isoenzyme compositions in tissues

The liver and muscle have different isoenzyme compositions. Distinct muscle-type phosphofructokinase, aldolase, enolase and pyruvate kinase enzymes are not present in liver and vice versa. Glycogen phosphorylase is another example. Glucokinase is present in the liver but absent from muscle. These differences reflect the different metabolic requirements of the tissues.

enzymes. Enzyme multiplicity may arise as a result of various factors.

Genetic factors

- **Multiple alleles at a single genetic locus**: the heterozygous individual with two different allelic variants (one each on the maternally and the paternally derived chromosome) will produce two different types of enzyme subunits. If the enzyme is composed of multiple subunits, an individual heterozygous for the genes of some or all of the subunits will be capable of assembling a greater variety of types.
- **Multiple genetic loci**: the organism may produce one protein with a given enzyme function in one tissue, and a different protein that catalyses the same reaction in a different tissue. Gene expression varies from tissue to tissue and at varying times in the overall development, from foetus to adult and even with ageing in the adult. Multiple gene loci produce differences in isoenzyme profile.

Secondary or post-translational alterations in isoenzymes

Enzyme subunits can be modified to produce a range of composite enzymes from the same gene complex. Only part of the enzyme subunit may be involved.

Apparent multiplicity

Artefacts or apparent isoenzymes from the same enzyme or proenzyme can be created under differing conditions of extraction and storage conditions. Only permanent forms are considered to be true isoenzymes.

Aldolase is encoded at three genetic loci. In muscle, aldolase A has two subunits, Aα and Aβ. The transition from Aα to Aβ is by slow deamination of an asparagine residue near the carboxyl terminus. The post-translational process may be tissue specific, creating differences in tissue isoenzymes. For example, pyruvate kinase is a tetrameric enzyme. Its activity is inhibited when the enzyme is phosphorylated. The predominant isoform in the liver is designated L and its activity is modulated by phosphorylation. Two other isoforms are less susceptible to phosphorylation. In this way, hormone action inhibits utilisation of glucose by the liver (by phosphorylation of the L isoenzyme) when the blood glucose level is low and the substrate is more urgently required by other tissues, such as brain and muscle.

Coenzymes and prosthetic groups

Many enzymes require coenzymes such as nicotinamide-adenine dinucleotide (NAD)/NADH or coenzyme A (CoA), and the prosthetic groups, the metal ions, haem groups and vitamin-derived cofactors. These extend the specificity of the enzymes. The covalent attachments of certain prosthetic groups allow the transfer of intermediates in a reaction between the active sites of multienzyme complexes, which is called the swinging arm system.

KEY POINTS

1. Metabolism is in part dependent on the structure of the cell. Structure and functions are distributed between cells, and chemicals move between compartments by specific transport mechanisms. The cell compartments include the nucleus, cytosol, mitochondria, endoplasmic reticulum, Golgi apparatus, lysosome and peroxisome. The nucleus contains the genes for the synthesis of cellular proteins. Cytosol is an aqueous phase containing many of the enzymes catalysing metabolic reactions. The mitochondria include the enzymes that function to transport oxidatively metabolised nutrients. The endoplasmic reticulum is involved in protein synthesis.

2. The strands of DNA within the nucleus are polymers of deoxyribonucleotides; strands of RNA are polymers of ribonucleotides. Each unit consists of deoxyribose covalently linked to bases, adenine and guanine (purines), and cytosine and thymine (DNA) or uracil (RNA) (pyrimidines). The reading of the code of the DNA and RNA is in triplets of any three of these bases, the codon. The order of any three of these bases determines the amino acid sequence of proteins produced by the DNA molecule.

3. Stretches of DNA in the chromosome are genes; much of the remainder of the sequences between genes has no known function. Other sequences, while not transcribed to proteins, act as regulatory elements by facilitating the binding of functional proteins to the DNA strand.

4. The number of protein-encoding genes is between 26 000 and 31 000, the correct figure is probably 31 000; of these, some 740 genes are non-protein-coding RNAs involved in cellular function.

5. The DNA sequence that is encoded for protein synthesis is initially transcribed into mRNA. mRNA may undergo splicing, which enables one gene to encode for several proteins. The mRNA passes from the nucleus, enters the cytoplasm and becomes available to act as a template for the synthesis of protein. Amino acids required for protein synthesis are provided by specific transfer RNAs.

6. Proteins synthesised in the cell are subsequently sorted or trafficked to other parts of the cell or other organs.

7. Isoenzymes (isozymes) are protein enzymes that are identical in all respects to the prime functioning enzyme, but differ in functional efficiency by virtue of small but important amino acid variations from the other isoenzymes in that family. The range of enzymes provided by the genetic configuration is individual to each person. Hence, the metabolic pathways in normal, abundant and deficient dietary states will be dictated by the enzyme amounts and activity, in turn, will depend on the isoenzymes or enzyme separation in the individual's cells or organs.

8. Enzyme activity may be regulated by three mechanisms: enzyme synthesis and degradation; conversion from an inactive to an active form, and changes in the concentration of metabolic intermediates. The activity of an enzyme is described by the Michaelis–Menten equation.

THINKING POINTS

1. The question 'are you a man or a mouse?' is more complex than the original questioner intended. Discuss from a molecular biological point of view.
2. Take any series of reactions and the enzymes involved, trace their genetic origin and, if they have isoenzymes, look at how such isoenzyme functional variation may affect a reaction.
3. Look at how these reactions are dependent on the availability of cofactors, e.g. minerals and vitamins, which are nutritional influences on reaction function.

FURTHER READING

Berger, S.L. (2000) Gene regulation, local or global. *Nature*, **408**, 412–14.

Denton, M. and Marshall, C. (2001) Protein folds. Laws of form revisited. *Nature*, **410**, 417.

Doolittle, R.F. (1995) The multiplicity of domains in proteins. *Annual Review of Biochemistry*, **64**, 287–314.

Kay, L.E. (2000) *Who Wrote the Book of Life? A History of the Genetic Code*. Stanford University Press, Stanford CA.

Kramer, A. (1996) The structure and function of proteins involved in mammalian pre-mRNA splicing. *Annual Review of Biochemistry*, **65**, 367–409.

Levitt, M., Gerstein, M., Huang, E., Subbiah, S. and Tsia, J. (1997) Protein folding: the end game. *Annual Review Biochemistry*, **66**, 549–79.

Lewin, B.(1997) *Genes VI*. Oxford University Press, Oxford.

Nelson, D.L. and Cox, M.M. (eds) (2000) *Lehninger's Principles of Biochemistry*, Nelson, D.L. and Cox, M.M. (eds). Worth, New York.

Perham, R.N. (2000) Swinging arms and swinging domains in multifunctional enzymes. Catalytic machines for multistep reactions. *Annual Review Biochemistry*, **69**, 961–1004.

Ringrose, L. and Paro, R. (2001) Gene regulation. Cycling silence. *Nature*, **412**, 493–4.

Stern, D.L. (2000) Evolutionary biology. The problem of variation. *Nature*, **408**, 529–431.

WEBSITES

www.hupo.org   Human Proteome Organisation

NUTRITION AND GENETICS

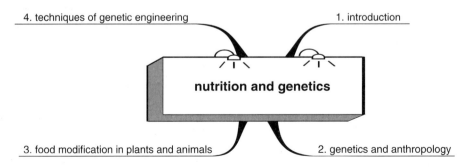

Fig. 7.16   Section outline.

INTRODUCTION

It is very difficult to identify the molecular biological basis of many of the diseases that have been attributed to poor or excessive nutrition. The establishment of the HGP is of great importance for the nutritionist whose interest is interindividual variation, interaction with the environment and hence requirements and sensitivities to different nutrients and food ingredients.

As gene identification translates into gene function and the structure of gene products, there is much to be learnt about biochemical pathways and their regulation, which are of great relevance to nutrition. The metabolic process by which each nutrient is converted to energy or to structure and other functions will be individual and dependent on the efficiency of the isoenzyme complexes in the metabolic pathways. This individual metabolic response will be genetically determined (Figure 7.17). Major nutrients (glucose, fatty acids, amino acids) and minor nutrients (iron, vitamins) are involved with hormones in the regulation of gene expression. All nutrients are involved in some manner in the control of gene expression and post-translational events. In each section where relevant the nutrient–gene interaction will be mentioned.

Variations in the genome structure and resultant protein allosteric variations will dictate the differences in an individual's ability to metabolise individual nutrients, and this will in part dictate the well-being of that individual. The effect of a single gene mutation on an individual's metabolic response to a nutrient may be obvious, although not always so. The effect of such mutations, which is increased when several genes are involved, may be considerable. In addition, there are the complicating actions of secondary and tertiary modifiers and other coincidental nutritional factors. All contribute to a complicated interplay between the genome and diet, where the impact of inheritance may be low and several dietary factors involved.

The enzyme and isoenzyme differences become important when there is an excess or a deficiency of a nutrient, in which case the important differences, and hence vulnerabilities, of individuals will be exposed. Starvation adversely affects individuals regardless of their genetic makeup, but it is much more complicated to understand the response of individuals and different populations to a sufficiency or an excess of food. The population eating the food will be of different genetic constitution and the food eaten by different populations will be of differing constitution. Stark examples of populations being exposed to a radically new diet format are provided by the Aborigines of Australia, the Polynesian Islanders and the Native Americans changing from their accustomed traditional diet to a European-type diet. It is recommended by some that we revert to hunter–gatherer type diets from 40 000 years ago, yet our alleles may be more in accord with our current diet. The cultural element of taste also has to be taken into the equation.

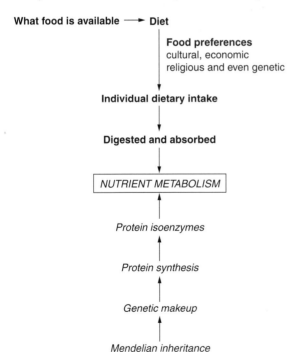

Fig. 7.17 Nutrition and the molecular basis of metabolism. Bold: environmentally determined; italic: genetically determined.

FURTHER READING

Simopoulis, A.P. (1999) Genetic variation and nutrition. *Nutrition Review*, **57**, S10–19.

Symposium (2002) Post-genomic opportunities for understanding nutrition. *Proceedings of the Nutrition Society* **61**, 401–603.

GENETICS AND ANTHROPOLOGY

By looking at mtDNA, which is passed through the maternal line, it is possible to follow mutation patterns and the pattern of the movement of peoples thousands of years ago. Mitochondrial DNA studies have not undermined the hypothesis that modern human beings developed in Africa 100 000 years ago and displaced other human species. Some of these peoples migrated through Asia and on into Australia some 60 000 years ago, and on into the Americas 15 000–35 000 years ago. Alternative theories suggest multiple evolutionary sources. Neanderthals have a central place in human evolution, but a mtDNA study on a preserved specimen showed that Neanderthal man and modern man probably evolved independently. A theory was famously tested when Thor Heydahl and his Koni-Tiki expedition sailed from South America to the Pacific Islands to demonstrate that ancient peoples could have undertaken same journey to colonise those islands. However, the mtDNA evidence is that the Polynesians migrated from Asia. The DNA work does not explain the interesting and similar sculptures found in the Pacific Islands and South America. The population of Iceland, who have been isolated from cross-breeding with other populations, are being recruited into a gene–disease study. Their gene pool is uncontaminated by other races marrying into their stock. The number of such studies will no doubt increase.

Long lines of inheritance can be followed in, for example, the Jewish priestly caste, the Cohanim, who can be shown to have been descended in a close father-to-son tradition over 80–130 generations.

An ethical point is that such studies may on occasions show that the child's apparent father may not be the biological father. Such cases may occur in between 1 and 30% of instances, depending on the mores of a society.

FURTHER READING

Ward, R. and Stringer, C. (1997) A molecular handle on the Neanderthals. *Nature*, **388**, 225–6.

Harding, R.M., Fullerton, S.M., Griffiths, R.C. *et al.* (1997) Archaic African and Asian lineages in the genetic ancestry of modern human. *American Journal of Human Genetic*, **60**, 772–89.

Wong, K. (1999) Is out of Africa going out of doors? *Scientific American*, August, 7.

FOOD MODIFICATION IN PLANTS AND ANIMALS

The hunter–gatherers from whom we are descended would have been experts at recognising safe and nutritious sources of food. The experienced gatherer would be able to maximise the reward from a food-searching expedition. Once farming began, those same skills would be used to develop and raise prime examples of vegetables, fruit and animals for meat. Similarly, dairy produce would be obtained from good yielding stock. So the science of breeding began, and the development of farm plants and animal stock that best suited the local environment. These developments were even more favourable if they were resistant to disease and climatic changes. New breeding stock was sometimes found by chance. A strain was placed on the relationship between production and need when the population increased and concentrated in towns and cities. The needs of the farmer, large and small are somewhat different from those of the gardener or allotment holder. Other elements then became important in the choice of food plants and animals, e.g. shelf-life, nutritional quality and cooking properties.

All of these evolutionary and breeding changes took place over the many years necessary for the breeding process to take place and further time for these new-fangled plants and animals to gain acceptability. The somewhat haphazard nature of this process changed with a number of factors.

- The long voyages of exploration and trade began the trafficking of new plant and animal foods across previously inaccessible seas and land masses.
- A generation of breeders appeared, whose skills, goals and objectives for producing new varieties were enhanced by the new science of Mendelian genetics.

- The science of nutrition became established, and goals for good food became identified.
- The population explosion required increased production of food.
- As the social structure and prosperity in many parts of the world changed, the population came to expect clean, delicious and nutritious food.
- The expectation of an increasingly educated population is that the food they eat must be free of infection and not contaminated by unwholesome applied chemicals, pesticides, herbicides, fungicides and radioactivity.

The requirement of various sectors of society for food has varied:

- Some require cheap, easily accessible food available in a convenient manner.
- Some strive for greater yields from less land.
- Some require pure food, free from contamination of whatever kind.
- Some require foods that are dictated by beliefs or faith.
- Some want industry to provide food in a readily accessible manner, regardless of its methods.
- When the system is unable to meet demand, a new look is taken at the types and production of food.

The pressures created by these needs have led to factory farming and the development of genetically modified (GM) foods: no longer evolution, but farming revolution. The major difference in approach is that the breeder takes a holistic approach and selects a favourable trait. This is a slow process and can only apply to species able to mate with each other or in plants able to tolerate interbreeding or the application of grafts. Coincidentally, sometimes unwanted traits may also appear, as can happen in closely bred families, e.g. hip disorder in some dog breeds go hand in hand with desirable features in other respects. The modifiers of genes, genetic engineers, have single strategies and aim to retain the essential features of the species and add in one identifiable gene change. This logic depends on the single change having no other add-on consequences.

Genetically modified foods

The first series of agricultural biotechnology food

Genetically modified foods

These are created by the direct introduction of desirable characteristics by the artificial transfer of genes or synthetic DNA into an organism. A genetically modified organism or GMO has therefore been altered in a way that does not involve mating or conventional genetic recombination. The first generation of GMOs was altered for traits encoded in one gene, e.g. herbicide, insecticide or virus resistance. The modifications are becoming more sophisticated to alter metabolic pathways and hence the food quality and nutrient value of the new crop.

products was not regarded by the industry as being radically different to existing foods. Some of the products are genetically modified to be resistant to pesticides or to make their own pesticides. Pesticide resistance allows a farmer to use a pesticide for weed control without killing the food crop.

Biotechnology has also been used to produce transgenic animals, in which a foreign gene or DNA material is inserted into the animal genome to produce a 'transgenic' animal with altered characteristics, e.g. the insertion of genes which confer increased yields of meat or milk with reduced cholesterol or fat content. Examples of such genetically modified animals include sheep cloned from embryonic cells (Dolly the sheep), Japanese high beef-yielding cattle and rapidly maturing fish for fish farming (Figure 7.18).

Animal products include rennin or chymosin, which was previously produced from rennet from the calf's stomach wall but is now largely produced by engineered *Escherichia coli* bacteria. Bovine somatotrophin synthesised by bacterially engineered microorganisms or growth hormone can increase milk production. It is possible to increase the vitamin A content of canola oil. The saturated fat content of oil-producing plants may be reduced for human foods or increased to make soaps. Fruit could be engineered to contain vaccines. Complex changes in metabolic pathways are being contemplated.

This is a highly controversial area of nutrition with powerful and persuasive arguments being made by both sides. The key point is that the total consequences of a contemplated action must be understood and evaluated before the action is undertaken.

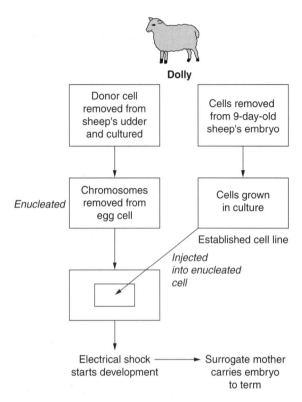

Fig. 7.18 Cloning of animals. Sheep enucleated cells are combined with egg cells from an embryo to produce embryos that grow into cloned offspring.

TECHNIQUES OF GENETIC ENGINEERING

Transformation

Genetic transformation is the transfer of DNA from one plant or species into another. Recombinant DNA (rDNA) is used to manipulate DNA from one cell from one species and to add this to cells from another species. rDNA is a fragment of DNA that has been placed in a cloning vector by splicing, which enables the rDNa to be replicated and transcribed in its new cell. The rDNA may be directly added to a cell, or forced into the cell or a carrier used to transfer the genetic material. Some microbial cells can directly transfer DNA from cell to cell. The cell cultures resulting from such trans-

fers can then be grown using tissue-culture techniques to produce whole plants and, more recently whole animals. The transferred genes may be switched on (expressed) or suppressed to meet the cell circumstances in which they are operating. Such engineering changes for plants are called transformations (Figure 7.18).

The technique is somewhat different for monocotyledons, e.g. maize and wheat. Here, a biolistic method is used, in which the plant tissue is bombarded by foreign DNA which enters the plant cell genome. When dicotyledons are infected by *Agrobacterium tumefaciens*, the *Ti* gene of the bacterium is transferred from the bacterium into the plant cells and portions of the gene then enter the plant genome. These genes can be substituted for plant genes of choice. Often two genes are used, one containing the target gene bordered by plasmid DNA and the other containing *vir* genes, which encode proteins which facilitate the movement of the target gene into the plant genome. The disadvantage of this method is the contamination of the added gene with other DNA.

Alternatively, large fragments of DNA can be made using yeast and artificial bacterial chromosomes, which can then transform plant cells using particle bombardment.

Marker genes

When genes encoding desired novel traits are transformed, marker genes are also included to identify and aid the selection of successfully transformed cells. Selection genes enable the transformed cell to grow on a medium, e.g. having resistance to antibiotics allows the cells to grow in an enriched antibiotic medium. These selection genes may persist into the completed transformed plant. Another group of marker genes, the reporter genes, provide colours and other identifying features and readily identify transformed cells.

The expression of plant genes is regulated by active promoter sequences that are placed next to the transferred gene. A common promoter is the 35S cauliflower mosaic virus (35S CaMv). These promoters allow the expression and activation of genes.

The addition of amino acid sequences to the gene products directs their transport to specific organelles.

Suppression of expression

Transgenic DNA is antisense to the endogenous target gene and this property can be used to suppress the target gene's expression. There are other ways in which expression can be suppressed, e.g. by identical gene sequences within the genome. The mechanism of this suppression is complex. Ribozymes, which are RNA molecules with enzymatic activity, are used to produce resistance to viruses.

Safeguarding and enhancing gene expression

It is important that the inserted DNA is expressed. This is achieved by specific DNA sequences that bind nuclear proteins.

Chimeraplasty

This is the phenomenon in which DNA, flanked by methylated RNA, is taken up by the host cell; this can cause a very specific mutation in the gene codons.

Terminator technology

Terminator technology prevents embryo formation in plants grown from commercial seeds. The farmer is unable to use seeds from the first year's crop to grow the next year's crop, and has to buy a new stock. The gene may encode sterility, growth impairment or inhibition of disease resistance. This terminator gene is suppressed during the first passage of the development of the seed and the plant.

Agronomical traits

Herbicide resistance
Resistance to the non-selective herbicides glyphosphate and glufosinate ammonium has been introduced into soyabeans, tomatoes, corn, oilseed rape (canola) and wheat. Such herbicide tolerance is intended to improve weed control, so that when the crop is sprayed, the crop is resistant to the herbicide and in that way selectivity is introduced.

Glyphosphate inhibits the plant enzyme 5-enolpyruvyl-3-phosphoshikimic acid synthase, which is involved in the synthesis of aromatic amino acids, vitamins and other secondary plant metabolites. The inhibition effect is achieved by the introduction of genes encoding for enzymes with reduced affinity for glyphosphate or enzymes that degrade glyphosphate.

Glufosinate ammonium inhibits plant glutamine synthetase activity. The inhibition of this enzyme leads to an accumulation of ammonia in the plant. The introduced protective gene converts the herbicidal form of the glufosinate ammonium (l-phosphinothricin) into the inactive form. The sulfonylurea and imidazoline classes of herbicide both inhibit the same enzymatic step in the synthesis of branched-chain amino acids. Transfer of a resistant gene from a goose grass gives resistance to this herbicide.

Insect resistance
Three-quarters of commercial chemical pesticides act as inhibitors of acetylcholine esterase and sodium pump systems.

Biological insect controllers include *Bacillus thuringiensis* (Bt), which produces a protein toxic to insects (Cry toxins). Each strain of Bt produces a unique toxin. The Cry proteins are produced as protoxins which are released in the intestine of the insect and bind to specific Cry toxin receptors. This leads to cell disruption and death. Genes that express the production of cry1Ab and cry1Ac are added to plants to control the European corn borer and tobacco budworm, respectively.

Toxic proteins accumulating within a plant can confer protection against herbivores. These proteins include ribosome-inactivating proteins, antifungal proteins, proteinase and amylase inhibitors, and carbohydrate binding proteins (lectins). Proteinase inhibitors are naturally present in legumes and cereals. The cowpea trypsin inhibitor gene has been used in a number of crops to confer insect resistance.

Virus resistance
While there are no certain ways to create a plant free from viral infection, resistance can be created by introducing viral sequences into the plant genome. The cloning of a virus coat into the plant's genome gives added resistance to viral infection to that plant.

Fungal resistance
The addition of genes to plant genomes that synthesise antifungal metabolites, e.g. phytoalexins, confers effective protection from fungal infection, especially if the metabolite originates from a plant species different to the one being protected. Fungal walls are also susceptible to the action of chitinases and other hydrolytic enzymes, so the plant may be induced to produce these enzymes.

Tolerance to environmental conditions
The tolerance of plants to drought, high-salinity environments, freezing and excess water is a problem in agriculture, and survival under these conditions is complicated and involves multiple gene action. Genetic engineering to allow plants to accommodate to these conditions is a major challenge.

Yield improvement

Plant growth is influenced by light and light-sensitive receptors. For example, the ratio of phytochrome A to phytochrome B is important in light and shade conditions. By engineering an increase in phytochrome A, denser cropping and increased yields are possible. Dwarf plants direct more of their energy into crop production.

Quality traits
The deletion, suppression and enhancement of genes involved in the synthesis of oils, proteins carbohydrates and micronutrients will generate plants specifically meeting agricultural and nutritional needs.

THINKING POINT

Look at the arguments for and against the application of genetic engineering to food products.

FURTHER READING

Domoney, C. (1996) Improvement of crop quality by genetic manipulation. *British Nutrition Foundation, Nutrition Bulletin*, **20** (Suppl.), 266–75.
EC Directive 90/220/EEC (OJL117) (1990), *Genetically Modified Foods*. Article 2, 8 May, pp. 15–27.
Lurquin, P.F. (2001) *The Green Phoenix: A History of Genetically Modified Plants*. Columbia University Press, New York.

WEBSITES

www.rikilt.wageningen-ur.nl/News/text.report.html New developments in crop biotechnology and their possible implications for food product safety (Kleter, G.A., Noordam, M.Y., Kok, E.J. and Kuiper, H.A.).
www.ncbe.rdg.ac.uk   Genetically modified food.
www.agbioworld.com   Genetically modified crops: demystifying the science.
www.nuffield.org/bioethics/publications/modified-crops/rep0000000075.html Genetically modified crops: the ethical and social issues (Nuffield Council on Bioethics Reports).
www.greenpeace.org   Greenpeace website.

MOLECULAR BASIS OF DISEASE

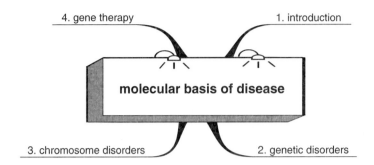

4. gene therapy 1. introduction

molecular basis of disease

3. chromosome disorders 2. genetic disorders

Fig. 7.19 Section outline.

INTRODUCTION

Medical genetics has enabled scientists and clinicians to study the aetiology of non-infective disease at the cellular and molecular levels. Many conditions are now recognised as belonging to a group of conditions, in which changes in the genetic material are either entirely or partially responsible for the pathology.

The interpretation of human pedigree patterns is complex and beyond the scope of this book (see McKuisick, 1998, for further details).

Mendelian disorders are caused by a mutation at a single genetic locus. Gene mapping precisely locates the disease locus on a chromosome and then searches for cloned sequences within the gene to identify how this differs from the advantageous gene.

Mutations in DNA sequences cause changes in phenotype. It may be difficult to identify the evolutionarily relevant mutations. Many mutations have no noticeable impact on an organism, implying that the loss of an enzyme may not always have apparent consequences for function or survival. Many evolutionarily relevant mutations are outside the protein-encoding regions. DNA regions that encode genes also contain long lengths of neutral variations that have no effect on the phenotype.

Phenotypic variation is nevertheless a common feature of human disease resulting from a single gene mutation. The effects of such mutations are even greater in the relatively few conditions that involve several genes. The actions of secondary and tertiary modifiers and environmental factors also have an effect. There is thus a complicated interplay between the genome and environment in multifactorial disorders, in which the impact of inheritance may be low and several environmental agents may be involved.

To identify a gene-dependent condition, the Mendelian characters or disorders are used as genetic markers to follow a small section of chromosome through a pedigree. Ideally, a marker should have a known chromosomal location, be highly polymorphic, show codominant inheritance and be measurable by blood tests. Genetic heterogeneity implies a clinically similar condition produced by different genes or different mutations in the same gene. In practice, a number of gene mechanisms may be involved.

More than 10 000 human genes have been catalogued in Online Mendelian Inheritance in Man (OMIM), which documents inherited human diseases and their causal gene mutations. Approximately 1000 single genes are associated with an increased susceptibility to a disease or a disorder (Table 7.3).

Approximately half of the diseases of the first year of life are related to defects in gene-encoding enzymes. The developing foetus is protected from such defects by access to the mother's metabolic system through the placenta. The baby is normal at birth and the inborn errors of metabolism present only after the infant is totally dependent on its own metabolism.

Table 7.3   Disorders caused by mutations of genes

Type of disorder	Dominant or recessive	Peak age of onset
Enzyme	Primarily recessive	First year of life
Modifiers of protein function	Recessive or dominant	Early adulthood
Receptors	Recessive or dominant	First year of life and adulthood
Transcription factors	Largely dominant	*In utero*

In mammals, genes found next to each other rarely share common functions, but often have a common evolutionary history. Segments of DNA that encode for a protein region that has a function, e.g. a domain, are most likely to retain their sequence through the evolutionary process. Genes that are tightly linked, that is clustered in the same region of the chromosome in one species, tend to be tightly linked in other species. The majority of sex-related genes, which determine gender, are found in the X chromosome.

New mutations occur in the human population at a rate of 1–100 mutations each generation. Duplication has been a major reason for changes in genes during vertebrate evolution. Hundreds of human genes are direct inserts or transferred from bacteria. Sex chromosomes differ in their mutation pattern during the formation of eggs and sperm, with mutations occurring most frequently in males. This may be because the female has two X chromosomes balancing each other, whereas in the male the single X and Y chromosomes are unbalanced.

Mutation rates can be calculated from the rates at which identified genes are eliminated by natural selection and created by mutation. Most mutations for autosomal recessive conditions occur undetected in normal heterozygotes and may be transmitted by phenotypically normal carriers over many generations before appearing in an affected person.

The HGP allows rapid identification of candidate genes for many conditions and functions, and makes it easier to study diseases of unknown biochemical malfunction. The identification programme first maps the chromosomal region containing the gene by linkage analysis in affected families and then searches for the gene itself. The sequencing of the genome has also allowed an understanding of the mechanisms wherein common chromosomal deletion syndromes occur.

The HGP has identified and mapped some 1.4 million examples of single nucleotide polymorphism (SNP). SNPs reflect past singular event mutations, and follow a change in one base in the DNA. Individuals differ from each other by about one base pair per thousand SNPs. Individuals sharing a variant allele have a common evolutionary heritage. The variation in SNP is least in the sex chromosomes. Every permutation of SNP will occur somewhere in the 3 billion base pairs of the human genome in the 6 billion individuals alive today.

It is easier to identify a population with a particular disadvantaged gene and disease expression than to study populations who are vulnerable or resistant to environmental factors such as a deficiency or excess of dietary constituents, tobacco smoking or alcohol consumption. The tension between the gene and its outside environment is called an interaction. In many studies, whether case–control or cohort studies, the environmental side of the gene–environment interaction may be incorrect; that is, the wrong environmental factor is studied or the measurement is faulty. There is sometimes a subjective element to the choice of the environmental factor. The definition of interaction is seldom made. Statistically, gene–environment interaction occurs when the effect of the genotype on the disease only occurs when a particular environmental situation prevails, e.g. alcohol intake or taking the oral contraceptive. Some progress has been made in identifying factors determining an individual response to alcohol, in that some conditions are less marked or absent in lifelong abstainers. Venous thrombosis is rare in young women who do not take the contraceptive pill, increased four-fold in the entire population of women who use the oral contraceptive, and increased eight-fold in those women who take the oral contraceptive and also have the Arg506Gly (Leiden) mutation in the blood-clotting factor V gene.

A genetic basis to a condition, physical attribute or disease may be determined by:

- **The DNA sequence**: The δ-globin gene was discovered on chromosome 11 during DNA sequencing studies. The nucleotide sequence suggests that the transcribed protein is a member of the β-globin family.
- **A definable protein abnormality**: α_1–antitrypsin was discovered as a serum protease inhibitor. Absence of this enzyme was shown to be associated with pulmonary emphysema and cirrhosis of the liver. This has been mapped to chromosome 14.
- **A disease entity**: cystic fibrosis has been shown by its familial occurrence pattern to be a genetic disease. Linkage analysis has implicated a gene on chromosome 7.

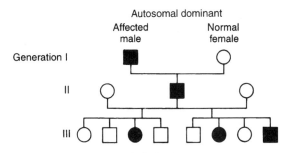

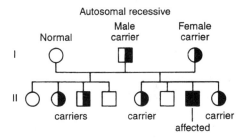

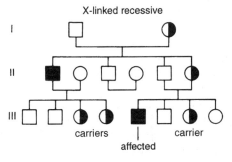

GENETIC DISORDERS

When there is a mutation or change in a gene or chromosome, which is associated with a disease or vulnerability or variation from the expected, that gene or chromosome is often named after that disease or vulnerability or variation. This implies that the gene or chromosome is the cause, but this is not the case. It is only when there is a variation or mutation in the gene or chromosome from the healthy form that the association applies.

Some neurological diseases, e.g. Huntingdon's chorea and fragile X syndrome, have similar genetic abnormalities in that there is a lengthening of tracts of repeat DNA sequences. This 'repeat instability' may arise during the repair of damage to DNA.

Mendelian disorders

These single-gene defects or single-locus disorders (Figure 7.20) result from a mutant allele or a pair of mutant alleles at a single locus. Such changes can be inherited or arise *de novo* through a mutation. When an allele is dominant or recessive, alleles may result in dominant or recessive conditions, respectively. Modern geneticists suggest that these conditions are not attributable to dominant or recessive genes, but rather that the consequent phenotypes

Fig. 7.20 Families with Mendelian single-gene defects. Autosomal dominant: half of the offspring, whether male or female, are affected in the third generation. Autosomal recessive: when a carrier mates with a carrier, two of the children are carriers and one child is affected. In contrast, when a carrier mates with a non-carrier, two of the children are carriers. X-linked recessive: the characteristic is carried by the mother; in the third generation the daughters but not the sons of the affected male are carriers. Among the children of the female carrier, half of the sons are affected and half of the daughters are carriers.

are dominant or recessive. The inheritance is either autosomal dominant, autosomal recessive, autosomal codominant or X-linked inheritance, dominant or recessive. Y-linked traits occur less commonly.

Vocabulary

Autosomal dominance: a dominant trait that is carried on the autosomal chromosomes.

Codominant: both alleles contribute to the phenotype, with either being dominant.

Penetrance: the degree to which a genotype is expressed phenotypically in a population of gene carriers.

Recessive allele: is hidden in the phenotype of a heterozygote by the presence of the dominant allele

X-linked: the trait is carried on the X-chromosome

Autosomal dominant conditions
In these disorders, usually:

- both homozygotes and heterozygotes manifest the condition
- affected individuals have an affected parent
- the risk is 1 in 2 for each child of one affected and one unaffected parent
- both genders are equally affected

- both genders are equally likely to transmit the condition.

Variable expression, non-penetrance or mutation may affect the degree of severity the condition. Even a dominant disease may show variable expression. Non-penetrance may result in a person with no signs of the condition carrying the genes from an affected parent and producing an affected child.

Autosomal recessive conditions
These diseases are determined by a single autosomal locus. The condition manifests only in people who are homozygous for the abnormal allele (aa). The parents of affected children are phenotypically normal carriers (Aa). When the two parents are heterozygous for a particular phenotype, the offspring stand a 25% chance of being normal, 50% of being heterozygotes and 25% of showing clinical expression of the condition. Each child has a 1 in 4 risk of being affected. The distinctive features are as follows.

Familial diseases associated with gene changes (locus by chromosome number p short arm, q longarm: gene)

Cystic fibrosis: a condition of abnormal mucous secretions in lungs and other organs resulting in chronic bronchial infection and gastrointestinal abnormalities, due to an abnormal chloride channel (7q: CFTR).

Duchenne muscular dystrophy: a muscular weakness, initially affecting the upper legs and arms, slowly becoming more general in distribution. Increased blood creatinine kinase concentrations are a feature (Xp21: dystrophin).

Familial combined hyperlipidaemia: a common, familial condition associated with a raised blood cholesterol or triglycerides or both. Genetically heterogeneous (1q; HYPLIP) or even (11p: HYLIP).

Haemoglobinopathies: conditions associated with changes in the chemistry of haemoglobin that affect oxygen carriage or the lifespan of the red blood cell. Alpha-1 locus (16p: HBA1) and beta locus (11p: HBB).

Haemophilia A and B: conditions with abnormal blood coagulation, due to a failure to produce blood clotting factor VIII (Xq: factor VIII) or factor IX (Xq: factor IX).

Huntington's disease: a neurological disease manifesting in middle age with chorea (involuntary jerky movements), dementia and later seizures (4p: Huntintin).

Phenylketonuria: abnormal metabolism of phenylalanine, due to phenylalanine-4-monooxygenase deficiency. Affected babies are born with normal intellect, but as the concentrations of phenylpyruvate increase the intellect declines (12q: phenylal hydrox).

Polyposis coli: multiple polyps in the colon which predispose to cancerous change (5q: APC).

X-linked hypophosphataemic rickets: reduced blood phosphate concentrations, inherited through the X-chromosome, leading to abnormal bone structure and other problems of calcium/phosphorous metabolism (Xp: PHEX).

Source:
www.ncbi.nlm.nih.gov/Omim/searchomim.html

- Phenotypically normal parents may have one or more affected children.
- Unless an affected person mates with a carrier, all of the children are unaffected.
- Both gender are affected equally.
- The condition may often be demonstrated biochemically, e.g. the haemoglobinopathies, cystic fibrosis, phenylketonuria and sickle cell anaemia. Other conditions, e.g. Friedreich's ataxia, are not demonstrated biochemically.

Autosomal codominant

This is the simplest form of Mendelian inheritance. The characteristics are determined by a single genetic locus with two alleles (alternative forms of a gene Aa) located on one of the autosomes (any chromosomes except for the sex chromosomes, X and Y). In the heterozygote Aa, both alleles are expressed. The homozygote form is AA or aa, each of which shows a different phenotype. Many biochemical variants, e.g. isoenzymes (different types of the same enzyme), are codominant. Examples are:

- blood groups, ABO, rhesus factor
- red cell enzymes, acid phosphatase, adenylate kinase
- cell-surface antigens, human leucocyte antigen (HLA) systems.

X-linked inheritance

In X-linked inheritance, the males are affected and the condition is carried on by the unaffected or very mildly affected females. If conception results in a male foetus, then the mother provides the X-chromosome and the father the Y-chromosome. If the conception results in a girl, then the abnormal gene is carried on one X-chromosome and the female will pass one of the X-chromosomes to her daughter, who will be heterozygous, the same as her mother. The other normal gene will compensate for the abnormal gene. In the next generation, 50% of boys born of the heterozygous female will manifest the disease as they have no compensating X-chromosome. An affected male will produce heterozygous daughters but normal sons, who will only receive his normal Y-chromosome. An example is glucose-6-phosphate dehydrogenase deficiency.

The specific features are as follows.

- The disease affects mainly males.

- Affected males have unaffected parents but may have affected maternal uncles.
- The disease is transmitted by carrier women who are usually asymptomatic, half of the sons of a carrier are affected and half of the daughters are carriers.
- The children of an affected male are unaffected, but all of his daughters are carriers.
- The daughters of an unaffected man and a carrier woman have a 50% chance of being carriers, as did their mothers.

> The variability in X-linked conditions may result from the suppression of one of the female X-chromosomes, achieved, in part, by methylation of a dinucleotide (termed lyonized). Which X-chromosome is inactivated is random but persists throughout the life of that cell line. Some genes in the tip of the short arm of the X-chromosome may escape inactivation and are expressed, e.g. Duchenne muscular dystrophy or haemophilia A and B.

X-linked dominant inheritance is not common. X-linked hypophosphataemic rickets, which occurs only in females but is believed to be lethal in males, is an example of a disease inherited in this way.

Somatic genetic disorders

Mutations in somatic cells may occur in tumour cells, and involve alterations in large groups of genes. A gene often observed to be affected in tumour formation is the *p53* gene, a tumour suppressor gene found on the short arm of chromosome 17. A series of cancers has been found that have alterations in regions of the chromosomes within the malignant cell.

Mitochondrial disorders

An extreme form of non-Mendelian inheritance occurs when the genotype of only one parent is inherited and the other is permanently lost. This contrasts with Mendelian genetics where the contribution of both parents is equally inherited.

Locus heterogeneity: a term applied when an apparently single clinical disease is caused by either of two or more separately located genes. For example, an increased risk of breast cancer is associated with the *BRCA1* gene on chromosome 17p. However, only a proportion of breast cancers can be attributed to this mechanism.

Intralocus heterogeneity: different mutations or deletions within a single gene may cause different phenotypes.

Intrafamily heterogeneity: a situation in which the disease manifestations and clinical course are very variable, even within a family with the same inherited gene defect. This variability may be due to the action of two or more modifying genes.

Anticipation: refers to the severity of the disease increasing with successive generations.

Genomic imprinting: a deletion on a chromosome results in a different clinical consequence in males and females.

Interfamily heterogeneity: between families there is a great variation in disease phenotype, but the disease within families is remarkably constant. Any heterogeneity in such conditions is due to intralocus differences rather than being due to two separate but closely linked genes.

It is likely that differential methylation that is sex specific at the gamete level causes this variation in expression in genes on the X-chromosome. The Barr body is the X-chromosome that has been inactivated by methylation.

Haplotypes and linkage disequilibrium: a disease mutation can occur when a particular cluster of individual genetic attributes occurs, e.g. female, blood group, HLA-A type. This would allow a prediction of the point on the chromosome at which the mutation has occurred.

Usually the mother's genotype is preferentially or solely inherited. This maternal inheritance occurs because the genes of the mitochondria are inherited entirely through the ovum and not through the sperm. In mammals mtDNA appears to mutate more rapidly than nuclear DNA.

Multifactorial disorders

These disorders occur when a phenotypic characteristic is revealed in an individual with a genetic predisposition, by a particular environmental situation. Such associations are demonstrated by twin, sibling or family studies. This genetic predisposition, which results from the interaction of multiple genes, is important in the understanding of conditions that are often attributed entirely to an outside influence, e.g. nutrition. A predisposition is highlighted by the interaction with an environmental precipitant, e.g. the response to alcohol by men and women in different racial groups: following the drinking of alcohol, Mongol races flush owing to an accumulation of blood acetaldehyde. Other examples are insulin-dependent diabetes, hypertension, colonic cancer and manic–depressive disorders.

CHROMOSOME DISORDERS

These are much less common than allele-based conditions. They are the result of the loss, gain or abnormal arrangement of one or more of the 23 pairs of chromosomes and are, in general, the result of a numerical or structural mutation in the parent's germ cell. Polyploidy, in which multiples of 23 chromosomes occur, is most frequently observed in spontaneously aborted infants, with triploidy 69 and tetraploidy 92 chromosomes. Aneuploidy, in which a single chromosome is lost or gained, usually results when a chromosome fails to separate during cell division. The resulting child may have all aneuploid cells or have a mosaic of normal cells and some with an aneuploid chromosome complement. Aneuploidy results in either trisomy, an extra chromosome, or monosomy, the loss of a chromosome. Examples are

- Down's syndrome: chromosome 21 trisomy
- Klinefelter's syndrome: sex chromosome 47, XXY
- Turner's syndrome: chromosome 45, X.

Chromosomal breakage may result in translocation with complex genetic consequences.

GENE THERAPY

Gene therapy is an emerging subject, with the goal of replacing the products of defective genes with functioning genes. Two issues are important at present: efficacy and toxicity. Weakened viruses have been used as vectors to carry the gene into the genome, but these viruses may be less innocuous than believed and can cause adverse inflammatory and even fatal responses. Successfully transferred genes may have a short effective life and activity.

KEY POINTS

1. Many genetic diseases are associated with alterations in the previously health-promoting genetic material.
2. Mendelian disorders are those in which there is a single-gene defect or single-locus disorder. These result from a mutant allele or a pair of mutant alleles at a single locus.
3. Chromosome disorders result from the loss, gain or abnormal arrangement of one or more of the chromosomes.
4. Multifactorial disorders occur when a phenotypic characteristic is revealed by a particular environmental situation, in a person with a genetic predisposition caused by the interaction of many genes.

THINKING POINT

How many conditions can you think of that are classically attributed to nutrition and have a significant, even dominant, genetic component to their aetiology?

FURTHER READING

Bernlohr, D.A., Simpson, M.A., Hertzel, A.V. and Banaszak, L.J. (1997) Intracellular lipid-binding proteins and their genes. *Annual Review of Nutrition*, **17**, 277–303.

Brenner, S. and Miller, J.F. (2001) *Encyclopedia of Genetics*. Academic Press, New York.

Clayton, D. and McKeigue, P.M. (2001) Epidemiological methods for studying genes and environmental factors in complex diseases. *Lancet*, **358**, 1356–60.

Connor, M. and Ferguson-Smith, M. (1997) *Essential Medical Genetics*, 5th edn. Blackwell Scientific Publications, Oxford.

Emery, A.E.H. and Rimoin, D.L. (1997) *Principles and Practice of Medical Genetics*, 3rd edn. Churchill Livingstone, Edinburgh.

Girard, J., Ferre, P. and Foufelle, F. (1997) Mechanism by which carbohydrates regulate expression of genes for glycolytic and lipogenic enzymes. *Annual Review of Nutrition*, **17**, 325–52.

Horwitz, M. (2000) *Basic Concepts in Medical Genetics*. McGraw-Hill, New York.

Jimenez-Sanchez, G., Childs, B. and Valle, D. (2001) Human disease genes. *Nature*, **409**, 853–5.

Jump, D.B. and Clarke, S.D. (1999) Regulation of gene expression by dietary fat. *Annual review of Nutrition*, **19**, 63–90.

McKuisick, V.A. (1998). Mendelian inheritance in man. *Catalogues of Human Genes and Genetic Disorders*. Johns Hopkins University Press, Baltimore, MD.

Olson, A.L. and Pessin, J.E. (1996) Structure, function and regulation of the mammalian facilitative glucose transporter gene family. *Annual Review of Nutrition*, **16**, 235–56.

Redei, G.P. (2001) *Genetics: An Encyclopedic Dictionary*. Academic Press, New York.

Sanderson, I.R. and Naik, S. (2000) Dietary regulation of gene expression. *Annual Review of Nutrition*, **20**, 311–38.

Sinden, R.R. (2001) Neurodegenerative diseases. Origins of instability. *Nature*, **411**, 757–8.

Towle, H.C., Kaytor, E.N. and Shih, H.-M. (1997) Regulation of the expression of lipogenic enzyme genes by carbohydrate. *Annual Review of Nutrition*, **17**, 405–33.

WEBSITES

www.ncbi.nlm.nih.gov.Omim   Online Mendelian inheritance in man, listing and gene-dependent human disease

http://homophila.sdsc.edu Online Mendelian inheritance in man, listing and gene-dependent human disease

www.rochegenetics.com Roche genetics education programme

TESTS TO IDENTIFY GENES

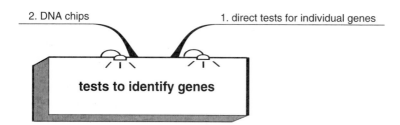

Fig. 7.21   Section outline.

DIRECT TESTS FOR INDIVIDUAL GENES

Gene deletions

Following some mutational changes the gene may cease to function because of either a total or partial deletion. These changes are not detectable cytogenetically but are demonstrated by a failure of a probe to hybridise to the DNA.

Direct detection of point mutations

Short probes, some several hundred or thousand nucleotides long, are used, which will hybridise to any sequence with 95% or greater accuracy. This hybridisation is very precise and does not happen if there is even a small degree of mismatching. This enables the singular elements within a genome to be identified.

To map the nucleic acid sequence at a molecular level, the DNA molecule is divided into varying lengths at defined points using restriction enzymes.

Ribonuclease A cleavage
Single base mutations in both cloned and genomic DNA sequences can be detected by cleavage at mismatches in RNA:DNA duplexes with ribonuclease A. A single-stranded RNA probe is synthesised from a cloned DNA fragment applicable to the mutated region. This probe is then hybridised to its complementary sequence in cloned and genomic DNA sequences or amplified by the polymerase chain reaction (PCR). The resulting RNA:DNA duplex can then be used to identify mismatch positions.

The lengths of nucleotides produced can be accurately analysed as short sequences of double-stranded DNA. DNA is cut into short sequences by a range of restriction enzymes, each of which has a target zone in a duplex DNA of about 4–6 base pairs long. The enzyme cuts the DNA at every site at which its target sequences occur. After the DNA molecule has been cut with suitable restriction enzymes into distinct fragments, these are separated, on a molecular weight basis, using gel electrophoresis. Restriction mapping uses overlapping fragments that have been created by different enzymes, each splitting the DNA at a different point. A difference in restriction maps between two individuals is called a restriction fragment length polymorphism (RFLP). Restriction markers identify genetic loci and hence mutations. This allows the relevant genetic loci to be placed on a gene map even if the abnormal gene or its protein or function is not known at that time. From such basic information diagnostic tests or even isolation of the gene can be developed.

Every individual has a unique constellation of restriction sites; such a combination of specific regions is called a haplotype. The use of DNA restriction analysis to identify individuals has been named 'DNA fingerprinting'. One way of using RFLP is the lod score. RFLP can also be used to place genes on a genetic map and is used to map genomes and, in particular, the human genome. The use of yeast strains with known genetic translocation mapping has enabled chromosomal regions to be identified and mapped using hybridisation techniques.

DNA hybridisation

The hydrogen bonds that hold the double helix of DNA together can be disrupted by heat or high salt concentration, so that the strands are separated (denaturation). Restoring the double helix restores the original properties of the DNA. This technique can be used to isolate DNA segments. The nucleic acid sequence is identified by a recombination technique to a complementary nucleic acid sequence by a zip-like effect. When nucleic acids from different sources but similar sequences join together, they anneal with each other. This phenomenon is called hybridisation, e.g. between parts or lengths of DNA and RNA. The ability of two nucleic acid preparations to hybridise gives a precise test for complementary sequences, since only complementary sequences can form a duplex structure.

It is possible to compare the nucleotide sequence of a gene with the amino acid sequence of a protein and determine either the amino acid sequence of the protein or the nucleotide sequence corresponding to that protein primary sequence, i.e. whether they are collinear, that is correspond, and whether or not the gene is responsible for the synthesis of the protein. The restriction map of DNA will match exactly the amino acid map of the synthesised protein. There are, however, extra regions in the DNA not represented by protein synthetic products.

Messenger RNA always includes a nucleotide sequence that corresponds exactly with the protein product. The gene may include additional sequences that lie within the coding region interrupting the sequences that represent the protein, exons represented in the mRNA and introns missing from the mRNA.

The chromosome carrying a genetic trait is identified by genetic analysis. The gene is tracked to a region of the chromosome by genetic characterisation of individuals with grossly abnormal chromosomes. The search continues at a molecular level for the gene within the region that can be associated with the disorder. Once a particularly susceptible gene is isolated, it is possible to search for a sequence in the allele of that gene which is associated with that disorder.

Another technique, blunt-end ligation, relies on the ability of the T4 DNA ligase to join together two blunt-ended DNA molecules, i.e. molecules lacking any protruding single strands. When DNA has been cleaved with restriction enzymes, which cut both strands at the same position, blunt-end ligation can be used to join the fragments directly together.

Cloning of specific genes requires the identification, or characterisation, of particular regions or sequences of the genome. It is now a routine procedure to obtain the DNA corresponding to any particular gene. The purpose of cloning is to insert DNA into a suitable system and amplify this DNA. Cloning a fragment of DNA allows indefinite amounts to be produced from even a single original molecule. A clone is a number of cells or molecules that are all identical to an original ancestral cell or molecule. The cloning of DNA uses the ability of bacterial plasmids and phages to continue to function after additional sequences of DNA have been incorporated into their genomes. The phage or plasmid is called a cloning vector. Such an insertion generates a hybrid or chimeric plasmid or phage. These chimeras can thereafter be replicated in the bacteria. Copies of the original foreign fragment can be retrieved from the continuing generations of bacteria. A probe is needed that will react with the target DNA, e.g. a known protein product with mRNA coding for the protein. It may also be possible to identify mRNA in the cytoplasm that represents a particular unknown gene product. This is important in disorders where the abnormal gene product is not known. If the mode of expression of the foreign DNA is being studied then the foreign DNA must be inserted into the plasmid in an appropriate orientation.

To obtain and study a particular gene, the order of events used in cloning is reversed. The genome is cloned first, and clones containing a particular sequence are selected. Vectors carrying DNA from the genome itself are called genomic or chromosomal DNA clones. Cloning an entire genome, as opposed to specific fragments, is called a shotgun experiment. The genome is broken into fragments, which are put into a cloning vector to generate a population of chimeric vectors. A set of cloned fragments is used to form a genome library. As new probes are found they can be tested against the library collection of grouped fragments. An alternative method with mRNA is to prepare single-strain DNAs from the entire mRNA populations

Cloning of specific genes

The cloning vector DNA is cleaved at predefined sites. A restriction enzyme is used with a single target site in a non-essential part of the DNA vector. Hybrid molecules are added at this split and then the sequence is rejoined with the added material now part of the original DNA. Non-essential DNA can be replaced by foreign DNA. The foreign DNA fragment is joined to a cloning vector by a reaction between the ends of the fragment and gap in the DNA vector. Thereafter, the DNA is replicated to increase the amount of material or to express a particular sequence. Critical to such a system is that the inclusion of the new sequence does not upset any essential function. Plasmid genomes are circular, so included DNA is added to the circle. These can be kept indefinitely and isolated according to size by gel electrophoresis. Long, non-circular genes can also be used.

Synthesis of duplex DNA

A primer is annealed to the poly(dA). The enzyme engages in the usual 5'–3' elongation, adding deoxynucleotides one at a time. The product of the reaction is a hybrid molecule consisting of a template RNA strand paired with a complementary DNA strand. The original mRNA is degraded by alkali, which does not affect DNA. The product is a single-stranded DNA that is complementary to the mRNA. The hairpin at the 3' end of the single DNA provides a primer for the next step, in which *E. coli* DNA polymerase I converts this single-stranded DNA into a DNA duplex.

and to produce a single-strand DNA library. These can be stored and tested when a new probe becomes available.

A particular genome clone can be selected from the library by colony hybridisation. Bacterial colonies carrying chimeric vectors are lysed on a nitrocellulose filter. The DNA is denatured *in situ*, fixed and hybridised with a radioactively labelled probe. A genome clone needs only to carry some of the probe's sequence to react with it.

Chromosome walking

A clone may be isolated that is believed to contain the known gene or a region of interest. Sections of the chromosome are hybridised with clones from the reference library. It is possible to study both long and short lengths and regions of the genome by systematically moving along the chromosome. This is known as chromosome walking.

Copying messenger RNA onto DNA

To isolate a particular mRNA, two cell types are needed, one that expresses the RNA and one that does not. This technique uses subtractive hybridisation. The mRNA of the target cell line is used as a substrate to prepare a set of single-strand DNA molecules corresponding to all of the expressed genes. This is then hybridised with all of the mRNA of another closely related cell. The sequences that are common to both cell types are removed. After discarding all of the DNA sequences that hybridise for the other mRNA, those that are left are regarded as peculiar to that cell and can be characterised. This technique has been used to isolate clones in the T-cell receptor, but not in the closely related B-lymphocyte.

To identify a DNA sequence that represents a particular protein, the responsible mRNA is used as the starting point. Reverse transcription allows synthesis of duplex DNA from the mRNA. This is particularly easy if the mRNA carries a poly(A) tail at the 3' end.

Digested strands of DNA are separated on gel electrophoresis. DNA is denatured to give single-stranded fragments, which are transferred from agarose gel to a nitrocellulose filter, where the fragments are immobilised. This system is known as *Southern blotting*. The DNA fragments are separated and those corresponding to a particular probe are isolated directly from a digest of the clone DNA. DNA immobilised on nitrocellulose can be hybridised *in situ* with a radioactive probe. Only those fragments complementary to a particular probe will hybridise and can be identified by autoradiography. *Northern blotting* is used for RNA and *Western blotting* for proteins.

An alternative procedure is dot blotting, in which cloned DNA fragments are spotted next to one another on a filter. The filter is hybridised with a solution containing the radiolabelled probes. The radioactive intensity of the dot corresponds to the extent to which the RNA is represented in the clone.

Polymerase chain reaction

This reaction requires a knowledge of the sequences on either side of the target region and allows such a region between two defined sites to be amplified. PCR enables sequences of interest to be selectively amplified even when there is an excess of unwanted DNA. A target sequence of up to 1 kb can be amplified 10^5–10^6-fold. A prerequisite is a unique flanking sequence, so that specific oligonucleotide primers can be used.

At present, direct detection is limited to well-understood disorders that are relatively homogeneous at the molecular level. A preparation of DNA, often just an extract of the whole genome, is denatured. The single-stranded preparation is annealed with two short primer sequences that are complementary to sites on the opposite strands on either side of the target region. DNA polymerase is used to synthesise a single strand from the 3'-OH end of each primer. The entire cycle can be repeated by denaturing the preparation and starting again. The number of copies of the target sequence grows rapidly, doubling with each cycle. Recently, the production of a DNA polymerase from a thermophilic bacterium has meant that the same enzyme remains active through the heating steps required for the denaturation–renaturation cycles, allowing a sequence to be amplified up to 4×10^6 times in 25 cycles. The length of the target sequence is determined by the distance between the two primer sites, up to 2 kb. If a replication event causes an error then this will also be amplified. This technique enables the identification of individual alleles in a genome and is a very powerful tool in modern molecular biology.

Polymerase chain reaction

Heat-stable DNA polymerase is used, and the reaction is run by putting a tube containing all the ingredients through perhaps 30 temperature cycles. After gel electrophoresis, genomic target sequences can be demonstrated and a search made for the presence or absence of target sequences.

DNA CHIPS

Rapid advances in genomics have led to the development of DNA chips which are microarrays, short DNA sequences immobilised on a surface. By determining which spots bind to mRNA extracted from a biological sample, an instant snapshot is obtained of the activity of thousands of genes at a time. Strands of RNA bind tightly and very specifically to mRNA with a complementary sequence. The mRNA is tagged with a fluorescent dye, making identification simple.

KEY POINTS

1. Specific probes are required to identify particular gene sequences; usually a messenger RNA which represents a particular protein is used.
2. Some apparently gene-dependent disorders have no known isolated and identified genetic locus or encoded protein product. Searching for these requires a number of physical methods, including *in situ* hybridisation, somatic cell hybridisation and gene mapping linkage analyses. Much of this information originates from family studies, where families with an identified genetic characteristic are studied for a series of markers or a candidate region of a chromosome.
3. Among many mutational changes, a gene may lose function owing to physical or partial deletion. These are demonstrated by the failure of a probe to hybridise to that particular DNA. To map the nucleic acid sequence at a molecular level, the DNA molecule is broken at defined points using specific restriction enzymes. It is also possible to compare the nucleotide sequence of a gene with the amino acid sequence of a protein and determine the amino acid sequence of the protein or the nucleotide sequence corresponding to that protein primary sequence. The technique of cloning a number of cells or molecules allows a genetic trait to be identified. The gene is tracked to a region of the chromosome by genetic characterisation of individuals with grossly abnormal chromosomes. The cloning of specific genes requires the identification or

characterisation of particular regions or sequences of the genome.

4. Digested strands of DNA or RNA or protein can be separated on gel electrophoresis; this constitutes the 'blotting' method of identification of RNA and DNA or protein.

5. The polymerase chain reaction (PCR) allows a region between two defined sites in the gene to be amplified. This is a powerful tool in allowing sufficient amounts of DNA to be developed for further analytical work.

THINKING POINTS

1. A wide range of techniques is being developed in genetics. How can these be used in nutrition? Are these methods of any use in isolation from the conventional nutrition methods?

2. How can genetics and nutrition progress together?

NEED TO UNDERSTAND

The array of methods available to identify an individual's genetic makeup, and their possible applicability to nutrition.

FURTHER READING

Lewin, B. (1997) *Genes VI*. Oxford University Press, Oxford.

Trayhurn, P. and Chester, J.K. (1996) Workshop on molecular biological techniques in nutritional science. *Proceedings of the Nutrition Society*, **55**, 573–618.

Part IV

Calculating the nutritional status of an individual

- Evaluation of dietary intake
- Measurements of energy
- Body composition

8

Evaluation of dietary intake

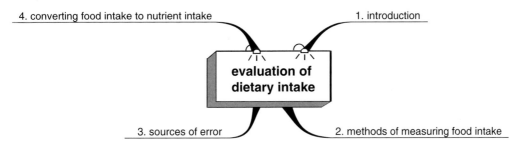

Fig. 8.1 Chapter outline.

INTRODUCTION

Data identifying food consumption are collected for a variety of reasons:

- to estimate the adequacy of dietary intake of the population
- to investigate the relationship between diet, nutritional status and health
- to evaluate nutritional education, intervention and food fortification programmes.

Information is obtained on food and dietary intake of individuals or groups of individuals, by methods either measuring food intake or converting food intake to nutrient intake.

METHODS OF MEASURING FOOD INTAKE

Population studies

Food supply data at the national level, using food balance sheets or food disappearance data, give crude information of the national availability of food commodities. From such data it is possible to give a picture of per capita availability of food, but the figure reflects food availability, not consumption.

Population studies have shown that dietary patterns can be grouped basically by the food sources of macronutrients. Countries differ in the types of carbohydrate staples that are available, primarily wheat, potatoes or rice. There are major differences in the sources of proteins (animal, vegetable and fish) and fats (predominantly animal fats, tropical oils, coconut palm, palm kernel oils and other vegetable fats). Populations that have more wheat or potatoes available also tend to have more animal fats and protein available, including beef, pork, milk, eggs and butter. Food sources of proteins are similar in these countries, but total fat availability is lower in Central and South American nations than in North America, European and Mediterranean countries. Central and South American countries have more carbohydrate and vegetable proteins, particularly rice, beans and grains. In Asia, rice is the predominant source of starch and the populations have more vegetable proteins available, particularly cassava, sweet potatoes, beans, nuts and grains.

The diet in Tanzania, Thailand and Sri Lanka consists of fats predominantly from animal sources and tropical oils, proteins derived from fish and vegetable sources, and carbohydrates from rice, fruit, vegetables and sugar. The diet in Cyprus and Finland is characterised by fats derived from animal and vegetable sources, protein from animal products, excluding fish, and carbohydrates from wheat, fruit, vegetables and sugar (Figures 8.2 and 8.3).

Extensive food and nutrition surveillance can be undertaken. Measurements of food intake over 7 days have been obtained, along with measurements, for example, of the height and weight of schoolchildren. Anthropometric and blood pressure measurements have also been obtained.

Community data

These data are made available by a variety of methods. They give community, socioeconomic and geographic information, and allow comparisons between different times and regions. Aggregate data based on surveys of groups of people rather than individuals can be used for community surveys of nutrient intake. These studies are usually based on the household rather than individuals, and give indications of the food consumption pattern in different communities. Regional and socioeconomic differences can thereby be highlighted. In such community surveys, four methods of measurement are used: food accounts, inventories, household recall and list recall.

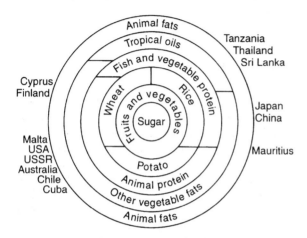

Fig. 8.2 Dietary patterns of a number of countries listed by food sources of macronutrients that are predominant in their respective food supply. (From Posner, et al., 1994, with permission.)

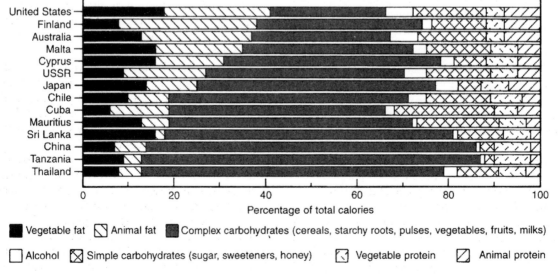

Fig. 8.3 FAO macronutrient data by animal structure/vegetable source, 1984–1986: vegetables, proteins and carbohydrates in the diet in a number of countries. (From Posner et al., 1994 with permission.)

Food accounts

The food account method is based on the household. The individual who is responsible for buying and preparing the food keeps a record of the quantities of food entering the house, including purchases, food from the garden, gifts, payment in kind and other sources. Such a survey assumes that there is no change in the average level of food stocks, but it is obvious that there will be variation within that period in the amount of food held within the house's food store. The Household Food Consumption and Expenditure Survey (the National Food Survey) has been completed on an annual basis in Great Britain for over 60 years. It started in 1940 by examining the nutritional quality of the diet of urban, working-class households, to follow the value of the wartime food rationing policy. By 1950, all sections of the population were surveyed and hence these reports give a comprehensive account of British food habits since 1950.

Inventories

The inventory method requires respondents to keep a record of all food coming into the house. A larder inventory is carried out at the beginning and end of the survey. The advantage of this method is that it gives a direct measure of the amount of food and nutrients available for consumption within a single household. This method, including the total purchases of food during the study period, is used in the National Food Survey.

Household record

In the household record method, the foods available for consumption, raw or processed, are weighed or estimated in household measures, allowing for preparation waste, etc. Food eaten by visitors is calculated and subtracted from the total. Allowance is made for food waste by either collecting the waste or estimating loss. This technique is best suited for populations in which most of the diet is home produced rather than preprocessed. It is the ideal method for unsophisticated societies.

In some communities, a group of people eat directly from a shared bowl of food, making measurement of the food intake of any one individual complicated. This can be overcome by careful studies that start from food preparation and continue to the meal, including watching the individuals eat.

List recall

This method requires recall of the amount and cost of food obtained for household use over a given period, from 24 h up to the more usual 1 week. In this way, an estimate of food costs and net household consumption of foods and nutrients can be obtained. This method is important in cases where most food is purchased rather than home produced.

Individual data

The individual measurement of food intake takes place under quite dissimilar circumstances. Precise studies are conducted in a metabolic unit with tight control of intake and output, with trained staff monitoring the project. Less controlled studies are carried out on active individuals collecting data, with collection being fitted into normal life. Clinical assessment of patients' dietary intake is even less easy and requires great skill.

Prospective records of food intake are more accurate than recollections of past intake. The weighed dietary record is regarded as the most accurate method of measuring intake. At its most precise, weighed portions of food are brought to the subject, the leftovers weighed, and urine and faeces collected under supervision. Outside such ideal conditions there are inherent problems. Weighing is an intrusion during the eating of a meal and shortcuts may distort results in the recorded eating pattern.

Several alternative methods have been devised for estimating food intake, e.g. written statements, portable tape recorders, and plastic models and photographs of food. Some methods include a combined tape recording and an electronic scale. The detailed manual coding of food records is being replaced by 'menu' computer programs based on food groups. The procedure includes placing food on an electronic balance and pressing the appropriate key, and nutrient intakes are then calculated directly by the computer, using the weight of food and the database. All such records require a high degree of co-operation from the individuals involved and validation is crucial to ascertain whether subjects are overreporting or underreporting.

A major source of error (up to 50%) is the estimation of portion size. The coefficient of variation may be in the order of 50% for foods, but less than 20% for nutrients. The error of estimation of the weight of food is probably random and will be reduced by increasing the number of observations.

Description, weighed and estimated records
Subjects can be taught to describe and give an estimate of food weighed before eating and then to record any leftovers. In such exercises it is important that the recipes are available and an information pool of average recipes is available, comparable to those of manufactured foods. Such records, either weighed or described estimates, are not as accurate as precise actual weighing, which is necessary if food composition tables are not available. In such a detailed process, raw ingredients, cooked foods, meals, snacks and the individual portions must all be weighed. Aliquots must be obtained for chemical analysis.

Diet histories
These methods rely on asking people to remember accurately the frequency and quantities of food eaten on previous occasions.

The length of time of a study may be important and it has been suggested that 3–4 days may be the optimum period, rather than the traditional 7 days. In some circumstances 2 day or even 1 day records may be sufficient. The period of observation necessary varies for different nutrients. The number of days necessary to classify 80% of subjects correctly into the extreme thirds of the distribution also varies. The 7 day record is probably sufficient to classify the distribution of nutrient intake of a population for energy and energy-yielding nutrients into three major groups. Longer periods are required for alcohol, some vitamins, minerals and cholesterol.

Interviews are best based on prepared protocols which allow for individual foods, set meals and variations in intake over time. Interviewer training is very important. The disadvantages are reliance on memory, interviewer bias and subject bias in response to being interviewed.

The diet history, like the questionnaire method, is a repeatable and relatively valid method. It covers significant periods and so compensates for the potential distortions due to week-to-week varia-

tions in diet. This is of particular importance for some nutrients, e.g. vitamins D and A.

A diet history usually consists of:

- a detailed interview to measure amounts and frequency (usually per month) of a wide variety of foods
- a cross-check food frequency list
- a 24 h recall
- a 3-day record (optional).

It is important that at least the first three elements are used.

For a *24 h recall*, individuals are asked a systematic series of questions to ensure recollection and description of all food and drink consumed in the 24 h before the interview, with an emphasis on food consumption meal-by-meal and looking for day-to-day and seasonal variation. Implicit in this method is that the interviewer is very familiar with the food habits of the local population. The 24 h recall is quick and easy to administer. The limitation is that it does not take account of day-to-day variation and differences between the weekday and weekend intake. Furthermore, individuals with low intakes tend to report higher than accurate intakes, and those with high intakes tend to report lower. There is consequently a reversion to the mean.

The advantages of retrospective methods are that they are quick, cheap, and independent of motivation and literacy. The disadvantages are that they rely on memory, observer bias is possible and there is no measure of day-to-day variation in the diet. These methods are of limited value in children under the age of 12 years, unless seen with their parents, and some individuals may wish to imply that they eat a better diet than they actually do. There are regional and cultural differences, and sauces and spices in some diets may alter the micronutrient intake.

Questionnaires
The administration of questionnaires is a widely used method for assessing diet. It is easy and cheap. Questionnaires may be self-administered or interviewer administered. The benefit of the former is that interviewer bias is eliminated. However, the questions must be very simple and unambiguous, and require the subjects to be able to read and write. Questions may be left unanswered and there may be

a low response rate. An interviewer-administered questionnaire ensures answers to more complex questions, completion of all questions and an explanation of problems. Questions are usually of the frequency and amount type (FAQ). Individuals are asked how often they usually consume an item of food or drink. Closed questionnaires have defined questions and demand an easily classified answer, whereas open questionnaires ask for comment. It can be appropriate for questions or questionnaires to be closed rather than open, in that the interviewer asks precisely the same questions of all subjects. Questionnaires range from simple to very comprehensive and may include from nine to 190 food items. The foods in the questionnaire should be the minimum number that includes the major sources of nutrients for the majority of subjects in that population.

Quantitative food frequency questionnaires can be used to estimate habitual intake of food items in epidemiological studies. Such questionnaires comprise questions on the frequency of consumption, which can be grouped into lists of foods with similar nutrient composition expressed as amounts or quantities per day, per week or per month. Portion sizes are given in everyday units such as slices, cups and spoonfuls.

These questionnaires are complicated and can be misleading through the omission of questions relating to other elements, which may be present in or absent from the food. These may include additives, contaminants, chemicals, natural toxins, and the nutritional effects of the method of food preparation and cooking.

Frequency categories should always be continuous, e.g. 'never', 'less than once per month', 'one or two times per month', 'three or four times per month' or 'more than three or four times per month'. These should be followed by a listing of the number of days per week on which the item is consumed. If the person answering the question is unable to find an appropriate answer then the sensitivity of the results will be reduced. It is important to define the contribution of 'within-subject error'. This method should be regarded as a semi-quantitative method of dietary assessment, although in expert hands can reach a degree of accuracy approaching that obtained with biomarkers and 7 day dietary diaries.

Questionnaires require a significant amount of development and validation, but have the advantage that they can be prepared for computer analysis.

Both diet records and diet histories have a number of practical limitations. When the different methods are compared most foods should appear in the same position in a hierarchy of measurements, say least to most, e.g. in the same quartile, compared with more accurate methods, e.g. weighed-food records. Sugar, cream products and vegetables are the foods most likely to be unreported, and bread, potatoes and fish overreported, contributing to the inaccuracies of the questionnaire method of obtaining nutritional information.

Dietary studies are most successful in societies that are simple in structure, closed communities, self-sufficient farming communities, long-distance seafarers and the very young. It is much more difficult to assess accurately the nutritional intake of a complex society with constant access to food.

Diet diaries and prospective weighed records have different strengths and weakness. Diet diaries may give a better picture of the long-term intake and also tend to give higher mean energy intakes. Independent markers of intake are essential for comparisons.

SOURCES OF ERROR

Systematic biases can creep into the process of obtaining dietary information. These include:

- insensitive or irrelevant measurements
- individual recall biases
- shyness about intrusive questions, or being watched
- responses that are intended to help the investigator
- answers that represent subjects' ideal diet rather than their actual diet
- knowledge of the study and responses that are helpful to the hypothesis.

Common errors associated with the collection of data on food intake include:

- omission of data on intermeal snacks, parts of meals, entire meals or entire days, either deliberately by the subject or in error

- recording of wrong amounts of foods
- incorrect identification of food
- recording of data on the wrong subject's form.

Errors may also be associated with the entry of data, including reading errors, wrong identification numbers, transcription errors, omission or double entry of data, or lines or segments of data being transposed. An important source of error is in biases in perception. The complex interaction between a subject and the interviewer may influence the data presented. This interaction will not be consistent: the responses of teenagers, and individuals with eating disorders, anorexia and obesity may influence the outcome. Under-reporting of food intake is a real problem; its prevalence may range from 18 to 54% of the sample and is very dependent on gender, body mass index and weight.

Error must be estimated so that allowance can be made in the final analyses. Histories of what people have eaten and drunk may be written, or recorded by word or visually. In other instances, trained field workers are necessary, and here the accuracy is very dependent on the individual. Much of this methodology depends on the sophistication of the society that is being studied.

Underreporting occurs because of lack of motivation, forgetfulness or a wish to please, especially in women or individuals with eating problems. Foods perceived as healthy are overreported, while less healthy foods and alcohol are underreported. These inconsistencies can be detected by the dietary information not correlating with an energy intake that would maintain body weight. The ratio of reported energy intake to basal metabolic rate (EI:BMR ratio) should exceed 1.27, the minimum value for health and survival.

The absoluteness of the results can be checked in two ways. One is to include markers of internal validity, which could include asking the subject for the same information in different ways, and to check for consistency. Biomarkers are measurements taken at the same time as the diet survey, whatever the method, and act as a guide to intake. The value of energy and nitrogen intake diet histories can be tested against 24 h urinary nitrogen excretion and the double labelled water method. The choice of biomarker can be very complicated.

Variables in identifying biomarkers for validation of dietary intake studies

- Is the biological sample the best one? Does the measurement give a valid answer, e.g. from urine, blood, serum or red blood cell? (e.g. folate or selenium)
- Is the measurement reliable? (e.g. vitamin A)
- Does lifestyle, e.g. vegetarian or meat-eating habit, affect the result? (e.g. vitamin B_{12})
- Is the biomarker metabolised and does the measurement represent intake or metabolic fate of the measured chemical? (e.g. flavonoids or carotenoids)
- Are there effects of interactions with other substances, e.g. in the intestine or in metabolic reactions? (e.g. Vitamins C and E)
- If the biomarker is metabolised, is the metabolism of the chemical fully understood?

CONVERTING FOOD INTAKE TO NUTRIENT INTAKE

The conversion of food consumption to nutrient intake requires computer software, a nutrient database and an appropriate program. A program should ideally accept data from diet histories, so that information on each food in a meal eaten is recorded and converted by the computer into constituent nutrients. There may be differences in the nutrient value imposed by the bioavailability of that food. The bioavailability of a nutrient is the proportion of that nutrient that is available for utilisation by the body. These techniques all have disadvantages in free-living populations.

Chemical analysis

Analysis of food may be necessary when the chemistry of a particular food is not available in a composition of food table or when no information is available on which foods are an important source of a nutrient or other food components of interest.

The *duplicate portion* technique is the most accurate and is the benchmark for other techniques. Its accuracy is dependent on obtaining a sample iden-

Table 8.1 Summary of dietary assessment methods

Type of method	Major strengths	Major limitations
Food record	Does not rely on memory Easy to quantify amounts Open-ended	High participation burden Requires literacy May alter intake behaviour
24 h dietary recall	Little respondent burden No literacy requirement Does not alter intake behaviour	Relies on memory Requires skilled interviewer Difficult to estimate amounts
Food frequency questionnaire	Relatively inexpensive Useful for nutrients with very high day-to-day variability, to estimate frequencies Does not alter intake behaviour	Relies on memory Requires complex calculations Requires literacy Limited flexibility for describing foods
Diet history (meal-based)	No literacy requirement Does not alter intake behaviour Open-ended	Relies on memory Requires highly trained interviewer Difficult to estimate amounts
Food habit	Rapid and low-cost Does not alter intake behaviour Open-ended	May rely on memory questionnaires May require a trained interviewer

tical to the food consumed by the subject under study. Such a study is complicated by intermeal snacks, or if insufficient food is prepared for a true duplicate to be obtained.

With the *aliquot sampling* techniques, the weights of all foods eaten and drinks taken are obtained and an aliquot, say 10%, is collected for analysis. However, errors can arise because of sampling techniques.

The *equivalent composite* technique is where the weights of all foods eaten and beverages drunk are recorded. At the end of the survey a sample of raw foods equivalent to the mean daily amounts of food eaten by an individual is analysed.

An alternative, less expensive method of measuring protein intake is the *24 h urinary nitrogen method*. The completeness of the urine samples is estimated by the *p*-aminobenzoic acid (PABA) check method. PABA is given orally at the beginning of the collection, and should reappear in the voided urine, indicating completeness of collection. Complete 24 h urine collections are an extremely useful validation measure in nutritional epidemiology. However, this method assumes a constant relationship between dietary protein intake and nitrogen output, and is dependent on protein intake, urinary nitrogen reflecting dietary protein intake is best at low protein intakes.

Mean energy intakes may be tested by physical activity questionnaires and the doubly labelled water method.

Body weight is also an important measurement from which estimates of BMR may be calculated.

Food composition tables

National epidemiological studies may look at nutrient intake as well as food consumption data. To be relevant to nutritional epidemiologists, food composition tables must encompass the following.

- Foods included in the table must be comprehensive and appropriate for the population studied. It is important that a food is described unequivocally and what is meant by a particular food is clearly apparent. This is easy for raw fruit and vegetables, but becomes more difficult for cooked dishes where the recipe may vary.
- The number of nutrients included in the table for each food must be sufficient for the study in question.
- The method of expression of amounts of nutrients must be specified.
- Nutritionally appropriate methods must be used for the estimation of each nutrient. It is important that there is standardisation of methods, and

these should include replicate analyses and analysis of reference materials provided by central bodies.

The disadvantage of using food composition tables and nutrient databases is that each value is the average of a limited number of samples analysed for each food. Sampling errors are large, especially for mixed food dishes and meals. These add to the total error and variation in results from dietary intake studies.

Analysis of individual foods

Differences in water content are a major cause of variation in the chemical measurement of nutrients. Therefore, foods containing a large amount of water are always subject to large variation. The least variable nutrient is probably protein. Estimates for energy, protein, fat, carbohydrate, monosaccharides and disaccharides are probably accurate within 10%. The vitamin and mineral content is much more speculative and less accurate.

KEY POINTS

1. Food consumption data are collected to identify whether the population is eating sufficiently well, to assess the relationship between diet, health and nutritional status, and to plan nutritional education, intervention and food fortification programmes.
2. A correct measurement of dietary intake is central to any nutritional epidemiological study. The validity of the results must be checked and error estimated so that allowances can be made in the final analyses.
3. Prospective records of food intake are more accurate than recall of past intake.
4. Various techniques have been described, including description, weighed and estimated records, measurement of intake, diet history, household data and inventory methods. Other methods include household records, list-recall methods and population studies and 7 day measurement of food intake, with anthropometric measures and blood constituents. Individual diet histories and 24 h recall are important assess-

ments of nutritional intake. The accuracy of food frequency questionnaires can be assessed.
5. The conversion of food consumption to nutrient intake is a complex process which requires chemical analyses of the various food constituents, the writing of food consumption tables and analysis of individual foods.

THINKING POINT

The measurement of dietary intake is important in clinical and epidemiological practice. Try one or two of the diet measurement systems and compare their accuracy over the same period.

NEED TO UNDERSTAND

It is important to understand the different methods of measuring dietary intake – national, community, household and individual – and the strengths and weaknesses of each method.

FURTHER READING

Bingham, S.A. and Nelson, M. (1991) Assessment of food consumption and nutrient intake. In *Design Concepts in Nutritional Epidemiology* (eds B.M. Margetts and M. Nelson). Oxford Medical Publications, Oxford University Press, Oxford, pp. 153–91.

Black, A., Welch, A. and Bingham, S.A. (2000) Validation of dietary intakes measured by diet history against 24 h urinary nitrogen excretion and energy expenditure measured by the doubly-labelled water method in middle aged women. *British Journal of Nutrition*, **83**, 341–54.

Brunner, E., Stallone, D., Juneja, M. *et al.* (2001) Dietary assessment in Whitehall II: comparison of 7d diet diary and food frequency questionnaire and validity against biomarkers. *British Journal of Nutrition*, **86**, 405–14.

Crews, H., Alink, G., Andersen, R., *et al.* (2001) A critical assessment of some biomarker approaches linked with dietary intake. *British Journal of Nutrition*, **86**, S5–35.

Holland, B., Welch, A.A., Unwin, I.D. *et al.* (1991) *McCance and Widdowson's The Composition of Foods*, 5th edn. Ministry of Agriculture, Fisheries and Food and The Royal Society of Chemistry.

Hudson, G.J. (1995) Food intake in a West African village. Estimation of food intake from a shared bowl. *British Journal of Nutrition*, **73**, 551–69.

Lissen, L., Heitmann, B.L. and Lindroos, L.K. (1998) Measuring intake in free-living human subjects: a question of bias. *Proceedings of the Nutrition Society*, **57**, 333–9.

Macdiarmid, J. and Blundell, J. (1998) Assessing dietary intake: who, what and why in under reporting. *Nutrition Research Reviews*, **11**, 231–53.

Nelson, M. (1995) Editorial – Can we measure what people eat? *Journal of Human Nutrition and Dietetics*, **8**, 1–2.

Posner, R.M., Franz, N. and Quatromoni, P. (1994) Nutrition and the global risk for chronic diseases: the Inter Health Nutrition Initiative. *Nutrition Reviews*, **52**, 201–7.

Rush, D. (1997) Nutrition screening in old people: its place in a coherent practice of preventive health care. *Annual Review of Nutrition*, **17**, 101–25.

Slater, J.M. (ed.) (1991) *Fifty Years of the National Food Survey* 1940–1990. HMSO, London.

West, C.E. and van Staveren, W.A. (1991) Food consumption, nutrient intake, and the use of food consumption tables. In *Design concepts in Nutritional Epidemiology* (eds B.M. Margetts and M. Nelson). Oxford Medical Publications, Oxford University Press, Oxford, pp. 101–19.

WEBSITES

www.fao.org   (1) Preparation and use of food-based dietary guidelines. (WHO/FAO 1996.6). (2) FAO Directory of international food composition tables

9

Measurement of energy

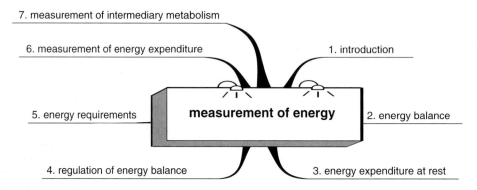

Fig. 9.1 Chapter outline.

INTRODUCTION

Energy is required continuously for cell repair and growth and intermittently for work, although intake of food to provide this energy is intermittent. There is loss of nutrient energy when food is converted to mechanical energy; about 65% is dissipated as heat.

Twelve people sitting talking in a room produce heat at 60 kJ/min, equivalent to a 1 kW electric fire.

Total energy expenditure (TEE) has three components:

- **Basal metabolic rate (BMR)**: at complete rest and without physical work (basal metabolism), energy is required for the activity of the internal organs and to maintain body temperature. This is the single largest contributor to TEE, at 60–70% of TEE. During sleep the overall metabolic rate approximates to the BMR.

- **Thermogenic component**: the energy expended through the physiological response following the ingestion of food, and exposure to cold or stimulants.
- **Physical activity**: only 25–35% of nutrient energy is used for mechanical work and less than 10% is for basic physiological activity, e.g. cardiac and respiratory contractions.

The energy requirement of an individual is the energy intake that will balance energy expenditure when the individual has a body size, composition and level of physical activity consistent with long-term good health, and will allow for the maintenance of economically necessary and socially desirable activity. In children and pregnant and lactating women, the energy level includes the energy need associated with the deposition of tissues and the secretion of milk at rates consistent with good health.

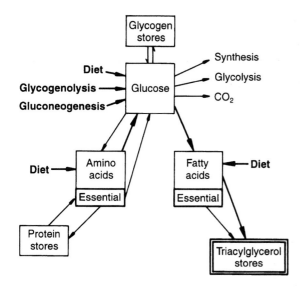

Fig. 9.2 Macronutrient interactions between glucose, amino acids and fatty acids.

References terms used for energy

Basal metabolic rate (BMR): the rate at which the body uses energy when the body is at complete rest; alternatively, BMR is the minimal rate of energy expenditure compatible with life. Values depend on age, gender and body weight.

Physical activity level (PAL): a multiple of BMR; the ratio of TEE (overall daily energy expenditure) to BMR.

Physical activity ratio (PAR): PAL and PAR are discussed later, in the section on energy requirements, and in Chapter 5.

Total energy expenditure (TEE): BMR × PAL.

ENERGY BALANCE

The regulation of body weight is dependent on a balance between nutrient intake and utilisation, although there are other important factors.

- The general principle of energy balance and hence body weight is:

  Energy consumed = Energy expended + Change in body store

- Amino acid oxidation adjusts to amino acid intake.
- Carbohydrate oxidation adjusts to carbohydrate intake.
- Fat balance is not regulated and nutrient excess goes into stores (Figure 9.2).
  - glycogen reserves are in the order of an average day's carbohydrate intake. The reserves are maintained at a balanced amount that prevents hypoglycaemia, but excess carbohydrates are channelled into lipid stores
  - fat balance does not appear to be regulated in the same manner. Fat oxidation and metabolism are not dependent on the fat content of the meal; fatty meals lead to fat accumulation and obesity.

ENERGY EXPENDITURE AT REST

BMR may be determined from the consumption of oxygen and excretion of carbon dioxide and urinary nitrogen, or from the heat production of the animal. Body size is a major factor in TEE and hence BMR. BMR is calculated using the body weight in kilograms/surface area in metres. The use of surface area of the body enables comparison of measurements of BMR in individuals of different size. The surface area is calculated from height and weight using nomograms. Body composition is also important, as the fat and lean components of the body have differing resting metabolisms. BMR is more closely related to lean body mass than to surface area. Gender differences are due to the associated, different, gender-related body composition. The energy expenditure varies with age, diet, climate and psychological stress.

Metabolic rate calculated from body weight alone can be used as an index of total energy intake for groups of individuals, assuming that the ratio of TEE to BMR is 1.6 on average, although this is not the case in sedentary individuals (Table 9.1). Rates of work or energy expenditure are calculated in watts (1 W = 1 kJ/s).

Changes in energy metabolism are due to the effect of and interactions between the environmental and biological factors that influence metabolism. The *Brody–Kleiber metabolic equation* attempts to predict the basal metabolism of all mammals regardless of size from their physical measurements, e.g. surface area. The arguments for the equation are:

- It is theoretically possible to define a mammal of unit mass from which the basal metabolism of all mammals can be calculated by a simple mathematical formula.
- A change in body mass has the same energetic effect regardless of species or individual differences in structure or body composition, i.e. $P = aM^b$, where P = basal metabolism, a = mass coefficient, M = body mass and b = mass exponent. $b = 0.75$ and $a = 70$ kcal/$M^{0.75}$ (mass in kilograms for mammals). Heat loss is proportional to body surface area.

This is an allometric approach and dates from a period in science when there was a desire to classify mathematically. There has been continuous debate on this question of the power-law exponent. These equations try to explain why a mouse uses six times more energy per unit body mass than a human. The energy demands of BMR comprise the energy demands of different cells, whereas maximal metabolic rate is determined by the high energy demand of muscles and the steps in the oxygen pathway through the energy supply cascade.

Body mass alters during life, and thus so too does the BMR (Table 9.1). It is therefore important to differentiate the quantitative from qualitative changes in mass. During neonatal growth there is a quantitative increase in mass associated with qualitative changes in body composition and form. In young adult life body composition and form remain fairly constant while mass continues to increase. In middle age body mass may increase owing to

Table 9.1 Equations for estimated basal metabolic rate (BMR) from body weight

Age (years)	BMR (MJ/24 h)	
	Male	Female
Under 3	0.249 wt − 0.127	0.244 wt − 0.130
3–10	0.095 wt + 2.110	0.085 wt + 2.033
10–18	0.074 wt + 2.754	0.056 wt + 2.898
18–30	0.063 wt + 2.754	0.062 wt + 2.036
30–59	0.049 wt + 3.653	0.034 wt + 3.538
Over 60	0.049 wt + 2.459	0.038 wt + 2.755

wt = body weight (kg).

The BMR of a 70 kg man is approximately 60–75% of the total daily expenditure, i.e. 6.3 MJ (1500 kcal)/day. This maintains normal body functions, temperature and the sympathetic nervous system. Resting metabolic rate (RMR) is measured in an individual at rest at a temperature that makes no demands on energy production over a period of at least 8–12 h after the last meal. Insulin, thyroid hormones and adrenaline also influence RMR. The BMR (in units of MJ or kcal/day) is measured under standard conditions, in the morning upon wakening after 12–18 h of rest and at an ambient temperature of 26–30°C. It is somewhat lower than RMR.

Determinants of metabolic rate that are invariable are: age, gender and genetic constitution. The variable elements are: the diet that antedated the test, body composition and weight, temperature, hormones, smoking, drugs and stress. Differences in RMR due to body composition can be corrected by relating the figures to fat-free mass. The reduction in metabolic rate in adults with age is a function of loss of lean tissue, and also the rate of decline of cellular metabolism. Women have a lower resting metabolic rate because of less lean tissue, although the measurement may be higher when measured as fat-free mass. The RMR in women falls before ovulation and rises by about 5% after ovulation.

increasing fat and retention of water, both of which are metabolically relatively inactive. In old age there may be a decline in body mass.

The actual metabolic mass of an animal during its lifetime results from a combination of processes reflecting various functional and structural transformations. The metabolic activity over a lifetime dictates the functional mass and composition of an animal. This metabolic activity varies during growth, pregnancy, lactation, illness, injury and senescence, but may be more constant during maturity.

REGULATION OF ENERGY BALANCE

In the regulation of energy balance, nutrient intake and energy (E) expenditure are related in the formula:

$$\Delta E = E_{in} - E_{out}$$

Inappropriately high intakes or low expenditure produce energy excesses, increase fat storage and result in a gain in body weight. E_{in} is the energy available for metabolism of the foods and E_{out} is formed from two components:

$$E_{out} = E_{exer} + E_{ther}$$

where E_{exer} is the energy available for metabolism of the foods lost from the body in urine and faeces, and E_{ther} is heat production (thermogenesis).

The thermic effect of physical exercise will vary according to the intensity of work performed and the duration of activity. A 70 kg man requiring a maintenance energy intake of 10.5 MJ (2500 kcal)/day will require 3.2 MJ (750 kcal)/day or 30% of these energy requirements for muscular activity. Clearly, the thermic effect of physical energy will be the most variable of all the components of E_{ther}. The metabolic efficiency of physical work is approximately 30%.

Adaptive thermogenesis is believed to account for no more than 10–15% of total energy expenditure, but may be important in the long term. This may be due to a change in RMR due to adaptation to environmental stress, e.g. temperature, food intake, emotional stress, and other factors. During undernutrition there is a progressive decline in the RMR. During overnutrition there is an increase in RMR in the order of 10–15%. These changes are in part due to sympathetic nervous system activity, adrenaline, thyroid hormones and insulin.

Thermogenesis is the increase above BMR caused by the thermic effect of food intake. It is a by-product of cellular and body maintenance, the thermic effect of food, the thermic effect of physical exercise, exercise heat production and the phenomenon of adaptive thermogenesis. The thermic effect of food is an increase in energy expenditure over the RMR following a meal. Heat is produced in response to an alteration in metabolic efficiency associated with changes in environmental conditions. The relative contribution of each to the TEE can be calculated. The effect of diet is complex and not well understood. All elements of diet are thermogenic. This is in part due to the energy required for digestion, absorption, transport, metabolism and storage of the ingested food. There may be other influences on the sympathetic nervous system by dietary carbohydrates. The thermic effect of food is said to be approximately 10% of calorie intake, although the effects of specific nutrients may vary. A complex network of dietary and hormonal factors acts to regulate diet-induced thermogenesis in humans.

In determining the response to food, the thermic effect of food is complex and not consistent, e.g. between obese and lean subjects. Part of the difference may be due to insulin resistance associated with obesity. It has been suggested that exercise plays a role in energy balance, both by expending energy and by regulating food intake. Aerobic fitness and the timing and size of a meal are determinants of the metabolic response to exercise, and account for some of the differences between lean and obese subjects.

The sympathetic nervous system and the indirect effects of adrenaline and noradrenaline may be involved in some of the changes. Thus, the type of nutrients in food, the substrates that result from the ingestion of that food, and the signal triggered by that food, all play a part in thermogenesis. Undoubtedly, fasting suppresses and sucrose stimulates sympathetic activity. In addition to insulin mediating glucose metabolism, thyroid hormones are important.

The effect on energy metabolism following carbohydrate overfeeding may result from energy requiring processes that are quite different from those induced by a mixed meal. This may result from differences in the metabolic fate of the carbohydrate. A proportion of ingested glucose, if in excess, is converted into lipid rather than oxidised or converted into glycogen. Lipogenesis from glucose is relatively inefficient. It is possible that the thermogenic effect of fat is mediated by free fatty acids or the hormones that are stimulated by such fatty acids.

It is probable that proteins produce a larger and more sustained thermic response than carbohydrate or fat. This may well reflect the energy cost of the synthesis of tissue proteins. Skeletal muscle is involved in more than half the total protein turnover, and the fasting-state fall in muscle synthesis can account for most of the change in whole body turnover. This has implications for energy expenditure and metabolic rate, which may reflect changes in protein synthesis.

ENERGY REQUIREMENTS

The total daily energy expenditure (TEE = BMR × PAL) is the sum of the BMR, the thermic effect of food eaten and the variable energy expended in physical activity. The TEE is expressed as a multiple of BMR and is affected by the PAL; therefore, it is necessary to know the gender, age and body weight and the intensity of the various activities of work and leisure, to calculate the BMR. The energy expended in physical activity varies.

Metabolisable energy is the sum of the energy required for body maintenance, activity, pregnancy, lactation and growth, and is affected by body weight and age.

Energy expenditure can be described as light, moderate or very hard:

- **Light work**: <170 W (2.5 kcal/min); it includes golf, assembly work, gymnastic exercises, bricklaying, and painting. (PAL for men = 1.55, women = 1.56).

Energy cost

The physical activity ratio (PAR) is an estimate based on the duration and type of physical activity. It is 1.2 × BMR for relaxation and 4 × BMR for gentle walking. Total energy activity for a day (the sum of the constituent PARs) is calculated by dividing the day into periods of activity, e.g. bed (8 h), working day (7–8 h for 5 days), with the remainder being variable. In this variable period PAR may vary over short or prolonged periods of activity. A PAR of 2 would apply to gentle domestic activities, 3 to gentle walking or village cricket, 4 to heavy housework, golf and DIY jobs, and 7 to exercise provoking breathlessness and sweating. Energy cost per hour may be expressed in megajoules (MJ) and, for a sample of activities, is: lying in bed, 0.2 MJ; watching television, 0.3 MJ; housework, 0.7 MJ; and walking, 0.9 MJ.

- **Moderate work**: 350–500 W (5–7.4 kcal/min); it includes general labouring with a pick and shovel, agricultural work, ballroom dancing and tennis (PAL for men = 1.78, women = 1.64).
- **Very hard work**: 650–800 W (10–12.5 kcal/min); it includes lumber work, furnace stoking, cross-country running and hill climbing (PAL for men = 2.10, women = 1.82).

Young children

Energy requirements for boys decline from 1.7 MJ (405 kcal)/kg/day at 3 years to 1.2 MJ (290 kcal)/kg/day at 9 years, and for girls from 1.6 MJ (385 kcal)/kg/day at 3 years to 1.1 MJ (255 kcal)/kg/day at 9 years.

Older children, adolescents and adults

A male weighing 74 kg, with an estimated average requirement for energy and a PAL of 1.4, uses approximately 10.6 MJ/day (2550 kcal/day). For a female weighing 60 kg, comparable figures would be 8 MJ/day (1900 kcal/day).

Pregnancy

Maintenance of a normal pregnancy requires energy for increases in tissue mass and metabolic activity. The increased tissue mass includes the uterus, foetus and placenta, increased blood volume and an increase of 2–2.4 kg of fat, which provides an energy reserve for lactation. The energy cost of the changes in tissue mass in women of 60 kg non-pregnant body weight during the whole of pregnancy is on average 167 MJ (40 000 kcal). The total increase in BMR over the duration of the pregnancy is in the order of 126 MJ (30 000 kcal), giving an overall total of about 293 MJ (70 000 kcal). However, it is unusual for the mother to take this increment in calories, and there is no apparent risk

Energy expended in physical activity

An estimate can be made of daily energy expenditure of groups, so that PAL is characterised by a description of lifestyle.

Daily activity expenditure = BMR × (Time in bed) + (Time at work × PAR) + (Non-occupational time × PAR)

to the mother or the foetus for failing to meet these additional requirements. It has been suggested that the increment in estimated average requirement EAR for pregnancy should be 0.8 MJ/day (200 kcal/day) above the pre-pregnant EAR only during the last trimester.

Women who are underweight at the beginning of pregnancy and women who do not reduce their activity may need more nourishment. Growing teenage mothers also need extra calories for their own growth as well as that of their baby.

Lactation

Women who are exclusively breast feeding until the baby is 3–4 months old have different requirements from those who are supplementing breast feeding. The gross energy content of breast milk is 280 kJ/100 g (67 kcal/100 g). The energy cost is in the order of 2.7 MJ (650 kcal)/day. It has been suggested that the additional energy requirement is in the order of 1.9–2.4 MJ (450–570 kcal)/day.

The elderly

The energy expenditure of the elderly is reduced, but in general so is physical activity. There is large variation between individuals. An active 70-year-old may have as high an energy expenditure as a sedentary 40-year-old. There is also a decline in the BMR, which is particularly affected by the reduction in the fat-free mass. In ageing, weight may remain steady but fat replaces lean tissue. In the old and very old (over 75 years), sickness and disability and a reduction in body weight (including lean mass) alter energy requirements. In estimating energy requirements in the elderly, a standard value for PAL of 1.5 BMR is useful, regardless of gender or whether the individual is housebound, in an institution or living at home.

MEASUREMENT OF ENERGY EXPENDITURE

Dietary survey

(See Chapter 8.) Comparisons with self-reporting using the doubly labelled water method indicate that individuals tend to underreport intake so that they approximate values to what they should be rather than what they actually are.

An activity diary will give an indication of energy expenditure, recording what the person was doing and for how long, e.g. walked the dog 20 min, watched television 30 min, jogged 30 min, went to the pub 120 min. These diaries tend to be somewhat inaccurate.

Heart-rate monitoring

This is a simple and inexpensive method for measuring TEE of large groups of people, and is a socially acceptable and sufficiently accurate method for estimating habitual TEE in free-living children to whom other methods are not acceptable. There is a significant decline with age in energy expenditure during physical activity and in duration of physical activity.

> Younger children (7–9 years) spend more time (470 min/day) engaged in physical activity than older children (12–15 years) (280 min/day). Boys spend approximately one-third more time (460 min/day) in physical activity than girls (320 min/day).

Calorimetry

This is the best method for measuring energy expenditure over a long period, although it is not a useful method for short-term measurements. Heat loss is measured, rather than heat production, so the result may be affected by heat storage.

Direct calorimetry
This measures heat produced and the excretion of water and carbon dioxide. It is the basis of the Atwater and Rosa respiratory chamber. Laboratory investigations using the whole-body direct calorimeter chamber and the water-cooled suit are validation methods, that are hardly used today.

Indirect calorimetry
This is now the most widely used technique. Heat production (metabolic rate) is determined from oxygen consumption and carbon dioxide production.

If the urinary excretion of nitrogen is also known, then the type and rate of fuel oxidation within the body can be calculated. Such measurements of oxygen consumption and carbon dioxide production may be derived from the respiration chamber or from portable respirometers. Oxygen consumption is proportional to energy and heat production. The ratio of excreted carbon dioxide to oxygen is peculiar to each major nutrient; the respiratory quotient for glucose oxidation = 1, for animal fat = 0.7 and for protein = 0.8. Measuring the urinary nitrogen enables the protein being metabolised to be estimated.

$$\text{Energy expenditure } = x\,O_2 + y\,CO_2 - z\,N$$

$$\text{and with constants } = 16.58\,O_2 + 4.51\,CO_2 - 5.90\,N$$

where x, y and z are constants, O_2 and CO_2 are the volumes of oxygen and carbon dioxide involved in respiratory exchange, and N is the amount of nitrogen excreted in the urine during the period of measurement.

Oxygen consumption can be measured over long periods in respiration chambers or into closed circuit systems, e.g. The Benedict Roth spirometer, the Douglas bag or the Max Planck respirometer.

Doubly labelled water method

This method is generally accepted as the most accurate technique for measuring energy expenditure over a defined period. It interferes minimally with free-living subjects, but is expensive and requires that intake equals expenditure. This method measures energy expenditure, which should equal intake in subjects maintaining weight. An oral dose of a known amount of $^2H_2{}^{18}O$ is taken and urine samples are collected daily over the next 15 days. Carbon dioxide production is measured as the difference in the water pool ($^2H_2$) and the bicarbonate and water pool (^{18}O). Changes in body weight and the water pool can be used to correct measured energy intake in relation to energy expenditure.

The TEE includes the energy cost of basal metabolism, physical activity, thermogenesis and the cost of synthesising new tissues.

Measurements in children
It is difficult to take measurements in children, especially in disease-compromised situations. Probably the best method is by the doubly labelled water method over as long a period as possible, e.g. 7–10 days. Gender and body weight are important variables. The total energy requirement of children can be calculated by adding estimates of the energy value of new tissue deposited during normal growth to the estimates of TEE obtained by the doubly labelled water method. Previous estimates of infant intake were problematic because of the difficulties estimating dietary intake. Physical activity is the difference between TEE and resting energy expenditure.

MEASUREMENT OF INTERMEDIARY METABOLISM

Studies in life are possible using stable safe isotopes, ^{13}C, ^2H, ^{15}N and ^{18}O.

Studies on intermediary metabolism in living people have been advanced by the use of ^{13}C nuclear magnetic resonance (NMR), especially for glucose in muscle glycogen, and brain glutamate neurotransmission and metabolism. Corrections have to be made for naturally occurring as opposed to enriched isotopes.

Stable isotopes and isotopomers

These isotopes are found naturally in small amounts in nature:

^{13}C, 1.1% of total carbon; ^2H, 0.015% of total hydrogen; ^{15}N, 0.37% of total nitrogen; ^{18}O, 0.20% of total oxygen.

These isotopes can be introduced into molecules to be positional or mass isotopomers.

- Positional isotopomers, e.g. [1-^{13}C]: glucose has seven possible mass ^{13}C isotopomers and 64 positional isotopomers.
- Mass isotopomers differ in the number of labels in the molecule, e.g. [^{14}N urea], or in mass spectrometry nomenclature: [^{14}N-^{15}N] or M urea, M1 urea, and [$^{15}N_2$] or M2 urea.

KEY POINTS

1. Energy is required continuously for cell repair and growth, but only intermittently for work. Food intake to provide this energy is intermittent.
2. At complete rest and without physical work (basal metabolism), energy is still required for the activity of the internal organs and to maintain body temperature. This is called basal metabolic rate (BMR). Basal metabolic rate = weight/surface area in metres^2. BMR in a 70 kg man is approximately 60–75% of the total daily expenditure, i.e. 1500 kcal/day. Determinants of metabolic rate that are invariable are: age, gender and genetic constitution. The variable elements are: the diet that antedated the test, body composition and weight, temperature, hormones, smoking, drugs and stress.
3. Heat loss is proportional to body surface area.
4. In the regulation of energy balance, nutrient intake and energy expenditure are related in the formula: $E = E_{in} - E_{out}$. Inappropriately high intakes or low expenditure produce energy excesses, increase fat storage and result in a gain in body weight. E_{in} is the energy available for metabolism of the foods and E_{out} is formed from two components: $E_{out} = E_{exer} + E_{ther}$, where E_{exer} is the energy available for metabolism of the foods lost from the body in urine and stools, and E_{ther} is heat production (thermogenesis).
5. The energy expenditure for light work (e.g. golf, assembly work, gymnastic exercises, brick laying, painting) is less than 170 W (2.5 kcal/min). That for moderate work (e.g. general labouring with a pick and shovel, agricultural work, ballroom dancing and tennis) is 350–500 W (5–7.4 kcal/min). That for very hard work (e.g. lumber work, furnace stoking, cross-country running, hill climbing) is 650–800 W (10–12.5 kcal/min).
6. The energy requirements of children vary with age. Pregnant and lactating women have increased energy needs.
7. Measurements of energy expenditure include heart-rate monitoring, direct and indirect calorimetry, and the doubly labelled water method.

THINKING POINT

The measurement of energy balance is one of the important measurements that have pointed the way in the development of an understanding of nutrition as a science. New techniques are now available that are more specific to particular metabolic pathways. How should these new and older methods interrelate?

NEED TO UNDERSTAND

Energy intake, expenditure and loss is a dynamic system that is constantly changing. Measurements need to be taken over time.

FURTHER READING

Baldwin, R.L. and Sainz, R.D. (1995) Energy partitioning and modelling in animal nutrition. *Annual Review of Nutrition*, **15**, 191–211.

Blaxter, K. (1987) *Energy Metabolism in Animals and Man*. Cambridge University Press, Cambridge.

Brockway, J.M. (1987) Derivation of formulae used to calculate energy expenditure in man. *Human Nutrition: Clinical Nutrition*, **41C**, 463–71.

Brunengraber, H., Kelleher, J.K. and Rosiers, C.D. (1997) Application of mass isotopomer analysis to nutritional research. *Annual Review of Nutrition*, **17**, 559–96.

Heusner, A.A. (1985) Body size and energy metabolism. *Annual Review of Nutrition*, **5**, 267–93.

Leibel, R.L., Edens, N.K. and Fried, S.K. (1989) Physiologic basis for the control of body fat distribution in humans. *Annual Review of Nutrition*, **9**, 17–43.

Livingstone, M.B.E. (1997) Heart-rate monitoring: the answer for assessing energy expenditure and physical activity in population studies. *British Journal of Nutrition*, **78**, 869–71.

Livingstone, M.B.E., Prentice, A.M. and Coward, W.A. (1992) Daily energy expenditure in free-living children: comparison of heart rate monitoring with the doubly labelled water method. *American Journal of Clinical Nutrition*, **56**, 343–52.

Nagy, K.A., Girard, I.A. and Brown, T.K. (1999) Energetics of free-ranging animals, reptiles and birds. *Annual Review of Nutrition*, **19**, 247–77.

Saltzman, E. and Roberts, S.B. (1995) The role of energy expenditure in energy regulation: findings from a decade of research. *Nutrition Review*, **53**, 209–20.

Schoeller, D.A. (1990) How accurate is self reported dietary intake? *Nutrition Reviews*, **48**, 273–9.

Schofield, C. and James, W.P.T. (1985) Basal metabolic rate. *Human Nutrition: Clinical Nutrition*, **39C**, (Suppl. I), 1–96.

Schulman, R.G. and Rothman, D.L. (2001) Measurements of intermediary metabolism. ^{13}C NMR intermediary metabolism: implications for systemic physiology. *Annual Review of Physiology*, **63**, 15–48.

Stubbs, R.J., Johnstone, A.M., O'Reilly, L.M. and Popper, S.D. (1998) Methodological issues relating to the measurement of food , energy and nutrient intake in human laboratory based studies. *Proceedings of the Nutrition Society*, **57**, 357–72.

Suarez, R.K. (1996) Upper limits to mass specific metabolic rates. *Annual Review of Physiology*, **58**, 583–605.

Symposium (1997): Mechanisms of Energy Compensation (1997). *Proceedings of the Nutrition Society*, **56**, 1–50.

Wagenmakers, A.J.M. (1999) Metabolic aspects of human nutrition at rest and during physical stress; recent methodological and technical developments. *Proceedings of the Nutrition Society*, **58**, 839–1033.

Weibel, E.R. (2002) Physiology. The pitfalls of power laws. *Nature*, **417**, 131–2.

Westerterp, K.R. (1998) Energy requirements assessed using the doubly-labelled water method. *British Journal of Nutrition*, **80**, 217–18.

Woo, R., Daniels-Kush, R. and Horton, E.S. (1985) Regulation of energy balance. *Annual Review of Nutrition*, **5**, 411–33.

World Health Organisation (1985) *Energy and Protein Requirements*. Report of the Joint FAO/WHO/UNO Expert Consultation. Technical Report Series 724. WHO, Geneva.

Zemel, B.S. Riley, E.M. and Stallings, V.A. (1997) Evaluation of methodology nutritional assessment in children: anthropometry, body composition and expenditure. *Annual Review of Nutrition*, **17**, 211–35.

10

Body composition

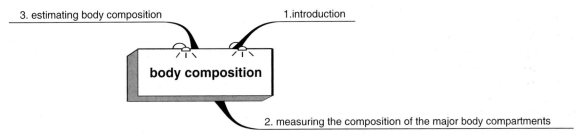

Fig. 10.1 Chapter outline.

INTRODUCTION

The body is not of constant composition, and is an assembly of different organs of differing composition. Body composition is affected by nutritional status and may be assessed by clinical examination. Conventional two-compartment models of body composition separate body weight into fat mass and fat-free or lean body mass.

The human body can be regarded as three compartments:

- cell mass (55% of the total weight), which is the active tissue, performing the work of the body
- extracellular support tissue (30% of the total weight), which supports the cell mass. This includes: (i) blood, plasma and lymph and extracellular fluid; and (ii) minerals and protein fibres in the skeleton and the connective tissue, including collagen.
- energy stores (15% of the total body weight) are predominantly held in adipose tissue, subcutaneously and around organs and some in glycogen.

Body composition and nutritional stores

- Lean body mass — Water and protein content of the body
- Fat — Energy stores
- Bone — Calcium and minerals

Most of the protein but only 1 kg of fat are essential cell components; the residual fat is storage.

The relative proportions will vary with a number of factors: age, gender, stage of development, physical fitness, hormonal status, pregnancy and even mood. In the embryo the proportion of water is higher than that in the mature animal:

- 28 week foetus: 88% water
- newborn baby: 75% water
- 2-month-old baby: 65% water
- 4 months to adult: 60% water.

The proportion of fat increases with age. In the elderly the amount of water slowly declines by small amounts.

MEASURING THE COMPOSITION OF THE MAJOR BODY COMPARTMENTS

The dilution principle

This measurement is based on adding a known amount of readily measurable substance Q into a body compartment of volume V which allows free and even distribution throughout the compartment. After a defined period the concentration of $Q(C)$ can be measured and then the volume can be calculated, using the equation:

$$V = Q/C$$

The requirements for the accuracy of such a measure are that Q readily diffuses throughout the compartment and that there is no metabolism of Q or binding to the walls or macromolecular component of that compartment.

Total body water

This can be measured by chemical methods, e.g. urea, antipyrine or ethanol. Alternatively, isotopic methods can be used, e.g. deuterium or tritium. The dilution is measured on a blood sample. The result is ideally expressed as the 'tritium' or 'antipyrine' space. This alerts the reader to the type of measurement, which may be different with each chemical. The usual result is 40 litres and accounts for 50–65% of body weight.

Extracellular water

Various substances have been used to measure extracellular water, including inulin, sucrose, sodium thiocyanate, sodium thiosulfate and isotopic bromide ions. Thiocyanate enters red blood cells, so a correction has to be made. The extracellular compartment usually accounts for 18–24% of the body weight.

Cell water and cell mass

If the total body water and the extracellular water have been measured, then the cell water can be calculated by difference. Approximately 70% of the total body cell mass is water, the cell mass will weigh 36 kg and represent 55% of the total body weight. Only half of the normal body weight is made of cells that are active in metabolism.

An alternative method is to use ^{40}K, the natural isotope of potassium which can be measured using a whole-body counter.

Body fat

The proportion of fat in the body can be measured by underwater weighing. The body volume is measured by displacement. The difference between the weight in air and the weight submerged in water is the volume of the displaced water. The volume corresponding to this mass of water is calculated by dividing by the density of water at the time of the underwater weighing. A drawback to this method is its inability to measure the density of the lean body mass.

The calculation uses Archimedes' principle, which states that the density d = mass/volume. The density of fat is 0.90, while that of the whole body is about 1.10. So, if x is the percentage of fat in the body,

$$\frac{100}{d_{body}} = \frac{100-x}{1.10} + \frac{x}{0.90}$$

$$x = \frac{495}{d_{body}} - 450$$

The density of the body can be measured by weighing first in air and then in water. If M is the mass of the body, and V the volume, then $d = M/V$. The measurement has to take into account the buoyancy of the lungs, which is measured by a nitrogen washout method.

Dilution principle for fat stores

Gases that are more soluble in fat than in water and that dissolve rapidly in body fat, e.g. ^{85}Kr or cyclopropane, have been used, without precision, to measure fat store.

Skeleton

The methods for assessing the size and composition of the bony skeleton are limited, but include:

- **biochemistry**: plasma calcium, urinary calcium; plasma alkaline phosphatase, plasma vitamin D, urinary hydroxyproline (collagen), calcium and phosphorus balance
- **radiology**: bone age, isotope bone scans; computed tomographic (CT) scanning
- **bone biopsy**.

ESTIMATING BODY COMPOSITION

The method used to estimate body composition will depend on the interest of the analyst. The anatomist will be interested in the size of organs, the physiologist in the components of cells, membranes and extracellular compartments, the nutritionist in fat, protein, water and mineral content, and the butcher in meat, fat and bone. A straightforward way to estimate any of these is carcass analysis. The results and the repeatability of such measurements are very limited. Non-destructive methods enable observations to be made over a period of time, and are more appropriate in human studies.

The normal composition of a 65 kg man is:

- protein: 11 kg (17%)
- fat: 9 kg (13.8%)
- carbohydrate: 1 kg (1.5%)
- water: 40 kg (61.6%)
- minerals: 4 kg (6.1%).

Of these, a proportion is storage tissue, predominantly fat. The fat store may range from 9 kg in this example to a significant proportion of overall body in weight in obese people. Available carbohydrate stores are meagre at 200 g. Approximately 2 kg of protein could be retrievable as energy, but with consequences to muscle mass. Only 10% of the body water can be lost without profound consequences for well-being.

Physical measurements

Height and weight
Possibly the most effective diagnostic examination is to look at the patient and to decide whether the patient is underweight, normal or overweight.

Height and weight are important indices of growth in children and adults. Life assurance company tables give acceptable weights for heights for adults. The measurement of children is recorded on height and weight velocity charts; that is, the changes over time are recorded. Up to the age of 3 years children's length is measured lying on a flat surface; over this age the standing height is recorded. Weight should be naked weight. Notes on the development of puberty are recorded on 'distance' charts, which note the advent of sexual and pubic characteristics.

Approximate measurements of muscle mass and body mass are made from the mid-arm circumference and triceps skin-fold thickness. The lower 10% of the range indicates significant underdevelopment. In the upper 10% of the range individuals can be regarded as obese.

Weight is judged in the context of the height of the individual. This relationship is contained in the Quetelet index or body mass index (BMI). This obesity index, uses weight (kg) and height (m) as weight/height^2:

- very obese: > 40
- obese: 31–40
- plump: 26–30
- acceptable: 20–25
- underweight: < 20.

Weight for age is expressed as a percentile of a reference population. In the first percentile are the lowest 10%, i.e. 90% are greater in that particular measurement. The 90% percentile means that these are the highest 10% in that measurement. Many malnourished children in developing countries are in the first percentile of these very Western-based charts, so a percentage of the median weight of the reference population is used. The indices are age dependent (60% weight for age is severe malnutrition in the infant but only moderate in the schoolchild).

Z-scores, that is standard deviation (SD) scores, have merit in the severely compromised child. The *Z*-score for weight for age is calculated by subtracting the median weight of the reference population at the child's age from the child's weight, and dividing by the SD of the weight of the reference population at that age.

The reference population commonly referred to has been taken from a North American population.

Reference data for growth and body composition of normal children

Reference tables should be race specific.

- Stature/length
- Weight
- Head circumference
- Growth increment
- Body mass index
- Circumference and skin-fold
- Leg length, arm length

Source: Zemel *et al.* (1997).

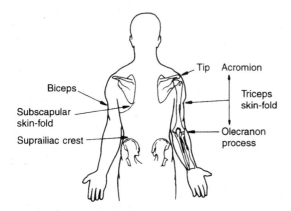

Fig. 10.2   Sites of measurement of skin-fold thickness.

Many of these children are overweight; therefore, the weight for age and weight for height are skewed above the median. Different SDs are used above and below the median. Height for age is normally distributed and therefore only one set of SDs is required. New percentile charts are being produced, but their implications will vary between age groups. A WHO Report suggests that the *Z*-score should be used universally in developing countries.

Body shape

As the majority of fat in the body is stored subcutaneously, *subcutaneous fat* can be measured by skin-fold callipers. There are various measures of skin-fold thickness (Figure 10.2):

- **triceps**: at a point equidistant from the tip of the acromion and the olecranon process
- **subscapular**: just below the tip of the inferior angle of the scapular

- **biceps**: at the midpoint of the muscle with the arm hanging vertically
- **suprailiac**: over the iliac crest in the midaxillary line.

Durnin and Womersley (1974) made measurements of skin-fold thickness and body density using underwater weighing and produced tables to enable calculation of the percentage of body fat weight from skin-fold measurements.

A line drawn between the L4–L5 lumbar disc space and the umbilicus is the clinical dividing point between the depots of fat. Skin-folds (subscapular, triceps, abdominal, thigh) and body circumferences (waist, i.e. the narrowest region between the bottom of the rib cage and anterior superior iliac spine; abdomen at the umbilicus; pelvis at the pubic symphysis; thigh; arm) have been used. X-rays, ultrasound and magnetic resonance imaging have also been used. The L4–L5 landmark produces optimal male–female separation for upper and lower body fat. Men have 53% of their fat in the upper body, while women have 46% in the upper body. There is wide individual variability in the relative amount of adipose tissue in the intra-abdominal visceral depots, and men have more of their adipose tissue in this compartment. Men have 79% of their fat in the subcutaneous region, while women have 92%; men 21% in the visceral area and women 8%.

Waist : hip measurements

Cardiovascular risk appears to be related to relative amounts of visceral adipose tissue, and not to the absolute amount of visceral tissue.

It is possible that total adiposity correlates directly with insulin production, and the waist–height circumference ratio correlates inversely with the fraction of insulin extracted by the liver. This may be due to increased concentrations of hepatic free fatty acids, which may interfere with hepatic catabolism of insulin and a provide a substrate for oversynthesis of very low-density lipoproteins.

Excess fat around the waist and abdomen (central obesity) is assessed by the waist:hip ratio. The level of the measurement varies immensely and it is important to record how the measurement was taken. The waist must be measured as defined above. The hip circumference might be defined as the maximum circumference of the midsection, taken at the maximum extension of the abdomen in front, the measurement at the iliac crest or the maximal diameter at the buttock or trochanteric region. A waist:hip ratio of greater than 1.0, rather than waist measurement alone, is a better predictor of a greater risk of diabetes and cardiovascular disease than excess fat around the hips and thighs. This is because there is a significant correlation between waist:hip ratio and intra-abdominal subcutaneous fat. This correlation does not extend to BMI.

This pattern of fat distribution is strongly associated with total body weight, except in the stocky southern Italian populations. Individuals with a predominantly central android or 'apple' distribution of fat have higher rates of atherosclerotic heart disease, stroke, hypertension, hyperlipidaemia and diabetes than individuals whose adipose tissue is distributed in a peripheral pattern, gynoid or 'pear'. The age of onset of obesity may also dictate the distribution of fat. There are gender differences in the way in which body fat is mobilised during weight loss. Men appear to lose weight in the abdominal area more readily than women, while women lose fat more readily from their hips.

Head and chest circumferences

In young children, head circumference is considered an index of brain development and is related to chest measurement, at the level of the third to fourth rib on the sternum insertion.

Muscle function

Hand dynamometry records the strength of squeeze. Unfortunately, this method is dependent on attention, motivation and culture, e.g. males may want to show how strong they are.

Biochemical and other tests

There are precise and important laboratory methods for measuring nutritional status for vitamins, and for electrolytes and trace elements; these are summarised in Chapters 16 and 18, respectively.

Electrolyte composition

The electrolyte composition of the extracellular and intracellular fluids is quite different (Table 3.1).

Table 3.1 Normal distribution of ions in intracellular and extracellular fluids (meq/litre)

	Intracellular	Extracellular
Cations		
Na	10	145
K	150	5
Ca	2	2
Mg	15	2
Total	177	154
Anions		
Cl	10	100
Bicarbonate	10	27
Sulfate	15	1
Organic acids		5
Phosphate	142	2
Proteins		19
Total	177	154

In the intracellular compartment, the major cation is potassium, whereas in the extracellular compartment the major cation is sodium. Considerable energy utilisation is required to maintain the electrolyte concentrations. Cellular activity in muscles, nerves or secretory cells requires changes in ionic concentrations. The control of the interior cell milieu is essential to life.

More general biochemical measurements assess plasma albumin and proteins. Albumin has a half-life of 20 days and is therefore a long-term indicator of nutritional status. A plasma albumin of under 25 g/l suggests severe malnutrition. However, plasma albumin may fall in other conditions, e.g. renal disease. Plasma proteins include transferrin and retinol binding protein, complement component (C3) and fibronectin, which have shorter half-lives and therefore reflect a more recent nutritional status. There is as yet no consensus as to which of these plasma proteins is the best to use for routine assessment.

Nitrogen loss can be measured in urine from the total urea in a 24 h urine collection, using the equation:

$$\text{Total nitrogen loss} = 24\,\text{h urinary urea} \times 0.035 + 2\,\text{g}$$

where 2 g indicates inevitable loss, e.g. in skin, hair and intestinal cells.

Metabolic measurements include plasma cortisol, glucose, interleukin-6 and albumin. Indices of inflammation include the white cell count, especially the neutrophil count and C-reactive protein.

Estimating lipid-free body mass
The estimation of body composition depends on the body being regarded as lipid-free body mass. The lipid-free mass can therefore be calculated from one measurement, e.g. water or potassium. It is assumed that this measurement is a constant figure. However, during growth it will alter in protein, water, glycogen, bone and electrolyte composition.

Water
This can be estimated using isotopes of hydrogen or oxygen. There is some metabolism of water, so the method overestimates values by 4% with hydrogen-labelled and by 1% with oxygen-labelled water.

Potassium
The stable isotope of potassium, ^{40}K, is used. This has a relatively high natural specific activity. Low background counts limit the precision of this method in large animals. An alternative method, which has the disadvantage of using radioactive ^{42}K, measures the dilution of an administered dose in the body potassium.

Neutron-activation analysis
This method allows the measurement in a non-destructive manner of the nine elements that account for 99% of body mass. The whole-body nitrogen can be measured with an accuracy higher than Kjeldahl analysis of the carcass. Similar accuracy is obtained for oxygen, sodium, phosphorus, chloride and calcium.

The total heat of combustion of body tissues can be calculated from the protein, lipid and glycogen content. These can be distinguished from the nitrogen and oxygen content; the ratios of carbon to hydrogen are relatively constant. Differences provide the potential for estimating energy stores.

Bioelectrical impedance and body composition
This method has the appearance of simplicity, although the physical realities of the system are complex. Simple bioelectrical impedance analysers measure a series of segmental resistances or impedances, the size of which is determined by

---

Magnetic resonance imaging (MRI)

Certain nuclei, e.g. H, possess spin and a magnetic moment. In a magnetic field the magnetic moment processes about the applied field direction at a frequency proportional to the intensity of the magnetic moment. By irradiating with electromagnetic energy at the resonant frequency, the procession angle can be increased. This energy is lost in relaxation of the spin-lattice. This alteration in spin energy can be received in a receiver coil and the different amplitudes of spin relaxations induced in the system can be recorded. The relaxation will vary in different chemical structures, e.g. it is prolonged in free water and shorter in water held in hydrated proteins. The major sources of protons of mobile molecules are the H nuclei in water and the CH of acylglycerol. Both proton density and relaxation time can be used to facilitate tissue discrimination.

---

skeletal dimensions. The method is cheap, easy to use and non-traumatic for the subjects.

Imaging
Imaging techniques based on ultrasound, X-ray, CT scans and nuclear magnetic resonance imaging (MRI) are used to estimate body composition. There is a good correspondence between cross-sectional adipose estimations by MRI images and carcass analysis.

Measurements in children

Specific tables for children for use with circumference measurements (mid upper arm, triceps) and subscapular skin-fold thickness) take into account the differing composition of young children. In puberty boys and girls grow quite differently, with boys increasing fat-free mass and girls increasing body fat.

KEY POINTS

1. The body is not of constant composition, and is an assembly of different organs of differing composition. Body composition is affected by nutritional status. This may be assessed by clinical examination.

2. Conventional two-compartment models of body composition separate body weight into fat mass and fat-free or lean body mass, the latter including viscera, muscles, organs, blood and bones.

3. Measurements of body composition include the use of the dilutional principles for total, extracellular and cellular water, body fat and a range of measurements for skeletal mass. Height and weight, body shape, subcutaneous fat, anthropometric measures and muscle function tests are also utilised. Biochemical estimations include electrolytes in extracellular and intracellular compartments, plasma proteins and urinary nitrogen.

4. Lipid-free body mass can be calculated from isotope-labelled water, potassium, neutron activation analysis, bioelectrical impedance, imaging or nuclear magnetic resonance imaging (MRI).

THINKING POINTS

1. Is the conventional two-compartment model of body composition the best way of regarding body mass? Would a model which classifies by turnover rate or which reflects clinical risks be better?

2. Height is regarded as an important measure of nutrition. Is this a suitable measurement in terms of nutrition?

NEED TO UNDERSTAND

1. The body consists of compartments which are readily measured. It is important to have an understanding of these compartments and their method of measurements.

2. It is also important to think of other methods which can develop in the light of modern nutrition.

FURTHER READING

Bagust, A. and Walley, T. (2000) An alternative to body mass index for standardizing body weight for stature. *Quarterly Journal of Medicine*, **93**, 589–96.

Bern, C. and Nathanail, L. (1995) Is mid arm circumference a useful tool for screening in emergency settings. *Lancet*, **345**, 631–3.

Durnin, J.G.V.A. and Womersley, J. (1974) Body fat assessed from total body density and its estimation from skinfold thickness. *Br J Nutrition*, **32**, 77–97.

Durnin, J.G.V.A., de Bruin and Feunekes, G.I.J. (1997) Skin thickness: is there a need to be very precise in their location? *British Journal of Nutrition*, **77**, 3–7.

Fogelholm, G.M., Kukkonen-Harjula, T.K., Sievanen, H.T. *et al.* (1996) Body composition assessment in lean and normal weight young women. *British Journal of Nutrition*, **75**, 793–802.

Fomon, S.J. and Nelson, S.E. (2002) Body composition of the male and female reference infant. *Annual Review of Nutrition*, **22**, 1–17.

Heymsfield, S.B., Wang, Z., Baumgartnet, R.N. and Ross, R. (1997) Human body composition: advances in models and methods. *Annual Review of Nutrition*, **17**, 527–58.

Jebb, S.A. (1997) Measurement of soft tissue composition by dual energy X-ray absorptiometry. *British Journal of Nutrition*, **77**, 151–63.

Jebb, S.A., Cole, T.J., Doman, D. *et al.* (2000) Evaluation of the novel Tanita body fat analyser to measure body composition by comparison with a four-compartment model. *British Journal of Nutrition*, **83**, 115–22.

Lean, M.E.J., Han, T.S. and Morrison, C.E. (1995) Waist circumference as a measure for indicating need for weight management. *British Medical Journal*, **311**, 158–61.

Nevill, A.M. and Holder, R.L. (1995) Body mass index: a measure of fatness or leanness? *British Journal of Nutrition*, **73**, 507–16.

Shann, F. (1993) Nutritional indices: Z, centile or percent? *Lancet*, **341**, 526–7.

Ulijaszek, S.J. and Kerr, D.A. (1995) Anthropometric measurement error and the assessment of nutritional status. *British Journal of Nutrition*, **82**, 165–77.

WHO Working Group (1986) Use and interpretation of anthropometric indications of nutritional status. *Bulletin of the World Health Organisation*, **64**, 6291.

Zemel, B.S., Riley, E.M. and Stallings, V.A. (1997) Evaluation of methodology for nutritional assessment in children: anthropometry, body composition and energy expenditure. *Annual Review of Nutrition*, **17**: 211–35.

Part V

Nutrients and non-nutrients

- Principles, amino acids and proteins
- Lipids
- Carbohydrates
- Dietary fibre
- Alcohol as a nutrient
- Vitamins
- Plant secondary metabolites and herbs
- Water, electrolytes, minerals and trace elements
- Non-nutritive components of food
- Agricultural chemicals in the food chain
- Drugs and nutrition

11

Principles, amino acids and proteins

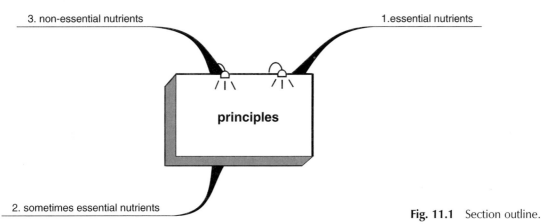

3. non-essential nutrients

1.essential nutrients

principles

2. sometimes essential nutrients

Fig. 11.1 Section outline.

ESSENTIAL NUTRIENTS

For a nutrient to be regarded as an essential contributor to the diet, that substance or group of substances must meet certain absolute criteria in human nutrition.

- There is no synthesis or absorption of that substance and the sole source is from the diet.
- An insufficiency of this nutrient leads to failure to thrive and ill-health, at all phases of life and function.
- Implicit in the concept of essential is that it is possible to define minimal dietary intakes of this nutrient to maintain health, at all stages of life and function.

This is a very complicated topic as there are caveats to such a simple triad of requirements. It is reasonable to regard the following as essential for life:

- ambient temperature
- oxygen
- water.
  Ambient temperature (between 0 and 30° C) is not a nutrient, but creates a climate where life is possible and food can grow. Oxygen is not a nutrient but is essential for existence. Water is also essential, but is not regarded as a nutrient.
- energy (calories)
- essential nutrients:
  - protein, nitrogen and essential amino acids
  - essential fatty acids

– vitamins
– trace elements.

Energy is derived from a mix of nutrients, primarily carbohydrates and fats, eaten in varying amounts depending on availability, individual taste and culture. There is a massive number of plant secondary metabolites that have varying properties as antioxidants and other functions, but are not seen as essential. Some essential nutrients, e.g. vitamin B_{12}, are synthesised by colonic bacteria but are not absorbed and are lost in the faeces.

SOMETIMES ESSENTIAL NUTRIENTS: NUTRIENTS THAT ONLY IN PART MEET THE CRITERIA OF BEING ESSENTIAL

In most circumstances dietary and metabolic sources are sufficient, but under conditions where there is increased demand, supplementation is necessary. There are limiting factors in the availability of such nutrients during increased demand, e.g. in the newborn baby, and during growth, pregnancy, and illness. The free exchange and provision of the necessary molecular components of the chemical are required, e.g. the correct carbon backbone, nitrogen or sulfate moieties. These nutrients have been called indispensable, conditionally indispensable, conditionally dispensable or dispensable, depending on the robustness of the provision of the nutrient. Indispensable implies the same as essential; the other terms are in decreasing degree of absolute need. Amino acids and polyunsaturated fatty acids come into this category.

NON-ESSENTIAL NUTRIENTS: NUTRIENTS THAT IN NO RESPECT MEET THE CRITERIA OF BEING ESSENTIAL

The chemical structure of nutrients in this category is freely exchangeable, both in synthesis and for metabolic needs, e.g. glucose, palmitic acid and glycine. However, they may, as carbohydrate or fat, be indispensable as contributors to the energy requirements of the body.

Some nutrients may have a status as essential from a social aspect, e.g. alcoholic beverages, chicken soup and chocolate cake. They do not enjoy the status of being essential in the nutritional sense, although some would argue that alcohol protects from coronary heart disease, and chicken soup is important in the care of the sick.

FURTHER READING

Cunnane, S.C. (2000) The conditional nature of the dietary need for polyunsaturates: a proposal to reclassify 'essential fatty acids' as 'conditionally-indispensable' or 'conditionally-dispensable' fatty acids. *British Journal of Nutrition*, **84**, 803–12.

Jackson, A.A. (1983) Amino acids: essential and non-essential? *Lancet*, **i**, 1034–6.

NUTRIENTS AND CHIRALITY

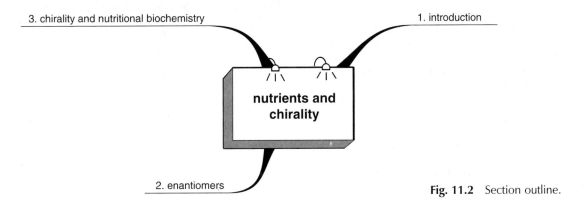

3. chirality and nutritional biochemistry

1. introduction

nutrients and chirality

2. enantiomers

Fig. 11.2 Section outline.

INTRODUCTION

Pasteur discovered the phenomenon of optical isomers of organic compounds. This led him to state that 'the forces of nature are not symmetrical'. He discovered that sodium ammonium tartrate could be divided into optically inactive and active crystals. These molecules were identical in physical properties except for the direction of rotation of polarised light. They had identical chemical properties except towards enzymes. Such variation in handedness is important in biology and even extends to pig's tails: 50% curl clockwise, 18% anticlockwise and 32% in both directions.

ENANTIOMERS

The two optical isomers are mirror images of each other. Kelvin called this phenomenon *chirality* (from the Greek word for hand) from the analogy of the mirror-image relationship between the left and right hand. Isomers that are mirror images of each other are called *enantiomers*. A mixture of equal parts of enantiomers is called a *racemic* modification and is optically inactive, the two enantiomers cancelling each other out.

When an enantiomer is reacted with a reagent that is itself optically active, the result will depend on which isomer is involved in the reaction; the other will be unaffected. The dominant product of the reaction results from the best stereochemical fit being selected. There are many examples of the differences in the activity of racemic isomers. The two isomers of omeprazole, the suppressor of gastric acid secretion, have different efficacies.

> The relationship between chirality and optical activity depends on the valencies of carbon being directed towards the vertices of a regular tetrahedron (Figure 11.3). The bonding of four different groups to the central atom gives two possible molecular structures, one of which is the non-superimposable mirror image of the other. Several chiral centres make for a series of optical compromises, which give rise to a series of asymmetrical molecules.

CHIRALITY AND NUTRITIONAL BIOCHEMISTRY

This phenomenon of chirality is important in nutritional biochemistry, since it affects many biochemical, pharmacological and metabolic processes. Every amino acid, with the exception of glycine, is optically active. All of these amino acids have the same configuration about the carbon atom carrying the alpha (α)-amino group. There are two enantiomers of amino acids, L and D. The L-α-

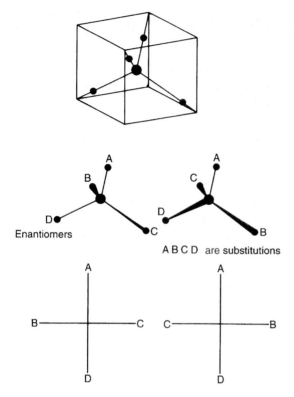

Enantiomers

A B C D are substitutions

Fig. 11.3 The two optical isomers are mirror images of each other. The bonding of four different groups to the central atom gives two possible molecular structures, one being the non-superimposable mirror image of the other.

their isomers. The C4, C5 and C6 sugars can be formed (in a theoretical sense) through the condensation of acetaldehyde to either glyceraldehyde or dihydroxyacetone. This gives a series of optically active monosaccharides; these differences are important biologically.

Proteins are constructed almost entirely from L-α-amino acids and nucleic acids from D-sugars. The chirality of the L-amino acids and D-sugars determines the chirality of the secondary structures of the right-handed polypeptide α-helix and the right-handed A- and B-forms of the DNA double helix. Some hormones may exist as isomers; a racemic mixture of a hormone may result in important differences in activity between the isomers, e.g. adrenaline.

> The difference in the smell of lemons and oranges is solely one of chirality: the smell of lemons is the L- and the smell of oranges the D-isomer of the same chemical (Figure 11.4). L-Asparagine tastes bitter and the D-form tastes sweet. Another chemical, carvone, tastes of caraway when in the L-form and of spearmint in the D-form.

KEY POINTS

1. Isomers are compounds that have the same molecular formula but different chemical structures.
2. Some molecules, because of their shape, are said to possess 'handedness' or chirality. Chirality exists when isomers differ in the arrangement of some of their atoms in space.
3. Molecules that are mirror images of each other are called enantiomers. They may differ biologically, especially in the manner in which they are attacked by enzymes.

amino acid is the naturally occurring form throughout the animal kingdom. The D-form is found in bacteria. When D-amino acids are ingested they are deaminated and lose their amino acid identity. Proteins and hence enzymes, being made of optically active amino acids, become optically active reagents. Enzymes are therefore very sensitive to the distinctions of chirality.

The L-form of the α-amino acid is metabolised in the body 20 times more rapidly than the D-enantiomers. This difference is dependent on the ease with which enzymes interact with the shape of the substrate. Polypeptides composed of the naturally occurring L-amino acids are stable compared with the corresponding D-enantiomers.

Monosaccharides are polyhydroxylated aldehydes, aldoses or ketones. The middle carbon of glyceraldehyde has four different substitutions which result in two enantiomers, a D- or an L-form, each with optical activity. D-Sugars are more stable than

THINKING POINT

Make a list of nutrients that may exist as isomers. What effect could such isomeric variation have on the metabolism of that nutrient?

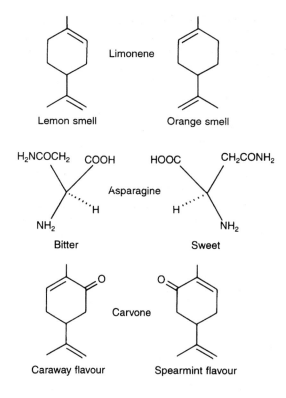

Fig. 11.4 Examples of the effect of chirality on physical attributes, smell, taste and flavour.

NEED TO UNDERSTAND

The metabolism of chemicals is determined by structure, isomeric form and chirality. This is central to metabolism.

FURTHER READING

Barron, L.D. (1997) From cosmic chirality to protein structure and function: Lord Kelvin's legacy. *Quarterly Journal of Medicine*, **90**, 793–800.
Solomons, T.W.G. (1996) *Organic Chemistry*, 6th edn, John Wiley & Sons, New York.

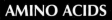

AMINO ACIDS

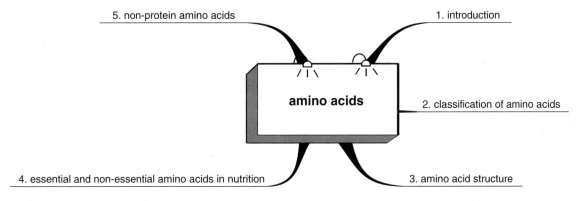

Fig. 11.5 Section outline.

Table 11.1 Amino acids

Amino acid	Abbreviation	Mass (Da)	Volume (Å³)	Occurrence in proteins (%)	Relative hydrophobicity (kcal/mol)
Polar R groups					
Asparagine	Asn	114	117	4.4	12.1
Glutamine	Gln	128	144	3.9	11.8
Serine	Ser	87	89	7.1	7.5
Threonine	Thr E	101	116	6.0	7.3
Tyrosine	Tyr (E)	163	194	3.5	8.5
Non-polar R groups					
Alanine	Ala	71	140	9.0	0.45
Cysteine	Cys (E)	103	109	2.8	3.6
Glycine	Gly	57	60	7.5	0
Isoleucine	Ile E	113	167	4.6	0.24
Leucine	Leu E	113	167	7.5	0.11
Methionine	Met E	131	163	1.7	3.8
Phenylaline	Phe E	147	190	3.5	3.15
Proline	Pro	97	123	4.6	n.a.
Tryptophan	Trp E	186	228	1.1	8.3
Valine	Val E	99	140	6.9	0.40
Charged R groups					
Aspartic acid	Asp	115	111	5.5	13.3
Glutamic acid	Glu	129	138	6.2	12.6
Lysine	Lys E	128	169	7.0	11.9
Arginine	Arg	156	173	4.7	22.3
Histidine	His	137	153	2.1	12.6

Mass: molecular weight minus that of water. E: essential amino acid; (E): facultatively essential. Occurrence: frequency of each amino acid residue in the primary structure of 207 unrelated proteins of known sequence. Relative hydrophobicity compared with glycine: the larger the value, the more hydrophobic the molecule.

INTRODUCTION

Twenty amino acids are important in human nutrition (Table 11.1). The side-chain of an amino acid determines its properties, and amino acids are classified by the chemistry of these side-chains (R group). The carbon to which the carboxyl is attached is the α-carbon. Amino acids have four different groups around the α-carbon, resulting in optically active L- or D-isomers or enantiomers. The L-forms are conjugated into proteins and biological systems. The D-form is found in the walls of bacteria and in some antibiotics, but not mammals. Dietary D-amino acids are deaminated during absorption and transported very slowly across membranes compared with the L-forms of the same amino acid.

At pH 7 amino acids may be negatively charged (aspartic acid and glutamic acid) or positively charged (lysine and arginine). The charge on others (histidine) is dependent on the pH. Asparagine and glutamine are polar, whilst being neutral.

CLASSIFICATION OF AMINO ACIDS

Amino acids can be grouped in a number of ways. They can be classified chemically based on structure (Figure 11.6) or nutritionally (Figure 11.7) or on increasing length of the side-chain (Figure 11.8).

Chemical classification

- mono-amino, mono-carboxylic amino acids: glycine (Gly), alanine (Ala), valine (Val), leucine (Leu), isoleucine (Ile)

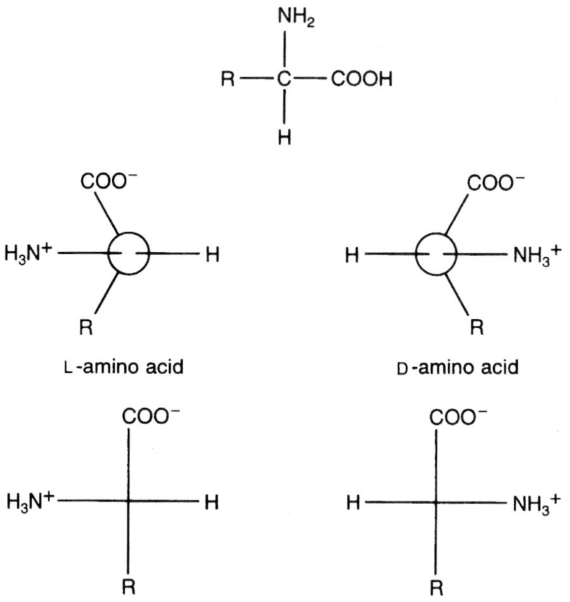

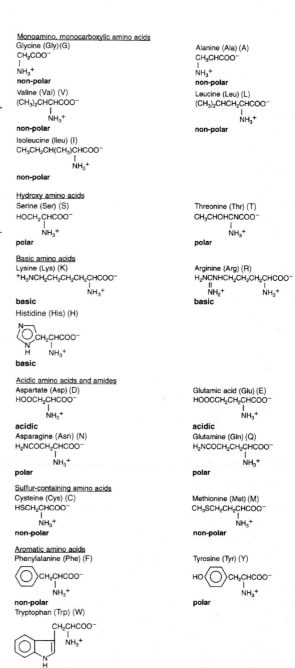

Fig. 11.6 Amino acids are classified by the substitution in the side-chain (R group). The carbon to which the carboxyl is attached is the alpha (α)-carbon. The side-chain determines the properties of the amino acids. The amino acids are optically active L or D isomers or enantiomers.

Fig. 11.7 Amino acids important in human nutrition showing full name and abbreviated name. The amino acids are listed as overall structure; non-polar or polar, basic or acidic. This gives a clue as to the function of the amino acids in proteins. Hydrophilic amino acids are found on the surface of proteins. Amino acids which are hydrophobic are found within the protein.

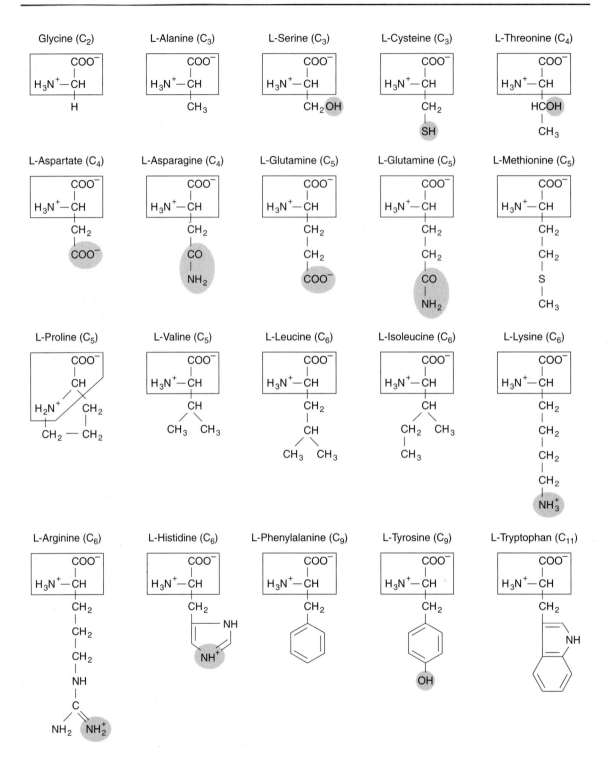

Fig. 11.8 Amino acids of increasing chain length. Side-chains of increasing complexity are attached to a basic structure (shown in box). The carboxyl group (C-1) and the carbon atom attached to the amino group (C-2) common to all amino acids are boxed. (Proline, with its ring structure, is an exception.) Polar groups are shaded.

- hydroxy-amino acids: serine (Ser), threonine (Thr)
- basic amino acids: lysine (Lys), arginine (Arg), histidine (His)
- acidic amino acids and amides: aspartic acid (Asp), glutamic acid (Glu), asparagine (Asn), glutamine (Gln)
- sulfur-containing amino acids: cysteine (Cys), methionine (Met)
- aromatic amino acids: phenylalanine (Phe), tyrosine (Tyr), tryptophan (Trp)
- imino acid: proline (Pro).

Functional classification

This separates the amino acids into four groups: polar, non-polar, acidic and basic. The polarity or non-polarity indicates how the amino acid will be incorporated into proteins, polar on the outside, non-polar in the interior of the protein. Amino acids may be charged or uncharged according to the pH of the environment.

Amino acids may undergo further reactions:

- enzymatic **acetylation** and **methylation**, usually of lysine: this suppresses positive charges forming on the amino group
- **phosphorylation**: the addition of a phosphate group to the hydroxyl group of serine or tyrosine and occasionally threonine
- **glycosylation**: the addition of a carbohydrate to an amino acid. A sugar may be attached to the amino group of asparagine to form an N-linked oligosaccharide. Occasionally a sugar may link to the hydroxyl group of serine or threonine to form an O-linked oligosaccharide.

The side-chain is the major factor in determining the transport system that is used by an amino acid. Among neutral amino acids, bulk and lipophilic properties of the side-chain are all important.

AMINO ACID STRUCTURE

Polar amino acids

These have no charge (see Figure 11.7). Examples are serine (Ser) and threonine (Thr). The side-chains are small, aliphatic, with a hydroxyl group which gives either hydrophobic or hydrophilic properties. The hydroxyls are somewhat polar, acting as hydrogen donators or acceptors. Threonine has a centre of symmetry of which only one isomer occurs naturally.

Asparagine (Asn) and *glutamine* (Gln) are the amide forms of aspartic and glutamic acid. They occur as amino acids in their own right and are incorporated into proteins. The amide groups are labile at extremes of pH, and hydrolyse to aspartic acid and glutamic acid. When present as an amino-terminal group in a peptide the glutamine may spontaneously alter its structure to the cyclic pyrolidone carboxylic acid.

Tyrosine (Tyr) is an aromatic (cyclic, benzene ring structure) amino acid residue that contributes to the ultraviolet absorption and fluorescent characteristics of proteins. The hydroxyl groups of tyrosine are relatively reactive and are readily nitrated and iodinated.

Non-polar amino acids

These are hydrophobic and interact with one another.

Glycine (Gly) is the simplest amino acid. It has no side-chain, is symmetrical and therefore does not exist in the D- or L-form. The presence of glycine in a polypeptide chain gives the chain flexibility.

Alanine (Ala), *isoleucine* (Ile), *leucine* (Leu) and *valine* (Val) are aliphatic residues that form a somewhat homogeneous class, having an inert side-chain and hydrophobic properties. The molecular surfaces and shapes are varied, giving a wide potential for forming a variety of polypeptide structures. Isoleucine has an extra centre of asymmetry, but in nature and therefore in the diet, only one isomer is involved in protein synthesis.

Methionine (Met) and *cysteine* (Cys) are sulfur-containing amino acids. The long alkyl side-chains of methionine produce a hydrophobic molecule that has a somewhat reactive sulfur grouping in the thioether group, which is especially vulnerable to oxidation. The thiol group of cysteine is extremely reactive, ionising at a slightly alkaline pH. Covalent disulfide bonds between cysteine residues occur in some proteins as cystine. Cystine is incorporated into proteins as cysteine, the disulfide bond developing later.

Phenylalanine (Phe) and *tryptophan* (Trp) are aromatic amino acid residues which contribute to the ultraviolet absorption and fluorescent characteristics of proteins. The aromatic ring of phenylalanine is very hydrophobic and chemically inert.

Proline (Pro) is a cyclic imino acid that has an aliphatic side-chain, without functional groups, which is bonded covalently to the nitrogen of the peptide group. In polypeptide structures the proline readily forms bends in the protein chain. Proline has no amide groups for hydrogen bonding; consequently, the protein structure is made rigid by the constraints placed on rotation by the cyclic five-membered ring. The 4-hydroxyproline derivative is important in the protein collagen.

Acidic amino acids

These owe their acidity to an extra carboxyl group.

The side-chains of *aspartic acid* (Asp) and *glutamic acid* (Glu) differ in having one or two $-CH_2-$ groups, each with a terminal carboxyl group. These are ionised at pH > 5 and are polar, and hence can chelate cations. The protonated forms may act as a hydrogen donor or acceptor, but rarely at neutral pH in proteins. The carboxyl groups are reactive, form esters with other amino acids and can be reduced to alcohols.

Basic amino acids

These include amino or imidazole groups.

The side-chain of *lysine* (Lys) is a hydrophobic chain of four methylene groups ($-CH_2-$) and an amino group, which is polar charged at biological pH. The non-ionised amino group readily undergoes acylation, alkylation, arylation and deamination reactions. The side-chain of *arginine* (Arg) has three hydrophobic methylene groups and a basic κ-guaninido group which is ionised.

The imidazole side-chain of *Histidine* (His) has special properties that are important in reactions requiring a catalyst. The tertiary amine has nucleophilic reactivity, important for enzymatic reactions. The imidazole group is free of steric hindrance. This is a strong base at neutral pH. In the non-

ionised form one N is an electrophile and the other a nucleophile; the donor and acceptor, respectively, for hydrogen bonding.

ESSENTIAL AND NON-ESSENTIAL AMINO ACIDS IN NUTRITION

Humans can synthesise some non-essential amino acids from glucose and ammonia, using the Krebs cycle or from free amino acids by transamination or reductive amination. However, amino groups are not transferred freely between all amino acids; there are nine amino acids (see Table 11.1) for which humans have no amination capability and therefore cannot synthesise. These are *essential* amino acids, which must therefore be provided in the diet and which were defined originally by Rose as those amino acids that must be included in the diet to ensure optimal growth. This is a concept fundamental to nutrition; nevertheless, all amino acids are essential in that a balanced intake of all amino acids is important in the body's economy. A diet of a sufficiency of the essential amino acids and an abundance of just one non-essential amino acids may not necessarily meet the body's needs.

There are few hints from chemical data to indicate why some amino acids are essential and others readily synthesised. Some essential amino acids are clustered in the family of amino acids with apolar R groups. Neither molecular volume, nor, as will be seen in the data presented elsewhere, the genetic code or triple codon for the essential amino acids gives any indication as to why an amino acid is essential.

Two other amino acids, tyrosine and cysteine, are *facultatively essential*. They are synthesised from

Facultatively essential amino acids

Tyrosine is synthesised from phenylalanine, while cysteine synthesis requires methionine (a sulfur provider) as a precursor, the remainder of the molecule being derived from serine. Phenylalanine and methionine are both essential amino acids. If their presence in the diet is at or below minimum requirement levels, then tyrosine and cysteine in turn become essential.

essential amino acids and become essential only if there is a deficiency of their precursor essential amino acid.

Conditionally essential amino acids require preformed carbon side-chains and substituted groups from other amino acids. Glycine, serine and cysteine may well function as an interrelated group, with the need for adequate provision of each. The requirements of the nitrogen cycles, e.g. glutamate cycle, may well increase the requirements for those particular amino acids involved in these cycles. Conditionally essential is a term that may be used in circumstances where an amino acid that is normally non-essential becomes required in large amounts, such as during an illness with added demands for that amino acid, e.g. glutamine.

The following factors may complicate amino acid requirements.

- A lack of a primary amino acid may limit the utilisation of other amino acids, leading to equal losses of carbon and nitrogen.
- A lack of non-essential amino acid could result in the deamination of essential amino acids to provide nitrogen.
- A lack of conditionally essential amino acids leads to problems in the balance of nitrogen and carbon substrates and the need for specific, if not essential, amino acids.

NON-PROTEIN AMINO ACIDS

Many of these are non-standard amino acids and are toxic. They are found in plants as unconjugated forms, but are most commonly found in legumes. Their toxicity can severely restrict the use of legumes as a dietary source of protein. The following list is not comprehensive:

- citrulline

$$CONH_2 \qquad H$$
$$| \qquad\qquad |$$
$$NH{-}CH_2{-}CH_2{-}CH_2{-}C{-}COOH$$
$$|$$
$$NH_2$$

- ornithine

$$H$$
$$|$$
$$NH_2{-}CH_2{-}CH_2{-}CH_2{-}C{-}COOH$$
$$|$$
$$NH_2$$

- gamma-aminobutyric acid (GABA)

$$CH_2{-}COOH$$
$$|$$
$$CH_2{-}CH_2{-}NH_2$$

- homocysteine

$$H$$
$$|$$
$$HS{-}CH_2{-}CH_2{-}C{-}COOH$$
$$|$$
$$NH_2$$

- 4-hydroxyproline
- 5-hydroxylysine
- 6-N-methyllysine
- γ-carboxyglutamate
- desomosine
- selenocysteine
- selenomethionine
- selenocystathionine
- canavanine
- indospicine
- homoarginine
- mimosine
- 3,4-dihydroxyphenylalanine
- β-cyanoalanine
- α,γ-diaminobutyric acid
- djenkolic acid.

KEY POINTS

1. Twenty amino acids are important in human nutrition. The amino acids have a variety of side-chains that provide a range of biological properties. The amino acids are classified by the nature of their side-chain. The L-forms are conjugated into proteins and biological systems. The D-form is found in the walls of bacteria and in some antibiotics, but not in mammals.

2. Humans can synthesise most of the amino acids from glucose and ammonia. These are called non-essential amino acids and can be synthesised via the Krebs cycle or from free amino acids by transamination or reductive amination.

There are eight essential amino acids, isoleucine, leucine, lysine, methionine, phenylalanine, threonine, tryptophan and valine, that humans cannot synthesise. Hence, these amino acids must be provided in the diet.

3. Tyrosine and cysteine are facultatively essential. They are synthesised from essential amino acids and only become essential if there is a deficiency of their precursor essential amino acid.
4. Some amino acids are conditionally essential, requiring preformed carbon side-chains and substituted groups from other amino acids, e.g. glycine, serine and cysteine may well function as an interrelated group, with the need for adequate provision of each. The requirements of the nitrogen cycles, e.g. glutamate cycle, may well increase the requirements for glutamate.
5. There are many other amino acids, of plant origin, which are at best not nutritional and which may be toxic.

THINKING POINTS

1. Amino acids are the building blocks for proteins.
2. The provision of these amino acids is limited by the eight essential amino acids and to a lesser extent by the facultatively essential amino acids.

NEED TO UNDERSTAND

The classification and types of amino acids.

FURTHER READING

D'Mello, J.P.F. (1991) Toxic amino acids. In *Toxic Substances in Crop Plants* (eds J.P.F. D'Mello, C.M. Duffus and J.H. Duffus). Royal Society of Chemistry, Cambridge.

Food and Agriculture Organisation/World Health Organisation/United Nations (1985) *Energy and Protein Requirements*. Technical Report Series, No. 724. WHO, Geneva.

Jackson, A.A. (1983) Amino acids: essential and non-essential? *Lancet*, **i**, 1034–7.

Lacey, J.M. and Wilmore, D.W. (1990) Is glutamine a conditionally essential amino acid? *Nutrition Reviews*, **48**, 297–309.

Reeds, P.J. (1990) Amino acid needs and protein storing patterns. *Proceedings of the Nutrition Society*, **49**, 489–97.

Young, V.R. and Bier, D.M. (1987) A kinetic approach to the determination of human amino acid requirements. *Nutrition Reviews*, **45**, 289–97.

WEBSITE

There are no dedicated sites but a search for 'amino acids' is rewarding.

PROTEINS

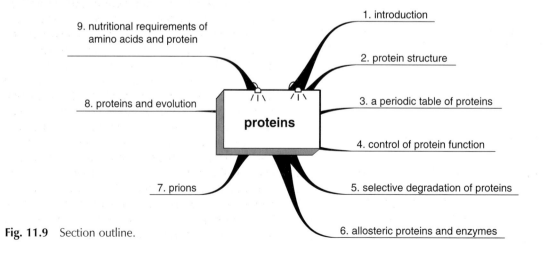

Fig. 11.9 Section outline.

INTRODUCTION

Proteins are high molecular weight polyamides, consisting of one or more chains of amino acids which then fold into a form that gives that protein a particular function. The molecular weight of proteins is measured in kilodaltons; one Dalton (Da) is the mass of one hydrogen atom, i.e. 1.6605×10^{-24} g. Proteins vary in size, from 1 to 1000 kDa, and length, with some extending to 2000 amino acid residues. The average protein has a molecular weight of between 24 and 37.5 kDa, which is 200–280 amino acid residues long. Proteins differ in their amino acid sequence rather than their amino acid content. With 20 amino acids available, each with a singular contribution to make to the structure, the number of permutations is enormous.

Proteins are present in all living tissues and are the principal material of skin, muscle, tendons, nerves and blood; they form enzymes and antibodies, and have a supporting role in molecular biology. There are more than 100 000 different types of protein in the body, and these form half of the dry weight of the body. Proteins are involved in every process in the body. Now that substantial understanding has been gained and information collected on the genome, the next phase is seen as understanding the proteome, the pattern of proteins produced by and present in a cell under particular conditions, protein expression and protein function. This will allow a database of all the proteins to be constructed.

The enzymatic activity of purely protein enzymes, i.e. those which do not involve coenzymes, is dependent on the chemical properties of the functional groups of the side-chain of nine amino acids:

- imidazole ring of histidine
- carboxyl groups of glutamate and aspartate
- hydroxyl groups of serine, threonine and tyrosine
- amino groups of lysine
- guanidinium group of arginine
- sulfhydryl group of cysteine.

The groups act as general acids and bases, and catalyse proton and group transfer reactions.

Metals, e.g. cobalt, iron, manganese, copper, zinc and molybdenum, function as cofactors in enzyme

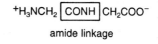

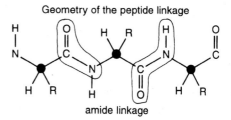

Fig. 11.10 Peptides are joined by amide linkages; the geometry of such an amide linkage is shown.

reactions. They are points of positive charge, which interact with two or more ligands and exist in two or more valency states.

PROTEIN STRUCTURE

Primary structure

A protein consists of a sequence of amino acids, unique to that protein, the sequence of which is called the *primary structure*. L-α-Amino acids can form peptides or protein structure by forming a peptide linkage between the amino groups and carboxyl groups, –NHCO–. The individual properties of the amino acids, with their varied size, shape and side-chains, contribute to very complex and functional protein structure.

Amino acids form peptides and proteins by linkage through a covalent peptide bond, between the carboxyl group at C1 of one amino acid and the amino acid group of C2 of another, to form a peptide. The backbone of the protein is an amide group, a carbonyl group connected by an α-carbon repeated many times (Figure 11.10). The α-carbon gives the chain its flexibility. Short chains up to 20 amino acids in length are peptides and the constituent amino acids are called aminoacyl residues. The condensation and formation of a peptide bond between the carboxyl group of one amino acid and the amino group of another (Figure 11.10) determines the eventual conformation of the protein. Subsequently, the polypeptide chain can take up secondary or tertiary protein structure.

Resonance

This is important in the peptide bond. The structure is a compromise between two resonating hybrids. In one, the C–N is a single bond with no overlap between the lone electron pair of the nitrogen and the carbonyl carbon. The other structure has a double bond between the amide nitrogen and the carbonyl carbon. All of the atoms directly connected to the C and N are held in a straight line, the amide plane. This amide link limits the number of orientations possible in the peptide chain and is important in determining the tertiary structure of proteins.

A polypeptide chain has an amino-terminal or N-terminal end, and a carboxy-terminal or C-terminal end. In describing protein structure there is a convention whereby the N-terminal amino acid residue (with the free amino group) is written on the left-hand side and the C-terminal amino acid residue (with the free carboxyl group) on the right.

Secondary structure

The amino acids in a protein, and their sequence in the primary structure, decide the shape and biological properties of that protein. The specific folding characteristics of a protein are determined by the amino acid sequence in the chain. Specific groupings of amino acids in a section of the protein result in biological properties that are individual to that protein, e.g. in an enzyme active centre. Collagen, as an extreme example, consists of one-third glycine and one-quarter proline.

When the primary structure is folded, a secondary structure results between residues close to each other. A sequence of amino acids will bend in a particular configuration, which is determined by the charges on the amino acids in that sequence, creating folds.

Extended polypeptide chains tend to develop a slight right-handed twist. All cross-over connections between proteins are right-handed. β-sheets of globular proteins (see later) are also always twisted in a right-handed format. Such twisted sheets form the backbone of protein structures. Proline is an important amino acid which creates an angle within a polypeptide chain.

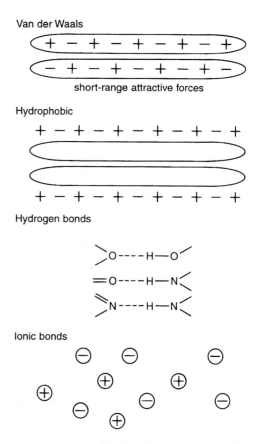

Fig. 11.11 Non-covalent bonds.

A major factor in the conformation of proteins is the presence of non-covalent bonds (Figure 11.11). These are usually created in an aqueous solution, the water forming a shell of ionic charges around and between molecules. Water is excluded from some parts of the protein structure, owing to hydrophobic effects. As a generalisation, amino acids that have side-chains that are hydrophilic, i.e. water soluble, are found on the surface of proteins. Amino acids that are hydrophobic are found within the protein (phenylalanine, leucine, isoleucine, valine, methionine). Glycine, alanine, serine, threonine and cysteine may be placed in the protein in a less well-defined position. Proline and cysteine are important in dictating peptide and protein structure. Proline's side-chain forms part of the main structure and its shape means that the direction of the main chain is altered by the formation of a bend. Cysteine can form a covalent –S–S–

disulfide bridge with another sulfur-containing residue, and this creates stable linkages.

The non-covalent bonds between different side-chains in different regions of the molecules, especially proteins, include the following.

- **Van der Waals' forces**: these are attractions between two adjacent atoms. They are weak reactions but are important in large molecular aggregations.
- **Hydrophobic interactions**: these occur between amino acids with apolar side-chains in response to the presence of water in soluble areas of the peptide chain. The hydrophobic amino acids tend to join together, to avoid contact with the aqueous environment and to form hydrophobic regions within the protein. The most hydrophobic of the amino acids, tryptophan, phenylalanine and tyrosine, are characterised by bulky aromatic side-chains. Leucine, valine and methionine are less strongly hydrophobic.
- **Hydrogen bonds**: these are weak electrostatic bonds that involve an amide H atom in the backbone of one amino acid residue being shared between two other atoms (both electronegative), such as a distant carbonyl oxygen or nitrogen residue. Groups in peptide side-chains can be H donors or H acceptors. One of each is required to form an H-bond. Liquid water may also interact with the NH and CO groups.
- **Ionic interactions**: these occur between oppositely charged side-chains and are modified by water. The basic amino acids, lysine, arginine and histidine, may interact with the acidic aspartic acid and glutamic acid. A basic amino acid may also react with negatively charged phosphate groups and nucleic acid groups. C- and N-terminal COO^- and N^+ can interact with each other and with side-chains.

The secondary structure describes the following functions.

- **Alpha (α)-helix**: in this formation, polypeptides form right-handed helical spirals, which are long rods in which each residue's carbonyl group forms a hydrogen bond with the amide NH group, four amino acids along the chain (Figure 11.12). The stability of the chain is dependent upon stable hydrogen bonds and tight packing when the chain folds. There is no free space in

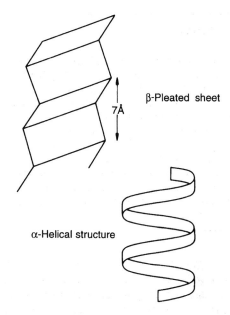

Fig. 11.12 Secondary structures: α-helix and flat β-pleated sheets.

the centre of the spiral. The side-chains project out from the helix. Amino acids vary in their readiness to adopt this configuration. Once the first spiral is established, consecutive spiral forms readily follow, through co-operative folding. Glutamic acid, methionine and alanine are associated with α-helix formation, whereas glycine, proline and asparagine are less frequently involved in such secondary motifs.

- **Beta (β)-sheets**: in this structure, two or more fully extended polypeptide chains, forming flat sheets, are brought together side by side. Hydrogen bonds form between the NH and carbonyl groups of adjacent chains (Figure 11.12). Amino acids with a branched or bulky side-chain or an aromatic ring (valine, isoleucine, tyrosine, leucine, phenylalanine, tryptophan) are commonly found in such conformations, unlike glutamic acid, aspartic acid and proline. Proline has no NH group and therefore cannot form hydrogen bonds.
- **Reverse or beta (β)-bends**: these are found in globular proteins. In such structures, reverses in chain direction occur, which give proteins their globular structure and special geometry. Such a

system is created by a carbonyl hydrogen bonding with an amide NH three positions along the chain. The amino acids proline, glycine, asparagine, aspartic acid and serine are particularly associated with such conformations. Glycine, being small, can readily form a flexible hinge. Proline has a more restricted and structurally prescribed formation which facilitates bend formation.

Tertiary structure

The tertiary structure of a protein is the most comfortable formation assumed by the chain. It is the structure with the lowest free energy and is therefore the most stable. Folding takes place in the endoplasmic reticulum, in water, along with dissolved cations and anions, which create an important environment for this folding process. The folding structure of a protein is determined primarily by the amino acid sequence, and between amino acids distant from one another (Figure 11.13).

The complicated formation and enormous range of shapes, and hence function, of protein come from the variation in distribution of surface localised charges and shape of charges on the amino acids. Cross-linkage through disulfide bonds or hydrogen bonds makes for the development of the tertiary structure of proteins. The sum of the charges will give the protein a net electrovalent charge in an electrical field. The final very tight packing of the protein is determined by tight, closely packed contacts between amino acid side-chains. This final phase gives each protein its unique three-dimensional shape. Proteins are the most tightly packed of any biological structure, which allows the protein to function, for example to arrange catalytic side-chains as in enzymes. Loose packing creates flexible hinges and conformational changes.

Most proteins are a mixture of hydrophilic and hydrophobic domains. The affinity of the peptides and proteins for water is called *hydrophilicity*, the converse being *hydrophobicity*. Proteins are in contact with water on their surface, i.e. the hydrophilic surface. The normal environment of proteins is water with a relatively high ionic strength created by salts in solution. Some proteins are not stable in pure water but require a modest ionic solution for stability.

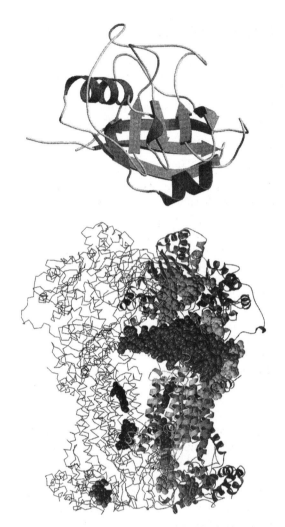

Fig. 11.13 X-ray structure pictures of proteins. Top: ribbon diagram of a cyclophillin protein with separate sheet and helix domains; bottom: complex dimer of bovine cytochrome bc1. (Reproduced with kind permission of P. Taylor and M.D. Walkingshaw.)

The hydrophobic sequences are buried in the interior of the protein, in a relatively water-free environment. Hydrophobic characteristics arise from a sequence of hydrophobic amino acids. Water molecules are generally excluded from the protein interiors. On the occasions when there is water in the protein interior, water forms an integral part of the protein structure. There are hydrophobic cavities in the protein, isolated from the aqueous bulk solvent. The water molecules

Ligands, active sites and receptors

The binding of small molecules to proteins may be important in forming and protecting or changing the structure of a molecule, with consequences for function and structure. Proteins may contain a cofactor such as iron or zinc. When a small molecule binds to a protein it is called a *ligand*. Such ligand arrangements are found with enzymes in which there is an active site with a catalytic reaction. When a small molecule binds to a specific site on the protein, there is a change in the protein conformation in such a way that the activity of the protein is altered.

An *active site* (Figure 11.14) is an area of the protein structure that facilitates the binding of a specific ligand through adsorption. If the protein is an enzyme then this region is an active site. If the region is larger, or involves transport or hormonal processes, then this region is called a *receptor*.

Implicit in the concept of active site is that the ligand is altered chemically in a catalytic process. A receptor will receive and pass on the ligand or a message will be activated, e.g. across a cell membrane. The formation and function of the active site depends on the positioning of specific amino acids in a particular formation. Reactive groups function as electrophiles or nucleophiles. Amino acid nucleophiles in the active site of enzymes include hydroxyl groups of serine and tyrosine, carboxyl groups of aspartate and glutamate, and sulfhydryl groups of cysteine.

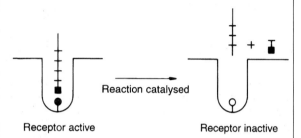

Fig. 11.14   Enzyme active sites, with the receptor active and after the reaction has been catalysed. The substrate enters the receptor site and attaches to an amino acid or other polar site. After the reaction the two products disengage and move from the site. The enzyme active site may be activated or inactivated by phosphorylation, which changes the bonding characteristics to a favourable or an unfavourable state.

attach by hydrogen bonds to polar groups of the protein. Such buried water molecules fill holes and pair with internal protein polar groups.

Water is a poor solvent for non-polar substances. Such substances have to force a cavity into which they can nestle; this is an energy-consuming exercise. Once the cavity has been formed, the solute will rearrange its bonds, so that the free energy of the system is minimised and stability returns. Such areas can occur in hydrophobic domains within the protein tertiary chain. Non-polar molecules tend to aggregate in water, so that the surface area of the cavity decreases.

The tertiary structure of a protein in general is found in two conformations.

- **Fibrous proteins** have elongated structures with the polypeptide chains extending to long strands. This is based on an α-helix or β-sheet. Such proteins provide structure in the cell or tissue, e.g. connective tissue.
- **Globular proteins** have a tertiary structure that is partially a helical secondary structure, with assemblies of polypeptide segments in the α-helix and β-sheet formation. Most enzymes have this format, as do those proteins involved in gene expression and regulation.

Quaternary structure

Some protein molecules are complexes of more than one polypeptide chain. Each chain with its tertiary structure forms a larger protein molecule. The resultant combination of subunits gives the quaternary protein structure. The advantage of such a system is that smaller lengths of polypeptides are able to function as a much larger unit. The possibility of error during protein synthesis is reduced, and such a complex system appears to be used when the molecular weight of the protein system exceeds 100 kDa.

Super-secondary structures (motifs of folds) are stable arrangements of several secondary structures and the connections between these structures. Polypeptides of several hundred amino acid residues

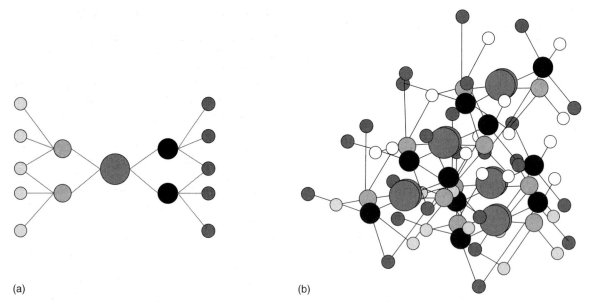

(a)   (b)

Fig. 11.15   (a) The perception of a group of proteins working together in a readily understood manner. (b) The reality of how proteins interact, as a co-ordinated, three-dimensional system. (Figure derived with permission from the editor of *Chiron*, Royal College of Physicians of Edinburgh.)

may fold into two or more stable globulin units called domains, which have very important roles in metabolism.

Complex motifs may be built up from simple units, series of βαβ loops, wherein the β-strands form a stable barrel (α/β). Each parallel β-segment is attached to its neighbour by an α-helical segment. Often, in enzymes, pockets are created which form a binding and regulatory site for cofactors or substrates. These large domains act in a co-ordinated protein–protein manner, and will signal to each other in a complex way. These mammoth systems involve over 1000 proteins acting in a synergistic manner, each augmenting and controlling the others like a well-tuned team (Figure 11.15).

Allosteric proteins are proteins consisting of more than one polypeptide chain. This quaternary structure exists in a number of alternative conformations and may therefore have different biological properties in each conformation. These allosteric proteins play an important role in both metabolic and genetic regulation. Such proteins are able to rotate freely around covalent bonds. The change in conformation requires alterations of non-covalent bonds.

Proteins with significantly similar primary sequences and similar functions belong to the same *family*. Such families have strong links with evolution and are helpful in tracing evolutionary trees.

A PERIODIC TABLE OF PROTEINS

If proteins fold in predictable ways, then it should be possible to classify proteins in a coherent manner rather than in biological families. This would enable a better understanding of proteins. The rational classification of proteins has been brought closer by systems, using computers, which break structures down to their basic forms. The folds of proteins can be classified. Similar proteins may be grouped together and idealised structures can be compared with known structures (Figures 11.16 and 11.17). Forms are developed in which the hydrogen-bonded links across a β-sheet impose a layer structure onto the arrangement of secondary structures in a protein domain. These layers are α-structures (packed α-helices) or β-structures (hydrogen bonded β-strands). In general, there are seldom

Examples of the diversity of protein function

Enzymes	Catalysts
Hormones	Growth hormone
Signallers	G-protein
Genetic controllers	Histone
Contractile proteins	Titin, tubulin, myofilament and similar proteins, found in muscles, cilia and sperm tail
Cytoskeleton	Protection
Transporters	e.g. lipoproteins, metal transporters
Cell membrane structure	Protective and barriers to chemical movements
Tubular cell membrane protection	e.g. gastrointestinal and lung mucus
Cell membrane channels	Ion channels
Cell membrane receptors	Receiving hormones for signalling and chemicals for function
Cell adhesion	Integrins
Immunological protection	Immunoglobulins
Silk	Spider silk is exceptionally strong
Hair	

Examples of protein control include:

- conformational change, as with haemoglobin, the oxygen transporter with or without oxygen or carbon monoxide
- molecular size reduction, the unmasking of an enzyme or hormone activity by loss of a peptide, from zymogen to enzyme, e.g. chymotrypsin or proinsulin
- feedback inhibition, by an accumulation of substrate or product on an enzyme
- toxic inhibition, a toxic chemical permanently or temporarily inhibiting an enzyme
- cofactor in enzyme activity, e.g. biotin in acetyl-coenzyme A carboxylase
- addition of non-amino acid or peptide moiety, e.g. methylation and DNA repair systems (methyl transferase)
- phosphorylation and protein kinase
- acetylation and cycloxygenase inhibition, and gene control through histone acetylation
- prenylation conjugation of a isoprene group (an intermediate in cholesterol biosynthesis) to a protein, e.g. ras oncogene, which is important in attaching the protein to a membrane
- carbohydrate side-chain creating glycoproteins, e.g. mucoproteins.

more than four layers in a domain and each layer is either predominantly a or b in type. αβ-Sheets have a twist, giving a staggered arrangement for the secondary structure elements in the outer layers. Sheets may also curl, producing a stagger between adjacent strands. All of these (twist, curl, stagger) result in the formation of a hydrogen-bonded cylinder or barrel. By considering flat sheets, cylinders, curled sheets, and partial barrels, a table can be constructed to clarify the situation. Layers of secondary structure (α and β) are combined to give globular protein domains. Proteins with all α- and β-proteins with internal repetitions are excluded, as they form propeller and triangular shapes.

CONTROL OF PROTEIN FUNCTION

The function of a protein is very varied, but is always under control. A protein may be structural, contractile, a transporter or an enzyme.

Denaturation

Proteins function in living systems in their native form in the tertiary format. Heating may denature the protein; loss of the tertiary structure leads to loss of function and often solubility. This is most vividly shown by the failure of a boiled fertilised egg to yield a chick. In nutrition and dietetics, most protein is in the cooked or denatured form, which is most readily digested in the gastrointestinal tract.

SELECTIVE DEGRADATION OF PROTEINS

Selective degradation of proteins is important in cellular activity, to remove misfolded proteins and to control protein activity. Proteins intended for proteolysis are marked by the amino acid at the amino-terminal end of the protein, e.g. arginine.

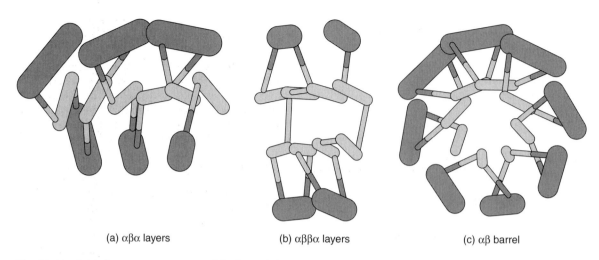

(a) αβα layers   (b) αββα layers   (c) αβ barrel

Fig. 11.16 Stick-figure representation of the basic forms of proteins. α-Helices are dark and drawn more thickly than the lighter β-strands. These αβα layers and barrel combinations can extend indefinitely. By manipulating these models almost all known globular protein domains can be generated. (With permission from W. Taylor and the Editor of *Nature*.)

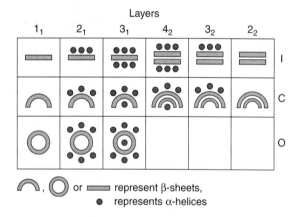

⌢, ◯ or ▭ represent β-sheets,
● represents α-helices

Fig. 11.17 Simplified layer structure of proteins. Layers of secondary structure: (β-sheets and α-helices. Most biological structures can be generated from three of these representations. (With permission from W. Taylor and the Editor of *Nature*.)

The response of the proteolytic system to these identified proteins is very specific. For instance, proteins may be marked with the small protein ubiquitin, which consigns the protein to degradation in the 26S proteasome complex.

ALLOSTERIC PROTEINS AND ENZYMES

Different allosteric protein and hence enzyme shapes are dictated by the DNA of the gene which encodes for that enzyme. The enzyme may be part of a family of isoenzymes, all of which catalyse the same reaction but with varying efficiency because of subtle differences in structure. The metabolic characteristics of an individual are determined by the translation by RNA into proteins and isoenzymes, which will be of varying potency and efficiency (Figure 11.18).

Co-operative substrate binding and modifications of enzymatic activity by metabolites may be features of some proteins with two or more structures that are in equilibrium. Such proteins are made up of several subunits, arranged symmetrically. The structures differ in the arrangement of the subunits and the number and energy of the bonds between them. In one situation, the subunits may be held together by strong bonds that would resist the tertiary change needed for substrate binding. In the other state these bonds would be relaxed. In the transition between them, the symmetry of the molecule would be preserved.

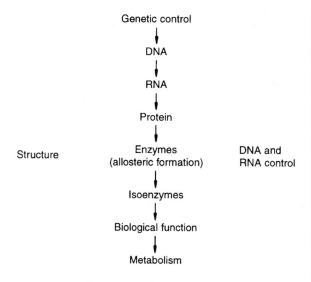

Fig. 11.18 Allosterism and enzyme activity.

The activity of allosteric enzymes is controlled by regulatory metabolites at a site separate from the substrate metabolised by the enzyme. This has the biological advantage that no direct interaction occurs between the substrate of the protein and the regulatory metabolite, and control is entirely due to a change in structure of the protein when it binds its specific effector. Such allosteric enzymes include glycogen phosphorylase and glutamine synthetase.

Glycogen phosphorylase

Glucose phosphorylase is the key enzyme in the control of glycolysis, the mobilisation of energy from glycogen. This complex allosteric protein is subject to activation and inhibition. Phosphorylase kinase is activated by phosphorylation of a pair of serine residues and inhibited by hydrolysis of the serine phosphate bonds. In muscle, phosphorylase kinase is activated by the release of calcium ions from the sarcoplasmic reticulum, which also stimulates muscle contraction. When activated, phosphorylase kinase catalyses the stepwise phosphorylation of glycogen, with the release of glucose-1-phosphate.

Most of the binding sites for substrates and effectors are widely separated. Despite this, binding of ligands to any of the sites can affect all of the others. A change in phosphorylation of serine-l4

Glycogen phosphorylase structure

The enzyme is a dimer (two identical subunits combined covalently) of a single polypeptide chain of 842 amino acid residues to which a pyridoxal phosphate is attached to lysine-680. Its unphosphorylated form, phosphorylase B, is inactive, but is activated by cyclic adenosine monophosphate (cAMP) when it reaches 80% of the activity of the phosphorylated form. This form, known as phosphorylase A, exhibits near-maximal activity without cAMP. Each of the two forms is subject to regulation by other factors. Phosphorylase B is partially activated by the weak effector inosine monophosphate (IMP) and phosphorylase A by glucose. Phosphorylase is a complex structure, each of its subunits consisting of two domains of a core of pleated β-sheets flanked by α-helices. The N-terminal domain includes the serine phosphate, the activating AMP and inhibiting glucose-6-phosphate (G6P) binding sites, the glycogen storage site and a small part of the catalytic site. The C-terminal domain complements the catalytic site and also contains the neighbouring site, where the inhibitory nucleosides and purines bind. In the enzyme dimer the two subunits are joined end-to-end in a small contact, making up no more than 7% of the surface area in the phosphorylase B and 10% in A. One side of the dimer is convex, with a radius of curvature matching that of the glycogen particle. It contains the entrance to the catalytic tunnel and the glycogen storage site. The side that faces away from the glycogen particle contains a regulatory phosphorylation site and the overlapping AMP and G6P binding sites.

induces a change from the weakly activated B to the inhibited A structure at the subunit boundary. Such a phosphorylation results in the burial and ordering of the amino-terminal 16 residues, the exposure and disorder of the carboxy-terminal five residues in phosphorylase A, and the reversal in phosphorylase B. This is accompanied by changes in hydrogen bonding. The dominant interaction is responsible for the allosteric transition. The tense structure (T) state is inactive and the active state is the relaxed state (R). The transition from the T to the R structure consists of rotation of one subunit relative to the other by 1°. Allosteric effects are provided by tower helices that tilt and slide relative to each other close to the active centre. These helices rigidly block access to the catalytic site, a polypeptide loop in the T structure. Displacement allows substrates, as well as additional cation side-chains, to move into the catalytic site. This converts the coenzyme phosphate from the monoanionic to the dianionic form, which is necessary for catalytic activity.

Phosphofructokinase

This is a further controller of glycolysis in cells. As in haemoglobin, co-operativity and feedback inhibition arise from a transition between two alternative quaternary structures, in which one pair of rigidly linked subunits rotates relative to the other and rearranges the relative bonds between them. The effector sites lie at the subunit boundaries where the allosteric transitions take place. In phosphofructokinase the catalytic sites span the subunit boundary where the allosteric transitions take place and are directly affected by the position of the boundary. The alterations in function are the result of changes in tertiary structure, comparable with a set of levers.

Signal peptides

These target proteins to effect secretion within cells and take part in protein–protein and protein–lipid interactions. Signal peptides have a common structure, a short positively charged amino-terminal region, a central hydrophobic region and a more polar carboxy–terminal region.

PRIONS

The PrP protein is found in many tissues, but has an important role in maintaining neural cell function. There are two normal variants of the protein in Caucasian populations. One has a methionine, the other a valine at the 129th amino acid. There are two copies of PrP in each cell. An individual may be homozygous (two PrP_{val} or PrP_{met}) or heterozygous (only PrP_{val} or PrP_{met}).

A prion is an infective protein similar in structure to PrP which may interfere with or substitute for the PrP protein. Prions are believed to be the infectious agents in the fatal transmissible spongiform encephalopathies. The prion causing scrapie

in sheep is different to the somewhat similar prions responsible for bovine spongiform encephalopathy (BSE) in cattle and Creutzfeldt–Jakob disease (CJD) in humans. Susceptibility to infection with prions may be enhanced in individuals homozygous for PrP_{val}. Other examples of prion diseases are listed in Table 4.1. The proteins involved have a poorly structured native conformation that is readily disturbed by genetic mutations, which leads to β-sheet structures. This change acts as a seed whereby normal protein adopts the abnormal conformation. There is an accumulation of abnormally folded proteins with age. The β-pleated aggregate is protease resistant.

The PrP gene does not differ between individuals in one species, but the shape of the protein encoded by that gene may differ and hence result in different prion diseases (strains). A species barrier limits the ability of a prion to spread from one species to another. Proteins other than PrP are involved in the spread of traits. The prion configuration may affect the spread of prions from one species to another. If there is a variety of prions in a species, then some of the prion configurations may affect transfer, i.e. be infective, while others may not.

PROTEINS AND EVOLUTION

Ancient conserved proteins

Cellular life is believed to have first appeared on the Earth 3.5 billion years ago. Since then the major biological kingdoms have separated. The separation of prokaryocytes and eukaryocytes probably occurred some 2 billion years ago. Plants, animals and fungi separated 1 billion years ago. Deuterostomes and protosomes separated some 670 million years ago. Despite this early separation it is generally believed that many organisms throughout the various kingdoms have conserved genes, proteins and portions of proteins with similar function, which are wholly or partially similar in their sequence.

These evolutionarily conserved proteins are called ancient conserved proteins, and may be conserved almost intact or in the functional domains of the protein. The amino acid sequence data from functionally similar enzymes from different kingdoms have been used to determine the subsequent divergence times of the major biological groupings. The difficulty in interpreting these protein clock studies is that different kingdoms have changed at different rates over these long periods and along different lineages.

Some portions of proteins have diverged significantly, and hence will be different in different creatures. Those regions where the similar portions persist are usually where there is greatest structural or functional significance. Ancient conserved proteins often persist as most or all of the single highly conserved protein or protein family, e.g. actin or histones; or not as the whole protein but in regions of the protein, i.e. specific domains or motifs, e.g. zinc finger DNA binding domains or enzyme active sites.

The term *homologous* is given to sequences or residues in encoded macromolecules with the same or similar residues at corresponding positions. In proteins this is used to imply a common evolutionary origin and gene structure, and not merely a similar protein structure.

The constant region is the region of a chain that is characterised by invariability of the amino acid sequence from molecule to molecule. Conserved or homologous proteins have regions that retain the same general fold and regions where the folds differ. The similar pieces are called the common core and include the major elements of secondary structure and peptides that form the active sites. Homologous proteins include the globins, cytochromes, serine proteases, dihydrofolate reductase, Cu-electron transport proteins, sulfhydryl protease, lysozyme and immunoglobulin domains.

Actin has the same amino acid sequence in the tomato, rabbit and human. Myosin is found in yeast and tomato, and binds to actin, tropomyosin, profilin and proteins that move mitochondria around the cell. The yeast gene *CDC28* encodes for kinases that initiate the cell cycle, and three such genes in humans have the same function. There is a gene in yeast that is analogous to the human cystic fibrosis gene.

The respiratory coenzyme cytochrome *c* has been found in more than 80 different species, which suggests a phylogenetic relationship. Similar usage of a protein by a variety of species includes the globins, the A- and B-chains of haemoglobin and myoglobin. Different proteins may evolve at different rates over time. The globin gene may be traced back 600 million years to an ancestral invertebrate. Gene evolution appears to owe much to gene duplication; one gene is conventional and retains the status quo, while the other gene may vary and can be amplified in response to changes in the environment.

NUTRITIONAL REQUIREMENTS OF AMINO ACIDS AND PROTEIN

Protein intake is relatively constant at 10–12% of energy intake and diminishes in parallel with the fall in energy that accompanies ageing. This may be a factor in muscle loss with age. A safe intake of protein should not be lower than 0.75 g/kg/day (WHO/FAO/UNO, 1985). Dietary protein provides nitrogen in an organic form for the renewal of amino acids for their various functions including proteins in cell walls, plasma proteins, muscles, enzymes and collagen. The amino acids of protein can be deaminated and may act as an energy source in their own right.

Dietary amino acid and protein requirements

Proteins differ in their biological quality, depending on the amounts and proportions of essential amino acids. A protein that is rich in all of the essential amino acids would score higher on the scale of biological quality than a protein deficient in one or more essential amino acids.

It is necessary to define protein and specific amino acid needs in diets with both abundant and deficient amounts of nutrients, including protein and specific amino acids. The protein requirement of all age groups should be based on the recommendations in the report of the FAO/WHO/UNO Expert Consultation, where the values were based on estimates and the amounts of high-quality egg or milk protein required for nitrogen (N) equilibrium as measured in nitrogen balance studies (Table 11.2). The estimated average intake of protein increases from 10.6 g/day at 4–6 months to 14.8 g/day at 4–6 years and 22.8 g/day at 7–10 years. In the male, protein requirement increases from

Table 11.2 Estimated average intake of protein by age, gender, pregnancy and lactation

	Protein intake (g/day)	
	Male	Female
4–6 months	10.6	10.6
4–6 years	14.8	14.8
7–10 years	22.8	22.8
11–14 years	33.8	33
50 + years	42.6	37
Pregnancy		+6
Lactation 0–6 months		+11
Lactation 6+ months		+8

33.8 g/day in 11–14-year-olds to 42.6 g/day in the over-50s. In the female, corresponding values are 33 and 37 g/day. Athletes may require more dietary protein depending on the muscle power required in the sport. Additions were made for growth, in infants and children, and in pregnancy and lactation additions were made to account for the growth of the foetus and to allow for adequate breast milk production. An addition should be made of 6 g/day for pregnancy and 11 g/day for lactation during the first 6 months, then 8 g/day after 6 months as the protein content of the breast milk begins to fall. There is relatively little change with age in the requirement for protein for maintenance, values falling from 120 mg (N)/kg/day at 1 year to 96 mg (N)/kg/day for adults. This assumed an efficiency of dietary utilisation of 70% during growth.

In the case of the elderly, the recommended nitrogen intake is the same as for younger adults, 0.75 g protein/kg/day. Daily protein intakes in the UK have tended to increase, to figures of 84 g for men and 64 g for women. There has been concern that excessive intakes of protein may be associated with health risks.

Dietary allowances have been defined as operational or factorial. *Operational* allowances define the amount of each amino acid that has to be eaten to keep bodily functions within normal or identified limits, e.g. maintenance of weight, amino acid concentrations and excretion of nitrogen in the urine. These are practical day-to-day nutritional issues. In human nutrition, outcome may be described, rather than defined, as normal, optimal, maximal and engendering well-being.

The amount of individual amino acids necessary to maintain protein balance may be different from that required for maximum rates of protein turnover, depending on age, gender, metabolic status and special conditions. The requirements of a baby, a teenage girl who is pregnant, an endurance athlete and an elderly person recovering from a stroke will thus be different.

Factorial allowances are based on an understanding of the underlying biology of the amino acid's metabolism. The rate and amounts required for the metabolism of each amino acid match the biological importance of the amino acid. An ideal is when the intake of the amino acid under study supports the requirements of a range of processes. This approach assumes a knowledge of the overall metabolism of the amino acid, alone and in the context of variable needs and amount of accompanying amino acids. Net protein turnover in the body is measured during growth, and in the mother and foetus during pregnancy, and the loss through secretion of protein, amino acids and non-protein nitrogen in milk. Loss of nitrogen in urine is also measured. This approach defines a minimum or obligatory need which by definition is less than the recommended dietary intake. In a factorial analysis of amino acid requirements the pattern of

The effect of gastrointestinal protein secretion becomes important in compromised nitrogen balance. In such circumstances, with mucoproteins and enzymes being lost to the body, losses of amino acids may be specific. This depends on the manner in which nitrogen is lost. If the nitrogen loss is due to amino catabolism and hence in the form of urea, then the loss includes all amino acids. If the loss is as specific proteins, then it may be accentuated and specific if there is an increase in particular amino acids in that protein. The amino acid composition of enzyme and mucous secretions that escape digestion in the small intestine and are degraded in the colon is different from that of proteins degraded metabolically. The non-essential amino acid:essential amino acid ratio in small intestinal protein secretions is 2:3:1, compares with 1:1 in the body proteins. Secreted intestinal mucus is particularly rich in threonine and cysteine. Continued loss of such enriched proteins from the gastrointestinal tract is significant, especially at times of dietary protein shortage.

necessary amino acids required is set by the pattern of different amino acid utilisation, for protein synthesis and other pathways.

It is difficult to achieve consensus between operational and factorial approaches. In the simplest factorial model the minimum amino acid needs are divided between net protein production and maintenance.

Estimation of the biological value of a protein

Nitrogen excretion
The nutritional value of a protein is measured by first establishing the rate of nitrogen excretion on a protein-free diet. Thereafter, known amounts of the protein being tested are added to the diet and the effects on nitrogen excretion measured.

$$\text{Biological value of a protein} = \frac{\text{Retained nitrogen}}{\text{Absorbed protein}} \times 100$$

If the protein provides all the needs for protein synthesis, at a rate equal to protein turnover, then the biological value will be 100. The standard is whole chicken egg protein.

If half the nitrogen fed is lost by excretion, then twice the required intake of that protein is necessary to achieve equilibrium.

Amino acid content
An alternative approach is to measure the amino acids in the protein. The figure can be compared with that of the egg protein standard.

$$\text{Amino acid score} = \frac{\text{mg of amino acid in 1 g of test protein}}{\text{mg of amino acid in 1 g of reference protein}} \times 100$$

Not all amino acids measured chemically are biologically relevant. There may be losses during cooking, e.g. lysine being vulnerable to cross-linking with other amino acids. The protein efficiency ratio (PER) is calculated as the weight gain per weight of protein eaten by young rats.

The biological value of protein is calculated with reference to growth in the young. The majority of individuals, however, are neither young nor growing, although it may be argued that the middle-aged

> Following an enriched protein diet, the enzymes that degrade amino acids are activated, especially in the liver. The priority is protein synthesis. This is reflected in the K_m of the catabolic and synthesising enzymes, with values for protein-synthesising enzymes being close to 10^{-3} mM and those for catabolising enzymes closer to 1 mM. Therefore, the catabolising enzymes only come into play during conditions of abundant amino acids.

and elderly are replacing tissue and their needs are probably similar to those in growth.

Amino acid regulation of protein turnover

Amino acid requirements include the maintenance of protein turnover above a certain limit, regardless of net protein retention. It is not yet clear whether protein turnover is regulated by the rate of supply of any amino acid or whether it is restricted to a limited number of amino acids. The physiological state of the subject may be a variable: age, growth, pregnancy or health.

Total body protein

This is a very important measurement as a reduction in values to under 80% of normal is a serious problem. Total body protein may be assessed from estimates based on the size of muscle masses, e.g. arm and leg, or indirectly from serum proteins or albumin, or by *in vivo* neutron activation analysis for total body nitrogen. These methods are either approximations or subject to substantial radiation risks. All such methods make assumptions, but dual-energy X-ray absorptiometry is a method of some utility.

Protein turnover

This is a measure of a continuous process. Single-point measurements that give an indication of protein status and separate what is regarded as normal from abnormal include somewhat old-fashioned measurements. They have been used clinically and are approximations. If the result is abnormal then there is protein negative balance, i.e. input is insufficient to meet the needs of the body. A normal result may not, however, mean that all is well. Methods include.

- measurements of the plasma concentration of total protein, albumin and transferrin
- a 3 day diet history of protein intake and 24 h urinary urea excretion (nitrogen × 6.25), which assumes that 16% of protein is nitrogen. The two measures should ideally equal each other.

Amino groups from amino acid metabolism are excreted as urea and ammonium ions. Excretion reflects the difference between breakdown and synthesis. 24 hour urinary hydroxyproline excretion is a measure of collagen breakdown. Creatinine excretion is a measure of muscle mass. 3-methylhistididine excretion reflects muscle myofibrillar loss. So, the total 24 h urinary nitrogen when compared with the 24 h dietary intake is a rough estimate of protein turnover. The approximation of this technique does not take into account the awkwardness of the procedure.

Tracer balance techniques
The use of radiolabelled amino acids requires a model system to enable calculations:

$$Q = I + B + N = S + M + C$$

where Q is the flux of the amino acid, I the dietary intake, B is the input from protein breakdown, and N is the input from *de novo* synthesis. The flux is equal to the incorporation of the amino acid into body protein, S, oxidation and other forms of metabolism, M. There is a small additional loss from the gastrointestinal tract as faeces (1 g N/day), skin (20 mg N/kg body weight) and non-measurable urinary uric acid (3 % of urinary nitrogen). Q can be calculated with the flux based on NH_3 (Q_A) or on urea (Q_u).

In human studies stable isotopes are used, e.g. ^{13}C and ^{15}N. The amino acid chosen is usually leucine, as this has one catabolic pathway and is predominantly metabolised in muscle. The amino acid can be given orally or more usually intravenously to achieve a plateau enrichment of the plasma. If leucine is used, its muscle metabolic product α-ketoisocaproic acid (KIC) is used for measurement, as it is a better indicator of intracellular leucine enrichment. Such methodology requires that:

- a steady-state plasma concentration of tracer is achieved
- the dose of tracer has no consequences for the metabolism of the tracer
- the labelled and unlabelled amino acids are metabolised identically
- no significant recycling of the isotope occurs
- the enrichment in plasma is representative of that at the site of protein synthesis.

Non-protein pathways of amino acid metabolism

It is not strictly correct to equate overall nitrogen balance with protein balance. Some items in the diet, especially human milk, contain significant amounts of non-protein nitrogen and amino acids, which are necessary for the synthesis of nitrogenous compounds not linked to overall protein metabolism. Haem and creatine are not recycled and are a drain on stores of methionine and glycine. An adult man requires 1 g glycine/day to support creatine and haem synthesis. On a protein-free diet, such a man would have to mobilise 1.5 g glycine from body stores.

Two aromatic amino acids (tyrosine and tryptophan) are important in hormone synthesis. Tyrosine forms thyroxine and the catecholamines, adrenaline and noradrenaline and tryptophan form serotonin.

Gastrointestinal protein loss

Faecal nitrogen losses have important effects on dietary nitrogen needs. Nitrogen fixation by gut flora results in a faecal amino acid pattern that is different to that of the dietary amino acids. There is substantial secretion of protein into the intestinal tract. Only a proportion is recycled in the small intestine. A large proportion of the protein passing through the ileum is of endogenous origin.

KEY POINTS

1. Proteins are high molecular weight polyamides, consisting of one or more chains of amino acids linked through covalent peptide bonds.

2. Proteins consist of a sequence of amino acids that is unique to each protein. The sequence is called the primary structure. Specific groupings of amino acids in one section of the protein give biological properties individual to that protein, e.g. in an enzyme active centre.

3. When the primary structure is folded a secondary structure results in an α-helix or β-sheet formation, created by free rotation around bonds.

4. A major factor in the conformation of proteins is the non-covalent bonds. The non-covalent bonds between different side-chains in different regions of molecules, especially proteins, include van der Waals' forces, hydrophobic interactions, hydrogen bonds and ionic bonds.

5. The tertiary structure of a protein is the structure with the lowest free energy and therefore the most stable form. It is found in fibrous proteins, which provide structure in cells and tissues. Globular proteins have an α-helical secondary structure, commonly found with most enzymes and proteins involved in gene expression and regulation.

7. A small molecule that binds to a protein is called a ligand. Ligand arrangements are found with enzymes in which there is an active site for a catalytic reaction.

8. Some protein molecules are complexes of more than one polypeptide chain and form a larger protein molecule, the quaternary protein structure, e.g. allosteric proteins. Alternative conformations of this quaternary structure have different biological properties, an important principle in metabolic and genetic regulation.

9. Different allosteric protein and enzyme shapes are dictated by the DNA of the gene encoding that enzyme. The metabolic characteristics of an individual are determined by the translation of RNA into different isoenzymes.

THINKING POINTS

1. The developments in nutrition for the future will come from an understanding of the role that allosteric proteins have on the metabolism of nutrients. Such exciting thoughts are currently being emphasised as giving a clue to disease processes.

2. Equally exciting is the thought of how nutrients are metabolised in different individuals and at different times. This will give insights into nutritional recommendations tailored to the person, not the community.

3. An optimum dietary intake of high-quality protein is important at all phases of life. Such an ideal intake may come from animal or vegetable sources, or both, and depends on education and access to food.

NEED TO UNDERSTAND

1. The structure and biological importance of the different amino acids, the L-form, the essential and indispensable amino acids, and the methods used to define their nutritional requirements.

2. The importance of proteins, their structure and types.

3. The concept of the allosteric proteins and the normal genetic variation that makes us both normal and different.

FURTHER READING

Carpenter, K.J. (1994) *Protein and Energy*. Cambridge University Press, Cambridge.

Cohen, F.E. and Prusiner, S.B. (1998) Pathological conformations of prion proteins. *Annual Review of Biochemistry*, **67**, 793–819.

Dean, P.M. (ed.) (1995) *Molecular Similarity in Drug Design*. Blackie Academic and Professional, London.

Doolittle, R.F. (1995) The multiplicity of domains in proteins. *Annual Review of Biochemistry*, **64**, 287–314.

Doolittle, R.F., Feng, D.-F., Tsang, S. *et al.* (1996) Determining divergence times of the major kingdoms of living organisms with a protein clock. *Science*, **271**, 470–4.

Food and Agriculture Organisation/World Health Organisation/United Nations (1985) *Energy and Protein Requirements*. Technical Report Series, No. 724. WHO, Geneva.

Food and Agriculture Organisation/World Health Organisation/United Nations (1989) *Joint FAO/WHO Expert Consultation On Protein Quality Evaluation*. FAO, Rome.

Frydman, J. (2001) Folding of newly translated proteins *in vivo*: the role of molecular chaperones. *Annual Review of Biochemistry*, **70**, 603–49.

Fuller, N.J., Wells, J.C.K. and Elia, M. (2001) Evaluation of a model for total body protein based on dual-energy X-ray absorptiometry: comparison with a reference four-component model. *British Journal of Nutrition*, **86**, 45–52.

Jeong, H., Mason, S.P., Barabasi, A.-L. and Oltvai, Z.N. (2001) Lethality and centrality in protein networks. *Nature*, **411**, 41.

Leibman, S.W. (2001) The shape of a species barrier. *Nature*, **410**, 161–2.

Levitt, M, Gerstein, M, Huang, E. *et al.* (1997) Protein folding: the end game. *Annual Review of Biochemistry*, **66**, 549–79.

Munro, A.W. Taylor, P. and Walkingshaw, M.D. (2000) Structures of redox enzymes. *Current Opinion in Biotechnology*, **11**, 369–76.

Perutz, M. (1990) *Mechanisms of Cooperativity and Allosteric Regulation*. Oxford University Press, Oxford.

Reeds, P.J. (1990) Amino acid needs and protein storing patterns. *Proceedings of the Nutrition Society*, **49**, 489–97.

Rennie. M.J., Edwards, R.H., Halliday, D. *et al.* (1982) Muscle protein synthesis measured by stable isotope techniques in man: effects of feeding and fasting. *Clincal Science*, **63**, 519–23.

Scheffner, M. and Whitaker, N.J. (2000) Cell biology. Proteolytic relay comes to an end. *Nature*, **410**, 882–3.

Stroud, M.A., Jackson, A.A. and Waterlow, J.C. (1996) Protein turnover rates of two human subjects during an unassisted crossing of Antarctica. *British Journal of Nutrition*, **76**, 165–74.

Taylor, W. (2001) A 'periodic table' for protein structures. *Nature*, **416**, 657–9.

Waterlow, J.C. (1995) Whole-body protein turnover in humans – past, present and future. *Annual Review of Nutrition*, **15**, 57–92.

Welch, W.J. and Gambetti, P. (1998) Chaperoning brain diseases. *Nature*, **392**, 23–4.

WEBSITE

www.hupo.org   Human Proteome Organisation

12

Lipids

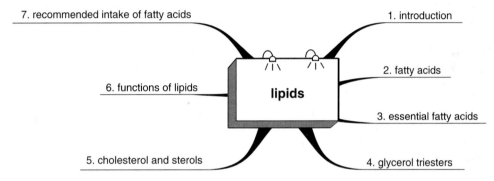

Fig. 12.1 Chapter outline.

INTRODUCTION

Fat is a heterogeneous mixture of lipids, predominantly triglycerides, but also including phospholipids, glycolipids and sterols. Triacylglycerols (triglycerides) are the principal dietary lipids which are stored in fat stores in humans and consist of esters of fatty acids, both saturated and unsaturated, and glycerol. Phospholipids contain phosphoric acid as a monoester or diester. Glycolipids contain between one and four linked monosaccharide residues joined through a glycosyl linkage to a lipid (diacylglycerol or sphingosine). Cholesterol, cholesterol ester and phospholipids are important in the structure of cell membranes, mitochondria, lysosomes and the endoplasmic reticulum. Lipids are important in providing insulation against the cold.

The principal dietary sources of fat are dairy products, meat, margarine and other fats, biscuits, cakes and pastries. Plant storage fats are present in nuts, cereal grains and fruits such as the avocado. Other dietary lipids include cooking fats, salad oils and mayonnaise. Eggs are a source of lipids, predominantly saturated and monounsaturated fatty acids, lipoprotein, triacylglycerols, cholesterol and phospholipids. Many foods contain structural fats, phospholipids and glycolipids, cholesterol and plant sterols. Eating brain as a food provides animal sphingolipids in the diet. Dairy products contain milk fat globule membranes. Green leafy vegetables contain galactolipids, and there are membrane lipids in cereal, grains, vegetables and fruit.

FATTY ACIDS (SEE TABLE 12.1)

Saturated fatty acids

Most saturated fatty acids are straight-chain structures with an even number of carbon atoms.

Table 12.1 Name, structure and occurrence of the most common fatty acids

	Name	Structure	Remarks
Saturated straight chain-acids			
C1	Formic acid (methanoic acid)	H·COOH	Occurs in human urine and many plant materials
C2	Acetic acid (ethanoic acid)	CH$_3$·COOH	Present in most biological materials. Formed from ethanol, by many species of aerobic bacteria and from pentoses, by some anaerobic species
C3	Propionic acid (propanoic acid)	CH$_3$·CH$_2$·COOH	Formed by bacterial decomposition of carbohydrates
C4	*n*-Butyric acid (butanoic acid)	CH$_3$·(CH$_2$)$_2$·COOH	Occurs in traces in many fats
C5	*n*-Valeric acid (pentanoic acid)	CH$_3$·(CH$_2$)$_3$·COOH	
C6	Caproic acid (hexoic acid, hexanoic acid)	CH$_3$·(CH$_2$)$_4$·COOH	
C8	Caprylic acid (octanoic acid)	CH·(CH$_2$)$_6$·COOH	Component of many fats
C10	Capric acid (decanoic acid)	CH$_3$·(CH$_2$)$_8$·COOH	Component of many animal and vegetable fats
C12	Lauric acid (dodecanoic acid)	CH$_3$·(CH$_2$)$_{10}$·COOH	Major component of vegetable fats (esp. laurel). In smaller quantities in depot fat of animals, milk fat and fish liver oils
C14	Myristic acid (tetradecanoic acid)	CH$_3$·(CH$_2$)$_{12}$·COOH	Component of almost all animal fats (1–5%) and vegetable fats, esp. milk fat, fish oils, palm oil and nutmeg
C16	Palmitic acid (hexadecanoic acid)	CH$_3$·(CH$_2$)$_{14}$·COOH	Widely distributed in nature. Present in almost all fats
C17	Margaric acid (heptadecanoic acid)	CH$_3$·(CH$_2$)$_{15}$·COOH	Occurs in traces in mutton fat
C18	Stearic acid (octadecanoic acid)	CH$_3$·(CH$_2$)$_{16}$·COOH	Found abundantly in important edible fats. Also occurs in vegetable fats
C20	Arachidic acid (eicosanoic acid)	CH$_3$·(CH$_2$)$_{18}$·COOH	Occurs in traces in many seed and animal fats
	Heneicosanoic acid	CH$_3$·(CH$_2$)$_{19}$·COOH	
C22	Behenic acid (docosanoic acid)	CH$_3$·(CH$_2$)$_{20}$·COOH	Present in traces in animal fats and seed fats. Constitutes 50% of the spleen cerebrosides in Gaucher's disease
C24	Lignoceric acid (tetracosanoic acid)	CH$_3$·(CH$_2$)$_{22}$·COOH	Component of sphingomyelins and of kerasin (spleen cerebroside in Gaucher's disease). Also found in some vegetable fats and bacterial and insect waxes
C26	Cerotic acid (hexacosanoic acid)	CH$_3$·(CH$_2$)$_{24}$·COOH	Occurs free and combined. In Chinese wax (cetyl ester), beeswax and wool fat
C28	Montanic acid (octacosanoic acid)	CH$_3$·(CH$_2$)$_{26}$·COOH	Component of montan wax, beeswax and Chinese wax
C30	Melissic acid (triacontanoic acid)	CH$_3$·(CH$_2$)$_{28}$·COOH	Occurs in beeswax

Table 12.1 *(Continued)*

	Name	Structure	Remarks
Monounsaturated fatty acids			
C10	*cis*-Δ^9-Decenoic acid	$CH_2 = CH(CH_2)_7COOH$	Occurs in butter and milk fats and sperm head oil
C12	Linderic acid (*cis*-Δ^9-dodecenoic acid)	CH_3-$(CH_2)_6CH = CH(CH_2)_2COOH$	Occurs in various seed oils, e.g. *Lindera obtusiloba*
C12	Lauroleic acid (*cis*-Δ^9-dodecenoic acid)	$CH_3(CH_2)_5CH = CH(CH_2)_3COOH$	Occurs in sperm head oil and blubber
C14	Myristoleic acid (*cis*-Δ^9-tetradecenoic acid)	$CH_3(CH_2)_3CH = CH(CH_2)_7COOH$	Occurs in milk fat and depot fat of many animals
C16	Palmitoleic acid (*cis*-Δ^9-hexadecenoic acid)	$CH_3(CH_2)_5CH = CH(CH_2)_7COOH$	Widely distributed in marine oils, depot and milk fats, animal fats and vegetable oils
C18	*cis*-Δ^6-Octadecenoic acid	$CH_3 \cdot (CH_2)_{10} \cdot CH = CH \cdot (CH_2)_4 \cdot COOH$	Occurs in seeds of aromatic plants [parsley, celery (petroselinic acid), etc.] and in some umbellate fats
C18	Oleic acid (*cis*-Δ^9-octadecenoic acid)	$CH \cdot (CH_2)_7 \cdot COOH = CH \cdot (CH_2)_7 - CH_3$	Most abundant of the unsaturated fatty acids. Present in nearly all natural fats (one-third of fatty acids of cow's milk; phosphatides). Occurs in traces in human urine
C18	Elaidic acid (*trans*-Δ^9-octadecenoic acid)	$CH_3 \cdot (CH_2)_7 \cdot CH = CH \cdot (CH_2)_7 \cdot COOH$	Formed by isomerisation of oleic acid
C18	*trans*-Vaccenic acid (*trans*-Δ^9-octadecenoic acid)	$CH_3 \cdot (CH_2)_5 \cdot CH= CH \cdot (CH_2)_9 \cdot COOH$	Occurs in many animal fats and vegetable oils
C18	Δ^{12}-Octadecenoic acid	$CH_3 \cdot (CH_2)_4 \cdot CH = CH \cdot (CH_2)_{10} \cdot COOH$	Occurs in partially hydrogenated peanut oil
C20	Gadoleic acid (Δ^9-eicosenoic acid)	$CH_3 \cdot (CH_2)_9 \cdot CH = CH \cdot (CH_2)_7 \cdot COOH$	*cis* and *trans* forms. In many fish and marine animal oils, vegetable oils, and brain phosphatides
C22	Cetoleic acid (Δ^{11}-docosenoic acid)	$CH_3 \cdot (CH_2)_9 \cdot CH = CH \cdot (CH_2)_9 \cdot COOH$	Occurs in various marine oils
C22	Erucic acid (*cis*-Δ^{13}-docosenoic acid)	$CH \cdot (CH_2)_{11} \cdot COOH = CH \cdot (CH_2)_7 \cdot CH_3$	Occurs in seed oils, esp. rapeseed oil
C22	Brassidic acid (*trans*-Δ^{13}-docosenoic acid)	$CH_3 \cdot (CH_2)_7 \cdot CH = CH \cdot (CH_2)_{11} \cdot COOH$	Formed by isomerisation of erucic acid
C24	Selacholeic acid (nervonic acid, *cis*-Δ^{15}-tetracosenoic acid)	$CH \cdot (CH_2)_{13} \cdot COOH = CH \cdot (CH_2)_7 \cdot CH_3$	Occurs in shark and ray liver oils, brain cerebrosides (nervone) and sphingomyelins
C26	Ximenic acid (Δ^{17}-hexacosenoic acid)	$CH_3 \cdot (CH_2)_7 \cdot CH = CH \cdot (CH_2)_{15} \cdot COOH$	Occurs in *Ximenia americana* (tallow-wood). A hexacosenoic acid is found with nervonic acid in brain cerebrosides

(Continued overleaf)

Table 12.1   (*Continued*)

	Name	Structure	Remarks
Polyunsaturated fatty acids			
C6	Sorbic acid ($\Delta^{2,4}$-hexadienoic acid)	$CH_3 \cdot CH = CH \cdot CH =$ $CH \cdot COOH$	Occurs as lactone in oil of unripe mountain ash berries
C18	Linoleic acid (*cis-cis*-$\Delta^{9,12}$-octadecadienoic acid)	$CH_3 \cdot (CH_2)_4 \cdot CH$ $\parallel$ $CH \cdot CH_2 \cdot CH$ $\parallel$ $CH \cdot (CH_2)_7 \cdot COOH$	Widely distributed in plant, esp. in linseed, hemp and cottonseed oils. Also in lipids of animals (component of phosphatides, etc.). Essential dietary component
C18	Hiragonic acid ($\Delta^{6,10,14}$-hexadecatrienoic acid)	$CH \cdot (CH_2)_2 \cdot CH = CH \cdot CH_3$ $\parallel$ $CH \cdot (CH_2)_2 \cdot CH = CH \cdot (CH_2)_4 \cdot COOH$	Occurs in sardine oil
C18	α-Linolenic acid ($\Delta^{9,12,15}$)	$CH \cdot CH_2 \cdot CH = CH \cdot CH_2 \cdot CH_3$ $\parallel$ $CH \cdot CH_2 \cdot CH = CH \cdot (CH_2)_7 \cdot COOH$	Occurs in many vegetable oils, esp. drying oils such as linseed oil. Also in traces in animal fats (phosphatides). Essential dietary component
C20	Timnodonic acid ($\Delta^{4,8,12,15,18}$-eicosapentaenoic acid)	$CH_3 \cdot CH = CH \cdot CH_2 \cdot CH = CH$ $\mid$ $CH \cdot (CH_2)_2 \cdot CH = CH \cdot CH_2$ $\parallel$ $CH \cdot (CH_2)_2 \cdot CH = CH \cdot (CH_2)_2 \cdot COOH$	Occurs in sardine oil, cod-liver oil, pilot whale oil and oil from *Squalus sucklei* (spiny dog fish)
C20	Arachidonic acid ($\Delta^{5,8,11,14}$-eicosatetraenoic acid)	$CH_3 \cdot (CH_2)_4 \cdot CH = CH \cdot CH_2 \cdot CH$ $\parallel$ $CH \cdot CH_2 \cdot CH = CH \cdot CH_2 \cdot CH$ $\parallel$ $CH \cdot (CH_2)_3 \cdot COOH$	Occurs in animal lipids (liver, phosphatides). Synthesised in animals from dietary linoleic acid
C-22	Clupanodonic acid ($\Delta^{4,8,12,15,19}$-docosapentaenoic acid)	$CH_3 \cdot CH_2 \cdot CH = CH \cdot (CH_2)_2 \cdot CH$ $\parallel$ $CH \cdot (CH_2)_2 \cdot CH = CH \cdot CH_2 \cdot CH$ $\parallel$ $CH \cdot (CH_2)_2 \cdot CH = CH \cdot (CH_2)_2 \cdot COOH$	Occurs in fish oils
C24	Nisinic acid ($\Delta^{4,8,12,15,18,21}$-tetracosahexaenoic acid)	$CH_3 \cdot CH_2 \cdot CH = CH \cdot CH_2 \cdot CH = CH \cdot CH_2$ $\mid$ $CH \cdot (CH_2)_2 \cdot CH = CH \cdot CH_2 \cdot CH = CH$ $\parallel$ $CH \cdot (CH_2)_2 CH = CH \cdot (CH_2)_2 \cdot COOH$	Occurs in tunny oil
Branched-chain fatty acids			
C4	Isobutyric acid (2-methylpropanoic acid)	CH_3 >$CH \cdot COOH$ CH_3	Occurs free in carob beans (*Ceratonia siliqua*), as ethyl ester in croton oil; also in faeces and as a product of enzymatic breakdown of proteins. Intermediate in metabolism of valine
C5	Isovaleric acid (3-methylbutanoic acid)	CH_3 >$CH \cdot CH_2 \cdot COOH$ CH_3	Occurs in root of valerian, tobacco leaves, volatile oils, depot fat of dolphins and porpoises, and as glyceride in human faeces. Formed from leucine in bacterial degradation of proteins. Intermediate in metabolism of leucine

Table 12.1 (*Continued*)

	Name	Structure	Remarks
C5	Tiglic acid (*cis*-2-methyl-Δ^2-butenoic acid)	$CH_3 \cdot CH = C \cdot COOH$ $\qquad\qquad\quad \mid$ $\qquad\qquad\quad CH_3$	Occurs in croton oil (glyceride), Roman cumin oil (esters) and geranium oils. Intermediate in metabolism of isoleucine

Hydroxy fatty acids

	Name	Structure	Remarks
C18	Ricinoleic acid (*cis*-12-hydroxy-Δ^9-octadecenoic acid)	$CH \cdot CH_2 \cdot CH(OH) \cdot (CH_2)_5 \cdot CH_3$ $\parallel$ $CH \cdot (CH_2)_7 \cdot COOH$	As glyceride, chief constituent of castor oil
C23	2-Hydroxytricosanoic acid	$CH_3 - (CH_2)_{20} \cdot CH(OH) \cdot COOH$	Component of normal brain cerebrosides to an extent of about 7% of total fatty acids
C24	Cerebronic acid (phrenosinic acid, 2-hydroxytetracosanoic acid)	$CH_3 \cdot (CH_2)_{21} \cdot CH(OH) \cdot COOH$	Component of cerebroside phrenosin (cerebron). About 15% of total fatty acids of brain cerebrosides
C24	2-Hydroxynervonic acid (2-hydroxy-Δ^{15}-tetracosenoic acid)	$CH_3 \cdot (CH_2)_7 \cdot CH =$ $CH \cdot (CH_2)_{12} \cdot CH(OH) \cdot COOH$	Component of cerebroside hydroxynervone (of which the isomeric Δ^{17}-acid is also a component). About 12% of total fatty acids of brain cerebrosides

(Reproduced from Geigy Scientific Tables, Ciba-Gergy Ltd, with permission.)

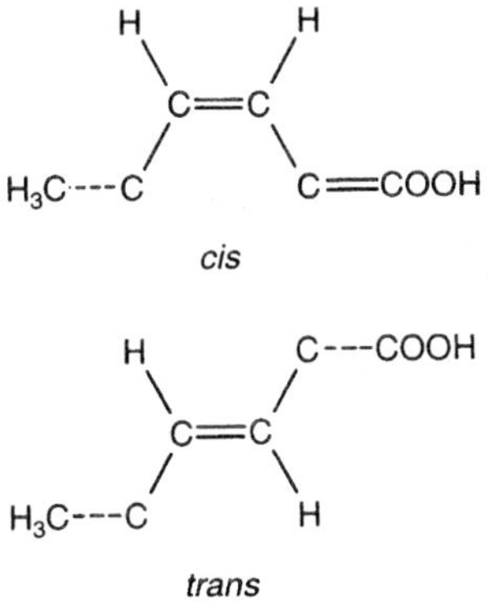

Fig. 12.2 Geometric isomerism in unsaturated fatty acids: *cis* and *trans*.

Saturated fatty acids have a basic formula $CH_3(CH_2)_n COOH$, where n can be any even number from 2 upwards. Almost without exception, dietary fatty acids are formed as even numbers of carbons in an unbranched chain. In naturally occurring lipids the number of carbons in the chain ranges from two to more than 30, the most common fatty acids being palmitic, $n = 14$, and stearic acid, $n = 16$.

Unsaturated fatty acids

Unsaturated fatty acids contain double bonds, and are of nutritional and biological importance. Removal of hydrogen bonds results in ethylenic double bonds, which are unsaturated. The hydrogen atoms on either side of the double bond in the fatty acid molecules are of *cis* or *trans* geometrical configuration (Figure 12.2). These are *stereoisomers*, in that the two forms differ in the arrangement of their atoms in space; *cis* means that the hydrogens are on the same side (the most common configuration for fatty acids in nature), whereas in *trans* the hydrogens are on the opposite side. This results in differing physical properties and response to enzymatic attack.

Monoenoic unsaturated fatty acids
These contain one unsaturated double bond. The more common have an even number of carbon atoms with chain length of 16–22 carbons and a double bond in the *cis* form, often in the delta-9 (Δ^9) position. A double bond causes restriction in the movement of the acyl chain at that point. The *cis* configuration introduces a kink into the

Nomenclature of polyunsaturated fatty acids

There are several nomenclature systems for the polyunsaturated fatty acids. The nomenclature may be based on the saturated parent acid, number of carbon atoms and position of the double bonds. The differences are dictated by whether the numbering is taken from the methyl or carboxyl (COOH) end.

Geneva system

Numbering from the carboxyl end gives the chemical nomenclature and is called the Geneva system. Numbering starts from the carbon 1 carboxyl group (Figure 12.3). For examples:

  oleic acid: *cis*-9-octadecaenoic acid
  elaidic acid: *trans*-9-octadecaenoic acid

A short-hand system indicates the number of double bonds, e.g. stearic acid C18:0, oleic or elaidic acid C18:1. The position of the double bond is given by *cis*-9, 18:1 (oleic acid), or *trans*-9, 18:1 (elaidic acid).

An important aspect of unsaturated fatty acids is the opportunity for isomerism, which may be either *positional* or *geometric*. Positional isomerism occurs when double bonds are located at different positions in the carbon chain. A 16-carbon monounsaturated fatty acid may have positional isomeric forms with double bonds at C7 and C9. These are called Δ^7 and Δ^9; the position of unsaturation is numbered with reference to the first of the pair of carbon atoms between the double bond.

Linoleic acid can be written as *cis* (Δ^{-9}), *cis*(Δ^{-12-18}:2) or (*cis, cis*)9,12-octadecadienoic acid, showing that it is an 18-carbon fatty acid with *cis* double bonds 9 and 12 carbons from the carboxyl end.

n-System

The alternative nutritional or biological system uses the prefix n, or historically ω. In this system the numbering is from the methyl end. The main dietary unsaturated fatty acid families are n-3, n-6, n-7 and n-9. This numbering system is determined by the position of the first double bond from the methyl carbon atom (Figure 12.3). This double bond determines the number of double bonds that can be inserted.

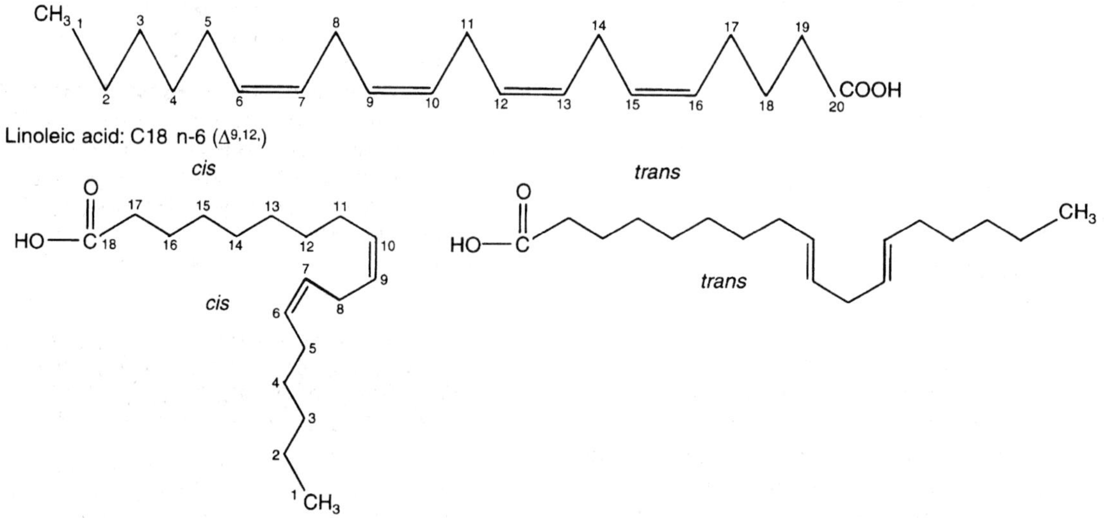

Fig. 12.3   Structure of polyunsaturated fats and numbering systems with the ω- or n-system used in nutrition and delta (Δ) or Geneva system for chemistry. Examples are given of arachidonic acid, C20, n-6, and linoleic acid, C18, n-6. The chemical numbering with the Geneva system is from the carboxyl group, so that the carboxyl group is 1 and the double bonds are indicated by the proximal carbon of the double bond, e.g. C20: the position of a *cis* or *trans* is indicated. The ω- or n-numbering is from the methyl end.

average molecular shape. This means that the *cis* form is less stable thermodynamically and has a lower melting point than the *trans* form.

Polyunsaturated fatty acids

These are derived from monoenoic fatty acids, the position of the second double bond being dictated by the synthetic processes. Mammalian enzymes may only remove hydrogen atoms between an existing double bond and the carboxyl group. Further desaturation has to be preceded by chain elongation. Unsaturated fats with one or more *cis* double bond are more common in natural lipids than are *trans*. The *cis* bond affects the linearity of the chain of methylene groups, in that the molecule folds back on itself. Polyunsaturated fats are susceptible to oxidation but are protected by natural antioxidants, e.g. vitamin E.

ESSENTIAL FATTY ACIDS

The essential fatty acids and their longer chain molecular products are necessary for the maintenance of growth, good health and reproduction. They are important in biological membranes and affect the permeability of the membrane to water, sugars and metal ions, as well as eicosanoid synthesis. All essential fatty acids are polyunsaturated fats, but not all polyunsaturated fatty acids are necessarily essential. Essential fatty acid activity depends on the presence of a *cis*-9, *cis*-12 methylene-interrupted double bond system. If the double bond is converted from *cis* into *trans* this essential biological activity disappears.

The process of desaturation and elongation is important in the tissue synthesis of some polyunsaturated fats. The parent unsaturated fatty acids are extended by alternate desaturation, i.e. the introduction of a double bond and chain-lengthening reactions. There are limited enzymes involved in these reactions and fatty acids from each family compete for the enzymes. Linoleic acid and α-linolenic acid are the preferred substrates. Arachidonic acid, the main product of the elongation and desaturation of linoleic acid, has essential fatty acid activity, but is only essential when insufficient amounts of its precursor, linoleic acid are available.

Humans and other animals are unable to insert double bonds into fatty acids at carbon position 12 and 15 towards the methyl end of the fatty acid chain; therefore, linoleic and α-linolenic acids cannot be synthesised and are essential desaturated fatty acids. There are three distinct, non-interconvertible families of fatty acid. Polyunsaturation is undertaken by three desaturases, Δ4, 5 and 6, which introduce double bonds between carbon atoms 4–5, 5–6 and 6–7. The fatty acids that have a double bond at n-3, n-6, n-7 and n-9 cannot be interconverted in animal tissues.

The parent substrates for desaturation are oleic, linoleic and α-linolenic acids. They give rise to a series of fatty acid families. The essential fatty acids all belong to the n-3 and n-6 groups, but not the n-7 or n-9 groups.

The *n-3 family* originates from α-linolenic acid n-3; α-linolenic acid: *cis, cis, cis*-9, 12,15 (C18:3) is the parent fatty acid. α-Linolenic acid (C18:3, n-3) can add methylene groups to increase the chain length to eicosapentaenoic acid.

C18:3,9,12,15
C18:4,6,9,12,15
C20:4,8,11,14,17
C20:5,8,11,14,17
C20:5,7,10,13,16,19
C22:4,7,10,13,16,19

The n-6 *family* originates from linoleic acid n-6; linoleic acid: *cis, cis*-9,12 (C18:2) is the parent fatty acid, with the n-6 numbering from the methyl end. Linoleic acid can be extended to gamma (γ)-linolenic and arachidonic acid (C-20:4, n-6).

C18:3,9,12,15
C18: 4,6,9,12,15
C20:4,8,11,14,17
C20:5,8,11,14,17
C20: 5,7,10,13,16,19
C22:4,7,10,13,16,19

The *n-9 family* originates from oleic acid n-9; a non-essential fatty acid family. Oleic acid (*cis*-9,C18:1) is the parent fatty acid. Oleic acid can increase the chain length to become eicosatrienoic acid.

C18:2,6,9
C20:2,8,11
C20:3,5,8,11

C22:3,7,10,13
C22:4,7,10,13

Deficiency of essential fatty acids in adults is rare, but has been seen in children fed virtually fat-free diets. The skin abnormalities were those previously seen in experimental animals, with dermatosis of the skin, increased water permeability, increased sebum secretion and decreased epithelial hypoplasia. The n-3 fatty acids (parent α-linolenic acid) are important components of brain and retinal lipid tissue. These fatty acids cannot be synthesised in the animal and their dietary provision may be particularly important in early life for brain development.

If there is a deficiency of essential fatty acids then non-essential fatty acids are preferentially metabolised. The endproducts of non-essential fatty acid extension cannot, however, function in cell membranes or in eicosanoid precursors. The ratio of eicosatrienoic acid (all *cis*-5,8,11; C20:3 from oleic acid) to arachidonic acid (all *cis*-5,8,11,14; C20:4 from linoleic acid) in the plasma (the triene:tetraene ratio) is an indirect biochemical index of essential fatty acid deficiency. The optimum ratio should be between 0.2 and 0.4. It is possible that *trans* fatty acids may influence the metabolism of essential fatty acids by inhibiting desaturases.

Conditionally indispensable fatty acids

At least 23 fatty acids are classified as essential. To some this is confusing and complex. The symptoms of essential fatty acid deficiency depend on age, nutrient intake and health status. The growing baby and growing infant have greater needs than the

---

Fatty acid deficiency

When animals are made deficient in fatty acids the body weight decreases, the heart enlarges and there is decreased capillary resistance. Cholesterol accumulates in the lungs, and endocrine organs alter, in that the thyroid gland shrinks and abnormalities in reproduction have been described in both sexes. The essential fatty acid activity of any one fatty acid is measured by restoration of normality of rats deprived of essential fatty acids. This consists of growth, restoration of water permeability and normality of skin.

Desaturation of fatty acids: the basis of essentiality

The initial desaturation introduces a double bond at position 6 into the first member of each fatty acid family. The desaturation enzyme is common to all of these processes. The order of affinity of the substrate for Δ^6-desaturase is 18:3 < 18:2 < 18:1. Linoleic acid is converted into arachidonic acid by this enzyme. If the absolute amount of linoleic acid is low or absorption is abnormal, then deficiency problems arise. Alternatively, deficiency may result from genetic disorders, e.g. a lack of specific desaturase enzymes. These include rare diseases such as Reye's syndrome and the Prader–Willi syndrome. There may also be reduced Δ^6-desaturase activity as a result of normal biological variation. γ-Linolenic acid bypasses this enzyme system. If the diet contains small amounts of linoleic acid but a massive amount of other fatty acids, the Δ6 desaturase system may be overwhelmed. If there is insufficient linoleic acid, then oleic acid is extended to a 20-carbon atom structure, *cis*-5,8,11-eicosatrienose, instead of arachidonic acid.

---

elderly. To some extent the problem with definition is solved by the use of the term polyunsaturated fatty acids (PUFAs), which is a collective term for both n-3 and n-6 fatty acids. There is interconversion within the n-3 and within the n-6 PUFAs, so each of the constituent n-3 and n-6 PUFAs is not essential in its own right. It has been suggested that the term conditional be introduced to define the varying need for these fatty acids.

Hydrogenation of fatty acids

An important effect on the fatty acid composition of food is industrial processing, particularly catalytic hydrogenation, which improves the stability and physical properties of the fat by reducing the overall fatty acid unsaturation. The total number of double bonds in the fatty acid molecule is reduced and the double bonds are shifted along the hydrocarbon chain.

The biohydrogenation of fats occurs commonly in the rumen of ruminants. Polyunsaturated fatty acids of plant origin, e.g. linoleic and α-linolenic acid, can undergo partial or complete hydrogenation by anaerobic rumen bacteria.

Trans fatty acids

Fatty acids with *trans* bonds may be monounsaturated or polyunsaturated, with *cis* and *trans* bonds within the same molecules. The biohydrogenation of fats in the rumen of ruminants can result in the production of *trans* fatty acids. In addition to occurring naturally, *trans* fatty acids can be formed during the partial hydrogenation of a *cis* unsaturated fatty acid. This can occur either biologically or industrially. Dairy product *trans* fatty acids are mainly C14 to C18, particularly vaccenic acid (*trans*-11, C18:1) and elaidic acid (*trans*-9, C18:1). Industrially produced *trans* fatty acids are more complex and more variable in type.

The *cis* double bonds can isomerise to produce fatty acids with one or more *trans* bonds, as well as acids with both *cis* and *trans* bonds. The double bond system, *trans*, may be separated by one or more methylene groups, or may be placed between adjacent pairs of carbon atoms. The centres of unsaturation are said to be *conjugated*.

Conjugated fatty acids

Conjugated linoleic acid is a collective term for a mix of geometric and positional isomers of octadecadienoic acid (18:2), where the double bonds are conjugated rather than separated by methylene as in linoleic acid.

In linoleic acid the arrangement is of a double bond followed by two single bonds then another double bond:

–C=C–C–C=C–

whereas in conjugated linoleic acid the arrangement is of two double bonds separated by one single bond.

–C=C–C=C–

This fatty acid is an intermediate in the conversion of linoleic acid to oleic acid by ruminant bacteria. It is of interest as a health-promoting fatty acid.

Cyclic fatty acids

These are uncommon but important metabolic inhibitors, and are found in many bacteria, plants and fungi.

Branched-chain fatty acids

Chain branch and substitution is noted by prefix br-16:0 for branched-chain hexadecaenoic acid or ho-16:0 for hydroxypalmitic acid. Bacteria are a source of branched-chain fatty acids which are usually saturated, although these can also occur in animal fats. The presence of a branched chain lowers the melting point. Butter fats, and bacterial and skin lipids contain significant amounts of branched-chain fatty acids.

Oxyacids

These are major components of surface waxes, cutin and suberin of plants.

Dietary fatty acids

Dietary lipids will contain saturated, monounsaturated and polyunsaturated fatty acids. The amount and type will differ from food source to food source.

- Mammalian animal storage fats are predominantly saturated (e.g. palmitic acid) and monounsaturated (e.g. oleic acid) fatty acids.
- Fats from ruminant animals contain monounsaturated (e.g. stearic acid) fatty acids as a consequence of the action of rumen desaturases.
- Milk fat contains a high proportion of saturated fatty acids with a chain length of 12 carbon atoms or less (C4–C8). Milk from cows, sheep and goats is relatively rich in short- and medium-chain fatty acids and *trans* and branched-chain fatty acids. The proportions vary throughout the season. Human milk is somewhat richer in oleic acid than is ruminant milk, and contains 7% of linoleic acid.
- Warm-blooded animal lipids are predominantly unsaturated C16, C18, C20 and C22 fatty acids with small amounts of short-chain C4 and C8 fatty acids. The saturated fatty acid palmitic acid (10–18% of the total fatty acids) and the unsaturated oleic acid predominate and are found in hard fats with a low melting point.
- Fish and marine animal oils are rich in polyunsaturated fatty acids of the n-3 family, including C20 and C22 with up to six double bonds (Table 12.2).
- In plant seeds oils, oleic acid and palmitic acid are predominant, with linoleic acid a minor

Table 12.2 Fatty acids in vegetable and fish oils

Vegetable oils	Fish oils
n-6	n-3
18:2 linoleic acid	18:3 α-linolenic acid
18:3	18:4
20:3	20:4
20:4 arachidonic acid	20:5 eicosapentanoenoic acid
22:4	22:5
22:5	22:6

component. A diet rich in linoleic (n-6) and α-linolenic acid (n-3 family) can thus be obtained by eating vegetable seed oils. Arachidonic acid (n-6) is not present in vegetable oils but is synthesised from linoleic acid; meat is a good dietary source. Erucic acid (C22:1) is the principal fatty acid in rapeseed oil, an important temperate crop despite the erucic acid being toxic to the myocardium (cardiotoxic). A new variety of rapeseed, cambra, contains only 2% erucic acid.

Dietary trans *fatty acids*
The British diet contains on average 6–7 g of *trans* unsaturated fatty acids, half of which come from industrial hydrogenation and the remainder from ruminant products.

Some 6% of the dietary fat intake in the British diet comes from *trans* fatty acids, in milk, butter and other dairy products, margarine, meat and meat products, fish, eggs and cereal-based foods. These important sources of *trans* fatty acids provide approximately half of the *trans* unsaturated fatty acids in the diet. Ruminant fat may also contain isomeric fatty acids.

Some seed oils have a significant fatty acid content of *trans* unsaturation, although this is not common. All green plants contain small amounts of *trans*-3-hexadecenoic acid.

Other important sources are the industrially hydrogenated fish and vegetables oils, used in the manufacture of margarine, frying oils, shortenings and specialty products.

Hydrogenated fish oils may yield longer chain *trans* monoenoic acids, C18 to C22. Vegetable oils producing *trans* acid include soya bean, rapeseed, sunflower seed and palm kernel. Soya bean oil may contain 30–50% of *trans* fatty acids of the C18 series, particularly *cis,trans*- and *trans,cis*-dienoic acid.

In general, *trans* fatty acids do not possess essential fatty acid activity; a small amount in the diet is unlikely to cause any pathology.

GLYCEROL TRIESTERS

The glycerol triesters are the esters of glycerol, substituted at the three alcohols to form three distinct classes of lipid: triacylglycerol, phospholipids and waxes. The principal substitutions in the glycerol esters are fatty acids.

> Glycerol (1,2,3-propanetriol) is the alcohol present in the natural triester glycerides, phospholipids and waxes. The formula of glycerol is:
>
> $HOCH_2CHOHCH_2OH$
>
> 1 CH_2OH
> |
> 2 $CHOH$
> |
> 3 CH_2OH

> In triacylglycerols of vegetable origin the C2 position is esterified to a C18 unsaturated fatty acid; in pig triacylglycerols the C2 position is occupied by palmitic acid. In rodent fats the distribution is random. Many other natural triacylglycerols have an unsaturated fatty acid in the C2 position. The C1 position is usually occupied by a saturated fatty acid. Over 50% of the triacylglycerol fatty acids are unsaturated and 16:0 fatty acid is the most common saturated fatty acid.

Triacylglycerols

These are esters of glycerol and fatty acids (Figure 12.4). The distribution of fatty acids in the C1, C2 or C3 position varies. The numbering C1, C2, C3 is based on a conventional L-configuration, when this notation is used the letters sn (stereospecific numbering) are used. This distribution of fatty acids gives a wide range of fatty acid ester triacylglycerols from different sources.

The type and quantity of dietary fatty acids are important in determining the proportions of fatty acids in the ester. On average, the fatty acid composition of triacylglycerides is approximately

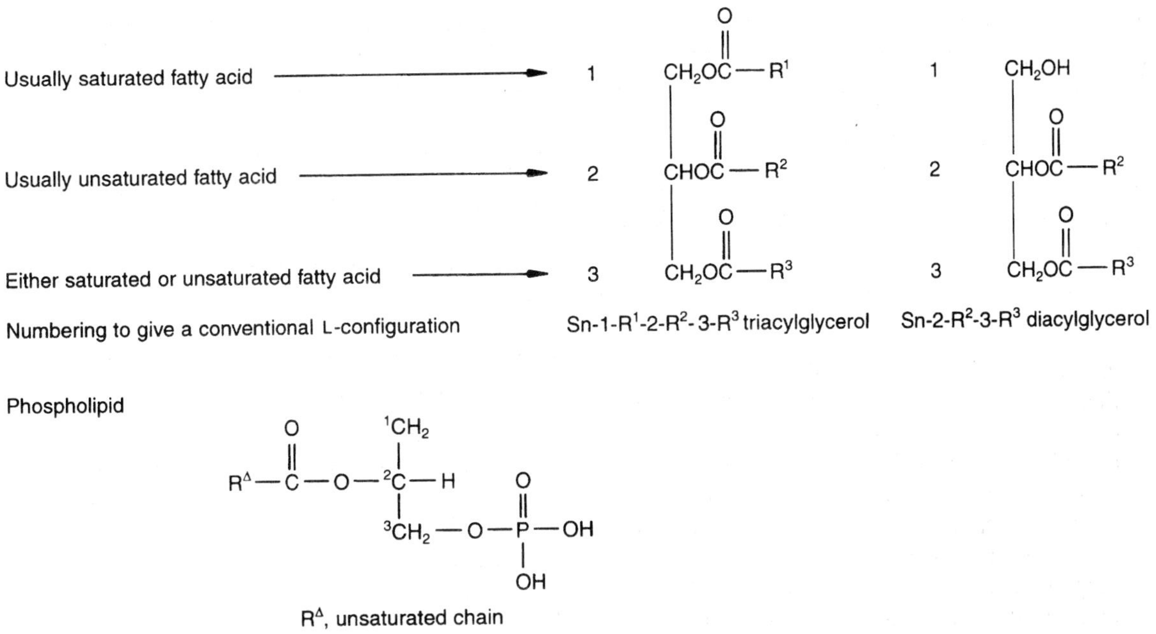

Usually saturated fatty acid ⟶ 1

Usually unsaturated fatty acid ⟶ 2

Either saturated or unsaturated fatty acid ⟶ 3

Numbering to give a conventional L-configuration

$$
\begin{array}{l}
1 \quad CH_2OC\!-\!R^1 \ (=O) \\
2 \quad CHOC\!-\!R^2 \ (=O) \\
3 \quad CH_2OC\!-\!R^3 \ (=O)
\end{array}
$$

Sn-1-R^1-2-R^2-3-R^3 triacylglycerol

$$
\begin{array}{l}
1 \quad CH_2OH \\
2 \quad CHOC\!-\!R^2 \ (=O) \\
3 \quad CH_2OC\!-\!R^3 \ (=O)
\end{array}
$$

Sn-2-R^2-3-R^3 diacylglycerol

Phospholipid

$$
R^\Delta\!-\!C(=O)\!-\!O\!-\!{}^2C(H)\!-\!{}^1CH_2
$$
$$
{}^3CH_2\!-\!O\!-\!P(=O)(OH)\!-\!OH
$$

R$^\Delta$, unsaturated chain

Fig. 12.4 Triacylglycerol: structure of acylglycerols and phospholipids.

20% palmitic acid, 7% palmitoleic, 50% oleic and 10% linoleic acid.

Medium-chain triglycerides prepared from coconut oil contain C8:0 and C10:0 fatty acids. They are important in clinical nutrition as they are readily hydrolysed by pancreatic lipase and pass to the liver in the portal vein as fatty acids. This provides a ready form of energy to patients with problems in digesting triglycerides, which may lead to steatorrhoea.

Physical properties of triacylglycerides
The physical properties of acyl lipids are affected by the individual fatty acids. The melting point of the triacylglycerides is important. Cell membranes do not function when the fatty acids are crystalline. For mammals the critical temperature is 37°C and for poikilotherms anything from −10 to over 100°C, the difference between the requirements of a warm and cold living environment. *Trans* fatty acids in triacylglycerols pack together more closely than those of *cis* isomers and this affects the melting point. A *trans* bond has little effect on the conformation of the chain, although the physical properties are much closer to those of a saturated fatty

acid. Oleic acid with one *cis* bond in the chain has a melting point of 13°C, whereas elaidic acid, the *trans* isomer of oleic acid, has a melting point of 44°C.

Phospholipids

These are derivatives of phosphatidic acid, esterified with phosphoric acid on the C3 position and with fatty acids on the Cl (usually saturated) and C2 (unsaturated) positions. Phosphatidyl inositols are esters of a cyclic derivative of glucose. The cardiolipins (phosphatidylglycerol and diphosphatidylglycerols) are esters of phosphatides with an additional glycerol and are predominantly linoleic acid esters. Sphingomyelins contain a dihydroxy amine, sphingosine.

Wax esters

These are esters of long-chain fatty acids with long-chain fatty alcohols, with the formula R′COOR″. These waxes are found in some bacteria, the oil of the sperm whale, the flesh oils of several deep-sea

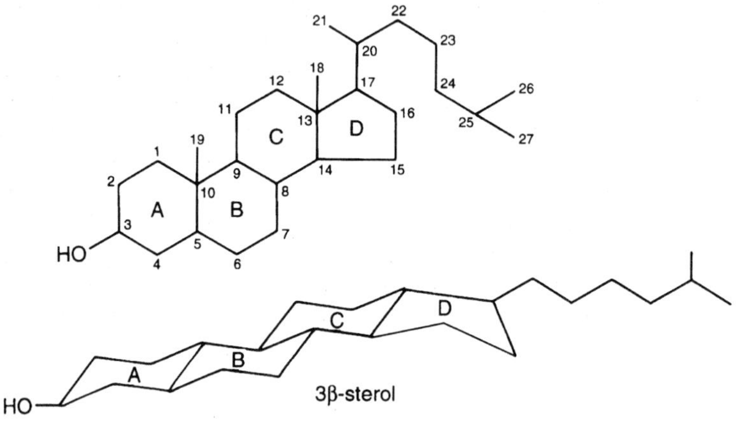

Fig. 12.5 Structure of cholesterol showing the numbering system and the flat, geometric structure of the molecule.

fishes and zooplankton. They are poorly hydrolysed by the pancreatic lipase of the human digestive system and are of little nutritive value.

CHOLESTEROL AND STEROLS

The sterol ring system is an important hydrophobic structure and is widespread through biology. The alcohol moieties can form esters with fatty acids.

Cholesterol (Figure 12.5) is found in all animal tissues and is a structural component of cell walls and membranes, and a precursor of bile acids, adrenal and gonadal hormones, and vitamin D. It can accumulate in atheromatous lesions of arterial walls.

Cholesterol belongs to the family of steroidal alcohols containing between 27 and 30 carbon atoms. All possess the 17-carbon cyclopentanophenanthrene ring. All contain a 3-β-hydroxyl group and an endocyclic double bond, usually in the 5,6 position, with a side-chain which has varying degrees of saturation and unsaturation. Cholesterol exists as the free sterol or as esters with fatty acids. The more common sterols are found in higher animals and plants, with the exception of ergosterol, found in yeasts. Sterols may, however, be found in fungi, algae and marine invertebrates. Other sterols include:

- coprostanol (5-β-cholestanol), 5-β-cholestan-3β-ol
- stigmasterol (24-α-ethylcholesta-5:22-dien-3β-ol): widely distributed in plants, but only calabar and soya beans contain sufficient to serve as sources
- ergosterol (24-β-methylcholesta-5:7:22-trien-3β-ol): occurs in yeast, together with 5-α:6-dihydroergosterol. Ergosterol contains one more carbon atom than cholesterol
- lumisterol (9-β:10-α-ergosterol), pyroergocalciferol (9-α:10-α-ergosterol) and isopyroergocalciferol (9-β:10-β-ergosterol)
- ergocalciferol (vitamin D$_2$), 5,6-*cis*-ergocalciferol and 5:6-*cis*-cholecalciferol (vitamin D$_3$), the natural vitamin D of fish oils: derived from 7-dehydrocholesterol by ultraviolet irradiation
- brassicasterol (24-β-methylcholesta-5:22-dien-3-β-ol): occurs in rapeseed oil
- campasterol (24-α-methylcholest-5-en-3-β-ol): obtained from rapeseed oil, soya bean oil and wheat germ oil
- spinasterol: a 7:22 diene found in spinach and alfalfa
- sitosterol: the five sitosterols are the most widely distributed plant sterols. β-Sitosterol (24-α-ethylcholest-5-en-3β-ol) is the principal sterol of cottonseed and calycanthus oil and is also found in soya bean oil, wheat germ oil, corn oil, rye germ oil, cinchona wax and crêpe rubber
- fucosterol and sargasterol: found in freshwater green and brown algae. Fucosterol is 24-ethyli-

denecholest-5-en-3β-ol and sargasterol is the 20-α-methyl isomer

- mycosterols: are sterols originating in fungi and include zymosterol (5-α-cholesta-8:25-dien-3β-ol). Acosterol and fecosterol are minor sterols with double bonds at the 8:9 position and episterol has the double bond at the 7:8 position. Marine sterols vary from species to species; gastropods have cholesterol as the principal sterol, whereas pelecypods (bivalves) contain a complex of C28 and C29 sterols. These include chalinasterol [24(28)methylene-cholesterol], which is found in sponges, oysters, clams and sea anemones.

FUNCTIONS OF LIPIDS

Lipids have structural, storage and metabolic functions, although individual lipids may have several different roles at different times, or even simultaneously.

Structural lipids

Lipids play an integral part in biological membranes. The importance of lipids in such barriers lies in their ability to prevent the movement of water and other molecules, at surfaces and in membranes, between one environment and another.

All living cells contain a membrane providing a structure in which many metabolic reactions take place. In mammals the lipids involved are the glycerophospholipids and unesterified free cholesterol, while in plants the glycosylglycerides are predominant, especially in the chloroplasts. The importance of the compounds involved in membranes is the distribution of the hydrophilic groups close to hydrophobic groupings. These are called amphiphilic structures.

The composition of lipid molecules on either side of many membranes (membrane asymmetry) is quite different. In lipids that are esters of fatty acids the hydrocarbon chain of the fatty acid is the hydrophobic moiety. The esterified fatty acid chain plays a major part in determining the physical properties of these lipids. An increase in the number of double bonds determines the degree of unsaturation and lowers the melting point of the acyl chains. Within families of saturated fatty acids the melting point is also lowered as the chain length decreases or when the chain is branched.

The membranes of storage organs, e.g. adipose tissue, the liver, muscle and kidney mitochondria, contain n-6 fatty acids, particularly arachidonic acid. Nervous tissue, the retina and the reproductive organs have a substantial content of longer chain fatty acid with five or six double bonds (arachidonic and docosahexaenoic acid) derived from both the n-3 and n-6 families. Brain and nervous tissue lipids are significantly in the form of sphingolipids, the alcohol being sphingosine rather than glycerol. The brain in the newborn baby is 12% of body weight, whereas it is 2% of the adult's weight. The brain is 12% lipids, the composition of which differs in grey matter, white matter and myelin. One-fifth to one-third, however, is phospholipid tissue, and the cholesterol content is between 0.7 and 1.6%, depending on the brain tissue. The provision and synthesis of lipids, including cholesterol in the brain and nervous tissue, are important in the growing foetus, baby and infant, significantly in late intrauterine life and early infancy.

The biosynthesis of eicosanoids (which includes prostaglandins) requires the PUFA arachidonic acid, of the n-6 family.

The structural lipids that are eaten as part of animal and plant tissues are phospholipids and glycolipids. They are, by the nature of their role in the cell, enriched in PUFAs.

Storage lipids

In humans the main reservoir of lipids is adipose tissue. Milk fat is an energy store for the benefit of

> Carbohydrate stores provide only half as much energy per gram as lipid stores and contain an equal amount of water. When lipid stores are metabolised more metabolic water is released per gram, but less per molecule of adenosine triphosphate (ATP), compared with carbohydrate (0.132 water molecules compared with 0.12, respectively).

the newborn mammal, and the egg-yolk lipids are a store for the developing chick embryo. Lipids are in a dynamic state and constantly being broken down, removed from the tissue or replaced. Lipids transported as lipoproteins are taken into tissues where they may, depending on the requirement of the body, be stored as energy reserves in the adipose tissues, incorporated into the structural lipids of membranes or oxidised to supply energy.

Lipids consumed as food are derived from the adipose tissues of animals, fish and seed oils. The high energy density of triacylglycerols makes them ideal as long-term fuel stores and resources. The fatty acid composition of storage lipids is very variable and depends on the composition of the diet.

The storage fats of monogastric animals are influenced by the fat content of their diet. The adipose tissue of ruminants is determined by the bacteria of the rumen, with the production of saturated and monounsaturated acids, although unusual fatty acids, both *trans* and branched, are also produced. If the diet of pigs and poultry is derived from carbohydrates, then the subsequent synthesis of fat results in predominantly saturated and monounsaturated fats. The inclusion of vegetable oils such as soya bean oil in their diet can increase the linoleic acid content of the carcass.

Fish oils are obtained from either (i) lean fish, e.g. cod, in which reserve oils are stored as triacylglycerols in the liver; or (ii) fatty fish, e.g. mackerel, in which the oils are stored in the flesh. The fatty acids are dependent on season and diet, but are predominantly PUFAs, n-3 type, of 20 or more carbons in length.

Storage triacylglycerols used commercially in seed oils come from fleshy fruit, e.g. the exocarp of the olive or seed endosperm of rape. The fatty acids vary with seed source; in rapeseed oil oleic acid predominates, whereas lupin and evening primrose contain γ-linolenic acid.

Lean meats contain arachidonic acid (20:4,n-6). The storage fats in meat are largely saturated and monounsaturated fatty acids. Plant leaf fatty acids are predominantly palmitic acid, palmitoleic acid, oleic acid, linoleic acid and α-linolenic acid.

Only 12 oil-bearing seeds are important commercially, and only two of these are used for industrial purposes, linseed oil (rich in α-linolenic acid) and castor oil (ricinoleic acid, a laxative).

RECOMMENDED INTAKE OF FATTY ACIDS

Adults

Dietary expert committees have recommended that the fat content of the diet should be reduced to 30–35% of energy, unsaturated fatty acids should be increased and saturated fatty acids should provide only 10% of food energy. A Report of the British Nutrition Foundation Task Force in 1992 suggested that this is achievable by eating fewer meat products, dairy products and baked foods, and more oily fish (herring, mackerel, sardine and salmon), fruit, vegetables and wholemeal cereals. Saturated fat should be replaced by starch in the form of bread, cereals, fruit and vegetables.

The properties of *trans* fatty acids and their contribution to the diet are not fully understood, although COMA (the UK Committee on Medical Aspects of Food and Nutrition Policy) suggested that they should not contribute more than 2% of total fat intake.

The body stores of essential fatty acids are measured indirectly. The target ratio of unsaturated to saturated blood conjugated fatty acids should be more than 0.45, even approaching 1.0, with a mixture of n-6 and n-3 polyunsaturated fats and monooleic acid. The n-3 *cis* PUFAs should provide 0.2% of total energy intake and n-6 1.0%, and *cis*-monounsaturated fatty acids should provide 12% of daily total energy intake. The target is a plasma cholesterol concentration of less than 5.2 mmol/l (200 mg%).

Intakes of essential fatty acids in Great Britain have been suggested to be 10 g/kg of food/day (2% energy intake) of n-6 fatty acids and 1–2 g/day of n-3 fatty acids. The main daily dietary sources of n-6 fatty acids are vegetables, fruits and nuts (3.0 g), cereal products (2.6 g) and vegetable oils (2.4 g). The main sources of n-3 fatty acids are vegetables (0.4 g), meat and meat products (0.3 g), cereal products (0.3 g) and fat spreads (0.3 g). Most adult Western diets provide 15–18 g of essential fatty acids and, in general, healthy individuals have body reserves of 1000–2000 g in their adipose tissue.

Babies

Human milk is rich in linoleic acid (C18:2), and is important for the development of infants and their brain structure. The linoleic acid content of milk lipids varies in amount (3–12%), depending on maternal dietary intake and possibly smoking habit. α-Linolenic acid (C18:3) makes up 0.4% of human milk and docosahexaenoic acid (DHA 22:6) 0.2%. Infant formula feeds do not always meet these requirements.

Pregnant and lactating women

Requirements in these women are similar to other adult recommendations.

n-6/n-3 Polyunsaturated fatty acid ratios

In human milk the ratio of n-6 to n-3 PUFAs is in the order of 11:1. In practice, the important ratio is of the essential fatty acids, linoleic acid (n-6) to α-linolenic acid (n-3) (see text describing fatty acid nutrients). These two compete for the enzyme Δ6-desaturase; the ideal ratio is not known, but in adults a ratio of 5:1 has been recommended.

Monounsaturated fatty acids

An intake of total monounsaturated fats of 15% (oleic acid 12%) of total energy intake has been recommended for adults. All of these dietary proposals should be accompanied by an adequate intake of antioxidants, e.g. vitamin E, selenium, ascorbic acid and β-carotene. Vitamin E intake is linked to unsaturated fatty acids, especially linoleic acid, and is stored in similar locations. The dietary recommendation is 0.4 mg vitamin E/g linoleic acid.

Other lipids

The other lipids, e.g. cholesterol, are adequately synthesised by the body, and there are no dietary requirements for these.

KEY POINTS

1. Dietary fat is a heterogeneous mixture of lipids, predominantly triglycerides, but also phospholipids and sterols.
2. Fatty acids have a basic formula $CH_3(CH_2)n-COOH$, where n can be any even number from 2 upwards. Unsaturated fatty acids are important nutritionally and biologically. There are several nomenclatures for the unsaturated fatty acids which may be based on the saturated parent acid, the number of carbon atoms and position of the double bonds. The differences are dictated by whether the numbering is taken from the methyl or the carboxyl end.
3. The four main dietary unsaturated fatty acid families are n-3, n-6, n-7 and n-9. This numbering system is determined by the position of the first double bond from the methyl carbon atom.
4. The essential fatty acids and their longer chain molecular products are necessary for the maintenance of growth, good health and reproduction. The essential fatty acids all belong to the n-3 and n-6 groups, linoleic acid (n-6) and α-linolenic acid (n-3). The fatty acids that have a double bond at n-3, n-6, cannot be synthesised by humans and are therefore essential in the diet.
5. Glycerol (1,2,3-propanetriol) is the alcohol present in the natural triester glycerides, phospholipids and waxes.
6. Lipids have structural, storage and metabolic functions, although individual lipids may have several different roles.
7. Structural lipids are important at surfaces and in membranes, functioning as barriers between one environment and another. Such barriers can exclude water and other molecules.
8. Food fats are the storage fats of animals and plants. The high energy densities of triacylglycerols make them ideal as long-term fuel sources. The fatty acid composition of storage lipids is very variable and depends on the composition of the diet.
9. Cholesterol is a structural component of cell walls and membranes, and a precursor of bile

acids, adrenal and gonadal hormones and vitamin D. It can also accumulate in atheromatous lesions of arterial walls. Cholesterol belongs to the family of steroidal alcohols containing between 27 and 30 carbon atoms, and exists as the free sterol or as esters with fatty acids.

10. The more common sterols are found in higher animals and plants, with the exception of ergosterol, found in yeasts. Sterols are also found in fungi, algae and marine invertebrates.

11. The fat content of the diet should be 30–35% of the dietary energy content. Unsaturated fatty acids should replace saturated fatty acids and provide 10% of food energy. The ratio of unsaturated to saturated fatty acids should be more than 0.45, even approaching 1.0; a mixture of n-6 and n-3 polyunsaturated fats and mono-oleic acid should be a target. Human milk is rich in linoleic acid (C18:2, n-6), and is important for the development of infants.

THINKING POINTS

1. Fatty acids are important as energy sources, but the essential fatty acids are also indispensable as precursors of biologically important chemicals.
2. It is important to sustain an adequate intake of essential fatty acids.
3. Fatty acids as triacylglycerols are important energy stores.
4. Sterols are synthesised by the body and are important in cell-wall membrane structure and as hormones.

NEED TO UNDERSTAND

The difference between essential fatty acids and those fatty acids that are substantial energy sources.

FURTHER READING

Cunnane, S.C. (2000) The conditional nature of the dietary need for polyunsaturates: a proposal to reclassify 'essential fatty acids' as 'conditionally-indispensable' or 'conditionally-dispensable' fatty acids. *British Journal of Nutrition*, **84**, 803–12.

Gurr, M.I. and Harwood, J.L. (1991) *Lipids*. Chapman & Hall, London.

Kritchevsky, D. (2000) Antimutagenic and other effects of conjugated linoleic acid. *British Nutrition Bulletin*, **25**, 25–7.

Willett, WC., Stampfer, M.J., Manson, J.E. and Colditz (1987) *Trans Fatty Acids*, British Nutrition Foundation, London.

WEBSITES

www.acsh.org/nutrition/index.html   American Council on Science and Health Nutrition

www.lipidsonline.org   Lipids online

13

Carbohydrates

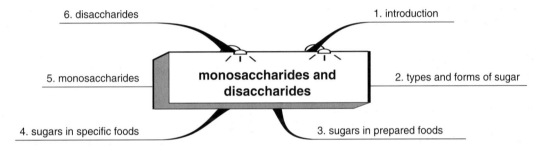

6. disaccharides

1. introduction

5. monosaccharides

monosaccharides and disaccharides

2. types and forms of sugar

4. sugars in specific foods

3. sugars in prepared foods

Fig. 13.1   Section outline.

INTRODUCTION

Carbohydrates are an important source of energy in all human diets. The amount in the diet varies according to the economy, the range being 40–80% of calorie intake. Carbohydrates are synthesised from carbon dioxide and water. The primary structures are monosaccharide sugars (Figure 13.2), which may dimerise to disaccharides, e.g. sucrose, or polymerise extensively to form polysaccharides, e.g. cellulose, pectin and hemicellulose. In humans, carbohydrates are central to energy utilisation as glucose and to storage as starch, a polymeric carbohydrate.

TYPES AND FORMS OF SUGAR

Sugars give sweetness to food. Sugars, either are naturally present or added, supplement the flavour of foods that are not particularly sweet in themselves, e.g. milk, fresh vegetables, sauces, canned vegetables, mayonnaise, breakfast cereals, and canned and packet soups. They are also important in soft drinks.

Sugars contribute to existing flavours and generate new flavours. They can be used by yeast and bacteria as a substrate in fermented products. Sugars can also have a preservative action in jam and contribute to the shelf-life of cakes.

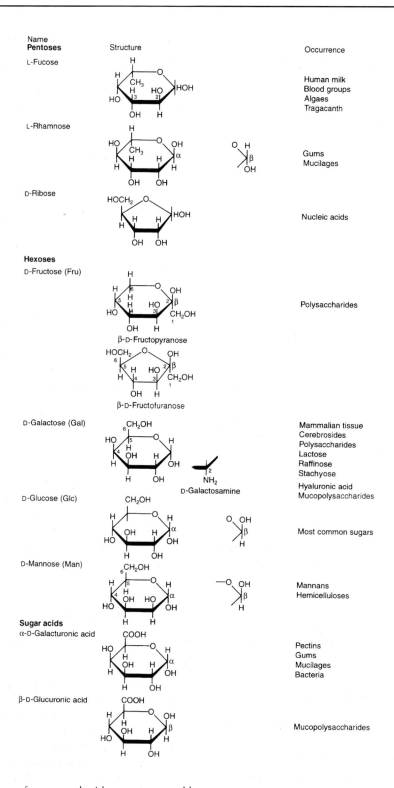

Fig. 13.2 Structure of monosaccharides, pentoses and hexoses.

Sugar occur in various ways in food:

- from natural constituents of such foods as fruit, milk, vegetables and honey
- as an essential ingredient of prepared foods, preserved sweets, chocolates and cakes
- as an optional additive such as sucrose added to tea, coffee and other foods.

The attraction of sucrose is in the amount that can be taken, whether as a concentrate or diluted in the bulk of food.

Cane sugar

Sugar cane is grown in tropical countries between 25° north and south of the equator. The crop takes some 9–18 months to grow to a height of 3–5 m, and ripens during the cooler and drier parts of the year. This is a very energy-efficient crop, three times as efficient as potatoes and seven times as efficient as wheat. Four endproducts of sucrose manufacturing are obtained:

- **raw sugar**: subsequently converted to refined syrup and sugar
- **cane molasses**: the non-crystallisable residue from the production of raw sugar which is used for cattle feed, fermented to alcohol or converted into rum or fuel. It can also be used for growing yeast and may be cleaned up, as treacle
- **bagasse**: cane fibre used for fuel, paper and board
- **filter press mud**: used as fertiliser.

Raw sugar is converted into refined sugar by removing the colour and residual impurities.

Beet sugar

Beet sugar is a temperate crop which is very energy efficient in growth. The sucrose is extracted by diffusion from the roots after slicing the beet. The endproducts are:

- **sucrose**: usually refined, white and ready for consumption
- **beet molasses**: normally fermented and used for cattle feed
- **beet pulp**: used for animal feed.

Another source of sugar is gur or gaggary, which is made in West Africa, India and Pakistan. This is a crude mixture of sucrose, crystals and syrups obtained by extracting and concentrating sugar cane juice in an open pan over a fire. The juice is concentrated and solidified in coconut shells or wooden moulds. Variants on this include panella and khandsari sugar.

Other speciality sugars

- **Demerara sugar** is a golden-brown sugar produced in Demerara, Guyana. It contains residual molasses, giving flavour and slight moisture. London Demerara is a brand name for white sugar with added molasses. Muscovados or Barbados sugar contains molasses to give a treacle flavour.
- **Caster sugar** has smaller crystals than ordinary granulated sugar, and icing sugar is a finely powdered sugar produced by granulating sugar through a hammer mill.
- **Lump sugar** is a soft, crystalline mixture of refined and partially refined cane sugar.
- **Transformed sugar** is a patented process (Tate & Lyle) which has reduced bulk, is non-sticky, and is used in dry mixing and vending packs.

Other sugars

Glucose is made from a high-conversion glucose syrup. The amount of added glucose consumed in the diet is small. Fructose and maltose may be obtained from high fructose and high maltose syrups. Lactose is extracted from whey, a by-product of cheese manufacture. Most lactose is consumed as milk.

Syrups and mixtures

During the course of the manufacture of sucrose, several sucrose syrups are produced.

- **Molasses**: in the production of sucrose, impurities and lime are removed and a clear solution is obtained, which is then concentrated. Sugar crystals and a mother liquor, called molasses, when partially refined and blended, produce treacle. Golden syrup is prepared from a mixture of by-products of sugar cane refining, which are further refined, decolourised and concentrated.

- **Invert syrup**: this is a mixture of glucose and fructose in equal parts. When (+)-sucrose is hydrolysed by dilute aqueous acid or by the action of the enzyme invertase (from yeast) the result is equal amounts of D-(+)-glucose and D-(+)-fructose. This hydrolysis is accompanied by a change in the sign of optical rotation from positive to negative, the reaction is called the inversion of (+)-sucrose. The levorotatory mixture of D-(+)-glucose and D-(+)-fructose is called invert sugar. It has a chemical composition like that of honey, but without any of the congeners that give honey its particular flavour. Invert syrup is sweeter than sucrose syrup and is used in the food industry, especially in brewing. It is derived from warming a solution of sucrose with a mild acid, e.g. citric acid. Invert syrup differs from sucrose syrup, in that it is sweeter on a molar basis, less viscous, more water absorbent and more readily fermented. [See the section on monosaccharides for an explanation of D- and (+)-forms.]
- **Glucose syrups**: these are made from starch from either maize, potato, wheat or cassava. These contribute 16% of the sugars and syrups consumed. The starch is hydrolysed by acid or by enzymes. Partially hydrolysed products, called maltodextrins, are several glucose units in length and provide bulk without sweetness. These are spray-dried powders which readily retrograde and have poor storage properties in syrup form. When further treated with enzymes they produce glucose and other sugars. Maltose rather than glucose is the main endproduct when different enzymes are used.
- **High-fructose syrups**: these are made from glucose syrups in which 94% of the dissolved sugars is glucose. They are high-conversion glucose syrups. To convert the glucose to fructose, the syrup is diluted and treated with an enzyme which converts the glucose into a mixture of glucose and fructose in the ratio of 52:42. It is possible to separate this by chromatography into high-glucose and high-fructose fractions. A high-fructose fraction has the benefit of greater sweetness in relation to bulk.

The world production of sugar is approximately 100 million tonnes, 55% from sugar cane and 45% from sugar beet. Sugar cane is a very important crop in many tropical and subtropical countries.

SUGARS IN PREPARED FOODS

Bulk and texture

In sweets, jams and cakes, sugars are an important part of the food and provide the characteristic taste, texture and flavour.

Sugars form an important part of the characteristics of cakes and sweets, and effect crispness, crunchiness, a feeling of softness, lightness, chewiness, etc. In cakes made with sugar, air is trapped in the mixture when sugar is creamed with fat. When the mixture is baked, the gelling of starch is delayed and this increases the temperature at which the egg coagulates. In this way, trapped air expands and the mixture rises fully before the heat sets the system. The texture of biscuits results from the particular formulations and baking conditions used. The sugars are usually solid and crystalline, and this makes the texture close and crunchy.

Preservation

High concentrations of sugars prevent the growth of bacteria and moulds, in part because of inhibition of the availability of water to the bacteria. Sugar-reduced products may have to be kept refrigerated or have a very reduced life after opening. Traditional preservation methods use either sugar or salt. Jams and marmalade contain 60% dissolved solids, most of which is as sugars, partly from the fruit and partly added.

Browning reaction

Sugars can undergo two major types of browning reaction. If sugar is heated, browning occurs, called caramelisation. There is also a heat-induced reaction between sugar and the amino acids of the proteins in food, known as the Maillard reaction (see Sugar–protein interactions, later in this chapter).

SUGARS IN SPECIFIC FOODS

- **Cereals and cereal foods**: there may be little or no added sugars in some cereal foods, e.g. bread. Sweet biscuits contain 25% sugar and some breakfast cereals require sugar to give particular flavours.
- **Milk and milk products**: sugars make up approximately 5% of milk solids in whole milk, 5% in skimmed milk and 52% in dried skimmed milk. Lactose is substantially less sweet than other sugars. Sucrose is added to sweetened condensed milk, primarily to act as a preservative. Ice-cream contains 14% of added sugars; soft ice-cream substantially less. These sugars provide bulk, sweetness and texture. Fruit yoghurt contains approximately 9% of added sucrose.
- **Fruits**: most edible fruits are rich in sugars, e.g. 9% (86% of the dry weight) in eating apples; 64% (82% dry weight) in raisins.
- **Canned fruit**: the liquid or syrup is sucrose syrup or sugar-rich fruit juices. The strength of the syrup depends on the fruit and sourness. The amount of sugar is added to help preserving characteristics of the product. The high sugar content in canned fruit helps to conserve colour, flavour and texture, as well as sweetness.
- **Vegetables**: the energy content of vegetables comes from sugars, which range from 2–9% of the weight.
- **Preserves, sweets and chocolates**: sugars are major components in jam and milk chocolate, and are also essential to the flavouring of caramel and toffee.
- **Beverages**: sugars are added to soft drinks to make them sweet. The added sugars are traditionally sucrose and glucose syrup, but fructose and fructose syrup are also used.
- **Alcoholic drinks**: sugars may be present in sherries and beers, either as small amounts (1–3%), or as major ingredients, as in sweet sherry (7%) and liqueurs (up to 30%).
- **Cakes, pastries and puddings**: these are rich in sucrose or glucose syrup and fructose syrup. They constitute 16% of shortbread, 31% of sponge cake and 12% of blancmange.
- **Processed meat products**: small amounts of sucrose are added to corned beef and luncheon meat to make the products softer.

Table 13.1   Chemistry of simple natural carbohydrates and their derivatives

Monosaccharides
Glucose
Fructose
Mannose
Xylose
Galactose
Disaccharides
Sucrose
Lactose
Maltose
Derivatives of monosaccharides and disaccharides
Hydrogenated derivatives (or sugar alcohols)
Sorbitol
Mannitol
Polymers of glucose
Dextrose
Amino sugars
Galactosamine
Mannosamine
Acids

Aldonic acid C1 OOH	*Uronic acid* C6 OOH
Gluconic acid	Glucuronic acid
	Galacturonic acid
	Mannuronic acid

Lactone
Gluronolactone
Acidic sugar
Acetylneuraminic acid

MONOSACCHARIDES

Monosaccharides chemically are either polyhydroxyaldehydes (aldoses) or polyhydroxyketones (ketoses). Carbohydrates have optically active centres of asymmetry, chiral centres. There are two optically active forms, dextrorotatory and laevorotatory, depending on the direction that they rotate plane-polarised light (Figure 13.3). The symbol D or (+) is used for dextrorotatory rotation and L or (−) refers to laevorotatory rotation. Such rotation is tested with a solution of the compound and the rotation of the plane of polarised light, measured through the solution. In a mixture of equal amounts of the D- and L-forms, the two rotations cancel each other out; this is known as a racemic mixture.

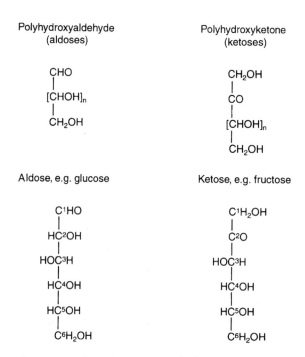

Polyhydroxyaldehyde (aldoses)

CHO
|
[CHOH]$_n$
|
CH$_2$OH

Polyhydroxyketone (ketoses)

CH$_2$OH
|
CO
|
[CHOH]$_n$
|
CH$_2$OH

Aldose, e.g. glucose

C^{1}HO
|
HC^{2}OH
|
HOC^{3}H
|
HC^{4}OH
|
HC^{5}OH
|
C^{6}H$_2$OH

Ketose, e.g. fructose

C^{1}H$_2$OH
|
C^{2}O
|
HOC^{3}H
|
HC^{4}OH
|
HC^{5}OH
|
C^{6}H$_2$OH

Fig. 13.3 The designation of dextrorotatory and laevorotatory is based on the structure of polyhydroxyaldehyde (aldoses) and polyhydroxyketone (ketoses).

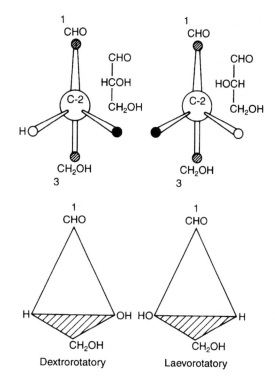

Dextrorotatory   Laevorotatory

Fig. 13.4 The structure of carbohydrates is based on glyceraldehyde. This gives the dextrorotatory or laevorotatory properties. Dextrorotatory D- is called D series; this applies if the secondary alcohol farthest away from the principal function, e.g. aldehyde, keto, carboxyl group, has the same configuration as D-glyceraldehyde.

An understanding of the stereochemistry of sugars is based on configurational properties. For common sugars the prefix *n* or *z* is used for the area of asymmetry most remote from the aldehyde or ketone end of the molecule. The reference compound is glyceraldehyde (Figure 13.4). C4, C5 and C6 sugars are derived from glyceraldehyde or dihydroxyacetone by the stepwise addition of formaldehyde. Aldehydes can form hydroxyl compounds with the carbonyl group. If a molecule of water is added the result is an aldehyde hydrate. If a molecule of alcohol is added the product is a hemiacetal; adding a second alcohol molecule produces an acetal. Sugars often form intramolecular hemiacetals; they do this readily in water, so the resulting compounds form a five- or six-membered ring.

> The α-designation for the D-series means that the aldehydal C1 hydroxyl group is on the same side of the structure as the ring oxygen, and β indicates the reverse. For the L-series the opposite is the case.

> Substitution at the equatorial position is easier because there is less chance of steric hindrance with other substitutions. The most stable conformation is the chair form, which results in the maximum number of substitutions in the equatorial position. The furanose ring is non-planar and can exist in more than one conformation.

Glucose exists in two different forms: α-D-glucose and β-D-glucose. The carbons of the hexoses are numbered as shown in Figure 13.5.

When the sugar is dissolved in water the hemiacetal is in equilibrium with the straight-chain hydrated form. The straight-chain form, which usually represents only a small fraction of the total, can convert to either hemiacetal, α or β. The conversion of one stereoisomer to another in solution is referred to as mutarotation. Hemiacetals with five-

Cyclic structures

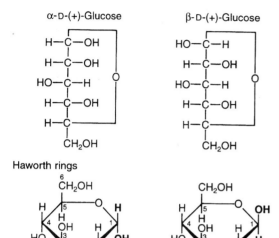

α-D-(+)-Glucose

β-D-(+)-Glucose

Haworth rings

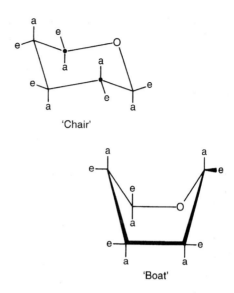

'Chair'

'Boat'

Fig. 13.7 The 'chair' and 'boat' structure of hexoses. a-orientated substitutions are axial; e-orientated substitutions are equatorial.

Chair structures

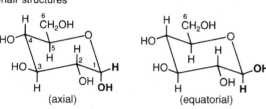

(axial)   (equatorial)

Fig. 13.5 Glucose exists in two isomeric forms, anomers, which differ in the configuration of C1. These are represented by cyclic structures, the Haworth rings or the chair structures.

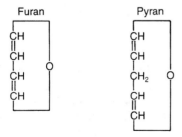

Furan   Pyran

Fig. 13.6 Carbohydrates: the general structures of the ring form are based on the C4 furanoses and the C5 pyranoses. The carbohydrate structures are analogous to the heterocyclic compounds furan and pyran.

membered rings are called furanoses and those with six-membered rings are called pyranoses (Figure 13.6). In general, the pyranose form dominates.

Another way of showing the structure is the Haworth projection. The alternative and most frequently used conformations are the 'chair' and 'boat' forms, in which the atomic groups of the ring carbons are either perpendicular to the plane of the ring, i.e. axial, or parallel to the plane of the ring, i.e. equatorial (Figure 13.7).

Glucose is readily methylated in the α- or β-position. Such derivatives of glucose are called glucosides, and those of galactose are galactosides. The most stable conformation is one where the bulkiest group, –CH$_2$OH, occupies an equatorial position (Figure 13.8). Of all D-aldohexoses, β-D-(+)-glucose is able to conform to a shape in which every bulky group is in the equatorial position. This may explain why β-D-(+)-glucose is the most common organic chemical in nature.

Glycosidic linkage

A glycoside is an acetal formed by the interaction of an alcohol with the carbonyl of a carbohydrate; the link between the sugar and an alcohol is a

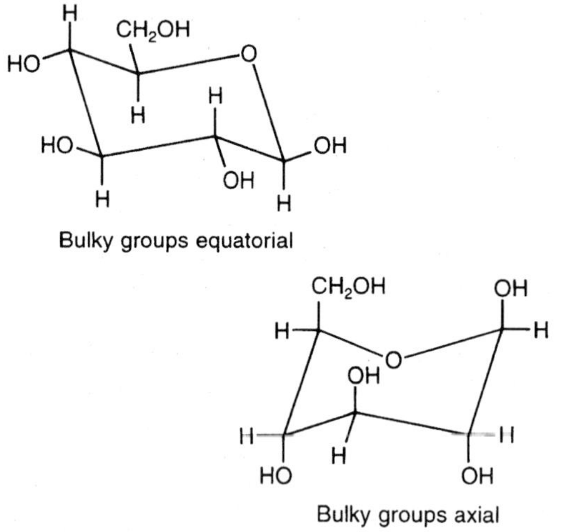

Bulky groups equatorial

Bulky groups axial

Fig. 13.8 Glucose, showing the two geometric forms. When the bulky groups (CH$_2$OH) are equatorial (in the plane of the molecule) the configuration is stable. When such groups are axial (at right angles) to the plane of the molecule, the molecule is less stable.

If the linkage is glycosidic on one side only, then suffixes -osido and -ose are used

If the linkage is glycosidic on both sides, then the suffixes -osido and -oside are used

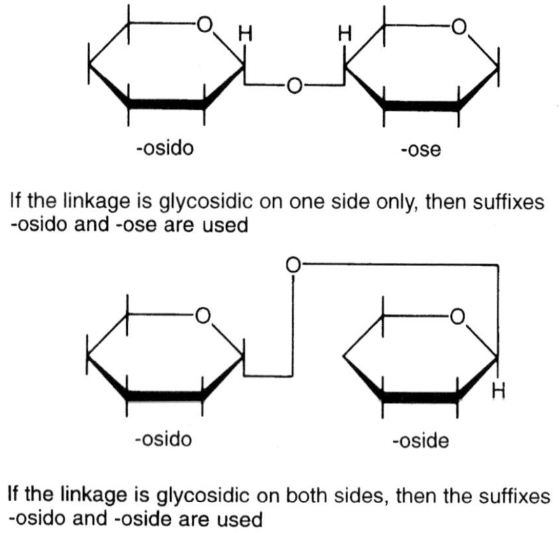

Fig. 13.9 Oligosaccharides are joined by glycosidic linkages.

glycosidic bond (Figure 13.9). A glycoside can be formed with an aliphatic alcohol, phenols and hydroxycarboxylic acids, as well as with another sugar. Glucose can form a glycoside with the alcohols of another glucose in the α- and β-conformation. Monosaccharides can link through glycosidic bonds to form disaccharides and larger carbohydrate structures. Thus carbohydrate acetyls are formed, i.e. O-R, where R is a sugar.

DISACCHARIDES

Maltose has the structure 4-O-(α-D-glucopyranosyl)-D-glucopyranose. Both halves of the molecule contain the six-membered pyranose ring. Maltose is a disaccharide joined by a glycosidic bond between the C1 carbonyl of one D-(+)-glucose molecule and the C4 (providing the -OH as an alcohol) of a second D-(+)-glucose molecule with an α-(1–4) glycosidic linkage (Figure 13.10). The C1 carbon determines the configuration of the linkage, as this is the active carbon and hence α. The second D-(+)-glucose is an α-D-glucosopyranosyl group. Maltose has a free aldehyde group and is therefore a reducing sugar.

Reducing sugars

Carbohydrates that can reduce Fehling's, Benedict's or Tollen's solution (complexed cupric solutions) are known as reducing sugars. All monosaccharides, whether aldose or ketose, are reducing sugars. Most disaccharides are reducing sugars, with the exception of sucrose. Sucrose is a non-reducing sugar because it does not contain a free aldehyde or ketone group, being a β-D-fructoside and an α-D-glucoside. In contrast, lactose, which has reducing properties, is a substituted D-glucose to which a D-galactosyl unit is added. The D-(+)-glucose unit has a free aldehyde group for oxidation.

Cellobiose is a disaccharide formed from two D-(+)-glucose molecules. These are two pyranose rings and a glycosidic linkage to the –OH on C4. The D-glucose units are connected by a β- rather than an α-linkage. (+)-Cellobiose is 4-O-(β-D-glucopyranosyl)-D-glucopyranose.

Lactose is a reducing sugar, a disaccharide of D-(+)-glucose and D-(+)-galactose joined through a β-linkage. Lactose is a substituted D-glucose in which a D-galactosyl unit is attached to one of the oxygens, a galactoside not a glucoside. The glycosidic linkage involves an α-OH at C4. Lactose is 4-O-(β-D-galactopyranosyl)-D-glucopyranose.

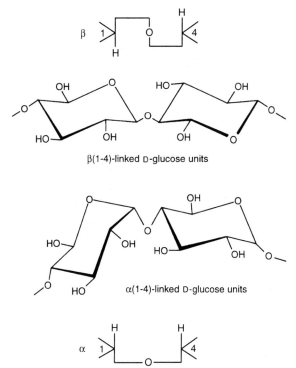

Fig. 13.10   1–4-Linked glucose units: β- and α-linkages.

Sucrose is a non-reducing sugar consisting of a D-glucose and a D-fructose unit joined by a glycosidic linkage between C1 of glucose and C2 of fructose. Sucrose is a β-D-fructoside and an α-D-glucoside, a D-glucopyranose and a D-fructofuranose. Sucrose may be regarded as α-D-glucopyranosyl-β-D-fructofuranoside or β-D-fructofuranosyl-α-D-glucopyranoside.

The structures of the most common disaccharides are shown in Figure 13.11.

KEY POINTS

1. Monosaccharides are either polyhydroxyaldehydes (aldoses) or polyhydroxyketones (ketoses) with optically active chiral centres. The two forms of the molecule are described as dextrorotatory (D or +) or laevorotatory (L or −), depending on the direction in which they rotate plane-polarised light. A mixture of equal amounts of the D-and L-forms is known as a racemic mixture.
2. Monosaccharides include α-D-glucose, fructose, mannose, xylose and galactose. Monosaccharides form intramolecular hemiacetals, so the resulting compounds form a five-(furanose) or six-membered (pyranose) ring. Carbohydrates that can reduce Fehling's, Benedict's or Tollen's solution (complexed cupric solutions) are known as reducing sugars.
3. Monosaccharides can link through glycosidic bonds to form disaccharides and larger carbohydrate structures. Disaccharides include sucrose (glucose and fructose), lactose (glucose and galactose) and maltose (glucose and glucose).
4. The commercial interest in sucrose results in its being available in a variety of forms. There are many commercially advantageous effects of sugar in prepared foods.

THINKING POINT

The structure of the monosaccharides gives much less flexibility than amino acids in forming polymers. From what you have read, why is this?

NEED TO UNDERSTAND

Monosacccharides provide the basic structure for important structural polysaccharides, structures and energy provision throughout nature. It is important to understand the stereochemistry of the monosaccharides and how structures can be formed.

FURTHER READING

British Nutrition Foundation Task Force (1987) *Sugars and Syrups*. British Nutrition Foundation, London.
Dobbing, J. (ed.) (1989) *Dietary Starches and Sugars in Man: A Comparison*. ILSI Human Nutrition Reviews. Springer, London.
Eriksson, C. (ed.) (1981) *Maillard Reaction in Food*. Pergamon Press, Sweden.

Name	Structure	Occurrence
Lactose (4′-[β-D-galactopyranosido]-D-glucopyranose)	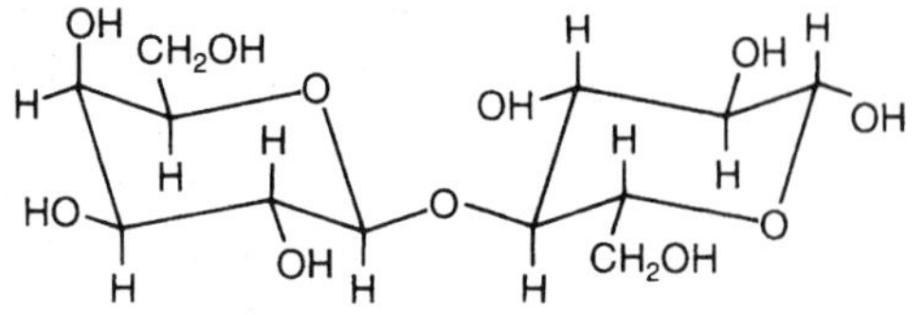	Constituent of mammalian milk (4–8%). Only faintly sweet
Maltose (4′-[α-D-glucopyranosido]-β-D-glucopyranose)	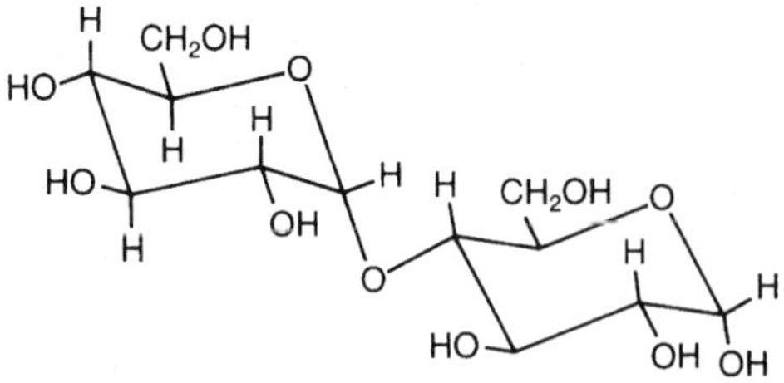	Breakdown product of starch and glycogen arising in the course of digestion. Found free in some plants (barley) and in honey
Sucrose (saccharose, cane sugar, beet sugar, α-D-glucopyranosido-β-D-fructofuranoside)	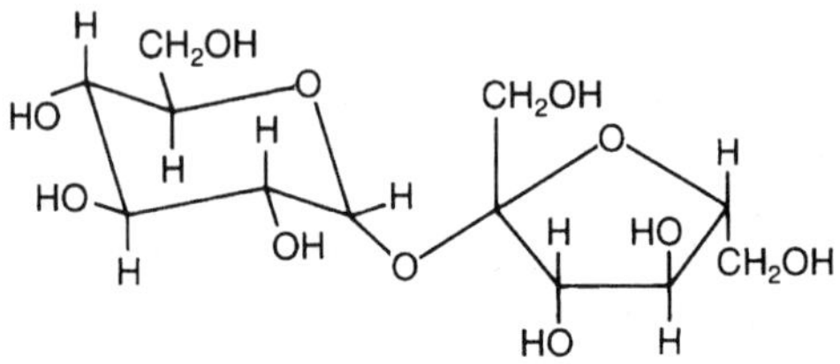	Almost universal in the vegetable kingdom

Fig. 13.11 Disaccharide structures. (Reproduced from Geigy Scientific Tables, Ciba-Geigy Ltd, with permission.)

POLYSACCHARIDES

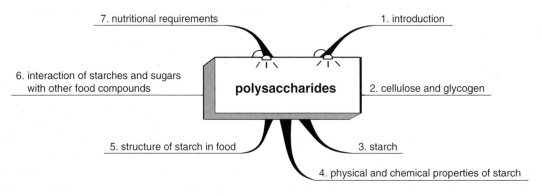

Fig. 13.12 Section outline.

INTRODUCTION

In biology most carbohydrates exist as high molecular weight polymers. Polysaccharides are simple sugars connected by glycosidic bonds. The sugars involved are D-glucose, D-mannose, D- and L-galactose, D-xylose, L-arabinose, D-glucuronic acid, D-galacturonic acid, D-mannuronic acid, D-glucosamine, D-galactosamine and neuraminic acid.

CELLULOSE AND GLYCOGEN

Cellulose is a major structural polysaccharide, providing approximately half of plant carbon, and consisting of polymeric glucose joined by a β-(1–4) type glycosidic linkage. D-Glucose, in the chair form of a pyranose ring, is a rigid structure and is characteristic of cellulose as an extended polysaccharide chain. Cellulose has a molecular weight of 50 kDa or greater, forming chains that join together as bundles, with a diameter of 100–250 Å with approximately 2000 chains in such a bundle.

Glycogen is the major polysaccharide for energy storage in animal cells. It is an α-(1–4) homopolymer, highly branched with an α-(1–6) linkage occurring every 8–10 glucose units along the backbone, with short side-chains of approximately 8–12 glucose units each (see Figure 13.13).

STARCH

Starch is the major polysaccharide for energy storage in plant cells. It is an α-(1–4) homopolymer with occasional α-(1–6) linkages at branch points. They differ in their chain lengths and branching patterns. Starch occurs both as unbranched amylose and as branched amylopectin (Figure 13.13). Amylopectin has α-(1–6) branches, but these occur at every 12–25 glucose residues and with longer side-chains, 20–25 glucose units long. An α-(1–4) configuration is much more susceptible than the β-(1–4) linkages to degrading enzymes. Starch is the main food reserve in plants and is a very important source of energy in human nutrition. During photosynthesis starch is stored in specialised parts of the plant as granules, e.g. tubers (potato), kernels (maize) and grains (wheat). The shape, size and composition of the granules are dependent on the amylose:amylopectin ratio. Starch is widely used in traditional human foods, but new uses are constantly being developed by new technologies. Starch-derived maltodextrins, polyols and non-digestible starch derivatives are used as fat replacers. The world production of starch is in the order of 20–25 million tonnes per year, 10–20 million tonnes of which are used for food purposes. In contrast, the world production of sucrose is in the order of 100 million tonnes per year, 99% of which is used in foods.

An α-(1–4)-linked unit in a polyglucose, e.g. amylose, results in a natural turning of the chain to form a helix. Such a helix wound round the molecule of iodine gives the characteristic blue colour of the amylose–iodine complex. Amylopectin and iodine give a red–brown colour.

Amylose is a linear unit with glucoses joined by α-(1–4) linkages and is insoluble in cold water. Because of the tetrahedral structure of the carbon atom and the α-(1–4) linkage, the natural form of starch is a helical structure with a turn every six glucose units. Amylose consists of between 200 and 2000 glucose units, depending on the source.

Amylopectin is a branched structure with glucose joined by α-(1–6) linkages at the branch point, and α-(1–4) linkages in the linear sections (Figure 13.13). The polymer contains between 10 000 and 100 000 glucose units, but no helical structure exists. Amylopectin is insoluble in cold water but is soluble in hot water. It does not readily become retrograded, and on cooling may form a loose gel.

PHYSICAL AND CHEMICAL PROPERTIES OF STARCH

Starch is present in the plant in the form of microscopic granules surrounded by a phospholipid membrane. The granules are insoluble in cold water. Within the granule, amylopectin forms a branched crystalline pattern, with the linear amylose dispersed through the amylopectin. The amylopectin lattice can be described as three forms:

Name	Structure	Occurrence
Amylopectin (α-amylose)	Highly branched molecule composed of several hundred unit-chains, each of which comprises 20–26 α(1—4)-linked glucose residues; the unit-chains are interlinked by glycosidic bonds from the reducing group to C6 of a glucose residue in an adjacent chain: 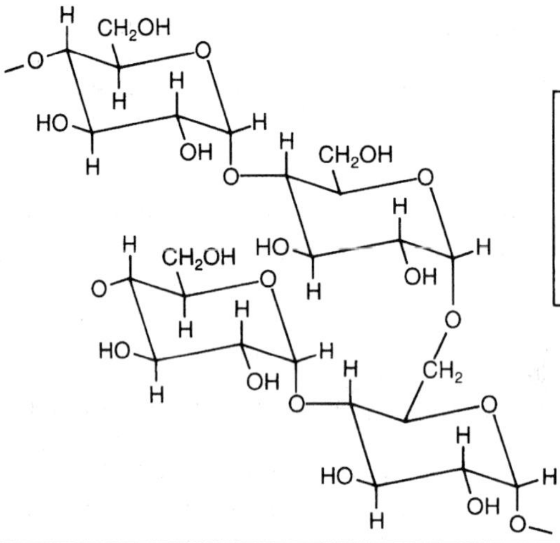 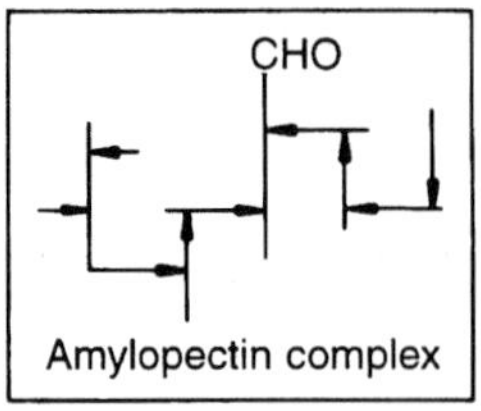	Main constituent of starch (usually c. 80%)
Amylose (β-amylose)	Essentially a linear chain of α(1—4)-linked glucose residues: 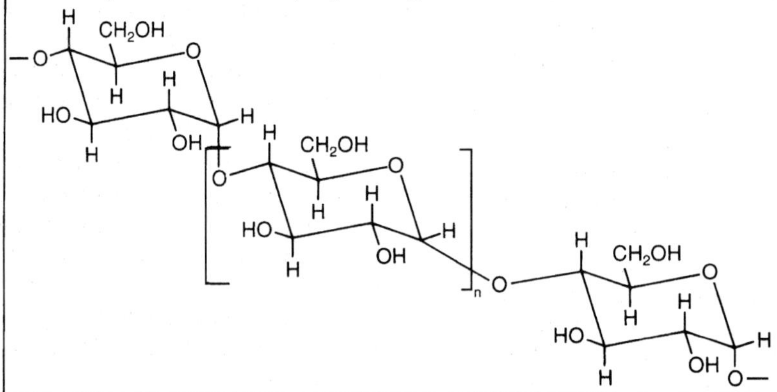	Constituent of starch (c.20%). Absent in some starches, e.g. that of 'waxy' maize (corn)

Fig. 13.13 Structure of starch: amylopectin and amylose. (Partly reproduced from Geigy Scientific Tables, Ciba-Geigy Ltd, with permission.)

- **type A**: chain length 23–39 glucoses with additional crystalline structures in between; found in cereals
- **type B**: chain length 30–44 glucoses, interspersed with water; found in raw potato and bananas
- **type C**: chain length 26–29 glucoses, a mix of type A and B; found in peas and beans.

In general, types B and C are resistant to enzyme digestion.

Gelatinisation

As a starch granule is heated in water the water is absorbed, the granule structure is altered by the

Table 13.2 *In vitro* nutritional classification of starch

Starch	Occurrence	Digestion in small intestine
Rapidly digestible starch	Freshly cooked starchy food	Rapid
Slowly digestible starch	Most raw cereals	Slow but complete
Resistant starch		
Physically inaccessible starch	Partly milled grain and seeds	Resistant
Resistant starch granules	Raw potato and banana	Resistant
Retrograded starch	Cooled, cooked potato, bread and cornflakes	Resistant

Source: Englyst and Kingman (1990).

loss of crystallisation of amylopectin, and the starch takes up a random formation. This is followed by swelling, hydration and solubilisation. The viscosity increases until the viscous solution of starch paste is formed, a process called gelatinisation. There is a thickening owing to the formation of a starch network which binds the swollen granules together. There are also changes in crystalline melting and starch solubilisation. The point of initial gelatinisation and the range over which it occurs are governed by starch concentration, method of observation, granule type and heterogeneity within the granule population. The extent of gelatinisation depends on the amount of water available.

- *Rapidly digestible starch*: heating starch in water results in a soluble preparation. In dilute solutions (< 1%) a precipitate forms; at high concentrations a gel is produced, which excludes water from the starch–water matrix, in a process called synersis. This gelatinised digestible starch is readily and rapidly digested by the enzymes of the gastrointestinal tract.
- *Slowly digestible starch*: this consists of physically inaccessible amorphous starch and raw granules with type A and C crystalline structures.

The gelatinisation temperature is a characteristic of the starch source, and varies between 72°C for waxy corn and maize starch, and 85°C for wheat starch. Gelatinised starch is susceptible to amylase digestion. On cooling, this gelatinised starch undergoes retrogradation.

Retrogradation

Starch retrogradation is a process which occurs when the molecules of gelatinised starch begin to associate again in an ordered structure. In its initial phases two or more starch chains may form a simple junction point, which may then develop into a more extensively ordered region. Retrogradation occurs in two steps:

1. Aggregation of the polysaccharide chains with phase separation into polymer-rich and polymer-deficient phases (gelation).
2. Slow crystallisation of the macromolecules in the polymer-rich phase.

The length of time taken for these phases depends on the concentration and chemistry of the starch. The whole process may take 2–30 days. Retrogradation occurs more readily at low temperatures, a process particularly marked at concentrations of 50–60% gels. Eventually under favourable conditions, a crystalline structure appears. Retrograded starch is not hydrolysed by amylase and belongs to the family of resistant starches (Table 13.2). At higher temperatures and reduced water the type A structure dominates at lower temperatures and in an excess of water the type B, less enzymatically digestible structure forms.

Starch paste

Pure amylose has a lower hot viscosity than pure amylopectin and therefore the amylopectin:amylose ratio is important in dictating the viscosity of the starch. Starch paste has properties of clarity, viscosity, texture, stability and taste that depend on the degree of gelatinisation. The starch granules do not swell and become viscous below 65°C. Starch paste may be affected by the production processes that affect the intragranular hydrogen bond, important in keeping the granule intact during gelatinisation. Processes such as prolonged heating, exposure to high temperature, too much stirring during and after cooking, and exposure to specific pH conditions all reduce starch paste function. Freezing and thawing also have profound effects on starch paste and increase retrogradation. Modified starches provide stability under processing conditions and freeze–thaw conditions. Various granular starch modifications may be made:

- **Cross-linked starches**: these may result from exposure to phosphate or adipate.
- **Stabilisation**: stability may be made a feature of the starch granule by adding large molecular weight substituent groups, e.g. acetate and hydroxypropyl. This weakens the intermolecular and intramolecular hydrogen bonds within the granules, and reduces the temperature of gelatinisation of the starch.
- **Precooked starches**: these become viscous in water without heating. Precooking of starch occurs by extrusion of native granules at low water content.
- The phosphate content of native starch, that is, chemically linked phosphorus, can also affect the physical properties. The amount of phosphorus may be very small, varying from 0.03% in waxy corn or maize starch to 0.06% in potato starch.

Converted starches
Modified starches can be produced which give the same viscosity at 15–20% concentration as the native starch of 5% concentration. This is possible through an internal hydrolysis reaction which is applied to the starch granule. These starches have improved textural properties with a firm gel.

Substitution of native starches with cyclic dicarboxylic acid anhydrides produces *hydrophobic* starches, used in beverages, emulsions, clouding agents, flavour encapsulation, vitamin protection, salad dressings and creams.

Enzymatic cycling processes using the enzyme cyclodextrin glucanotransferase gives cyclodextrins. Several glucose monomers are joined together into a circular cone with a hydrophilic rim at the top and bottom, and a hydrophobic region in the middle that can bind and hold molecules in the cavity. Such a structure is used by manufacturers to retain odours and flavours in foods.

Chemical and enzymatic hydrolysis of starch

The process occurs in two stages, liquefaction and saccharinification.

1. **Liquefaction**: gelatinisation and consequent reduction in viscosity allows access to the enzymes and, as the viscosity reduces, allows high concentrations of starch to be used.
2. **Saccharinification**: the enzymatic hydrolysis reaction with enzymes, including β-amylase and amyloglucosidase, can be stopped at a predetermined point, giving a mixture of starch hydrolysis products of defined molecular weight. The product is called dextrose equivalent (DE). It depends on the degree of hydrolysis of the starch and is a measure of the dextrose content. Starch is 0 DE and dextrose 100 DE.

DE is a somewhat imprecise measurement, and gives no information on the composition or properties of the product.

Hydrolysis products of starch
- **Maltodextrins**: there are starch hydrolysis products with a DE of 20.
- **Dried glucose syrups**: starch hydrolyses with a DE > 20 and when spray-dried is called dried glucose syrup. They are usually found in the ratio range of 30–60 DE. Above 60 DE the dried material is hygroscopic and difficult to keep dry.
- **Maltose syrups**: when β-amylase is used in the hydrolysis process, maltose is the main product.
- **Hydrolysates**: these are glucose syrups with a very high DE, 80–98.

STRUCTURE OF STARCH IN FOOD

Starchy foods are usually heated to make them palatable, and they may also be dried or frozen to increase ease of preparation in the domestic kitchen, to improve palatability and to extend shelf-life. All of these preparations have an effect on the functional and nutritional properties of starch (Tables 13.2 and 13.3).

Bread has a moisture content of 35–40%, which is close to the optimum condition for starch

Table 13.3 *In vitro* digestibility of starch in a variety of foods

	% RDS	% SDS	%RS
Flour, white	38	59	3
Shortbread	56	43	t
Bread, white	94	4	2
Bread, wholemeal	90	8	2
Spaghetti, white	55	36	9
Biscuits, made with 50% raw banana flour	34	27	38
Biscuits, made with 50% raw potato flour	36	29	35
Peas, chick, canned	56	24	19
Beans, dried, freshly cooked	37	45	17
Beans, red kidney, canned	60	25	15

Source: Englyst and Kingman (1990).
The values are expressed as a percentage of the total starch present in the food. RDS: rapidly digestible starch; SDS: slowly digestible starch; RS: resistant starch; t: trace.

crystallisation. Amylose retrogrades rapidly and within hours of cooking. In contrast, staling is a slow process which involves change in the physical form of amylopectin. In addition, water moves through the bread from the crumb to the crust. There is also a decrease in the proportion of soluble starch and in the starch's ability to swell in cold water. However, none of these factor affects the susceptibility of these starches to α-amylase hydrolysis.

Resistant starch

Resistant starch is not susceptible to intestinal and pancreatic enzymatic digestion. Such starch may be resistant because:

- the starch is physically inaccessible to enzymatic digestion, e.g. grains, seeds and dense, processed starch
- the starch is granular
- retrograded amylose has formed during cooling.

Although these processes make the starch resistant to human digestive processes, it is still susceptible to colonic bacterial attack.

The development of resistant starch may occur during food processing, the baking of bread, cooling and storage. Amylose forms a strong retrograded starch, stable to 120°C, while amylopectin retrograde starch can be disrupted by gentle heating. When stale bread is reheated the retrograded amylopectin, which was the cause of the staling, reverts to the native form. The amount of resistant starch in foods is influenced by the water content, pH, temperature and duration of heating, and the number of heating and cooling cycles, freezing and drying.

In bread, resistant starches form immediately after baking and remain stable during storage. In contrast, resistant starch production in boiled potatoes is time dependent; freshly cooked potatoes contain < 2% resistant starch, but this increases during cooling to about 3%. Reheating may reduce the degree of retrogradation, but on cooling the amount of resistant starch increases further. Similar changes may be found with wheat starch.

There is a rough correlation between the amylose content and the yield of resistant starch following cooking and drying. Waxy starch forms very little resistant starch, whereas high-amylose starch forms over 30% of resistant starch.

The processing conditions can affect the amount of gelatinisation, and the level and type of retrogradation of starch. Quick-cooking rice has a porous structure and a grain that hydrates very rapidly. Non-sticky grains result from controlled retrogradation of gelatinised starch. Par-boiling modifies the physical, chemical and textural characteristics of the rice, and reduces the leaching of vitamins, proteins and starch from the grain into the cooking water. The rice grains are steeped and steam-dried, resulting in gelatinisation of the starch granules which are held in a proteinaceous matrix without damaging the starch granules. In contrast, the retrogradation of starch in cooked rice may result in a tough and rubbery product.

Another processing technique that affects gelatinisation and the general physicochemical properties of rice is the use of extruder cookers which separate amylose and amylopectin, affecting starch stickiness, expansion, carbohydrate solubility and digestibility. The starch granules may be disrupted with partial starch breakdown and increased levels of resistant starch, depending on the relative amylose:amylopectin content of the original preparation.

INTERACTION OF STARCHES AND SUGARS WITH OTHER FOOD COMPOUNDS

Starch–protein interactions

Protein interacts with starch molecules on the granule surface, which alters the granule's physical properties. These interactions are important in bread and pasta production. Dough is a coherent viscoelastic mass. Bread is a physically unstable colloidal system. Protein in the dough forms a matrix in which the starch granules are separated at high concentrations. These starch granules gelatinise in part during baking and the glutinous matrix coagulates to form bread with its characteristic structure. The degree of gelatinisation of starch is very dependent on the moisture content and temperature, and also on the type of wheat products used.

Pasta is made from durum semolina, which is very hard because of its high protein content. During extrusion, protein forms a protective coating around the starch granule. There is partial starch gelatinisation and the coagulated protein forms a fibrillar structure. The starch granules gelatinise and swell until the cells are filled. It is only when the cells are broken and the starch is freed that a sticky product is produced.

Sugar–protein interactions

Sugars in the baking of dough alter the texture of the resulting bread by delaying the gelatinisation of starch and the denaturation of proteins. The reactions during baking include the Maillard reaction, occurring when wheat cereal products are toasted.

Starch–lipid interactions

Fatty acids and monoglycerides (less commonly with lecithin and not with acylglycerols) can form inclusion compounds with amylose, when the hydrocarbon of the lipid is placed within the helical cavity of amylose. This is because the bulky shape (steric hindrance) of the acylglycerols pre-

The Maillard reaction

This takes place when reducing sugars, e.g. glucose, fructose or lactose, are subjected to heat in the presence of protein. The reaction is an initial condensation between an amino acid group and a carbonyl group to form a Schiff base and water. After this, there is cyclisation and isomerisation in acidic conditions (Amadori rearrangements). The result is a 1-amino-l-deoxy-2-ketose derivative. Aldopentoses are more reactive than aldohexoses which, in turn, are more reactive than disaccharides. The important reaction is with lysine, with a loss of 42–66% of lysine depending on the sugars and protein. Other amino acids that may be involved in the Maillard reaction are tryptophan, arginine and histidine. Sucrose does not react, but may be degraded by heat, producing molecules that can react with free amino acids. This is particularly marked in dry heating. It can also result in a loss of nutritional qualities of the protein in baked food. Such losses are particularly marked in biscuits, which are dry-heated.

vents entry to the starch helix. The quantity of lipids also affects the ability of starch to retrograde. Amylopectin may form complexes with fatty acids, but to a much lesser extent than amylose.

Cereal starches form inclusion complexes with monoacyl lipids. The latter are present in the cereal complex with 15–20% of the total amylose. Monoglycerols are used to prevent retrogradation of amylose. They also have important effects on the physical properties and cooking properties of starch.

Starch–sugar–mineral interactions

Cations in general have little affinity for starch and glucose syrups at neutral pH.

NUTRITIONAL REQUIREMENTS

Sugar

Sugar or sucrose is a readily available source of energy. Sucrose intake varies from country to country. In the UK it is recommended that the average intake of non-milk extrinsic sugar (i.e. other than milk lactose) should not exceed 60 g/day or 10% of the total dietary intake. This nomenclature of non-milk sugars refers primarily to sucrose.

In 1987, the daily sucrose intake in the UK was 104 g/person, providing 14% of the body's energy intake. Honey and glucose, at 16 g/person/day, provided 2% of the body's energy intake, and lactose, at 23 g/person/day, a further 3%. On average, 26 g of sucrose was eaten per person per day as packaged sugar. Breast- or bottle-fed infants obtained 40% of their energy intake from lactose. For preschool children, 25–30% of daily food energy was provided by the daily intake of sugars. Older children and adults tended to take less sugar.

Starches

It has been recommended that starches should provide the balance of dietary energy not provided by the whole protein, fat and non-milk extrinsic sugars; that is, on average, 37% of total dietary energy for the adult population. The same principle should be applied to children over 2 years old.

Such calculations are for starch that is digestible in the small intestine, but not resistant starch.

KEY POINTS

1. In biology most carbohydrates exist as high molecular weight polymers. These polysaccharides are simple sugars connected by glycosidic bonds.
2. Cellulose is a major structural polysaccharide and accounts for approximately half of the carbon found in plants. Cellulose consists of polymeric glucose with a glycosidic linkage of the β-(1–4) type.
3. The two major polysaccharides for energy storage are starch in plant cells and glycogen in animal cells. They differ in their chain lengths and branching patterns. Glycogen is highly branched, with an α-(1–6) linkage occurring every 8–10 glucose units along the backbone, with short side-chains of approximately 8–12 glucose units

each. Starch occurs both as unbranched amylose and as branched amylopectin.
4. The chemical and physical changes associated with gelatinisation and retrogradation have important consequences for food production and intestinal absorption.
5. Starch is hydrolysed by the enzyme amylase. Starches that are not hydrolysed by amylase are resistant starches.
6. Starch, proteins or lipids may interact to form aggregates.
7. Starches should provide the balance of dietary energy not provided by the whole protein, fat and non-milk extrinsic sugars; that is, on average, 37% of total dietary energy for the adult population.

THINKING POINTS

1. The polymeric sugars are important sources of energy and structure in the organism.
2. Starch is an energy source with varied physical properties, allowing for a wide range of cooking products.

NEED TO UNDERSTAND

1. The carbohydrate polymers are dependent on α- and β-linkages. These linkages dictate the polymer's resistance to animal and bacterial enzymatic digestion.
2. The polymers are important because of their physical properties and as stores of carbohydrate energy.

FURTHER READING

Annison, G. and Topping, D.L. (1994) Nutritional role of resistant starch. *Annual Review of Nutrition*, **14**, 297–320.

Asp, N.-G., van Amelsvoort, J.M.M. and Hautvast, J.G.A.J. (1996) Nutritional implications of resistant starch. *Nutritional Research Review*, **9**, 1–31.

Atwell, W.A., Hood, L.F., Lineback, D.R. *et al.* (1988) The terminology and methodology associated with basic starch phenomena. *Cereal Food World*, **33**, 306–11.

British Nutrition Foundation Task Force (1990) *Complex Carbohydrates in Foods*. Chapman & Hall, London.

Dobbing, J. (ed.) (1989) *Dietary Starches and Sugars in Man: A Comparison*. ILSI Human Nutrition Reviews. Springer, London.

Englyst, H.N. and Kingman, S.M. (1990) Dietary fiber and resistant starch, a nutritional classification of plant polysaccharides. In *Dietary Fiber* (eds D. Kritchevsky, C. Bonfield and J.W Anderson). Plenum Press, New York, pp. 49–65.

Kunz, C., Rudloff, S., Baier, W. *et al.* (2000) Oligosaccharides in human milk: structural, functional and metabolic aspects. *Annual Review of Nutrition*, **20**, 699–722.

Southgate, D.A.T. (1976) *Determination of Food Carbohydrates*. Applied Sciences Publishers, London.

Van Loo, J., Cummings, J., Delzenne, N. *et al.* (1999) Functional food properties of non-digestible oligosaccharides: a consensus report from the ENDO project (DGXII AIRII-CT94-1095). *British Journal of Nutrition*, **81**, 121–32.

WEBSITE

www.inspection.gc.ca/english/bureau/labels/guide

14

Dietary fibre

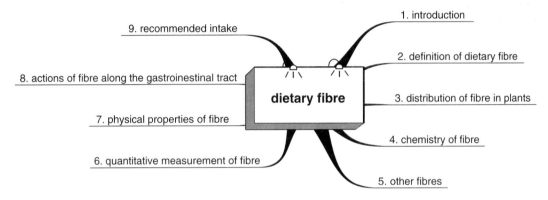

Fig. 14.1 Chapter outline.

INTRODUCTION

Dietary fibre is a member of a family of dietary complex carbohydrates that have individual and

Complex carbohydrates that have been included as fibre

Cellulose	Chitin and chitosan
Chondroitin sulfate	Cutin
Dextrin (resistant)	Fructan
Fructooligosaccharide	Galactooligosaccharide
Gums	Hemicellulose
Inulin	Maillard products
Maltodextrin (resistant)	Mucilage
Modified cellulose	Novel fibres
Oligofructose	Pectin
Polydextrose	Resistant starch
Saponin	Wax

diverse actions. The chemistry of individual polymers cannot, however, identify or predict the biological action in the gastrointestinal tract. Each fibre is peculiar in its biological action, and is affected by extraction, physical format and processing. One way of classifying dietary polysaccharides is to include polymers that exceed 20 sugar residues as dietary complex carbohydrates. Another name for dietary fibre is non-starch polysaccharides (NSP).

All of these materials are polymeric carbohydrates and lignins, which together form the plant cell wall and are not digested as they pass through the upper gastrointestinal tract.

DEFINITION OF DIETARY FIBRE

The definition of dietary fibre has proved to be difficult, largely because the renewed interest was generated by epidemiological observations rather

Name	Structure	Occurrence
Dextrans	$\alpha(1-6)$-Linked glucose residues in branched or straight chains, for instance: 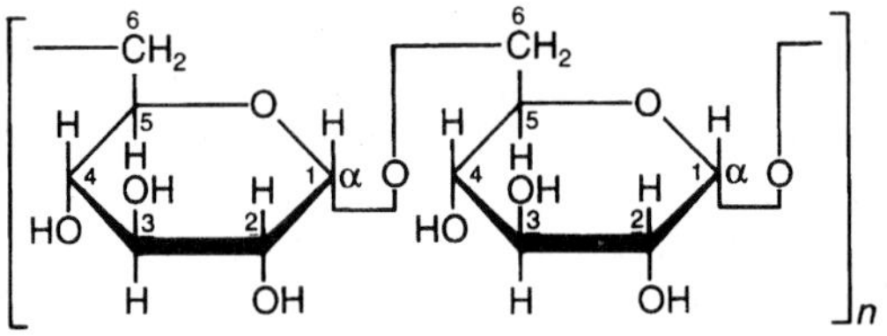 	
Glycogen (liver starch)	Highly branched molecule resembling amylopectin and consisting of unit chains of $\alpha(1-4)$-linked glucose residues interlinked by $\alpha(1-6)$-glycosidic bonds: 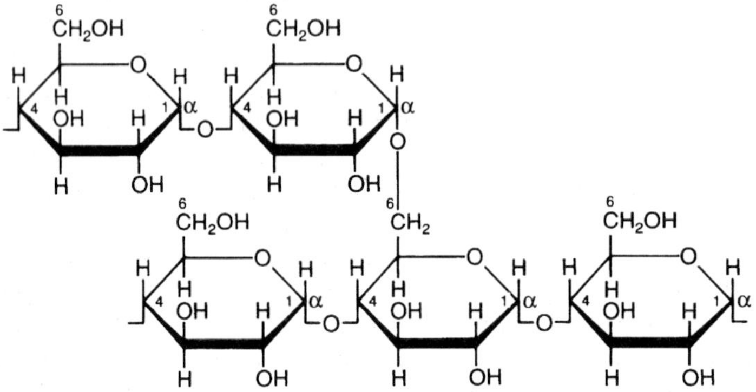 	Reserve carbohydrate of animal tissues. Converted in muscle to lactic acid during glycolysis. Also present in yeast
Pectic acid (pectins)	Linear chain of $\alpha(1-4)$-linked D-galacturonic acid residues: 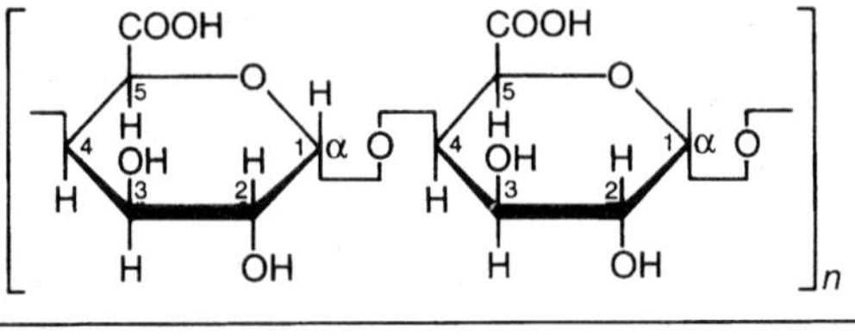 	Important cell-wall constituent of plants. Occurs as Ca salt or methylester
Cellulose	Linear chain of $\beta(1-4)$-linked glucose residues: 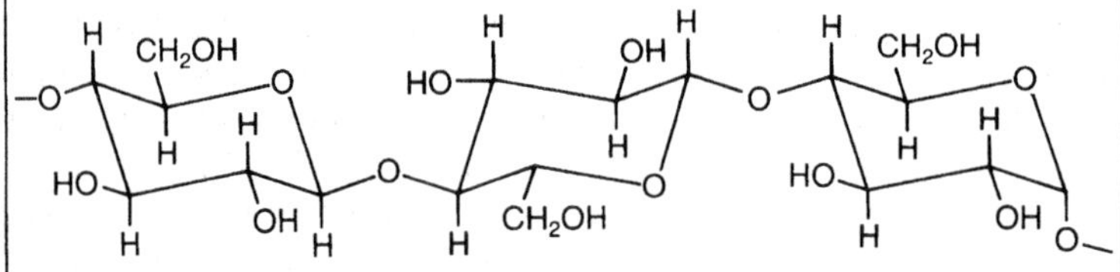 	Chief structural polysaccharide of plants. Also found in algae, bacterial membranes, and as tunicin in some lower animals. Not digested by human

Fig. 14.2 Structure of dextrans, glycogen, pectin and cellulose. (Partly reproduced from Geigy Scientific Tables, Ciba-Geigy Ltd, with permission.)

than experiments. Trowell and Burkitt observed that health problems endemic in Western countries were rarely seen in Africa, where they had worked as clinicians. They claimed that the difference lay in the diet, especially in the amount of roughage, a term that was subsequently changed to dietary fibre, that is, more fruit and vegetables. This caused some resistance in the minds of others, as fibre implies a material from which rope can be made. A clear definition and method of analysis would facilitate recommended intakes and labelling. As will be shown later, there are other considerations. Different fibres have varying effects along the gastrointestinal tract, so to limit the definition to one physiological function has problems. Fibre is said to protect against a number of conditions, from hiatus hernia to colonic cancer, coronary heart disease, obesity and haemorrhoids, and different fibres may have varying protective effects. Many interesting products, have been manufactured that may be cheap and useful, but may not readily be defined as fibre.

An early definition of dietary fibre by Hugh Trowell was the skeletal remains of plant cells that are resistant to digestion (hydrolysis) by human enzymes. Later, skeletal remains was changed to plant polysaccharides and lignins. A recent North American definition separates fibre into two groups, which together add up to total dietary fibre.

- Dietary fibre consists of non-digestible, intact, naturally occurring plant polysaccharides and lignin.
- Added fibre consists of isolated, non-digestible carbohydrates that have beneficial physiological effects in humans.

The persisting problem defining dietary fibre is that dietary fibre acts as a sponge along the gastrointestinal tract and, as such, its properties are affected by the manner of processing before ingestion.

DISTRIBUTION OF FIBRE IN PLANTS

Considerable anatomical differences exist between and within economically important plant groups and their fibre constituents. These differences occur in the cell wall and could be important in determining the diversity of actions in the gastrointestinal tract of sundry dietary fibres.

Dietary fibre in naturally occurring foods consists of plant cell walls, the structure of which differs not only among plant species but also during normal development within one species or even a single cell. The composition of the cell wall is dependent on the plant species, the tissue type, the maturity of the plant organ at harvesting, and to some extent post-harvest storage conditions. Non-carbohydrate components of plant cell walls may also influence the nutritional properties of the plant dietary fibres, e.g. proteins, lignin, phenolic esters, cutin, waxy materials and suberin.

Parenchymatous tissues are the most important source of vegetable fibre. The vascular bundles and parchment layers of cabbage leaves, runner beans, pods, asparagus stems and carrot roots are relatively immature and only slightly lignified on harvesting, and hence are readily digested. Soft fruits such as strawberries and raspberries contain very little dietary fibre but abundant amounts of water. Lignified tissues are of greater significance in cereal sources such as wheat bran and oat products. Cereals contain very low levels of pectic substances, but there is substantial arabinoxylan in wheat, and β-glucan in barley and oats. The distribution of polysaccharides within the plant tissue also varies. Much of the β-glucan in oats is concentrated in the cells of the outermost layer of the seeds, whereas the β-glucans in barley are more evenly distributed.

CHEMISTRY OF FIBRE

An important aspect of the plant cell wall is the interlocking of water-soluble polysaccharides to form water-resistant biological barriers. Many of the constituents of the plant cell wall, hemicelluloses and pectins, are soluble in water after extraction. This solubility, which is unmasked by extraction processes, contrasts with the insolubility of the complex polysaccharide of the intact cell wall (Figure 14.2).

Cellulose is the backbone of the plant cell wall and is a polymer of linear β-(1–4)-linked glucose molecules, several thousand molecules in length (Figure 14.2). Cellulose occurs largely in a crystalline form in microfibrils, coated with a monolayer of more complex hemicellulosic polymers held tightly by hydrogen bonds. These are embedded in a gel of pectin polysaccharides. The cellulose microfibrils are coated with a layer of xyloglucans bound by hydrogen bonds, and this enables the insoluble cellulose to be dispersed within the wall matrix.

Hemicelluloses contribute to the rigidity of the cell wall. The important hemicelluloses are xyloglucans, xylans and b-glucans. Substitution of the hydroxyl group at C6 with xylose, as in xyloglucans, confers increased solubility in alkali and water. Xyloglucan is a linear $(1–4)$-β-D-glucan chain substituted with xylosyl units, which may be further substituted to form galactosyl-$(1–2)$-β-xylosyl or fucosyl-$(1–2)$-D-galactosyl-$(1–2)$-β-D-xylosyl units.

The *pectins* act as biological glues, cementing plant cells together. The precise function of pectins within the cell wall is unclear, but they are closely associated with calcium homoeostasis. Most pectins are probably derived from the primary cell wall and appear to be soluble only after calcium ions are removed. The principal cross-linkage is provided by the helical $(1–4)$-β-D-galactosyluronic groups from adjacent polysaccharides (Figure 14.2), and condensation with calcium converts soluble pectin into rigid 'egg-box' structures. The extent of calcium cross-bridging or esterification through aromatic linkages, and the degree of branching and size of neutral sugar side-chains influence gel flexibility, cell-wall porosity and interaction with hemicellulosic polymers.

The *glycoproteins* within the cell wall provide extensive cross-linkages across the different polysaccharide components of the cell wall and form a network with the cellulose microfibrils within a hemicellulose pectin gel.

Gums and mucilages

The plant gums and mucilages are a poorly defined group of exudates from plants. Mucilages are gums dissolved in the juices of the plant. Plant gums are a heterogeneous group of complex, branched heteropolysaccharides. They are obtained from plants, often occurring as a reaction to injury. Mucilages are associated with seeds and are very water soluble. They are functionally important in seeds in dry areas: the mucilages bind water so that after rain the plant can rapidly grow and pass through the

cycle to produce a new seed and so survive the next drought.

Some plant polysaccharides are harvested from the plant and purified before use as processed food components or for therapeutic use. These are often soluble polysaccharides and include:

- **guar gum** (mol. wt 0.25×10^6): a linear, non-ionic galactomannan
- **gum karaya** (mol. wt 4.7×10^6): a cylindrical complex polysaccharide, partially acetylated and highly branched with interior galacturonorhamnose chains, to which are attached galactose and rhamnose end groups. Glucuronic acid is also a component
- **gum arabic** (mol. wt $0.5–1.5 \times 10^6$): a complex acidic heteropolysaccharide based on a highly branched array of galactose, arabinose, rhamnose and glucuronic acid. Uronic acid residues tend to occur on the periphery of an essentially globular structure
- **gum tragacanth** (mol. wt $0.5–1 \times 10^6$): a complex gum with two major components, bassorin and tragacanthin, composed of arabinose, fucose, galactose, glucose, xylose and galacturonic acid.

These gums and mucilages are used as additives by food manufacturers, and as such may contribute less than 2% of a food.

OTHER FIBRES

- Chitin and chitosan: constituents of the arthropod exoskeleton and fungal cell walls. Chitin is a $(1,4)$-linked *N*-acetyl-D-glucosamine, with glucose derivatives forming a long chain. Chitoson is the *N*-deacetylated product of chitin
- chondroitin sulfate: a constituent of animal connective tissue, formed of repeating units of glucuronic acid linked to *N*-acetyl-D-galactosamine
- cutin: a constituent of the plant cuticle
- dextrin (resistant): an indigestible intermediate formed during the partial breakdown of starch
- fructan: a linear or branched fructose polymer
- galactooligosaccharide
- inulin: a constituent of chicory and Jerusalem artichoke; a β-$(2,1)$-linked fructose polymer with a glucose at the end of the molecule

- maltodextrin (resistant): an indigestible intermediate formed during the partial breakdown of starch
- modified cellulose
- oligofructose: a constituent of onions, bananas, lettuce and wheat; an indigestible intermediate formed during the partial breakdown of inulin
- polydextrose: a synthesised glucose polymer
- resistant starch
- saponin: a plant glycoside
- wax: esters of long-chain saturated and unsaturated fatty acids.

QUANTITATIVE MEASUREMENT OF FIBRE

There are two approaches to the analysis of dietary fibre: gravimetric methods and gas–liquid chromatography (GLC). Gravimetric methods measure fibre by weighing an insoluble residue after chemical and enzymatic solubilisation of non-fibre constituents. The remaining protein is assayed and subtracted from the original weight. GLC methods require the enzymatic breakdown of starch and the separation of the low molecular weight sugars, acid hydrolysis to free sugars, conversion to alditol acetates, and finally separation and measurement of neutral monomers with GLC, together with determination of uronic acid and lignin. The GLC methods enable the nature of the carbohydrate to be determined in more detail.

PHYSICAL PROPERTIES OF FIBRE

The main action of dietary fibre is due to its physical properties. Dietary fibre acts as a sponge along the entire gastrointestinal tract, holding water and the solutes in the water, and therefore retarding absorption of these solutes and solution. Fibre also binds trace metals and bile acids, which can alter sterol turnover. These physical properties are modified in the colon, where the bacteria ferment the fibre and the breakdown products, e.g. short-chain fatty acids become important.

An important function of insoluble fibres is to increase viscosity in the intestinal contents. Other polymeric components of the diet (proteins, gelatinised starch), mucous glycoproteins liberated from the epithelia, and particulate material present in chyme (such as insoluble fibre or hydrated plant tissues) will also contribute to a lesser extent to overall viscosity. The viscosity of these substances in the intestine is sensitive to changes in ionic concentration due to intestinal secretion or absorption of aqueous fluids.

Vegetables undergo structural changes during cooking and mastication, e.g. cellular disintegration. The cells after cooking are ruptured and the cell contents lost. The grinding of foods before cooking and ingestion may also have pronounced effects on fibre action. Cell walls may be disrupted and the reduced particle size of some fibre preparations, such as wheat bran, may decrease the biological efficacy. The effect of other cooking processes, e.g. Maillard reactions, are not known.

ACTIONS OF FIBRE ALONG THE GASTROINTESTINAL TRACT

The four major effects of dietary fibre on gastrointestinal activity (Figure 14. 3) relate to:

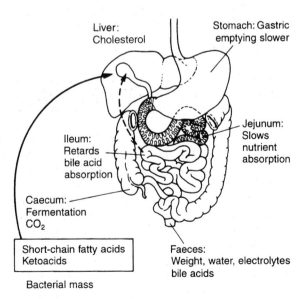

Fig. 14.3 Action of dietary fibre (non-starch polysaccharides) along the gastrointestinal tract.

- the rate of gastrointestinal absorption
- caecal fermentation
- faecal weight
- sterol metabolism.

Rate of intestinal absorption

There are two main components to the role of dietary fibre in the upper gastrointestinal tract: to prolong gastric emptying time and to retard the absorption of nutrients. Both are dependent on the physical form of the fibre, and in particular its viscosity.

The inclusion of viscous polysaccharides in carbohydrate meals reduces the postprandial blood glucose level concentrations in humans. There appears to be no correlation between the rate of gastric emptying and postprandial concentrations of blood glucose.

Diets that have a substantial complex carbohydrate content tend to be bulky, and require longer to eat. In one experiment the time taken to eat a whole apple took longer (17 min) than that required for purée (6 min) or apple juice (1.5 min) in equicaloric amounts.

Gastric emptying is affected by the physical nature of the gastric contents as well as the chemistry of the components. Isolated viscous fibres tend to slow the gastric emptying rate of liquids and other solids. Gastric emptying for a fibre on its own may be quite different to that when ingested along with other dietary constituents such as fat and protein. The gastric emptying time for different fibre sources is variable.

Rates of release of nutrients from dietary fibre in the intestine are influenced by factors such as the intactness of tissue histology, the degree of ripeness, and the effects of processing and cooking.

There is no evidence to suggest that viscous polysaccharides inhibit transport across the small intestinal epithelium. It is more likely that their viscous properties inhibit the access of nutrients to the epithelium. Two mechanisms bring nutrients into contact with the epithelium. Intestinal contractions create turbulence and convection currents, which mix the luminal content, bringing material from the centre of the lumen close to the epithelium. Nutrients then have to diffuse across the thin, relatively unstirred layer of fluid lying adjacent to the epithelium. Increasing the viscosity of the luminal contents may impair both convection and diffusion of the nutrients across the unstirred layer. In the case of isolated polysaccharides such as guar gum, the slowing of nutrient absorption appears to be a function of viscosity.

In the case of whole plant material the influence on absorption appears to be due to the inaccessibility of nutrients within the cellular matrix of the plant. The effects on absorption can be minimised by grinding the food before cooking or by thorough chewing; both processes open the cellular structure.

Inadequate mixing of luminal contents by soluble polysaccharides due to increased viscosity may also slow the movement of digestive enzymes to their substrates.

Viscous polysaccharides tend to delay small bowel transit, possibly owing to resistance to the propulsive contractions of the intestine. In rats most of this delay is secondary to alterations in ileal motility, with transit through the upper small intestine little affected.

Complex carbohydrates, particularly those that possess uronic and phenolic acid groups or sulfated residues, such as pectins and alginates, may bind magnesium, calcium, zinc and iron. However, there are other constituents of plant cells, e.g. phytates, silicates and oxalates, that also chelate divalent cations. The binding of minerals may be reduced by acid, protein, ascorbate and citrate.

The reduction in absorption of minerals and vitamins could, in theory, have adverse nutritional consequences, particularly in populations eating diets inherently deficient in these nutrients; that is, in malnourished individuals or fastidious health food-conscious communities, where diets may be marginal in micronutrients but high in fibre. Children are particularly vulnerable to such diets. Customary Western diets contain levels of minerals and vitamins in excess of daily requirements. Mineral balance studies have indicated that for people on nutritionally adequate diets, the ingestion of mixed high-fibre diets or dietary supplementation with viscous polysaccharides is unlikely to cause mineral deficiencies.

The ingestion of dietary fibre may affect drug absorption in two ways: by reducing gastric emptying or inhibiting mixing in the small intestine. Viscous polysaccharides delay the absorption of paracetamol. Quite separately, if a drug enters the enterohepatic circulation any bacterial metabolism of the drug may be altered by coincidental fermentation of fibre, and thus the half-life of a drug may be increased or decreased. An example of this is digoxin, which has a narrow therapeutic range and is passively absorbed in the small intestine, and so is affected by gastric emptying or decreased small intestinal absorption. Digoxin is also reduced in the colon to an inactive metabolite, which is absorbed or excreted in faeces.

Substrate for caecal fermentation

The colon may be regarded as two organs, the right side a fermenter, the left side affecting continence. The right side of the colon is involved in nutrient salvage, so that dietary fibre, resistant starch, fat and protein are utilised by bacteria, and the endproducts absorbed for use by the body.

The colonic flora is a complex ecosystem consisting largely of anaerobic bacteria, which outnumber the facultative organisms by at least 100:1. The colonic flora of a single individual consists of more than 400 bacterial species. The total bacterial count in faeces is 10^{10} to 10^{12} colony-forming units/ml. Despite the complexity of the ecosystem, the microflora population is remarkably stable. Although wide variations in the microflora are found between individuals, studies in a single subject show the microflora to be stable over prolonged periods. There is some attraction in identifying individual bacteria. It is, however, more profitable for physiological and nutritional studies to regard the caecal bacterial complex as an important organ in its own right, complementary to the liver in the enterohepatic circulation.

The caecal bacterial flora are dependent on dietary and endogenous sources for nutrition. There are variations in the amounts of substances passing through the intestine from the ileum, with an inverse relationship between caecal bacterial metabolism and upper intestinal nutrient absorption. Dietary fibre has an influence on bacterial mass and enzyme activity. The consensus view is that while the caecal bacterial mass may increase as a result of an increased fibre content in the diet, the types of bacteria do not alter.

The process whereby a compound is bacterially dissimilated in the caecum under anaerobic conditions is complex and varied, leading to partial or complete decomposition, with the endproducts being:

- absorbed from the colon to be utilised as nutrients
- absorbed and re-excreted in the enterohepatic circulation
- excreted in the faeces.

The colon is part of the excretion system provided by the liver and biliary tree, i.e. the enterohepatic circulation. Poorly water-soluble chemicals of molecular weight of about 300–400 Da are excreted in the bile having been made more water soluble through chemical conjugation with glucuronide, sulfate, acetate, etc., or made physically soluble by the detergent properties of bile acids. These may be endogenous, e.g. bile acids, bilirubin and hormones, or exogenous, e.g. drugs, food additives and pesticides. They pass unabsorbed through the small intestine. In the caecum these biliary excretion products, and also unabsorbed dietary constituents, e.g. resistant starch, fat, proteins and mucopolysaccharides secreted by the intestinal mucosa, are fermented by the bacterial enzymes. The fermentation process of biliary excretion products removes those substitutions that have increased water solubility and facilitated biliary excretion. The bacterial metabolic products are less water soluble. Some of the endproducts of the fermentation of biliary excretion compounds are reabsorbed, metabolically altered, reconjugated in the liver and excreted in bile; hence, an enterohepatic circulation is established.

The effects of dietary fibre in the colon may be summarised in terms of:

- susceptibility to bacterial fermentation
- ability to increase bacterial mass
- ability to increase bacterial saccharolytic enzyme activity
- water-holding capacity of the fibre residue after fermentation.

Enlargement of the caecum is a common finding when some dietary fibres are fed, and this is now believed to be part of a normal physiological adjustment. Such an increase may be due to a number of factors, e.g. prolonged caecal residence of the fibre, increased bacterial mass or increased bacterial endproducts.

The fermentation of fibre yields hydrogen, methane and short-chain fatty acids. Hydrogen is readily measured in the breath and has a diurnal variation, with a nadir at midday and an increase in the afternoon. Diverse sources of fibre influence the evolution of hydrogen in different ways. Disaccharides generate hydrogen more rapidly than trisaccharides which, in turn, evolve hydrogen more quickly than oligosaccharides. More complex carbohydrates may not be fermented as rapidly and may require induction of specific enzymes before they can be utilised.

Methane-producing organisms are said to be strict anaerobes. There is a wide diversity in the proportion of individuals who exhale methane in their breath, varying in different healthy adult populations from 33 to 80%. The breath methane status of an individual remains stable throughout the day and over prolonged periods, yet faeces from healthy individuals, regardless of breath methane excretion status, will always produce methane. This suggests that all individuals produce methane, but a critical level must be produced for methane to spill over into the breath.

It has been shown that considerable methane excretion only takes place when sulfate-reducing bacteria are not active. The metabolic endproduct of dissimilatory sulfate reduction is thought to be toxic to methanogenic bacteria. When sulfate is present, sulfate-reducing bacteria have a higher substrate affinity for hydrogen than do methanogenic bacteria.

Some non-absorbed carbohydrates, e.g. pectin, gum arabic, oligosaccharides and resistant starch, are fermented to short-chain fatty acids (chiefly acetic, propionic and n-butyric acid), carbon dioxide, hydrogen and methane. The production of short-chain fatty acids has several possible actions on the gut mucosa. All of the short-chain fatty acids are readily absorbed by the colonic mucosa, but only acetic acid reaches the systemic circulation in appreciable amounts. Butyric acid is metabolised before it reaches the portal blood, and propionic acid is metabolised in the liver. Butyric acid appears to be used as a fuel by the colonic mucosa, and *in vitro* studies of isolated cells have indicated that the short-chain fatty acids and butyric acid in particular are the preferred energy sources of colonic cells. Short-chain fatty acids are potent stimulants of cellular proliferation, not only in the colon but also in the small intestine. The absorbed short-chain fatty acids are used in metabolic processes throughout the body, e.g. metabolised into the glycerol of hepatic glycerides and into amino acids.

Short-chain fatty acids are the predominant anions in human faeces. They are derived by fermentation of complex carbohydrates, resistant starch and NSP.

> The caecal fermentation of 40–50 g of complex polysaccharides will yield 400–500 mmol total short-chain fatty acids, 240–300 mmol acetate, and 80–100 mmol of both propionate and butyrate. Almost all of these short-chain fatty acids will be absorbed from the colon. This means that faecal short-chain fatty acid estimations do not reflect caecal and colonic fermentation, only the efficiency of absorption, the ability of the fibre residue to sequestrate short-chain fatty acids, and the continued fermentation of fibre around the colon, which presumably will continue until the substrate is exhausted.

The absorption of short-chain fatty acids from the colon in humans is concentration dependent and associated with bicarbonate secretion. Bicarbonate is secreted in the colon during short-chain fatty acid absorption, a process independent of the chloride–bicarbonate exchange. It is possible that there is an acetate–bicarbonate exchange at the cell surface, but the precise mechanism is not understood. There is a stimulatory effect of short-chain fatty acids on sodium absorption from the colonic lumen, tied to the recycling of hydrogen ions. The non-ionised short-chain fatty acid crosses into the cell, where it dissociates, and a hydrogen ion is moved back into the lumen in exchange for sodium. Thus, short-chain fatty acids provide a powerful stimulant to sodium and water absorption.

The presence of bacteria in the colon produces an 'organ' of intense, mainly reductive, metabolic activity. This is in contrast to the liver, which is oxidative. The intestinal flora perform a wide range of metabolic transformations on ingested compounds. The major enzymes involved in these activities include azoreductase, nitrate reductase, nitroreductase, β-glucosidase, β-glucuronidase and methylmercury-demethylase. The action of fibre on the activity of these enzymes may be species dependent and animal studies are not always predictive of the action in humans.

Faecal weight

Faeces are complex and consist of 75% water; bacteria make a large contribution to the dry weight, the residue being unfermented fibre and excreted compounds. There is a wide range of individual and mean faecal weights. In a study in Edinburgh the individual variation was between 19 and 280 g over 24 h. The amount of faeces excreted varies quite markedly from individual to individual and by any one individual over a period of time, although why such variation occurs is unknown. Of the dietary constituents, only dietary fibre influences faecal weight.

The most important mechanism by which dietary fibre increases faecal weight is through the water-holding capacity of unfermented fibre. However, fibre may also influence faecal output by another mechanism. Colonic microbial growth may be stimulated by the ingestion of such fermentable fibre sources as apple, guar or pectin. This is an uncertain route, as there is not always an increase in faecal weight as a result of eating these fibres. There may also be an added osmotic effect of products of bacterial fermentation on faecal mass, although this is not as yet a well-defined contribution.

One of the major functions of the colon is to absorb water and produce faeces that can be voided readily and at will from the rectum. The ileum contains a viscous fluid, the viscosity being created by mucus and water-soluble fibres, whose molecular weight, degree of cross-linkages and aggregation will determine the viscosity. If the viscosity increases to a certain point, peculiar to the constituent macromolecules, then a sol or hydrated carbohydrate complex will result. The sol will be coherent and homogeneous.

The concentration of ileal effluent in the caecum and colon is the result of the absorption of water. This might be expected to create a gel. Faeces are not a gel, however, but a Plasticine-like material, heterogeneous without viscosity, and made up of water, bacteria, lipids, sterols, mucus and fibre. In the caecum there is therefore a marked physical change, in part as a result of bacterial activity, in part by the presence of bacteria themselves. The

solid structure of faeces is lost in watery diarrhoea. The mechanism of this change, whether physiological or pathological, is unknown but some of the steps involved are described below.

In the colon, water is distributed in three ways:

- free water that can be absorbed from the colon
- water that is incorporated into the bacterial mass
- water that is bound by fibre.

Faecal weight is dictated by:

- the time available for water absorption through the colonic mucosa
- the incorporation of water into the residue of fibre after fermentation of the fibre
- the bacterial mass.

Wheat bran added to the diet increases faecal weight in a predictable linear manner and decreases intestinal transit time. The increment in faecal weight is independent of initial weight. Wholemeal bread, unless of a very coarse nature, has little or no effect on faecal weight. The particle size of the fibre is all-important, coarse wheat bran being more effective than fine wheat bran. The greater the water-holding capacity of the bran, the greater the effect on faecal weight. The effect of the water binding by wheat bran is such that in addition to an increase in faecal weight, other faecal constituents, namely bile acids, which do not increase in absolute amounts, are diluted by faecal water and hence their concentration decreases. The increment in faecal weight per gram of wheat bran varies in different populations. For most healthy individuals, an increase in wet faecal weight, depending on the particle size of the bran, is generally in the order of 3–5 g/g fibre. However, in individuals with irritable bowel syndrome and symptomatic diverticulosis, the increment is in the order of 1–2 g wet weight/g fibre. This suggests that there is a difference in the handling of the fibre in the intestine in these conditions.

Bacteria are an important component of the faecal mass. It is not known what percentage are living and what percentage are dead and as such are being voided. The fermentation of some fibres results in an increase in the bacterial content and hence faecal weight. Other fibres, of which pectin is an important example, are fermented without any such effect. It is possible that some fibres which increase stool weight in association with an increased bacterial mass do so because of an increase in excreted bacteria adherent to unfermented fibre.

The degree to which free water is absorbed from the colon will be affected by a number of factors, which are poorly understood. An increase in the short-chain fatty acid concentration of faeces appears to be related to an increased output of faecal water, which may suggest that under some circumstances short-chain fatty acid absorption is less efficient and in part determines faecal output. This concurs with the view of Hellendoorn (1978), who suggested an important role for fibre fermentation products on stool weight and transit time. The demonstration that short-chain fatty acids were absorbed rapidly in the colon suggested that they play no part in determining faecal output. However, it would appear that there is continued fermentation of some complex carbohydrates, e.g. ispaghula, in the distal colon. Under these circumstances the faecal short-chain fatty acids may influence faecal water osmolality, absorption and stool weight.

The effect of fibre on faecal weight may be calculated as:

$$\text{Weight of faeces} = W_f(1 + H_f) + W_b(1 + H_b) + W_m(1 + H_m)$$

where W_f, W_b and W_m are, respectively, the dry weights of fibre remaining after fermentation in the colon, bacteria present in the faeces, and osmotically active metabolites and other substances in the colonic contents that could reduce the amount of free water absorbed; and H_f, H_b and H_m denote their respective water-holding capacities (i.e. the weight of water resistant to absorption from the colon, per unit dry weight of each faecal constituent).

Alterations in sterol metabolism

Dietary fibre has been shown to have an effect on sterol metabolism. This effect is not simple and may be indirect or direct.

Indirectly, dietary fibre may displace fat from the diet, or increased polyunsaturated fats are frequently eaten in conjunction with the fibre. The direct effect of fibre on sterol metabolism may be through one of several mechanisms:

- altered lipid absorption
- altered bile acid metabolism in the caecum
- reduced bile acid absorption in the caecum
- indirectly by short-chain fatty acids, especially propionic acid, resulting from fibre fermentation.

An important action of some fibres is to reduce the reabsorption of bile acids in the ileum, and hence the amount and type of bile acid and fats reaching the colon. Bile acids may be trapped within the lumen of the ileum, either because of a high luminal viscosity or because they bind to the lignin. A reduction in the ileal reabsorption of bile acid has several direct effects. The enterohepatic circulation of bile acids may be affected. In the caecum, bile acids are deconjugated and 7α-dehydroxylated. In this less water-soluble form bile acids are adsorbed to dietary fibre in a way that is affected by pH and is mediated through hydrophobic bonds, thereby increasing the loss of bile acid in the faeces. The consequence of this is that the enterohepatic pool is initially reduced. The precise relationship between the proportions of ileal and caecal absorption of bile acids is difficult to estimate. This variable is dependent in part on the amount and type of fibre. A further complication is the bacterial colonisation of the ileum stimulating caecal bacterial activity. Approximately 25% of the body pool of cholic acid and 50% of chenodeoxycholic acid pass into the caecum to be either absorbed or excreted in faeces. This may be renewed by increased synthesis of bile acids from cholesterol which, in turn, reduces body cholesterol.

The fibres that are most effective in influencing sterol metabolism (e.g. pectin) are fermented in the colon, as demonstrated by an increased breath hydrogen production. It is unlikely that the physiological effect is due entirely to adsorption to fibre in the colon. This is in contrast to the important sequestrating effect of fibre in the ileum. There may be an alteration in the endproducts of bile acid bacterial metabolism that are absorbed from the colon and return to the liver in the portal vein, modulating either the synthesis of cholesterol or its catabolism to bile acids. Alternatively, it is probable that bacteria bind bile acids in the colon after the initial deconjugation and dehydroxylation to be excreted in faeces.

Other fibres, e.g. gum arabic, are associated with a significant decrease in serum cholesterol without increasing faecal bile acid excretion.

RECOMMENDED INTAKE

This is not precisely defined. An intake of 30 g/day has ben suggested but then one could question how much of what sources of fibre, cereal, fruit or vegetable. Whatever is decided, a wide range of sources should be the rule. The five plan for fruit and vegetables would be a good start.

KEY POINTS

1. Dietary fibre is a term for the family of dietary complex carbohydrates and lignins in plant cell walls. Alternative names include roughage and non-starch polysaccharides (NSP). These plant cell-wall polymeric carbohydrates and lignins are not digested in the upper gastrointestinal tract.
2. These complex carbohydrates have individual and diverse actions along the gastrointestinal tract. The chemistry cannot, however, identify or predict the biological action of individual fibres in the gastrointestinal tract. Each fibre is peculiar in its biological action, and is affected by extraction, physical format and processing.
3. In the upper gastrointestinal tract the physical properties of dietary fibre are important in slowing the rate of absorption of nutrients.
4. Some dietary fibres may alter sterol turnover, usually by increasing faecal bile acid excretion.
5. Some dietary fibres increase caecal bacterial growth and metabolism.
6. Some dietary fibres increase faecal weight through a combination of the water-holding capacity of the fibre not fermented by bacteria, bacterial growth, and the osmotic effect of bacterial fermentation products in the colonic lumen.

THINKING POINT

Try to define dietary fibre. Is dietary fibre essential, conditionally indispensable, conditionally dispensable or none of these?

NEED TO UNDERSTAND

1. Whilst the definition of dietary fibre is ill defined, the physiological functions are well defined.
2. Fibre moves along the gastrointestinal tract as a sponge, slowing gastric emptying and retarding absorption from the intestine, and the residue surviving bacterial degradation in the caecum is the major determinant of stool weight.
3. Fermentable fibres also have an effect on cholesterol turnover.

FURTHER READING

British Nutrition Foundation Task Force (1990) *Complex Carbohydrates in Foods*. Chapman and Hall, London.

Eastwood, M.A. (1992) Physiological effect of dietary fiber. *Annual Review of Nutrition*, **12**, 19–35.

Guarner, F. and Malagelada, J.R. (2003) Gut flora in health and disease. *Lancet*, **361**, 512–19.

Hellendoorn, E.W. (1978) Fermentation as the principal cause of the physiological activity of indigestible food residue. In *Topics in Dietary Fiber Research* (ed. G.A. Spiller). Plenum Press, New York, pp. 127–216.

Kritchevsky, D., Bonfield, C. and Anderson, J.W. (eds) (1990) *Dietary Fiber*. Plenum Press, New York.

McCleary, B. and Prosky, L. (eds.) (2001) *Advanced Dietary Fibre Technology*. Iowa State Press, Ames, IA.

Symposium on 'The Nutritional Consequences of Complex Carbohydrates' (1996) *Proceedings of the Nutrition Society*, **55**, 863–943.

Trowell, H., Burkitt, D. and Heaton, K. (1985) *Dietary Fibre, Fibre-depleted Foods and Disease*. Academic Press, London.

Vahouny Dietary Fibre Symposium (2003) *Proceedings Nutrition Society*, **62**, 1–249.

WEBSITE

www.nap.edu/catalog/10161.html National Academy of the USA

15

Alcohol as a nutrient

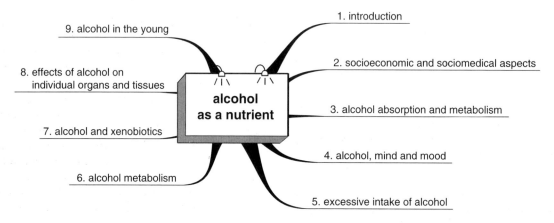

Fig. 15.1 Chapter outline.

INTRODUCTION

Alcohol is an interesting dietary component to discuss in detail. This simple molecule can be used as a model to underline the different modalities of nutrition, manufacturing, social, genetic predisposition and gender differences in metabolism, nutritional value and the consequences of excess. The popularity of alcohol results from its effects on mood and an induced sense of well-being. The ingestion of alcohol is a social activity; a meeting, occasion or function is better enjoyed by many in the relaxing ambience coincidental with the consumption of alcohol.

Ethanol provides 7 calories per gram. The full extent of how much energy is provided with an alcoholic drink varies with the beverage, from the sugars accompanying beer to the pure alcohol of vodka.

The use of yeast to ferment carbohydrates from fruit, grain, vegetables and other food sources for the production of alcohol is an age-old custom. Great skill is employed in developing different forms of alcoholic drinks, wines, fortified wines, beers and spirits. Some carbohydrate sources, such as in the starches in cereal grains, require preparation (malting) before fermentation, to convert the starch in maltoses. A by-product is carbon dioxide, which produces the 'head' on beer and the bubbles in champagne. The limiting factor in alcohol production is the amount of sugar available to the fermentation process, and the final alcohol content is around 5% in beers and 11% in wines. To achieve the greater alcohol concentration in spirits the solution is distilled to 40%, as in whisky, gin and brandy.

Alcohol strengths

Beer 50 g/litre
Wine 110 g/litre
Spirits 400g/litre

Proof: an old, crude measure of measuring the alcohol content of spirits involved soaking gunpowder in an alcoholic drink. If the gunpowder would still explode on being fired, then the spirit was more than half alcohol. In the Britain, Canada and Australia proof is 57% alcohol; in the USA proof is double the alcohol content, i.e. 40% brandy is 80% proof.

In assessing alcohol intake an empirical *unit* has been defined, equivalent to 8–10 g of ethanol. A unit is contained in: one single measure of spirits, one glass of wine, a measure of fortified wine, half a pint of beer or lager, or one small glass of sherry.

Because toxic substances such as methanol also concentrate in these drinks, the spirits are left in casks for prolonged periods to allow the noxious chemicals to filter out through the wood of the cask.

SOCIOECONOMIC AND SOCIOMEDICAL ASPECTS

Alcohol is used in widely diverse cultures, on occasions such as births, marriages, deaths and sporting events. In Britain, alcohol has traditionally been drunk in the home and in public houses or clubs. Increasingly, alcohol is enjoyed as part of a restaurant meal. Men drink alcohol more than women, in a ratio of approximately 2:1 depending on the venue. Some 3% of British adults drink every day, 34% weekly, 52% monthly and less than 10% less frequently than monthly. Alcohol is used by more than 75% of the Canadian population over the age of 15 years of age. Abstinence is looked at askance in many societies, yet alcohol excess is the root of much distress, social upheaval and violence.

In Western society, there is an ambivalent attitude towards alcohol. On the one hand it is a social facilitator, on the other hand its excessive use is associated with challenging sociomedical problems. Much of the Western social scene depends to some extent on the use and, in part, the cultured acclaim of the most perfect of these drinks. The comfortable feeling created by modest amounts of ethanol dispels potential anxieties in most of the population, including clinicians.

However, alcohol can lead to drunkenness, violence, motor vehicle driving offences, hooliganism, social degradation, impotence, marital disharmony, disease and brain atrophy. Both acute and chronic ethanol intake can impair work performance and decision making. There is an increased risk and severity of accidents associated with alcohol intake; however, fatigue may be a further risk factor in accidents and should never be underestimated.

In England and Wales 28 000 excess deaths a year may be directly attributable to alcohol abuse. In Britain it was estimated that alcoholism cost the country £1.7 billion in 1986. On average, at least 8 working days each year per head of population are lost through alcoholism. Most alcoholics work, and they have a three-fold increased risk of accidents over non-drinkers. Between 3 and 5% of staff in an average company, independent of seniority, will have an alcohol-related problem. Alcohol accounts for 5% of the energy intake in the USA, where the cost of the sick alcoholic amounts to over $100 billion a year. This does not include the distress to the family, society and workplace.

ALCOHOL ABSORPTION AND METABOLISM

Alcohol is taken by mouth and as there is no digestion is rapidly absorbed. Some alcohol is absorbed from the stomach, but most is absorbed in the proximal small intestine. The rate of absorption is dependent on gastric emptying time and hence, in general, on whether the alcohol is drunk alone or delayed with varying amounts and types of food. Eating before drinking alcohol reduces absorption rate even more. Alcohol is drunk because of its intoxicating effects. Such effects are dependent on blood alcohol concentration (BAC); the rate of rise in BAC rather than the decrease. The time of attaining maximum BAC will depend on the amount drunk and the rate of drinking. The excretion in breath [breath alcohol concentration (BrAC)] can be used to measure blood ethanol concentrations and is a ready roadside method used by the police to determine whether a person is legally considered safe to drive. The remainder is oxidised in the liver and other tissues. Maximum BAC is achieved some 30–60 min after drinking. When intake exceeds removal, the BAC will increase; when removal from the body exceeds intake then the BAC will decrease. BAC is measured as mg of ethanol/ 100 ml of blood (80 mg%) or as millimoles/litre (80 mg% is equivalent to 17 mmol/litre of blood). The rate of removal by metabolism is 6–10 g/h in a 70 kg person (120 mg of ethanol/kg body weight/h). Bctween 2 and 10% of ethanol absorbed is excreted unchanged by the kidneys and lungs. A pint (500 ml; 25 g alcohol) of beer takes 3 h to be eliminated from the body and a bottle of whisky (750 ml; 280 g alcohol) takes 1–2 days.

BAC is dependent on:

- gender
- age, height and weight
- pattern and chronicity of drinking
- type, number, size and alcohol content of drinks
- time when BAC is measured relative to:
  time of ingestion of alcohol and food
  time lapse since last drink of alcohol
  health status
  coincidental drugs and medications

Once absorbed, ethanol diffuses into all tissues, including the brain, fat tissues and the placental barrier to the foetus. The diffusion into fat tissues means that those with an abundance of fat have a buffering system to alcohol and its intoxicating effects, which will not be as great as the same intake in a lean individual. A pregnant mother exposes her baby to the toxic effects of alcohol when she drinks.

ALCOHOL, MIND AND MOOD

Short-term effects of alcohol intake

Alcohol is drunk for pleasurable- effects on the mind. The response is very variable from person to person and occasion to occasion. There is complex stimulation, behavioural and psychological arousal, and loss of inhibition. The response is also affected by the social atmosphere, previous drinking habits and the amount drunk.

A range of effects at different BACs may be:

20 mg/100 ml	mellow feeling, reduced inhibitions
50 mg/100 ml	noticeably relaxed, less alert, less co-ordinated
80 mg/100 ml	driving illegal, co-ordination definitely impaired
100 mg/100 ml	noisy, embarrassing, reduced reaction time
150 mg/100 ml	impaired balance, clearly drunk
300 mg/100 ml	consciousness threatened
400 mg/100 ml	unconscious, may die
500 mg/100 ml	lethal in many.

These responses will depend on many other effects, notably the frequency of ingestion of alcohol.

The need for nicotinamide adenine dinucleotide (NAD) during ethanol metabolism may deplete the tissues of NAD; two molecules are required for each ethanol molecule. If the glucose stores in the form of glycogen are insufficient then further problems with glucose homoeostasis may compound the problem and hypoglycaemia develop. This can occur 2–3 h after the alcohol intake starts and can lead to irritability and the deteriorating behaviour of heavy alcoholic episodes.

The phenomenon of the hangover is common. This may be due to a number of complicating factors, including acetaldehyde, hypoglycaemia, the diuretic effect of the alcohol, the dehydration caused by drinking and the loss of rapid eye movement (REM) sleep. If the alcoholic episode was extreme then the BAC may still be high many hours after alcohol ingestion has ceased.

Long-term effects of continuous heavy alcohol intake

The definition of heavy intake is very difficult and varies from person to person and with addiction and physical problems. Distinctions have to be made between intermittent binge drinking, with heavy bouts of intense drinking, and regular daily exposure to alcohol. Binge drinking is sometimes

Table 15.1 Comparison of the effects of alcohol consumption in men and women

| Effect | Weekly consumption (units) | |
	Men	Women
Safe	< 20	< 13
Risk increases with consumption	21–50	14–35
Hazardous	> 51	> 36

occupational; the individual may return from an intense period of alcohol-free work, enriched with money, wanting relaxation and fun and to get extremely drunk. Alternatively, people may drink regularly and never appear to be inebriated, yet their alcohol intake is very significant.

EXCESSIVE INTAKE OF ALCOHOL

Recognition of alcohol abuse

It is not routine for doctors to take an accurate ethanol intake history, and self-reporting individual notoriously underestimate intake. The safe limits of alcohol intake are different for men and women (Table 15.1) although there are individual differences, as discussed below.

Probably the best method for identifying alcohol abuse is the Michigan Alcohol Screening Test (MAST). This is a ten-question modification (devised by Pokorny *et al.*, 1972) of the original 25 weighted questions described by Selzer. Alternative methods of identifying excessive alcohol use include random measurements of BAC, BrAC and serum γ-glutamyltransferase activity. This enzyme activity is useful diagnostically, but may return to normal after about 5 years of heavy alcohol drinking.

A possible indicator of recent alcohol consumption is the measurement of 24 h urinary excretion of 5-hydroxytryptophol:5-hydroxyindole-3-acetic acid.

Morbidity and mortality

In many studies of ethanol-associated deaths, there is a suggestion of a U- or J-shaped relation

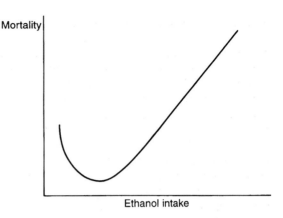

Fig. 15.2 The U- or J-shaped relationship between mortality and ethanol intake.

between ethanol consumption and mortality, the death rate in abstainers being higher than in those consuming 1–10 units a week (Figure 15.2). Life-long total abstainers from alcohol form a small section of the population, and this finding may be spurious and reflect an undue number of previously heavy drinkers now mortally compromised by ethanol, but abstaining in their terminal state. Other health hazards such as cigarette smoking may be more common in either group or, alternatively moderate drinking may be good for health, e.g. alcohol has effects on platelet function similar to aspirin, with benefits to the ageing vasculature. Crucial to the critical evaluation and interpretation of morbidity and mortality patterns in alcoholics, moderate drinkers and abstainers is a knowledge of their previous health record. Increasingly, in papers written in medical journals the authors must declare if they have any vested interests in the topic of the paper. It may be interesting and revealing if the alcohol consumption of the authors and hence their interest in the subject was recorded in alcohol-related papers.

In a general hospital in London, 12% of all admissions, 7% of admissions to a general surgical ward, and 26% of admissions to an overnight observation ward were alcohol related. Many of the admissions were young males.

In a 15-year follow-up study of 49 464 young Swedish Army conscripts, there was a strong association between alcohol intake and subsequent death rate. In soldiers drinking more than 250 g of alcohol a week (25–30 units), the risk of death rose to three times that of those with a moderate intake of 1–100 g per week (10–12 units). One-third of deaths were due to violence or suicide. The overall evidence is that there is a linear relationship between alcohol intake and morbidity, in contrast to the J-shaped relationship between alcohol and mortality described in some studies.

Alcoholism

Alcoholism occurs more frequently than by chance in some families. It is almost impossible to separate the influence of genetics and environment in studies of alcoholism. The reason for this is complicated, but genetic constitution, family influences, a shared environment with people with similar views on alcohol intake and various psychiatric abnormalities, depression, anxiety states and antisocial personality disorders have all been implicated. There is an interplay between predisposing genetic factors and protective factors, e.g. an innate or acquired dislike of alcohol, feeling unwell after drinking alcohol, a genetically based susceptibility to alcohol abuse or no access to alcohol.

Population genetic studies have included 'normal' drinking groups, population studies of alcohol metabolism, and genetic studies in twins and adopted children. A study in Copenhagen showed a four-fold increase in the incidence of alcoholism among male adoptees, adopted soon after birth. The shortcomings of these studies include adoptees being brought up with alcoholic parents, the studies having too few subjects, and potential bias in the recruitment of subjects.

The kinetics of ethanol and acetaldehyde metabolism, as a result of genetically determined variations in the enzymes involved, are responsible for individual and racial differences in alcohol drinking habits and acute and chronic reactions to alcohol. In addition, there is varied vulnerability to organ damage after chronic alcohol abuse. Although 5% of all people consuming alcohol develop alcohol addiction, only 20% of these develop cirrhosis. Such a variation has led to speculation that genetic vulnerability or even viral infections may also be implicated in the cirrhotic process.

Table 15.2 indicates the genetic and environmental determinants of the effects of differing levels of alcohol consumption.

Table 15.2 Genetic and environmental determinants of effects of differing levels of alcohol consumption

Genetic	Environmental
Personality Psychiatric predisposition	National, religious and family attitudes to alcohol
Pharmacogenetic, e.g. acetaldehyde concentrations	Cultural patterns of drinking
Culture	Continuous or bout drinking
End-organ vulnerability	Reaction of employers, spouse and family
Human leucocyte antigen-8 dependent	Vulnerability to accidents

ALCOHOL METABOLISM

The liver is the prime site is for alcohol metabolism and utilises three pathways, in different parts of the cell:

- **cystosol**: alcohol dehydrogenase (ADH)
- **endoplasmic reticulum**: microsomal ethanol oxidising system
- **peroxisome**: catalase.

Ethanol is metabolised through acetyl-coenzyme A (CoA) pathways (Figure 15.3), the first stage in fatty acid synthesis; this involves ADH, a rate-limiting step. Alcohol is metabolised in two phases:

$$CH_3CH_2OH + NAD$$
ethanol

alcohol dehydrogenase
$$\longrightarrow$$

$$CH_3CHO + NADH + H^+$$
acetaldehyde

$$CH_3CHO + H_2O + NAD$$
acetaldehyde

acetaldehyde dehydrogenase
$$\longrightarrow$$

$$CH_3COOH + NADH + H^+$$
acetate

ADH, which facilitates the reaction of an alcohol to aldehyde, is a very complicated enzyme family to classify. The branch of the family of ADH

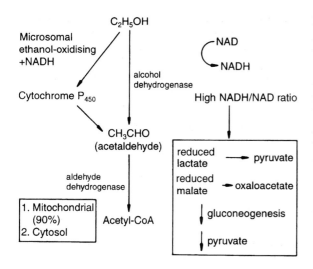

Fig. 15.3 Ethanol metabolism.

which oxidises ethanol to acetaldehyde is a cytosolic zinc-containing enzyme, a dimeric protein of two subunits, each of molecular weight 40 kDa. The enzyme has a broad substrate specificity, which includes the dehydrogenation of steroids, oxidation of glycols in the metabolism of noradrenaline and ω-oxidation of fatty acids. Human ADHs are encoded by at least seven genes and form at least five classes. The isozymes are differentially distributed in tissues, but have maximal activity in the liver. There are two active sites in ADH; one is based on a zinc atom which binds the ethanol molecule, the other is a NAD cofactor, which is the reactive site. The isozyme functional differences result from single amino acid changes that alter the configuration of the active sites, mainly for residues 48 and 93. The class IV ADH in the stomach predominantly expresses the sigma (σσ)-form. It is an active metaboliser of ingested alcohols. This gastric process determines up to 30% of the bioavailability of ethanol in humans. The reduced capacity for alcohol in women is in part due to a reduced gastric mucosal isoenzyme content.

Ethnic variations in alcohol dehydrogenase activity

There are a wide range of rates of ethanol metabolism due to there being at least four classes of

human ADH. The most important ADH isoform is class 1, with isoenzymes formed from three subunit chains, α, β and γ. The respective genetic loci are ADH1, ADH2 and ADH3. Polymorphism occurs with ADH2 and ADH3. The ADH3 isoforms are very similar in their kinetic constants. Various alleles occur for ADH2 (ADH2*1, ADH2*2, ADH2*3), the encoded enzymes of which vary in activity. ADH2 polymorphism is associated with alcohol problems. The isoenzyme encoded by ADH2*2 has a lower enzymatic efficiency than that encoded by ADH2*1. There is a positive relationship between alcoholic cirrhosis and the presence of the ADH2*2 allele.

Different mutant forms are found in various racial populations. The difference in ADH alleles is quite marked between Caucasians, Japanese, Chinese, Native Americans, Black Americans and Brazilians, which explains the racial differences in the effects of alcohol. African-Americans have slower rates of ethanol elimination than Caucasians.

In the ADH-mediated oxidation of ethanol, hydrogen is transferred from the substrate to NAD, forming the reduced form, NADH. The result is an excess of reducing equivalents in the hepatic cytosol as free NADH, as the system for the removal of NADH is overwhelmed.

Microsomal ethanol oxidising system

An accessory pathway comes into play at high ethanol concentrations, the microsomal ethanol oxidising system (MEOS). This is dependent on a specific cytochrome P450 activity. This system is increased in recently drinking subjects, i.e. it is induced by ethanol. While the cytochrome alcohol oxidase is a P450 IIEI system, it is possible that other isoenzymes have yet to be identified. MEOS has a relatively high K_m for ethanol (8–10 mM compared with 0.2–2 mM for ADH), hence the concentration differential. The clearance rate of some drugs, e.g. pentobarbital, increases from days to weeks. As this system also metabolises dietary carbohydrates, fats and proteins, the system is modulated by diet. Furthermore, the more rapid biotransferance of xenobiotics (substances that do not occur naturally, but that the body can metabolise) increases the vulnerability of the heavy drinker to the action of drugs.

Peroxisomal catalase is a possible but unproven pathway of alcohol metabolism in humans.

Alcohol dehydrogenase classes 1–5

There are at least of seven genes and five classes. They arise from eight different subunits, α, β_1, β_2, β_3, γ_1, γ_2, π and χ, as active dimeric isozymes. The isozymes differ in tissue distribution, but most have maximum activity in the liver. Classes 1–5 relate to products of five gene loci, class 1 by three closely related genes and each of the others by a single gene.

Those relevant to ethanol metabolism include:

class 1 (α, β, γ): wide range of substrates, including ethanol, bile compounds, sterols, neurotransmitters, retinol and mevalonate. Polymorphism occurs at ADH2 and ADH3, which encode β and γ

class 4 (μ, σ): gastric mucosal metabolism of ethanol and other dietary alcohols.

Aldehyde dehydrogenase isoenzymes

Many human ALDH isoenzymes have been identified. The human liver contains four major isoenzymes. One ALDH locus governs the synthesis of cytosolic $ALDH_1$ and a single $ALDH_2$ locus governs the mitochondrial $ALDH_2$. The two non-allelic genes $ALDH_{3a}$ and $ALDH_{3b}$ are involved in the synthesis of the $ALDH_3$ isoenzymes. $ALDH_1$ and $ALDH_2$ are basically similar, with a 65% degree of homology, but the sequences of the exon that includes the sequence for the signal peptide (17 amino residues) of $ALDH_2$ are not homologous.

Alcohol oxidation

All known pathways of ethanol oxidation produce acetaldehyde, which is converted to acetate by ADH. ADH also converts NAD to NADH. The rate-limiting factor is the reoxidation of NADH. The availability of ADH only becomes relevant in severe, protein malnutrition. The NADH/NAD ratio is important in liver metabolism during ethanol oxidation. There are also endogenous sources of acetaldehyde, e.g. as a result of the activity of:

- deoxypentosephosphate aldolases
- pyruvate dehydrogenase
- phosphorylphosphoethanolamine phosphorylase
- cleavage of threonine to acetaldehyde and glycine by a threonine aldolase.

More than 90% of acetaldehyde oxidation is in the liver, although there are genes for these enzymes in other tissues.

Aldehyde dehydrogenases
There are several aldehyde dehydrogenases (ALDH) in the cytoplasm and mitochondria of most species, although most of those with a low K_m activity, $ALDH_2$, are localised in the mitochondria. The tetrameric liver forms (NAD^+ specific) and dimeric forms of ALDH utilise either NAD or NADPH (nicotinamide adenine dinucleotide phosphate). The second duplicate level is dependent on their intracellular position, either cytosolic or mitochondrial. Mitochondrial metabolism of acetaldehyde is reduced with chronic alcohol consumption.

The acetaldehyde may bind covalently to liver microsomal proteins. This binding increases with long-term alcohol consumption and MEOS activity. A stable adduct (a new compound composed of the two compounds) is formed with the ethanol-inducible microsomal P450 IIEI, serum albumin and haemoglobin.

Acetaldehyde may also act as an antigen, with the generation of circulating antibodies against acetaldehyde-altered proteins and complement-binding acetaldehyde adducts that may contribute to the perpetuation or exaggeration of liver disease.

Aldehyde dehydrogenase variants
Individual and ethnic differences in rate of alcohol metabolism and clearance rates may be factors in the rate of production of acetaldehyde and the development of flushing reactions. The molecular difference between the two variants of ALDH is a single amino acid substitution, Glu→Lys, at position 14 from the N-terminal end. This enzyme variant, $ALDH_2$, results in a high blood acetaldehyde after ethanol ingestion, followed by flushing and an uncomfortable feeling. The ALDH gene is encoded by two alleles, ALDH2*1 and ALDH2*2; active and inactive, respectively. The latter is the dominant and therefore will limit the ability to consume large amounts of alcohol, and possibly increase the propensity to alcoholic liver disease.

Approximately 50% of Orientals, including the Japanese, have the inactive ALDH2*2 variant. Native Americans, a subset of the mongoloid races, experience flushing after drinking alcoholic drinks and yet alcoholism has been widely prevalent in this population. The role of acetaldehyde in flushing is not certain, although one mechanism may be through the release of histamine. Post-ethanol ingestion flushing is found in 5–10% of Caucasians, but is not associated with the ALDH variant.

ALCOHOL AND XENOBIOTICS

Interactions occur between xenobiotics and ethanol following acute ethanol consumption, which affects the metabolism of the xenobiotics. This results in an increased blood clearance of warfarin, phenytoin, tolbutamide, propranolol, rifampin and pentobarbital, and reduced clinical efficacy of these drugs. In chronic exposure to ethanol there are complex effects with drugs because of competition for common metabolic processes involving P450, interference with the supply of NADPH and inhibition of glucuronidation. All of these effects will alter the metabolism of drugs such as methadone, morphine and tranquillisers. Other drug metabolic processes such as acetylation and sulfation are unaffected. These alterations in the hepatic metabolic processes by ethanol result in an increased sensitivity to these drugs and other chemicals, sometimes with conversion to toxic metabolites, particularly those utilising the cytochrome P450 system, e.g. carbon tetrachloride, halothane, isoniazid and phenylbutazone. Ethanol also affects the metabolism of steroids, resulting in a reduction in blood testosterone concentrations. The metabolism of vitamin A and D is also altered.

Liver and alcohol

The activity of ADH in males is uniformly distributed throughout the liver. In females and older males ADH activity is increased at the perivenous zone. ALDH is uniformly distributed in all instances.

EFFECTS OF ALCOHOL ON INDIVIDUAL ORGANS AND TISSUES

Mouth

Clinical effects include enlargement of the parotid glands and alterations in parotid secretions.

Oesophagus

There is an increased incidence of dysmotility, reflux oesophagitis, Barrett's oesophagus and oesophageal cancer in heavy drinkers. Retching after a heavy alcohol session can lead to a Mallory–Weiss tear at the lower end of the oesophagus, haematemesis and other complications.

Stomach

Ethanol stimulates or inhibits gastric acid production depending on the chronicity of the usage, and the concentration and type of alcohol. Gastritis, peptic ulceration and duodenitis are important complications of ethanol ingestion, sometimes leading to haematemesis. The efficacy of H_2-blockers, e.g. cimetidine, and the healing of peptic ulceration are impaired by prolonged alcohol consumption.

Liver

Metabolic effects
Alcohol can cause an enlarged liver as a result of fatty infiltration. Serum concentrations of γ-glutamyltransferase are increased, possibly because of microsomal induction. Lipids accumulating in the liver originate from dietary lipids or from adipose tissue as free fatty acids, or may be synthesised in the liver. The deposition of fat in the liver occurs in two distinct patterns, which may coexist and are reversible. There may be an accumulation of large intracytoplasmic fat vacuoles with displacement of the nucleus, or the cytoplasm may show minute fat droplets, i.e. microvascular steatosis. One theory is that this hepatic fat deposition represents a malnutrition state similar to

Kwashiorkor, although these lesions can occur in the presence of an apparent sufficiency of nutrients.

Acetaldehyde can bind to the sulfhydryl groups of the cysteine residues in the microtubules. This acetaldehyde binding reduces the amount and turnover of hepatic glutathione, which is important in the scavenging of free radicals and protects against reactive oxygen species. A severe reduction favours peroxidation and may be facilitated by iron from ferritin.

Hepatic microtubules decrease in alcoholic liver disease. Microtubules promote the intracellular transport and subsequent secretion of proteins. Long-term alcohol intake delays the secretion of proteins, including albumin, transferrin and fatty acid binding proteins. The corresponding retention in the liver may also be important in the accumulation of fat in the liver.

Protein accumulation is associated with an increase in liver-bound water which, with the increased fat, enlarges the liver cells. This swelling has a distinct centrilobular distribution and alters key cellular functions by physically separating the reaction sites.

Hepatotoxicity

The zonal distribution of some enzymes is relevant to the selective, centrilobular toxicity. During alcoholic liver decompensation, acute hepatitis-like changes occur in the central zones of the hepatic acinus. Following chronic ethanol excess there is proliferation of the smooth endoplasmic reticulum, particularly in the centrilobular zone, and associated enzyme inductions. Chronic alcohol ingestion results in an increased consumption of oxygen, due

largely to increased mitochondrial reoxidation of NADH. In the liver this is associated with an increased oxygen gradient along the entire sinusoid length, so that necrosis occurs in zone 3 (also called perivenular or centrilobular). ADH is more concentrated in this region and therefore increased concentrations of acetaldehyde and exaggeration of the redox shift will prevail in the centrilobular acinar zones. There may be more ADH enzyme activity in the centrilobular zone, although this may be a result of ethanol ingestion.

Many of the toxic effects of ethanol are linked to its property of shifting the redox equilibrium towards a reduced state. Possible toxic mechanisms include increased triglyceride synthesis and mobilisation of fatty acids from fatty stores. Lipogenesis is increased, possibly by the elongation pathway or transhydrogenation by NADPH. This pathway is limited in its load-carrying potential and is readily overloaded. There is also an increase in hepatic α-glycerophosphate, which favours the accumulation of hepatic triglycerides by trapping fatty acids. The alteration in the NADH/NAD ratio depresses citric acid oxidation of two-carbon fractions and hence suppresses fatty acid oxidation (the major source of two-carbon fragments) and favours the accumulation of triglycerides. The partition of fatty acids between oxidation and esterification is determined in the outer membrane of the mitochondria, by the release of carnitine acyltransferase and glycerophosphate acyltransferase. An increase in the concentration of sn-glycerol-3-phosphate would favour esterification, and thus ethanol-induced fatty liver.

Ethanol increases the lactate/pyruvate ratio. Hypoxia increases NADH, which in turn inhibits the activity of NAD^+-dependent xanthine dehydrogenase and favours the xanthine oxidase pathway. Increased acetate from ethanol metabolism results in the accumulation of purine metabolites, e.g. uric acid. Oxygen radicals are produced, which are toxic to liver cells. Acetaldehyde, also derived from alcohol, may be a substrate for xanthine oxidase.

Pathological changes

Liver cells exposed to continuous flows of ethanol develop lytic necrosis. The cytoplasm contains clumps of refractile densely eosinophilic material, the alcoholic hyaline lines of Mallory, which are

---

Alcohol and the mitochondria

There are striking morphological and physiological alterations in the liver mitochondria in alcoholics, due directly to the effects of ethanol rather than to malnutrition. Changes include swelling, abnormal cristae, decreased respiratory capacity, reduced cytochrome *a* and *b* content and altered oxidative phosphorylation. There may also be altered function in the mitochondria, which decrease fatty acid oxidative processes as a result of changes in cellular membranes, plasma membrane glycoproteins and plasma membrane structure.

complex glycoproteins with antigenic properties. Polymorphs surround the necrosing liver cells. The portal zones show stellate fibrosis which, in the severely malnourished patient, can obliterate the hepatic venous radicals, heralding fibrosis. Unless ethanol consumption is stopped cholestasis and jaundice develop, which can progress to cirrhosis.

It is possible that alcohol itself may have a direct effect on collagen metabolism in the liver. Alcohol causes the proliferation of myelofibroblasts. In the final stages the collagen in the liver forms a network, dividing the residual liver into small regular nodules. Ethanol metabolism results in increased lactate production, consequent increased peptidylproline hydroxylase activity, inhibition of proline oxidase and increased collagen synthesis. With progression of fibrosis the regional hepatic tissue haemoglobin concentration and oxygen supply to the liver may decrease, enhancing the progression of the pathological process. The zonal nature of ethanol-induced liver disease is important in relation to fibrosis. Alcohol may promote fibrogenesis directly, resulting in pericellular, perisinusoidal and percentrilobular fibrosis which is coupled to an increased collagen messenger (mRNA). This process is shown diagrammatically in Figure 15.4.

The development of fibrotic distortion of the liver structure can lead to re-routing of the portal vasculature, the formation of varices at the lower end of the oesophagus and fundus of the stomach, and an increase in portal vein pressure. The variability of this further complication suggests that the regenerative nodules pressing on the efferent venous flow may be only partly responsible. Hepatocyte swelling may be a prime event in portal hypertension and fibrosis may be secondary.

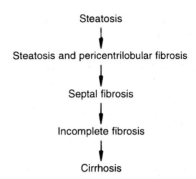

Fig. 15.4 The progression of alcohol-induced hepatic fibrosis.

Clinical effects

Alcoholic liver disease can lead to jaundice, fever, anorexia and right hypochondrial pain. There is a distinct mortality among individuals with such complications, which include acute liver failure.

The basis of treatment is abstinence from alcohol. Even in advanced cases the inexorable progression of the condition can be slowed by abstinence from alcohol.

Cirrhosis

A further complication of prolonged alcohol exposure is cirrhosis. If a 70 kg man drinks 210 g of alcohol per day for years then he has a 50% chance of developing cirrhosis. Initially, the liver may be uniformly nodular, but it may assume an irregular appearance with long-standing cirrhosis. The common signs of uncomplicated cirrhosis are weight loss, weakness and anorexia. Other signs include splenomegaly, ascites, testicular atrophy, spider naevi, gastrointestinal haemorrhage, gynaecomastica, palmar erythema and Dupuytren's contracture. Other complications include portal hypertension, hypoalbuminaemia and hypoglobulinaemia.

The complications of cirrhotic portal hypertension include ascites that may spontaneously become infected, bleeding from oesophageal and gastric varices, hepatic encephalopathy and hepatorenal failure. A transudate type of ascites with a low albumin concentration (< 250 g/l) may develop within the peritoneal cavity. A poor prognosis is reflected by ascites and extended prothrombin time.

Alcohol and liver collagen

The mechanism of the biosynthesis and degradation of collagen is not yet clear. Interstitial collagens are synthesised intracellularly as procollagens that contain extension propeptides at the carboxy ends of their three polypeptide chains. After secretion, there is conversion of procollagen and assembly into fibrils. Aminopropeptides of type I procollagen are released at an early stage of fibrillogenesis; those of type III are retained in collagen fibrils in the liver.

Pancreas

Pathological effects
Heavy alcohol intake is associated with chronic relapsing pancreatitis. A possible mechanism for pancreatitis is oedema or spasm of the papilla. Alternatively, the pathogenesis involves the precipitation of protein in peripheral pancreatic plugs. These plugs may calcify and thereafter block larger ducts, with resultant atrophy and fibrosis. A further extension of the problem is pancreatic pseudocyst formation and common bile duct obstruction. Pancreatic secretions become insufficient for nutrient digestion and malabsorption results.

Clinical effects
Acute relapsing pancreatitis can be extremely painful, but progressive loss of pancreatic function may be painless. Weight loss and steatorrhoea develop, with a reduction in fat-soluble nutrient absorption and an extension of the problem to a more general deficiency, e.g. vitamin D deficiency with consequent bone problems. A particularly brittle form of diabetes mellitus may develop.

Intestine

Alcohol may alter intestinal function. It may have a direct effect on transport, motility, absorption of nutrients, metabolism, circulation and cellular structure in the small intestine. The problem is compounded by pancreatic and hepatic insufficiency and dietary inadequacies, leading to deficiency conditions secondary to malabsorption of folic acid, pyridoxine, thiamin, iron, zinc and fat-soluble vitamin deficiency. Malnutrition is a major problem in these subjects, but may very readily, if temporarily, be corrected by abstention from alcohol, a good diet and vitamin supplements.

Endocrine abnormalities

Metabolic effects
Alcohol has effects on the endocrine system in a number of target organs, including the pituitary and hypothalamus. The peripheral metabolism of several hormones may be affected by alterations in hepatic blood flow, protein binding enzymes, cofactors or receptors, and malnutrition.

Clinical effects
Rarely, alcohol can cause a pseudo-Cushing's type of syndrome. Alcoholic hypoglycaemia can occur after prolonged fasting or malnutrition, which may on first sight be indistinguishable from a drunken state.

Cardiovascular system

Metabolic effects
Any protective influence of alcohol against coronary heart disease may be secondary to an increased high-density lipoprotein (HDL) concentration. However, the increase is in HDL_3, not the cardioprotective HDL_2. The apparent protective influence of light daily ethanol drinking is probably due to a consequence of multiple advantageous characteristics, such as acceptable blood pressure, mean body mass index and cigarette intake.

Clinical effects
Prolonged excessive ethanol intake may result in breathlessness, easy fatigue, palpitations, anorexia and oedema. These are caused by cardiomyopathy, cardiomegaly, arrhythmias, intraventricular conduction abnormalities, pathological Q waves and decreased voltages. Transmural cardiac infarction can occur in the absence of significant coronary artery disease. Alcoholic binges can result in fatal or incapacitating arrhythmias, usually supraventricular in nature. The consumption of alcohol is also associated with the development of hypertension.

Blood system

Alcoholic patients often have a red cell macroytosis (mean cell volume > 98 fl) due to a direct toxic effect on bone marrow (fl, femtolitres). Vitamin B_{12} and folate deficiency may be contributory factors, resulting from malabsorption, a folate-poor diet, the blockage of storage, methylfolate utilisation and increased renal loss. Quantitative and qualitative changes can occur in white cells with effects on resistance to, for example, respiratory infections.

Alcoholic thrombocytopenia is common, leading occasionally to disseminated intravascular coagulopathy. The reduced platelet count and function is a direct effect of alcohol toxicity. The mechanism may be mediated through shortened platelet survival, ineffective platelet function and decreased thromboxane A_2 release. It is also possible that the altered platelet function is partly responsible for the reduction in coronary thrombosis reported in moderate drinkers.

Musculoskeletal system

The incidence of osteoporosis is increased in alcoholics. The aetiology is complicated, but may result from malnutrition, lack of exercise (thought by some alcoholics to be a waste of drinking time), and alterations in endocrine status and absorption. Such osteoporosis may contribute to the five-to ten-fold increase in bone fracture rate, a rate not unrelated to the increased incidence of falling while drunk. Other complications include aseptic necrosis in the femoral head.

Gout
This occurs in alcoholics in whom there is an accumulation of purine metabolites, e.g. uric acid. It may also be related to the frequent obesity, hypertriglyceridaemia and activation of the xanthine oxidase pathways that occur in alcoholics.

Skeletal muscle myopathy
A proximal metabolic myopathy is reported in alcoholism. It selectively involves type II fast twitch glycolytic fibres and may result in a loss of 25% of muscle mass. This may relate to α-tocopherol availability.

Skin

Changes include facial oedema, rosacea and rhinophyma, all contributing to the rubicund face of the committed drinker. Other cutaneous changes include spider naevi and porphyria cutanea tarda.

Respiratory system

Clinical effects
Fractured ribs and pneumonia from inhaled vomit are common problems.

Central nervous system

Intoxication is an important consequence of alcohol drinking and follows the subjectively pleasant effects of the accumulation of alcohol in the blood and, more importantly, in the brain and nervous system. The brain adapts to continued exposure to ethanol, with larger amounts being required to obtain an equivalent effect. The adaptation leads to tolerance and thence to dependence.

The central tenet of the adaptation/tolerance/dependence hypothesis is that the central nervous system sets up an adaptive state that opposes the acute effect of the drug. Central neurones become more excitable, and this state becomes established and is only manifestly unstable when alcohol is withdrawn. Alcohol withdrawal results in central nervous system hyperexcitability. Other complications of withdrawal include tremulousness, seizures after some 17–48 h without alcohol and delirium tremens after 3–5 days. Such problems require careful evaluation, including the exclusion of cerebral trauma following a drunken fall, hypoglycaemia, and fluid and electrolyte problems.

Peripheral neuropathies and brain atrophy occur in prolonged drinking, in part owing to nutritional and particularly vitamin deficiencies. These include Wernicke–Korsokoff syndrome, which consists of nystagmus, ataxia and impaired memory due to thiamin deficiency, and resolves with replenishment of the vitamin. Alcoholic cerebellar degeneration, in its earlier stages, responds to thiamin. Nutritional amblyopia and pellagra, which present with depression and poor memory, respond to niacin. Pyridoxine deficiency may result in cerebral symptoms and signs.

There is a relationship between ethanol abuse and the incidence of haemorrhagic strokes, independent of other causes of stroke. The mechanism of this is obscure. In female drinkers there is an increased risk of subarachnoid haemorrhage.

Behavioural changes of a violent nature can occur in bout drinking, although these are probably associated with increased irritability and hypoglycaemia rather than central nervous system pathology.

Molecular basis of intoxication
The molecular basis of ethanol intoxication is not known. There is some evidence that the action is

through the same pathway as the barbiturates and benzodiazepines, whose major sites of action are the receptor protein for γ-aminobutyric acid (GABA), the major inhibitory neurotransmitter in the mammalian central nervous system.

Ethanol enters neuronal membranes and disrupts the packing of lipid membrane molecules. The anaesthetic effect of ethanol depresses neuronal activity by acting on receptors, e.g. $GABA_A$ and ion channels. Both processes involve depolarisation of the nerve cell membrane, in which Ca^{2+} is very important. Prolonged exposure to ethanol can cause neuronal death and brain damage. The mechanism appears to be damage by lipid peroxidation or activation of intracellular enzymes which break down membrane lipids and proteins.

Reproductive system

In men, ethanol leads to loss of sexual hair, initially increased and later decreased libido, reduced potency, testicular and penile shrinkage, reduced or absent sperm production and infertility. In women, chronic excessive ethanol intake leads to menstrual irregularities and shrinkage of the breasts and external genitalia.

Immune system

Disturbances in the reticuloendothelial system of the liver occur through interference with the mobilisation and activation of macrophages and their phagocytic activity. Cell-mediated immunity is also inhibited. These are direct toxic effects, in contrast to undernutrition which may also be associated with effects on immunoprotein production. Heavy intake of alcohol can also alter the production and turnover of B- and T-lymphocytes in the thymus and spleen. Alcoholic subjects may also have a leucopenia, reversible on stopping ethanol intake.

ALCOHOL IN THE YOUNG

Alcohol and the foetus

It has been suggested that there is no safe thres-

hold for drinking during pregnancy, and that ethanol and pregnancy are not safely compatible. The ingestion of more than 90 ml of absolute ethanol (six drinks) per day by the pregnant mother poses identifiable risks to the foetus. The peak alcohol concentration is more important than daily intake.

Foetal development

The placenta is a critical organ for foetal development. The placenta is a developed multifunctioning organ by 12 weeks of gestation. Ethanol and extraneous and metabolically created acetaldehyde affect placental growth, transport and metabolism. The delivery of oxygen to the foetus may be diminished by ethanol-induced reductions in prostaglandin metabolism, alterations in vascular tone in the placental blood flow, and foetal hypoxia.

Ethanol is well established as a teratogen. There are also indirect effects on the supply of essential nutrients, alterations in foetal immunity and possible mutagenic effects of paternal ethanol exposure.

Clinically, the foetal central nervous system is a major target organ for the deleterious effects of maternal ethanol ingestion. The mechanism is possibly through impaired protein synthesis and central nervous system cell division, and reduced cell number. Another postulate for poor brain growth is diminished tissue zinc. The foetal alcohol syndrome has characteristic features including poor intrauterine growth, distinctive facial structure and learning disabilities. These may also result from alcohol-related foetal injury. It has been calculated that in the USA this problem is responsible for some 11% of the total cost of the care for learning disabilities.

Alcohol and children

Drinking ethanol can lead to acute intoxication in children. It is characterised by hypoglycaemia, hypothermia and depressed respiration. Prolonged exposure may have effects on the child's physical development. There are significant effects on the upbringing of a child through excessive alcohol intake by the parents.

KEY POINTS

1. Ethanol is a nutrient the principal popularity of which is due to its effects on mood and an induced sense of well-being. Alcohol drinking is, in general, a social activity.
2. Alcoholic drinks are produced in many different forms. It is the constituents other than alcohol that give the beverage its particular taste.
3. Alcohol intake is measured by the unit; 1 unit is equal to 8–10 g of ethanol.
4. There is a U- or J-shaped relationship between alcohol intake and morbidity.
5. Alcoholism occurs more frequently in certain families. Cultural and genetic factors have been implicated.
6. Ethanol is metabolised initially by alcohol dehydrogenase to acetaldehyde, which is converted to acetate by the enzyme aldehyde dehydrogenase. The type, amount and distribution of isoenzymes of these enzymes affect the susceptibility to alcohol of women and some Mongol races.
7. Ethanol has destructive effects on all organs when drunk in excess, with consequences that affect the individual's health.

THINKING POINTS

1. Alcohol is the most commonly used substance influencing the mind and behaviour.
2. It is probable that everyone has a view on this substance, which is coloured by their own experience and usage of alcohol.
3. Alcohol has no essential nutritional value, and has enormous social value.
4. Is alcohol or a substitute mind-relaxing agent necessary? If so, what are the safe limits for different groups in the population?

NEED TO UNDERSTAND

How ethanol is metabolised in different gender and racial groups, and the consequences of their response to different alcohol intakes.

FURTHER READING

Feyer, A.-M. (2001) Fatigue: time to recognise and deal with an old problem. *British Medical Journal*, **322**, 808–9.

Fielding, B.A., Reid, G., Grady. M. *et al.* (2000) Ethanol with a mixed meal increases postprandial triacylglycerol but decreases postprandial non-esterified fatty acid concentrations. *British Journal of Nutrition*, **83**, 597–604.

Goodwin, D.W. (1985) Alcoholism and genetics – the sins of the fathers. *Archives of General Psychiatry*, **28**, 238–43.

Helmutt, K., Seitz, M.D. and Oneta, C.M. (1998) Gastrointestinal alcohol dehydrogenase. *Nutrition Reviews*, **56**, 52–60.

Kroke, A., Klipstein-Grobusch, K., Hoffman, K. *et al.* (2001) Comparison of self reported alcohol intake with the urinary excretion of 5-hydroxytryptophol:5-hydroxyindole-3-acetic acid, a biomarker of recent alcohol intake. *British Journal of Nutrition*, **85**, 621–7.

Lieber, C.S. (2000) Alcohol: its metabolism and interaction with nutrients. *Annual Review of Nutrition*, **20**, 395–430.

Lucas, E.G. (1987) Alcohol in industry. *British Medical Journal*, **294**, 460–1.

McCarver, D.G., Thomasson, H.R., Martier, S.S. *et al.* (1997) Alcohol dehydrogenase-2*3 allele protects against alcohol related birth defects among African Americans. *Journal of Pharmacology and Experimental Therapeutics*, **283**, 1095–101.

Murray, R.M., Clifford, C.A., Gurling, H.M.D. *et al.* (1983) Current genetic and biological approaches to alcoholism. *Psychiatric Developments*, **2**, 171–92.

Nicolas, J.M., Fernadez-Sola, J., Robert, J. *et al.* (2000) High ethanol intake and malnutrition in alcoholic cerebellar shrinkage. *Quarterly Journal of Medicine*, **93**, 449–56.

Palmer, T.N. (1991) *The Molecular Pathology of Alcoholism*. Oxford University Press, Oxford.

Philip, P., Vervialle, F., Le Breton, P. *et al.* (2001) Fatigue, alcohol and serious road crashes in France: factorial study of national data. *British Medical Journal*, **322**, 829–30.

Pokorny, A.D., Miller, B.A. and Kaplan, H.B. (1972) The brief MAST: a shortened version of the Michigan alcoholism screening test. *American Journal of Psychiatry*, **129**, 342–8.

Shaper, A.G., Wannamethee, G. and Walker, M. (1988)
Alcohol and mortality in British men: explaining the
U-shaped curve. *Lancet*, **ii**, 1267–72.

WEB SITES

www.druglibrary.org/schaffer/Library/studies/ledain/
    nonmed2b.htm
www.health.org
www.alcoholconcern.org.uk
www.ias.org.uk
www.scc.rutgers.cdu/alcohol_studies/alcohol
www.wineloverspage.com
www.history-of-wine.com
www.scotchwhisky.com

16

Vitamins

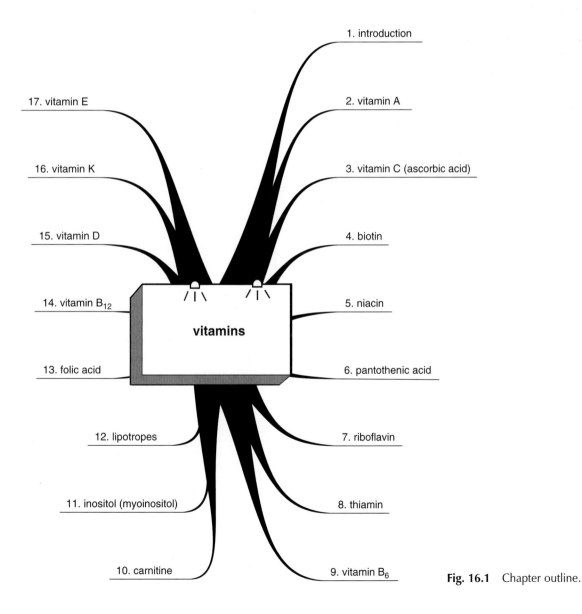

Fig. 16.1 Chapter outline.

INTRODUCTION

NOMENCLATURE AND CLASSIFICATION OF VITAMINS

As the vitamins were discovered each was identified with a letter. Once each vitamin had been isolated and its chemical structure identified, a specific chemical name became possible. Many of the vitamins, e.g. A, D, K, E and B_{12}, each consist of several closely related compounds with similar physiological properties.

The classification of vitamins may be as water and fat soluble, or according to function as blood forming, antioxidant, involved in energy or protein metabolism, or bone forming. These classifications are important from the historical perspective and belong to a brilliant period of discovery in nutrition. The deficiency conditions or diseases that brought vitamins to the attention of scientists were regarded as central to the action of the vitamins. The identification of the role of vitamins as coenzymes and with hormone-like actions supersedes all of these classifications.

Therefore, the vitamins are described individually, with the exception of the metabolically interconnected folic acid, vitamin B_{12}, choline and methionine system.

The water-soluble vitamins are vitamin C (ascorbic acid), vitamin B_1 (thiamin), nicotinic acid (niacin) and nicotinamide, riboflavin, vitamin B_6 (pyridoxine), pantothenic acid, biotin, folic acid and

vitamin B_{12} (cyanocobalamin). The fat-soluble vitamins are vitamin A (retinol), vitamin D (cholecalciferol), vitamin K and vitamin E (tocopherols). Vitamins may be single chemical entities, e.g. ascorbic acid, or consist of a family of closely related compounds, e.g. vitamins A, D, K, E and B_{12}.

> The vitamin B complex is a useful concept as the vitamins, while being unrelated chemically, often occur in the same foodstuff. The B vitamins are involved in intermediary metabolism, being coenzymes in the glycolytic, tricarboxylic acid and pentose pathways.

The classification of vitamins becomes more difficult as an understanding of their action increases. Vitamins may have actions that are important in blood formation (folic acid and vitamin B_{12}), as antioxidants (ascorbic acid and vitamin E), and in energy metabolism (thiamin, riboflavin and pyridoxine), bone formation (vitamin D) and protein metabolism (vitamins A and K). Some vitamins act specifically as coenzymes (Table 16.1). Nuclear receptors for vitamins A and D belong to the nuclear hormone receptor superfamily and act as ligand-inducible transcription factors.

The lipid-soluble vitamins have less easily defined functions. Vitamin D can be synthesised in the skin and has many similarities to a hormone, its influences extending further than its function in bone formation. Vitamin A, as a pigment–protein complex, acts as an absorber of light in the eye. Vitamins D and A act on a variety of receptors, which are now beginning to be understood. Vitamin K, important in clotting reactions, is also involved in the formation of γ-carboxyglutamate in a number

Tables 16.1 Vitamins as coenzymes

Vitamin	Coenzyme form	Function
Thiamin	Thiamin pyrophosphate	C-C and C-X bond cleavage
Riboflavin	Flavin mononucleotide	One- or two-electron transfer reactions
Pyridoxine	Flavin adenine nucleotide pyridoxal phosphate	Various reactions with α-amino acids
Nicotinic acid	Nicotinamide adenine dinucleotide (NAD)	
	Nicotinamide adenine dinucleotide phosphate (NADPH)	Hydride transfers
Pantothenic acid	Coenzyme A	Acyl group transfer
Biotin	Biocytin	Carboxylation reactions
Folic acid	Tetrahydrofolic acid	One-carbon transfers
Vitamin B_{12}	Deoxyadenosyl cobalamin	Rearrangements on adjacent carbon atoms

of processes that involve calcium and calcium-regulated metabolic processes.

FACTORS INFLUENCING THE UTILISATION OF VITAMINS

Bioavailability

Not all vitamins may be ingested in an absorbable form in the intestine, e.g. nicotinic acid derived from cereals is bound in such a way that it is not absorbed. Fat-soluble vitamins may be malabsorbed if the digestion of fat is in any way impaired.

Water solubility

The intestinal absorption of vitamins is by specific pathways, many of which are sodium dependent. In some instances, absorption includes chemical change, e.g. phosphorylation, which is a feature of the absorption process of riboflavin and pyridoxine.

Antivitamins

These are present in natural food. Several synthetic analogues of vitamins are highly poisonous, e.g. aminopterin, tesoxypyridoxine. These substances inhibit the activity of true vitamins and enzyme systems.

Provitamins

These, although not vitamins themselves, can be converted to vitamins in the body. Carotenes are provitamins of vitamin A, and the amino acid tryptophan can be converted to nicotinic acid. Vitamin D is synthesised in the skin by the action of sunlight on a derivative of cholesterol. Because vitamins have traditionally been regarded as dietary constituents, it is anomalous that vitamin D is synthesised in the skin in response to sunlight. In some respects vitamin D could better be regarded as a hormone.

Biosynthesis in the gut

The normal bacterial flora of the gut can synthesise some vitamins, e.g. vitamin K, nicotinic acid, riboflavin, vitamin B_{12} and folic acid. Because these are synthesised in the colon it may be that they are not nutritionally relevant, as they may not be absorbed.

Interaction with nutrients

An example of this phenomenon is a diet rich in carbohydrates and alcohol requiring additional thiamin for the body's metabolic requirements. Similarly, when there is a high intake of polyunsaturated fats, vitamin D requirements are increased.

KEY POINTS

1. Vitamins are organic substances that the body requires in small amounts for metabolism, and is incapable of synthesising, or does not synthesise in sufficient quantity for its overall needs.
2. Vitamins are not related to each other chemically, and differ in their physiological actions.
3. Vitamins may be classified as water or lipid soluble. The water-soluble vitamins are vitamin C (ascorbic acid), vitamin B (thiamin), nicotinic acid (niacin) and nicotinamide, riboflavin, vitamin B_6 (pyridoxine), pantothenic acid, biotin, folic acid and vitamin B_{12} (cyanocobalamin). The fat-soluble vitamins are vitamin A (retinol), vitamin D (cholecalciferol), vitamin K and vitamin E (tocopherols).
4. Vitamins may be single chemical entities, e.g. ascorbic acid, or comprise a family of closely related compounds, e.g. vitamins A, D, K, E and B_{12}.
5. Vitamins may have actions that are important in blood formation (folic acid and vitamin B_{12}) as antioxidants (ascorbic acid and vitamin E), and in energy metabolism (thiamin, riboflavin and pyridoxine), bone formation (vitamin D) and protein metabolism (vitamin K and A). Vitamins may also act in a general systemic manner as antioxidants, e.g. ascorbic acid and vitamin E.
6. Vitamins may act as enzymatic cofactors, have hormone-like actions on receptors or act as antioxidants.

7. As more is understood of their biological activity, many of the classifications of vitamins have become only of historical interest.

THINKING POINTS

1. Vitamins were discovered and characterised by the clinical signs of deficiency, e.g. ascorbic acid and scurvy. Now there is an increasing understanding of their biochemical function.
2. Should vitamins be reclassified, and if so how, e.g. cofactors, receptor hormone-like activity and other functions?
3. The recommended dietary intakes are dependent on a balance between need and toxicity.

NEED TO UNDERSTAND

1. Vitamins are essential and it is important to recognise where their essential activity is located in the metabolic processes.
2. The fat-soluble vitamins tend to have upper limits of daily intake, in contrast to the water-soluble vitamins.

FURTHER READING

Aranda, A. and Pascual, A. (2001) Nuclear hormone receptors and gene expression. *Physiology Review*, **81**, 1269–304.

Bates, C.J., Thurnham, D.I., Bingham, S.A. *et al.* (1991) *Design Concepts in Nutritional Epidemiology* (eds D.M. Margetts and M. Nelson). Oxford Medical Publications, Oxford.

Dietary Reference Values for Food, Energy and Nutrients for the United Kingdom (1991) Report on Health and Social Subjects, No. 41. HMSO, London.

Olmedilla, B., Granado, F., Southon, S., *et al.* (2001) Serum concentrations of carotenoids and vitamins A, E and C in control subjects from five European countries. *British Journal of Nutrition*, **85**, 227–38.

Traber, M.G. and Jialal, I. (2000) Measurements of lipid-soluble vitamins-further adjustment needed. *Lancet*, **355**, 2013–14.

VITAMIN A

INTRODUCTION

Vitamin A consists of a group of biologically active compounds closely related to the plant pigment carotene. The carotenoid family consists of approximately 100 naturally occurring pigments, which provide the yellow–red colour of many vegetables and some fruits. β-Carotene, a provitamin A, has widespread distribution in plants and is associated with chlorophyll. It is unique in that it is the only carotenoid in which both halves of the molecule are identical to retinol. Other carotenoids, e.g. xanthophyll, which is another yellow pigment associated with chlorophyll, and lycopene, the red pigment of tomatoes, do not have provitamin A activity.

The term 'retinol' means vitamin A alcohol, while vitamin A includes all compounds with vitamin A activity. One international unit of vitamin A is equivalent to 0.3 µg of retinol. In terms of biological activity, 6 µg of β-carotene is equivalent to 1 µg of retinol. Originally, vitamin A activity was

Retinol structure

The retinol molecule consists of a hydrocarbon chain with a β-ionone ring at one end and an alcohol group at the other. The usual form is the all-*trans* stereoisomer. An isomer with the *cis* configuration at the 11 or 13 position exists, but is less potent biologically. All carotenoids containing at least one unsubstituted β-ionone ring and a polyene side-chain containing at least 11 carbon atoms are potential precursors of vitamin A. The relative bioconversion of various retinoids to vitamin A varies.

Vitamin A_2 is 3-dehydroretinol. This has half the biological activity of retinol. It is extremely uncommon, occurring only in the liver of some Indian fish.

The terminal alcohol group of retinol can be oxidised to an aldehyde (retinal) or carboxylic acid group (retinoic acid). In foodstuffs the alcohol is usually esterified with fatty acid (retinyl esters).

described as international units, but now that crystalline retinol is available, international units, which are functional, are no longer necessary.

Retinol and carotene are soluble in fat but not in water; they are also stable to heat at ordinary cooking temperatures, but liable to oxidation and destruction if the fats turn rancid. Vitamin E can protect such oxidation. Retinol is also chemically changed by exposure to sunlight. Drying of fruit and food in the sun results in loss of vitamin A. Fish liver oils in clear glass lose their potency on exposure to light. Canned vegetables may retain their carotene over many years.

Retinol is present in milk, butter, cheese, egg yolk, liver and fatty fish. The liver oils of fish are the richest natural source of vitamin A. Carotenes are found predominantly in green vegetables associated with chlorophyll. The green outer leaves of vegetables are a good source of carotenes, whereas white inner leaves contain little. Yellow and red fruits and vegetables, particularly carrots, are good sources. Vegetable oils, with the exception of red palm oil, which is found in west Africa and Malaysia, do not contain vitamin A. Retinol is present in breast milk.

In a typical Western diet, about 15% of β-carotene and about 8% of other dietary carotenoids are converted to vitamin A in the intestinal mucosa. This varies between individuals and different food types. Carotenoids in fruit juices or oily solution are better absorbed than native carotene in carrots.

ACTION OF VITAMIN A

Vitamin A is essential for the growth and normal function of the retina, and the development of epithelial surfaces in the retina. Recent discoveries have shown that most actions of vitamin A in development, differentiation and metabolism are made possible by nuclear receptor proteins that bind retinoic acid, the active form of vitamin A.

The biological functions of the different molecular types of vitamin A and the retinoids, all-*trans*-retinal, 11-*trans*-retinal, 11-*cis*-retinal and all-*trans*-retinoic acid (T-RA), and *N-cis*-retinoic acid (C-RA) (Figure 16.2), act through specific interaction with a nuclear receptor protein.

The visual process

The photopigment rhodopsin is a receptor protein found in the retinal rod cells of all vertebrates and many invertebrates. Rhodopsin consists of a membrane-embedded protein, opsin, and a light-sensitive pigment group, retinal. Retinal absorbs light in the visible range (400–600 nm) and is found in two forms, an 11-*cis* form and a lower energy all-*trans* form. The 11-*cis* retinal is attached through a Schiff base linkage to a lysine residue in opsin and can absorb a photon of visible light (495 nm). The photon of light converts the 11-*cis* form to the *trans* form, which dissociates from the opsin. Following this, a sequence of biochemical, biophysical and physiological events occurs which, when summated into the visual cortex of the brain, is perceived as sight. The 11-*cis* retinal unbends and this causes a conformational change in the opsin. Possibly, the 11-*cis* retinal holds the opsin in a strained configuration which is released once the Schiff base linkage is broken. The message is amplified by cyclic guanosine monophosphate (cGMP) and the G-proteins.

Colour vision depends on pigments that absorb at different wavelengths: blue 420 nm, green 530 nm and red 560 nm. These are found in outer cone segments. It would appear that a single ancestral opsin duplicated twice to give a rod opsin and red and blue cone opsins. The different absorption spectra are due to three different opsins that bind retinal.

Biologically active acid derivatives of vitamin A are essential in a number of metabolic processes. The nuclear retinoid receptors belong to the steroid/thyroid receptor family of proteins, which act as ligand-dependent regulators of gene transcription. The vitamin A nuclear receptors consist of six members, three all-*trans* retinoic acid receptors (RARα, RARβ, RARγ) and three 9-*cis* retinoid acid receptors (RXRα, RXRβ, RXRγ). Other members of this family include the receptors for progesterone, oestradiol, glucocorticoids and 1,25-dihydroxyvitamin D_3. Retinoid signalling by the active forms of vitamin A, all-*trans*-retinoic acid and 9-*cis*-retinoic acid, is mediated by two groups of receptors, retinoic acid receptors (RARαβ and γ) and retinoid X receptors (RXRαβ and γ). These all have a highly conserved sequence-specific DNA binding domain and a ligand binding domain.

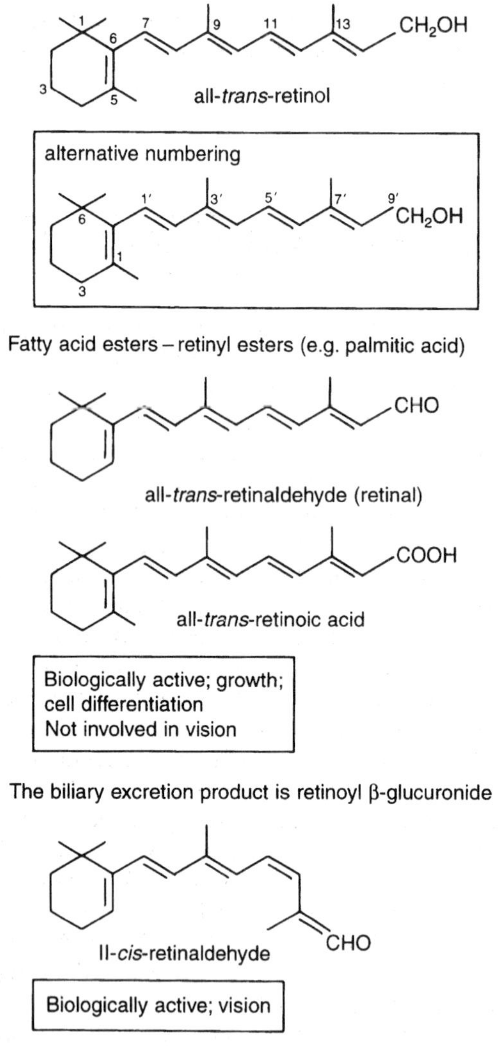

Fig. 16.2 Structure of substances with vitamin A activity: all-*trans* retinol, retinyl esters, retinal, retinyl β-glucuronide and 11-*cis* retinaldehyde.

Nuclear retinoid receptors

These receptor proteins are divided into functional domains. From the amino-terminal to the carboxy-terminal of the receptor, the A/B domain is either an immunogenic or a transcriptional domain. Region C is the DNA-binding domain which binds to a specific DNA sequence adjacent to the gene under regulation, which is stimulated to be transcribed; region D is a hinge or linker domain and region E is the ligand-binding domain conferring specificity upon the protein.

The high-affinity receptor proteins for retinoic acid (RAR and RAR with α, β, γ isoforms and two separate activating ligands, C-RA and T-RA) each have relative molecular masses of approximately 50 kDa. The receptors differ in their transcription activation domains. They are coded for by three different genes, which are expressed at different times and places during development and differentiation. Another group of retinoic acid receptors, the RXR 9-*cis*-retinoic acid, formed by cells from all-*trans*-retinoic acid, binds to RXR.

The RXR proteins participate in the activation of genes that are involved in development and differentiation. It is possible that RXR proteins act in metabolic regulation.

The retinoid receptors regulate the expression of genes. They act through cellular retinol binding protein type II. RAR also increases the binding of other receptors to and activation of their response elements. It is quite possible that RXR and the binding with N-*cis*-retinoic acid are central to intermediate metabolism with activation of enzymes, e.g. the medium-chain acyl-coenzyme A(CoA) dehydrogenase. It is also possible that 9-*cis*-retinoic acid and RXRα are necessary for the activation of the apolipoprotein A$_1$ synthesis in the liver.

These form dimers and bind to DNA, and regulate many developmental control genes including homeobox genes and growth factor genes. Gene transcription is induced by interacting with promoter sequences on the target gene, and modulated by nutritional and hormonal activity. The acid isoforms affect a wide diversity of biological systems, lymphoid cells, nerve and muscle cells, as well as developmental programmes. Retinoids have a role in the development of the the central body axis and limbs of the foetus. As an excess leads to gross abnormalities in the infant, the balance is important.

AVAILABILITY OF VITAMIN A

The first step in vitamin A metabolism is the absorption or uptake of retinol from the intestine.

Retinyl esters are hydrolysed in the small intestine by pancreatic hydrolases or an intestinal brush border hydrolase. The retinol is made more soluble by inclusion in a micellar system. Absorption requires a saturable passive carrier-mediated system.

β-Carotene is split by an enzyme in the small intestinal mucosa, β-carotene 15,15-oxygenase, yielding two molecules of retinol. Within the enteric cell, provitamin A carotenoids are oxidatively cleaved to produce retinal and apocarotenoids. Retinal is reduced to retinol.

After absorption, retinol is esterified with long-chain fatty acids. This reaction is catalysed by two microsomal enzymes:

- **lecithin**: retinol acyltransferase (LRAT), which uses the sn-1 fatty acid of phosphatidylcholine as the fatty acid donor
- **acyl-CoA**: retinol acyltransferase (ARAT), which uses acylated free fatty acids.

Retinol is carried from the intestine as retinyl palmitin in chylomicrons to be taken up by the liver.

The 11-*cis* isomer is found almost exclusively in ocular tissue and in a form not readily produced by vitamin A. Visual pigment regeneration requires the formation of 11-*cis* retinal and delivery to opsin (the visual cycle). Exposure to light leads to the formation of all-*trans* retinol in the photoreceptor and movement of the all-*trans* retinol through an extracellular compartment, the interphotoreceptor matrix, to the retinal-pigment epithelium. Here, in the dark *all*-trans retinol is metabolised to 11-*cis* retinal, which moves to the photoreceptors to bind to opsin. A retinal G-protein-coupled receptor similar to opsin binds all-*trans* retinal. This binding process coincides with the isomerisation to 11-*cis* retinal.

Vitamin A is stored as retinyl esters with long-chain fatty acids in animal tissues, especially the liver. Release from the liver is in the form of retinol; this circulates bound to a specific transport protein, retinol binding protein, which forms a complex with plasma pre-albumin. These can be measured by immunoassay. Concentrations are low in malnourished children. After ingestion, 8% of retinol is absorbed, 30–50% is stored in the liver, and 20–60% is conjugated and excreted in bile as a glucuronide. Stores of retinol are substantial, around 400 mg, and last for many months, even years.

There is almost certainly an enterohepatic circulation of retinoids, since retinoyl β-glucuronides and other retinoid metabolites are found in bile.

VITAMIN A DEFICIENCY

The clinical effects of vitamin A deficiency are usually seen only where the diet has been deficient in dairy produce and vegetables over a prolonged period, or in malabsorption syndrome.

Vitamin A is involved in the maintenance of epithelial surfaces, and a deficiency leads to epithelial metaplasia in the respiratory tract, mucous membranes (especially the eyes), gastrointestinal tract and genitourinary tract. The mucosa is replaced by inappropriately keratinised stratified squamous epithelium. In the skin, vitamin A deficiency results in keratinisation, which blocks the sebaceous gland with plugs, producing a condition known as follicular keratosis.

Vitamin A deficiency results in a reduction in the rhodopsin content of the rods of the retina, and this leads to night blindness. Epithelial surfaces undergo squamous metaplasia in vitamin A deficiency, that is, the cells become flattened and heaped one upon the other, with the surface being keratinised. This is particularly marked in the conjunctiva covering the sclera and cornea of the eye, and is known as xerophthalmia. This can lead to softening and destruction of the cornea and hence blindness.

Xerophthalmia

This is one of the most important deficiency diseases in the world. It is widespread in south-east Asia, the Middle East and Africa. It occurs in the first year of life among artificially fed infants, but is rare among breast-fed infants. If, however, the mother is deficient in vitamin A then the milk is also deficient, and hence the child has an inadequate intake of vitamin A. Dietary protein-calorie malnutrition compounds the problem. Xerophthalmia is common in young children, with a significant proportion becoming permanently blind.

Vitamin A deficiency may well worsen keratoconjunctivitis of other aetiologies, as with the measles infection. Initially, xerophthalmia occurs in the conjunctiva, but with more pronounced deficiency the cornea is affected, with a danger of corneal ulceration and permanent visual damage.

In vitamin A deficiency the epithelial cells of the cornea develop squamous metaplasia. Its clinical forms are:

- conjunctival xerosis
- corneal xerosis
- keratomalacia: leads almost certainly to blindness
- night blindness: an early symptom of vitamin A deficiency; may occur without any evidence of xerophthalmia
- xerophthalmic fundus
- corneal scars.

Treatment
Prophylaxis is necessary by teaching local populations to eat dark-green vegetables, which are rich in vitamin A. This is particularly important for pregnant women, weaning children, growing infants and adults.

Where xerophthalmia is endemic there may be merit in giving vitamin A prophylactically in capsule form or by fortification of foodstuffs with vitamin A in a water-soluble form, that is, added to table sugar or monosodium glutamate. It is said that a population should be regarded as being at risk of keratomalacia if more than 2% of the children have conjunctival xerosis or if 5% have a plasma retinol level of <100 μg/l.

Vitamin A (30 mg retinol daily, as oral halibut oil or intramuscular retinol palmitate) can be given for 3 days. Thereafter, retinol in the form of fish liver oil will prevent recurrence. The diet should be monitored, if possible, to ensure continued adequate vitamin A intake.

Vitamin A deficiency has also been suggested to be a possible risk factor for childhood illness and death. In the mountainous region of Nepal, Jumla, malnutrition is prevalent. A single oral dose of vitamin A (50 000–200 000 units, 15–60 mg, according to age) was given to children under 5 years old. In the treated group there was a 26% reduction in deaths resulting from diarrhoea, pneumonia and measles.

VITAMIN A EXCESS

An excess intake of food rich in carotenoids can result in a distinct orange–yellow colour of the skin, called hypercarotenaemia. The eyes do not become yellow. The persistence of this change in colour is dependent on continued intake of carotenoids.

Animal livers contain on average 1300–40 000 μg vitamin A/100 g. The liver of the polar bear is rich in retinol (600 mg/100 g liver). Eating the liver of the polar bear can cause drowsiness, headache, vomiting and excess peeling of the skin. Husky dog livers contain half this amount. Excess administration of retinol to young children can also lead to anorexia, irritability, dry, itching skin, coarse sparse hair and swelling over the long bones. Children are more sensitive than adults to a high retinol intake and great care should be taken in calculating the dosage.

There is also evidence that retinol is *teratogenic*. Consequently, it has been suggested that pregnant women or those who are trying to become pregnant should not eat liver or liver products and should not take vitamin supplements.

RECOMMENDED REQUIREMENTS

Adults

For the average adult the estimated average requirement (EAR) of 500 μg/day for a 74 kg male and 400 μg/day for a 60 kg female is reasonable. The lower reference nutrient intake (LRNI) is 300 μg/day for men and 250 μg/day for women; the reference nutrient intake (RNI) is 700 μg for men and 600 μg for women.

Infancy

The recommended daily amounts (RDAs) for infants are usually based on the vitamin A provided by breast milk. A daily intake of 350 μg retinol equivalents meets a young child's requirements, allowing for growth and maintaining liver stores. This means the EAR is 250 μg/day and the LRNI 150 μg/day.

Children

Children are growing and require vitamin A for the body stores. The recommended intakes are in the same order as for adults.

Pregnancy

In pregnancy extra vitamin A is required for the growth and maintenance of the foetus, to provide reserves and for maternal tissue growth. This is particularly important during the third trimester. An increment of 100 μg/day during the pregnancy, increasing the maternal RNI to 700 μg/day, should meet all requirements. A word of caution: there are dangers with large intakes of vitamin A (see below).

Lactation

The diet should contain an increment of 300 μg/day for milk production.

BODY STORE MEASUREMENTS

As vitamin A is stored in the liver in an esterified form, the liver content of the vitamin is the best measure of retinol status, although this is not a readily accessible measurement. Plasma retinol is an insensitive indicator of vitamin A status. Only during the latter stages of extreme deficiency does the plasma retinol fall below 0.70 μmol/l, while levels below 0.35 μmol/l indicate deficiency. Borderline values of 0.35–0.70 μmol/l may also be affected by inadequate protein intake, parasitic infestation, liver disease and other conditions.

The major markers of vitamin A status are plasma retinol and the relative dose–response (RDR) test. The control of retinol transport by retinol binding protein (RBP) is used as a functional test for retinol stores.

An alternative approach to the dose–response test is based on body size pool. Adequate vitamin A status is defined in terms of an adequate body pool, based on the amount of vitamin A in the liver, which contains the majority of vitamin A in the body. A liver retinol concentration of 20 μg/g tissue is the basis of the recommendations made by the Food and Agriculture Organisation (FAO) and the World Health Organisation (WHO).

Retinol dose–response test

In vitamin A deficiency there is a continuous synthesis of RBP which remains in the liver as apo-RBP. A blood sample is taken, a loading dose of retinol given, and a second sample of blood is taken after 5 h. The effects differ from the conventional loading test in that the plasma response is greater in deficient subjects.

Apo-retinol binding protein

The deficient liver protein readily combines with the incoming retinol and is excreted into the plasma. If the preloading concentration is increased by more than 20% this indicates a deficient liver retinol, below 20 μg/g. Little increase in plasma retinol is associated with a normal vitamin A status. The only biochemical marker for carotenoids is a plasma concentration that reflects short- to medium-term intakes.

There is a delay in biochemical change following treatment, which must be taken into consideration when estimating requirements.

KEY POINTS

1. Vitamin A consists of a group of biologically active compounds closely related to the plant pigment carotene. The carotenoid family consists of approximately 100 naturally occurring pigments, which provide the yellow–red colour of vegetables and some fruits.
2. The retinol molecule consists of a hydrocarbon chain with a β-ionone ring at one end and an alcohol group at the other. The usual form is the all-*trans* stereoisomer.
3. Vitamin A is essential for growth and normal function of the retina, and development of epithelial surfaces in the retina. The photopigment rhodopsin is a receptor protein found in the retinal rod cells. Rhodopsin consists of a membrane-embedded protein, opsin, and a light-sensitive pigment group, retinal.

4. Vitamin A and the retinoids act through nuclear receptor proteins, which regulate gene transcription.
5. Vitamin A deficiency is an important cause of eye malfunction, night blindness and xerophthalmia, a lesion of the conjunctiva and cornea. Other epithelial tissues, e.g. skin, are also affected.

THINKING POINTS

1. Vitamin A is essential for health, yet has clear toxic properties.
2. This has clear public health implications in supplementation programmes in malnourished populations.

NEED TO UNDERSTAND

1. Vitamin A belongs to a remarkable family of carotenes which have functions throughout biology.
2. The action of these lipid-soluble compounds is mediated through nuclear receptor proteins.
3. The action has similarities to a hormone, and vitamin A could almost be regarded as a dietary hormone.

FURTHER READING

Bonilla, S., Redonnet A., Noel-Suberville, C. *et al.* (2000) High-fat diets affect the expression of nuclear retinoic acid receptors in rat liver. *British Journal of Nutrition*, **83**, 665–71.

Clagett-Dame, M. and DeLuca, H.F. (2002) The role of vitamin A in mammalian reproduction and embryonic development. *Annual Review of Nutrition*, **22**, 347–81.

Dietary Reference Values for Food, Energy and Nutrients for the United Kingdom (1991) Report on Health and Social Subjects, No. 41. HMSO, London.

Levin, A.A., Sturzendecker, L.J., Kazmer, S. *et al.* (1992) *N-cis*-Retinoic acid stereoisomer binds and activates the nuclear receptor RXR. *Nature*, **355**, 359–61.

Li, E. and Norris, A.W. (1996) Structure/function cytoplasmic vitamin A-binding proteins. *Annual Review of Nutrition*, **16**, 205–34.

McCullough, F.S., Northrop-Clewes, C.A. and Thurnham D.I. (1999) The effect of vitamin A on epithelial integrity. *Proceedings of the Nutrition Society*, **58**, 289–93.

McLaren, D.S. and Frigg, M. (2001) *Sight and Life Guidebook on Vitamin A in Health and Disease*, 2nd edn. Task Force Sight and Life, Basel.

McLaren, D.S. and Frigg, M. (2001) *Sight and Life Manual on Vitamin A Deficiency Disorders (VADD)*, 2nd edn. Task Force Sight and Life, Basel.

Maden, M. (2000) The role of retinoic acid in embryonic and post embryonic development. *Proceedings of the Nutrition Society*, **59**, 65–73.

Mangelsdorf, D.J., Ong, E.S., Dyck, J.A. and Evans, R.M. (1990) Nuclear receptor that identifies a novel retinoic acid response pathway. *Nature*, **345**, 224–9.

Pepperberg, D.R. and Crouch, R.K. (2001) An illuminating new step in visual-pigment regeneration. *Lancet*, **358**, 2098–9.

Pfahl, M. and Chytil, F. (1996) Regulation of metabolism by retinoic acid and its nuclear receptors. *Annual Review of Nutrition*, **16**, 257–83.

Stevensen, C.B. (2001) Vitamin A, infection and immune function. *Annual Review of Nutrition*, **21**, 167–92.

Takase, S., Suruga, K. and Goda, T. (2000) Regulation of vitamin A metabolism-related gene expression. *British Journal of Nutrition*, **84** (Suppl. 2), S217–21.

Thurnham, D.I. and Northrup-Clewes, C.A. (1999) Optimal nutrition: vitamins and the carotenoids. *Proceedings of the Nutrition Society*, **58**, 449–57.

Wang, X.-D. and Russell, R.M. (1999) Procarcinogenic and anticarcinogenic effects of β-carotene, *Nutrition Reviews*, **57**, 263–72.

Wolf, G. (1998) Vitamin A functions in the regulation of the dopaminergic system in the brain and pituitary gland. *Nutrition Reviews*, **56**, 354–5.

Wolf, G. (1998) Transport of retinoids by the interphotoreceptor retinoic-binding protein. *Nutrition Reviews*, **56**, 156–8.

World Health Organisation/Unicef International Vitamin A Consultative Group Task Force (1988) *Vitamin A Supplements. Guide to their Use in the Treatment and Prevention of Vitamin A Deficiency and Xerophthalmia*. WHO, Geneva.

Yeum, K.-J. and Russell, R.M. (2002) Carotenoid bioavailability and bioconversion (2002) *Annual Review of Nutrition*, **22**, 483–504.

VITAMIN C (ASCORBIC ACID)

INTRODUCTION

Vitamin C (ascorbic acid) is a simple sugar with molecular weight of 176 Da. The important sources of the vitamin are fresh fruit and fruit juices; particularly rich sources are blackcurrant, guavas and green leafy vegetables. Liver and fresh milk are other sources. Vitamin C is lost by oxidation during cooking, particularly when boiled in water or cooked in deep fat. This oxidative process may be accelerated by traces of copper in an alkaline medium.

SYNTHESIS OF VITAMIN C

Many plant and animal tissues can synthesise vitamin C from glucose through intermediary L-gulonic acid and L-gulonolactone. This hepatic metabolism does not take place in humans, primates, guinea-pigs, an Indian fruit-eating bat, the red-vented bulbul and some birds. Consequently these animals, including humans, are susceptible to *scurvy*, through a deficiency of vitamin C. It is possible that there is modest synthesis of vitamin C in some humans, as not every sailor on long sea voyages developed scurvy.

Synthetic pathway of vitamin C

α-D-Glucose →→ UDP-D-glucuronate →
D-gluconate → L-gulonate → L-gulono-γ-lactone →
2-keto-L-gulonolactone → L-ascorbic acid

Humans, other primates, guinea-pigs and several other animals do not synthesise ascorbic acid as they do not possess the last enzyme required by the pathway, L-gulono-γ-lactone oxidase.

Ascorbic acid is converted to L-dehydroascorbate through the donation of two electrons (Figure 16.3). This requires:

- dehydroascorbate reductase, which uses reduced glutathione as a cosubstrate, resulting in ascorbate
- oxidised glutathione reductase, which uses NADPH for reduction of oxidised glutathione, may convert dehydroascorbate to ascorbate

The conversion of the lactone ring of L-dehydroascorbate to 2,3-diketo-L-gulonate requires an enzyme, lactonase. This enzyme is not present in humans. It may well be that other reducing agents such as glutathione, cysteine, tetrahydrofolate, tetrahydrobiopterin, dithiothreitol and 2-mercaptoethanol are used in place of ascorbate.

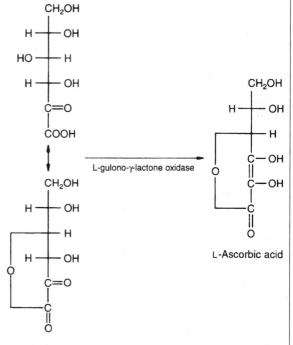

Fig. 16.3 Synthesis of 2-keto-L-gulonic acid to L-ascorbic acid is not possible in humans because of an absence of the enzyme L-gulono-γ-lactone oxidase.

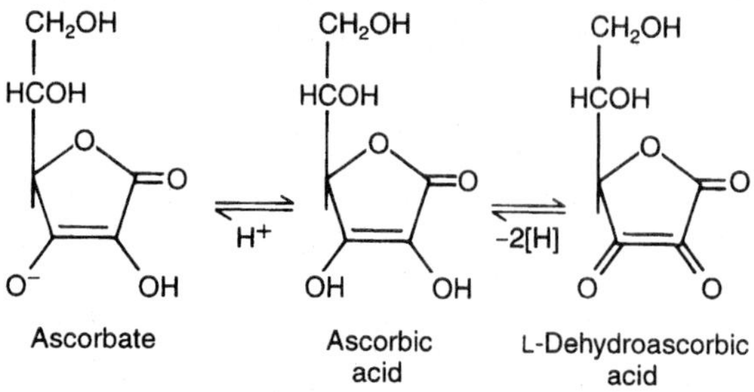

CH₂OH structures...

CH_2OH | $HCOH$ | Ascorbate

CH_2OH | $HCOH$ | Ascorbic acid

CH_2OH | $HCOH$ | L-Dehydroascorbic acid

Ascorbate $\underset{H^+}{\rightleftharpoons}$ Ascorbic acid $\underset{-2[H]}{\rightleftharpoons}$ L-Dehydroascorbic acid

Fig. 16.4 Structure of ascorbate, ascorbic acid and L-dehydroascorbic acid.

ACTION OF VITAMIN C

Vitamin C (Figure 16.4) is a powerful reducing agent and electron donor, and as such has a central role in the relative states of oxidation/reduction of other metabolically important water-soluble substances. It is a source of electrons for the reduction of oxygen and is a reducing agent which maintains elements in the reduced state. This is important in the intestinal luminal contents, wherein dietary iron in the ferric state is converted to the ferrous state. Ascorbic acid readily gives up an electron to convert Fe^{3+} into Fe^{2+}, which facilitates iron absorption.

Ascorbic acid is present in all tissues, especially the aqueous phase, and is important in synthetic processes and energy exchanges. It serves as a cosubstrate in a number of oxidoreduction reactions, acting synergistically with vitamin E. Urate, another water-soluble antioxidant, protects vitamin C. Interactions between iron and vitamin C are essential to iron metabolism in the body. Vitamin C is also involved in copper absorption and subsequent caeruloplasmin copper transport activity.

Ascorbic acid has an important role in a number of biological systems, in the synthesis of hormones, neurotransmitters, collagen and carnitine, and in the detoxification system through cytochrome P450 activity.

Enzyme reactions that require ascorbic acid include hydroxylations using oxygen with Fe^{2+} or Cu^{2+} as cofactors. The interaction between ascorbic acid and iron can increase the oxidative potential of iron, and iron acts as a pro-oxidant in the presence of ascorbic acid. The enzymes involved include the synthesis of hydroxyproline and hydroxylysine in pro-collagen. Ascorbic acid may be relevant in the hepatic microsomal mono-oxygenase system, which is important for steroid hormones and xenobiotics.

Other enzyme reactions that require ascorbic acid include:

- mono-oxygenases, which require copper, molecular oxygen and a reducing agent such as ascorbate. Ascorbate acts at the level of the metal to activate the oxygen, as in dopamine β-hydroxylase and peptidylglycine α-amidating mono-oxygenase
- a di-oxygenase reaction in which both atoms of a dioxygen molecule are entrapped into homogentisate, utilising 4-hydroxyphenylpyruvate dioxygenase.

All of the dioxygenases require ferrous iron, which is held in the ferrous state by a reducing agent, of which ascorbic acid is the most important. Other dioxygenases use α-ketoglutarate as a substrate and incorporate one atom of oxygen into succinate and one into a product of oxidation of the specific substrate, and require iron in the ferrous state, thus utilising ascorbate.

Dopamine β-hydroxylase is a final and rate-determined reaction in the conversion of tyrosine to noradrenaline. This is found in catecholamine storage vesicles in nervous tissue and in granules of the chromaffin cells of the adrenal medulla. The enzyme is formed from four identical subunits arranged as dimers joined by disulfide bonds, and contains 2–12 atoms of copper as Cu^{2+} per tetramer. Ascorbate is considered to be a reductant in the reaction. The adrenal medulla contains a very high concentration of ascorbate.

Many peptides, active as hormones, hormone-releasing factors and neurotransmitters, have a carboxy-terminal residue that is amidated. The amidation is catalysed by a copper-requiring enzyme that oxidatively cleaves the carboxy-terminal residue using molecular oxygen. The peptides that are amidated by this enzyme include bombesin, calcitonin, cholecystokinin, adrenocorticotropic hormone (ACTH), gastrin, growth hormone-releasing factor, α- and γ-melanotropin, neuropeptide, oxytocin, vasoactive intestinal peptide and vasopressin. The enzymes involved in the amidation are activated by the presence of ascorbate. Ascorbic acid appears to be involved in the conversion of 4-hydroxyphenylpyruvate to homogentisate in the oxidation of tyrosine to carbon dioxide and water.

Prolyl and lysyl hydroxylases are important in collagen formation. The known hydroxylases for collagen metabolism, prolyl 4-hydroxylase, prolyl 3-hydroxylase and lysyl hydroxylase, are all α-ketoglutarate-dependent dioxygenases that require ferrous iron. All require a reductant, the most effective being ascorbic acid. However, the main function of ascorbic acid may not be in the hydroxylation of prolyl and lysyl residues, but in protein biosynthesis.

The hydroxylation of other proline residues in elastin in the aorta and other tissues requires ascorbic acid. Ascorbic acid deficiency does not decrease elastin synthesis, but results in under-hydroxylation. It may also be involved in carnitine biosynthesis.

Carnitine is required in fatty acid metabolism for the formation of acylcarnitines that can cross mitochondrial and peroxisomal membranes. Acylcarnitines are required for the transport of fatty acids into mitochondria for oxidation. Two hydroxylation reactions are involved in the conversion of lysine to carnitine. Both enzymes require a reducing agent to keep the iron reduced.

The numerous metabolic requirements for ascorbic acid account for the many structural, regulatory, metabolic and immune disorders associated indirectly with scurvy. Ascorbic acid function may be to bring the iron constituent of enzymes, when oxidised, back to the active ferrous form.

AVAILABILITY OF VITAMIN C

Ascorbic acid is readily and rapidly absorbed in the small intestine, distributed in the blood and taken up by tissues to sustain metabolic functions. The plasma concentration (5% as dehydroascorbate) is related to dietary intake in a sigmoidal relationship (60–80 μmol/l on 100 mg/day) which plateaus at 1000 mg/day intake. Binding to proteins does not appear to be a central feature of vitamin C metabolism, although an association with albumin may be important. It is probable that the transport of

---

Tissue levels of vitamin C

High concentrations of vitamin C, between 1 and 3 mmol/kg, are found in the adrenal glands. There are high concentrations in all tissues at birth, which steadily reduce with increasing age. Tissue concentrations in the infant vary between 0.4 mmol/kg in the heart and 3 mmol/kg in the adrenal glands. This is in contrast to the middle-aged and elderly adult, where the concentrations range from 0.1 mmol/kg in the heart to 1.0 mmol/kg in the adrenals. There is good conservation of vitamin C by the kidneys, and urinary excretion only occurs when the plasma concentration exceeds 70 μmol/l. The rate of utilisation of vitamin C appears to be determined by the size of the vitamin C pool.

Other examples of vitamin C levels in various tissues, cells and fluids are:

- cervicovaginal tissue: 16 mmol/kg
- adrenal medulla: 10.5 mmol/kg
- monocytes: 8.0 mmol/kg
- brain: 1.3 mmol/kg
- aqueous humour: 1.0 mmol/kg
- tears: 0.77 mmol/kg.

---

ascorbic acid requires a membrane carrier and active transport that is probably specific to ascorbic acid. The body pool in a 70 kg adult is approximately 900 mg (5 mmoles).

Metabolism

A major pathway of ascorbic acid metabolism is to 2,3-dioxo-L-gulonate, which is further metabolised to oxalate and L-threonate. Ascorbic acid is excreted in the urine as the free ascorbic acid, dehydroascorbate, diketogulonate or oxalate. Excessive vitamin C intake (in g/day) may lead to the development of oxalate stones.

VITAMIN C DEFICIENCY

Scurvy

Scurvy is a nutritional disease resulting from prolonged subsistence on diets that do not include fresh fruit and vegetables. Scurvy tends to occur at the extremes of ages, in the young or in elderly people living in a socially isolated situation.

Aetiology
A lack of ascorbic acid is responsible for the characteristic disease. In addition to a dietary deficiency of vitamin C, the vitamin may have been destroyed by cooking.

Clinical signs
Haemorrhages, either large or microscopic, may occur anywhere in the body, including the gums, subcutaneous tissues, synovia of joints and beneath the periosteum of bones. Haemorrhages may also occur into the brain or heart muscle, with potentially fatal consequences.

There is failure of wound healing, and old wounds that have healed break down. Lind, a Scots naval surgeon who conducted the first clinical trial on the treatment of scurvy with fruit and lemons, said that the pathognomonic sign of the disease was the appearance of the gums, with the characteristic gingivitis. The gums, particularly in the region of the papillae between the teeth, are swollen and the scurvy buds may protrude beyond the biting surface of the teeth. The spongy gums are livid in colour and bleed readily. Superinfection is also a problem. Perifollicular bleeding around the orifice of a hair follicle is often found in the lower thighs and below the knees, but may appear on the buttocks, abdomen, legs and arms, followed by petechial haemorrhages which are not confined to the hair follicles. This must be differentiated from the follicular keratosis associated with vitamin A deficiency. In vitamin A deficiency there is a horny plug of keratin projecting from the orifice of the hair follicle, whereas in scurvy, there is a heaping up of keratin-like material on the surface around the mouth of the follicle, through which a deformed corkscrew hair projects. Other signs that have been described are ocular haemorrhages, particularly in the bulbar conjunctiva, Sjögren's syndrome (a loss of secretion of salivary and lacrimal glands), femoral neuropathy, oedema of the lower limbs, oliguria and psychological disturbances, hypochondria and depression. Anaemia, which may be normoblastic or megaloblastic, is a common finding. *Osteoporosis* may also occur in scurvy.

Vitamin C plasma concentrations

The white cell content of vitamin C is a good indication of ascorbic acid status, with an adequate dietary intake being suggested by a white cell level in excess of 0.85 mmol/l. Concentrations below 400 µmol/l suggest that there is a risk of scurvy. On a diet deficient in vitamin C, the plasma concentration falls from 110 to 70 µmol/l after 4 weeks, a concentration that is compatible with the appearance of scurvy.

Pathological effects
There is a failure of the body's supporting tissues to produce and maintain intercellular substances, and a defect in the capillary basement and the intracellular linkages between the endothelial cells. Wound healing and cartilage, bone and dentine growth are adversely affected. There is also a defect in the extracellular matrix where chondroblasts, osteoblasts and ondontoblasts lay down calcium. The matrix of collagen is important in bone and cartilage structure. The defect in scurvy is in the formation of collagen, which is an omnipresent support protein in the body. Collagen is assembled outside cells from pro-collagen, which is a coil with repeating glycine–hydroxyproline–proline units.

Hydroxyproline metabolism requires the enzyme proline hydroxylase, which is present in fibroblasts. This enzyme requires ascorbic acid for activation. Another observation is that scorbutic guinea-pigs have hypertrophy of the adrenal glands.

Scurvy in infants
Until the teeth have developed, gingivitis is not apparent but scurvy buds do occur. Bleeding is usually seen as a large subperiosteal haemorrhage over the long bones, e.g. the femur.

RECOMMENDED REQUIREMENTS

Adults

In the normal adult approximately 3% of the body pool of ascorbic acid, independent of size, is degraded each day. Leucocyte or buffy coat

Vitamin C: recommended intake

There is a sigmoidal relationship between vitamin C intake and plasma ascorbate concentrations. The recommendations for intake vary between expert committees. The variation in opinion is not unrelated to the definition of a normal vitamin status, and fulfilment and analytical measurement of that defined normality. Recommended intakes range from 40 to 200 mg/day. British recommendations are that the RNI is 40 mg/day, an LRNI of 10 mg/day for adults will probably prevent the development of scurvy and the EAR is 25 mg/day. An upper limit based on body saturation studies, not toxicity studies, suggests an upper limit of intake of 1–2 g/day.

vitamin C concentrations reflect tissue concentrations and there is a lower satisfactory limit of 0.09 µmol/10^8 cells, concentrations below which indicate deficiency. Plasma vitamin C concentrations reflect recent intake, and values less than 2 mg/l (11 µmol/l) indicate biochemical deficiency. While the necessary dietary intake of vitamin C has not been identified, dietary intakes of less than 10 mg/day are probably too small.

Pregnancy and lactation

The RNI should increase by 10 mg/day during the third trimester. During lactation an intake of 70 mg/day is probably satisfactory.

Children

Clinical scurvy has not been observed in fully breast-fed infants. The vitamin C content of breast milk varies from 170 to 450 µmol/l, which provides 25 mg/day. The LRNI for infants is 6 mg/day.

The elderly

There is no need routinely to increase vitamin C intake in the elderly, although as the diet of elderly people is not always ideal, vitamin C deficiency should always be considered.

Smokers

Smokers have an increased turnover of vitamin C and their intake should be increased to over 80 mg/day.

BODY STORE MEASUREMENTS

Ascorbic acid can be estimated in blood plasma or whole blood. Possibly the best index of vitamin C status is the white cell concentration of ascorbic acid.

There is a quantitative relationship between vitamin C intake and its levels in plasma (characteristically an S-shaped curve) and leucocytes. Vitamin C measurements, e.g. urinary vitamin C as a good mark of a high intake, are difficult because of the vitamin's instability.

The body can be saturated with approximately 5 g ascorbic acid, so in deficiency conditions 250 mg given orally four times a day should rapidly restore ascorbic acid concentrations. Alternatively, fresh fruit and vegetables, sprouting peas or extracts of pine needles are all that is required.

KEY POINTS

1. Ascorbic acid is a simple sugar with a molecular weight of 176 Da.
2. Ascorbic acid is a powerful reducing agent and an electron donor. As such, it has a central role in the relative states of oxidation/reduction of other metabolically important water-soluble substances.
3. Enzyme reactions requiring ascorbic acid are hydroxylations utilising oxygen with Fe^{2+} or Cu^{2+} as cofactors. The interaction between ascorbic acid and iron can increase the oxidative potential of iron, and iron acts as a pro-oxidant in the presence of ascorbic acid. The enzymes involved include the synthesis of hydroxyproline and hydroxylysine in pro-collagen, carnitine from lysine and the hepatic microsomal mono-oxygenase system, which is important for steroid hormones and xenobiotics.

4. A dietary deficiency of ascorbic acid results in scurvy.
5. Recommended requirements for vitamin C are defined for various ages and states.

THINKING POINTS

1. Vitamin C is essential for health, and is free from toxic properties.
2. This gives the vitamin enormous scope to be recommended for all manner of ailments.

NEED TO UNDERSTAND

1. Vitamin C is a powerful reducing agent and an electron donor, and also functions as a cofactor in hydroxylation enzymes which utilise iron and copper.
2. A dietary deficiency leads to scurvy.

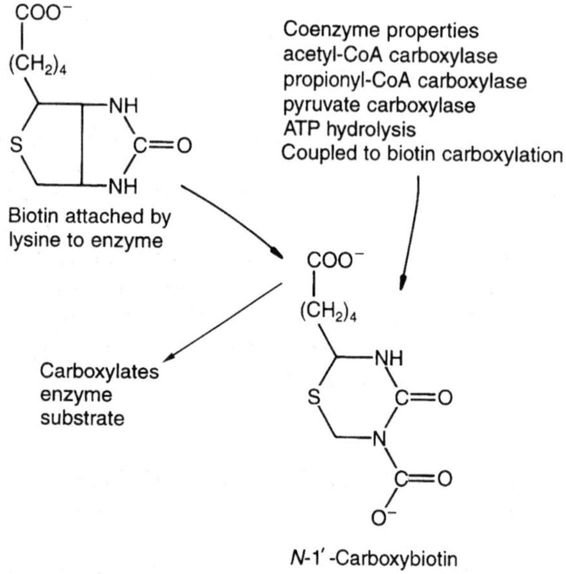

Fig. 16.5 Structure of biotin and its activity on the dependent coenzymes that are attached by lysine to the enzyme. ATP hydrolysis is coupled to biotin carboxylation.

FURTHER READING

Ausman, L.M. (1999) Criteria and recommendations for vitamin intake. *Nutrition Reviews*, **57**, 222–4.

Benzie, I.F. (1999) Vitamin C: prospective functional markers for defining optimal nutritional status. *Proceedings of the Nutrition Society*, **58**, 469–76.

Block, G., Henson, D.E. and Levine, M. (eds) (1990) Ascorbic acid (Foreword). Proceedings of a conference at NIH, Bethesda. *American Journal of Clinical Nutrition*, **54**(6, Supp.), vii.

Englard, S. and Seifter, S. (1986) The biochemical function of ascorbic acid. *Annual Review of Nutrition*, **6**, 365–406.

Sauberlich, H.E. (1994) Pharmacology of vitamin C. *Annual Review of Nutrition*, **14**, 371–91.

BIOTIN

INTRODUCTION

Biotin contains a ureido group in a five-membered ring fused with a tetrahydrothiophene ring with a five-carbon side-chain terminating in a carboxyl group. Its molecular weight is 244 Da (Figure 16.5).

Biotin is found in yeast, bacteria, liver, kidney, yeast extracts, pulses, nuts, chocolates and some vegetables. Most meats, dairy products and cereals are relatively poor sources. Liver, egg yolks and cooked cereals are rich sources of biotin, containing 20–100 μg/100 g, cow's milk contains 0.10 μmol/l and human breast milk contains 0.03 μmol/l of biotin, or less if the mother is deficient in biotin.

Another source of biotin is endogenous colonic bacterial synthesis. It is synthesised biochemically, by microorganisms, from pimelic acid, a seven-carbon dicarboxylic acid, L-alanine and L-cysteine.

ACTION OF BIOTIN

Biotin is a cofactor for the acetyl-CoA, propionyl-CoA and pyruvate carboxylase systems. These

Biotin in fatty acid synthesis

Propionyl-CoA carboxylase catalyses the carboxylation of propionyl-CoA to methylmalonyl-CoA, which is then converted to succinyl-CoA and enters the tricarboxylic acid cycle. Biotin is essential for the catabolism of propionic acid, which is derived from the intestinal flora, the catabolism of isoleucine, valine, methionine and threonine, the side-chain of cholesterol and the oxidation of odd-numbered fatty acids. 3-Methylcrotonyl-CoA carboxylase forms 3-methylglutacronyl-CoA from 3-methylcrotonyl-CoA in the catabolic path of leucine.

enzymes are involved in the synthesis of fatty acids, and in gluconeogenesis and carboxylation in this metabolic pathway. In the tissues, biotin is important in gluconeogenesis, especially in the liver and kidney, where oxaloacetic acid is utilised for the synthesis of glucose.

Acetyl-CoA carboxylase is found in the cytosol of the liver, where it catalyses the first step in the biosynthesis of fatty acids. The activity of this enzyme is important in the control of fatty acid synthesis. The carboxylases are synthesised as inactive apocarboxylases lacking biotin. Biotin binds to the apocarboxylases requiring the enzyme holocarboxylase.

Various types of enzymatic reaction are involved.

- All carboxylases involved in the fixation of carbon dioxide and requiring adenosine triphosphate (ATP) need biotin as a cofactor.
- Acetyl-CoA carboxylase catalyses the formation of malonyl-CoA from acetyl-CoA, bicarbonate and ATP. Malonyl-CoA is then used in fatty acid synthesis and fatty acid chain elongation.

Biotin binding

As a covalently bound cofactor in enzymes, biotin is a site for formation of a carboxylated intermediate, being bound to the enzyme by an amide linkage between the α-amino groups of enzyme lysine and carboxyl groups of biotin's valeric acid side-chain. The coenzyme function of biotin allows the carboxylation reactions to proceed by receiving the ATP-activated carboxyl group and transferring to the carboxyl acceptor substrate (Figure 16.5).

- Pyruvate carboxylase converts pyruvate to oxaloacetate, leading into the tricarboxylic acid cycle.

This feeds the tricarboxylic acid cycle, as well as providing a source of the carbon skeleton from the cycle necessary for the synthesis of the amino acids aspartate and glutamate.

AVAILABILITY OF BIOTIN

Little is known about the enteric absorption of biotin, but it is probably absorbed in the upper gastrointestinal tract. Raw egg white contains the protein *avidin* (molecular weight 68 kDa), which binds biotin with a high affinity. Ingestion of high amounts of avidin leads to the formation of biotin–avidin complexes and prevents the absorption of biotin. Denaturation of the avidin releases biotin.

In plasma, most of the biotin is bound to albumin and α- and β-globulin, but some is free. Biotin is stored in the liver and excreted as free biotin in the urine.

BIOTIN DEFICIENCY

Symptoms of biotin deficiency may include fatigue, depression, sleepiness, nausea and loss of appetite, muscle pain, hyperaesthesiae and paraesthesiae without reflex changes or other signs of neuropathy. These symptoms and signs are similar to those of thiamin deficiency. The tongue becomes smooth, with loss of papillae, the skin is dry with fine scaly desquamation, and anaemia and hypercholesterolaemia develop.

RECOMMENDED REQUIREMENTS

The dietary requirement of biotin is not known with certainty. The average intake in British men is 39 (range 15–70) µg/day and in women 26 (range 10–58) µg/day. It is estimated that biotin intakes of between 10 and 200 µg/day are safe and adequate.

The human neonate has higher biotin levels in the blood than those of adults, the biotin concentration of cord blood being 35–50% greater than that of maternal blood.

There are no indications that excess biotin can be harmful or toxic.

BODY STORE MEASUREMENTS

These are estimated by plasma biotin and lymphocyte propionyl-CoA carboxylase and its activation index (ratio of enzyme activity incubated with and without biotin) or urinary 3-hydroxy isovalerate.

KEY POINTS

1. Biotin contains a ureido group in a five-membered ring, fused with a tetrahydrothiophene ring with a five-carbon side-chain terminating in a carboxyl group.
2. Biotin is a cofactor for the acetyl-CoA, propionyl-CoA and pyruvate carboxylase systems. These enzymes are involved in the synthesis of fatty acids and involved in gluconeogenesis and carboxylation in this metabolic pathway.
3. Biotin is a covalently bound cofactor in enzymes, as a site for formation of a carboxylated intermediate, being bound to the enzyme by amide linkage between α-amino groups of enzyme lysine and the carboxyl group of biotin's valeric acid side-chain.
4. The coenzyme function of biotin allows carboxylation reactions to proceed by receiving the ATP-activated carboxyl group and transferring to the carboxyl acceptor substrate.
5. A dietary deficiency of biotin results in fatigue, depression, sleepiness, nausea and loss of appetite, muscle pain, hyperaesthesiae and paraesthesiae without reflex changes or other signs of neuropathy. The tongue becomes smooth with loss of papillae, the skin is dry with fine scaly desquamation, and anaemia and hypercholesterolaemia develop.

THINKING POINT

The binding of biotin to avidin is an interesting, not obvious, dietary cause of a specific nutrient being malabsorbed.

NEED TO UNDERSTAND

Biotin has an important coenzyme role in acetyl-CoA, propionyl-CoA and pyruvate carboxylase systems. The signs of deficiency are very non-specific.

FURTHER READING

Bender, D.A. (1999) Optimum nutrition: thiamin, biotin and pantothenate. *Proceedings of the Nutrition Society*, **58**, 427–33.

McMahon, R.J. (2002) Biotin in metabolism and molecular biology. *Annual Review of Nutrition*, **22**, 221–39.

Sweetman, L. and Nyahan, W.L. (1986) Inheritable biotin-treatable disorders and associated phenomena. *Annual Review of Nutrition*, **6**, 317–43.

Zempleni, J. and Mock, D.M. (2001) Biotin homeostasis during the cell cycle. *Nutrition Research Reviews*, **14**, 45–63.

NIACIN

INTRODUCTION

Niacin, or also known as nicotinic acid or vitamin B_3, has a molecular weight of 123 Da. It occurs as a pyridine derivative and is found in the body as an amide, nicotinamide (Figure 16.6).

Nicotinic acid is found in plants and animal foods in small amounts, with higher levels in meat, fish, wholemeal cereals and pulses. In many cereals, particularly maize and perhaps potatoes, the nicotinic acid is held in a bound, unabsorbable form. Nicotinic acid can be liberated from the bound form, niacytin, in an alkaline medium. In Central America

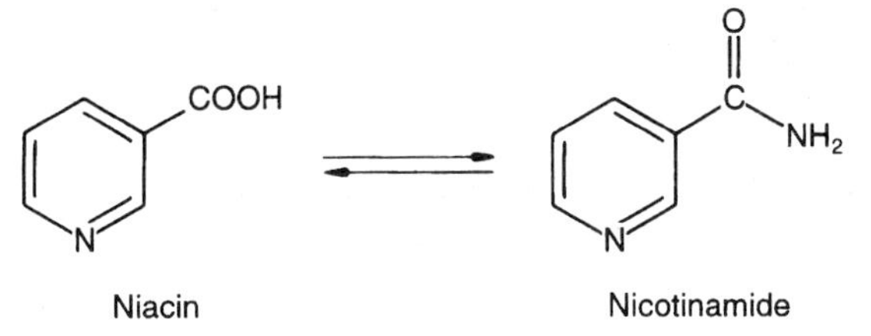

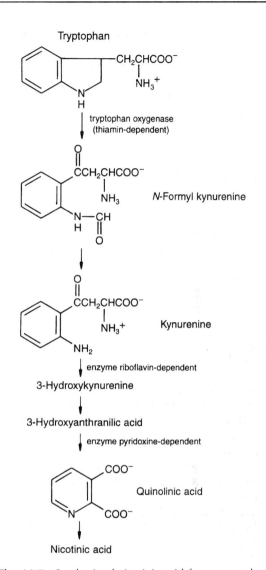

Fig. 16.6 Structure of niacin and nicotinamide.

maize is an important foodstuff. It is cooked with a thin paste of slaked lime, heated for 18 h and then eaten as tortillas. The prolonged heating liberates but does not destroy the bound nicotinic acid. Niacin leaches into the cooking water, which must also be consumed if the nicotinic acid is not to be lost.

SYNTHESIS OF NIACIN

Humans are not entirely dependent on dietary nicotinic acid as this vitamin can be synthesised from tryptophan.

The rate of conversion of tryptophan to niacin varies between individuals and at different times. Increased dietary intake of tryptophan results in a greater efficiency of conversion to niacin. The two enzymes involved in tryptophan metabolism, kynureninase and kynurenine hydroxylase, are vitamin B_6 and riboflavin dependent (Figure 16.7). Consequently, a deficiency in either of these vitamins may result in niacin deficiency, despite adequate intakes of tryptophan.

Approximately 60 mg of tryptophan in the diet is required to produce 1 mg of dietary nicotinic acid. The nicotinic acid equivalent, that is the nicotinic acid content plus 1/60th of the tryptophan content of the food or diet, is a good measure of the dietary intake, rather than the nicotinic acid content alone.

Fig. 16.7 Synthesis of nicotinic acid from tryptophan. The enzymes are thiamine, riboflavin and pyridoxine dependent.

ACTION OF NIACIN

Nicotinamide is a component of the coenzymes nicotinamide adenine dinucleotide (NAD^+) and nicotinamide adenine dinucleotide phosphate ($NADP^+$). NADP is also known as triphosphopy-

Typical reactions that require NAD^+ include alcohol dehydrogenase, glutamine dehydrogenase and glyceraldehyde dehydrogenase. NAD^+ acts as a true bound coenzyme in such reactions as epimerisations and aldolisations. Enzymes involved are UDP galactose-4-epimerase and S-adenosylhomocysteinase.

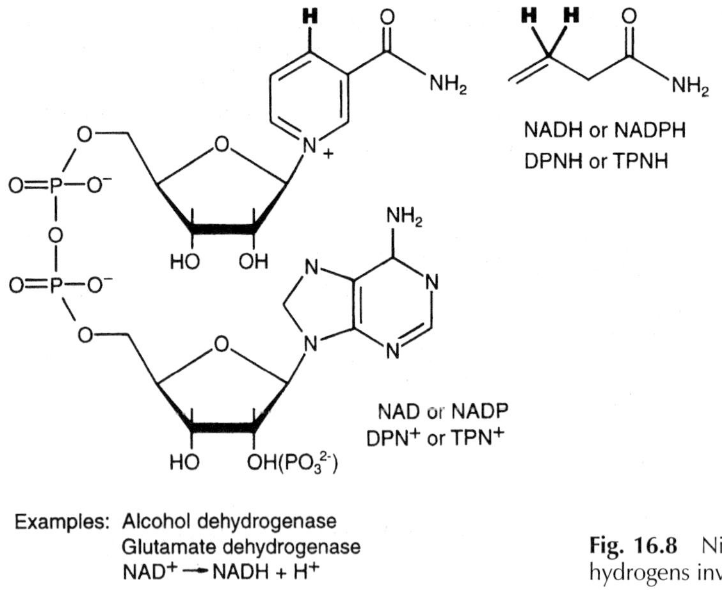

Examples: Alcohol dehydrogenase
Glutamate dehydrogenase
$NAD^+ \rightarrow NADH + H^+$

Fig. 16.8 Nicotinamide as a coenzyme, indicating the hydrogens involved in the coenzyme's activity.

ridine nucleotide (TPN^+). These coenzymes are electron carriers. In the reaction $NAD^+ \rightarrow$ NADPH, two electrons and a proton are accepted from the substrate which is being oxidised. NADH is then reoxidised, accepting O_2 with the reversal to NAD^+ and the formation of ATP NAD^+, a cellular electron carrier (Figure 16.8).

AVAILABILITY OF NIACIN

Free niacin is readily absorbed in the upper gastrointestinal tract. Nicotinic acid held in a bound form, niacytin, is not absorbed from the gastrointestinal tract. There is no apparent storage of this vitamin.

The vitamin is excreted as 5'-methylnicotinamide in the urine.

NIACIN DEFICIENCY

Pellagra

A deficiency of niacin results in pellagra, a disease found among poor populations living largely on maize, and possibly accompanied by protein-energy malnutrition, anaemia and deficiencies of thiamin and other vitamins.

Pellagra is a chronic and relapsing problem with a seasonal incidence, called the disease of the 3 Ds: dermatitis, diarrhoea and dementia. The latter two are usually found in more advanced cases and depression, rather than dementia, may be the problem. Pellagra became a common problem following the cultivation of maize, which was introduced into many countries as an easily grown crop in dry areas.

Aetiology

Pellagra is caused by a deficiency of nicotinic acid. Tryptophan, from which nicotinamide is synthesised in the body, is present in ample amounts in most dietary proteins, but not in zein, the chief protein in maize. To avoid pellagra, the maize must be eaten in conjunction with, for example, milk.

Pellagra is not found in central America because the maize is carefully cooked. Pellagra can occur in alcoholics and in patients who have been starved, as in malabsorption syndrome.

Hartnup's disease is a rare inbuilt inborn error of metabolism that resembles pellagra and is characterised by skin lesions, cerebellar ataxia and biochemical abnormalities, notably amino aciduria.

The problem is the transport of tryptophan which affects the absorption of the amino acid in the small intestine and the renal tubules.

Clinical features
The patient is underweight and there is increasing debility.

- **Skin**: an erythema develops, with the appearance of sunburn, with a symmetrical distribution over the parts of the body exposed to sunlight: the backs of the hands, wrists, forearms, face and neck. Areas exposed to mechanical irritation or trauma are particularly affected. The skin is initially red and slightly swollen, itchy and hot. In acute cases the skin lesions may progress to vesiculation and cracking, with exudates and ulceration. There may be secondary infection. In chronic cases the dermatitis is a roughening and thickening of the skin with dry scaling and brown pigmentation.
- **Digestive system**: diarrhoea may be present, as well as nausea and epigastric pain. The problem may be aggravated by parasites. There is angular stomatitis and cheilosis. The tongue is red, swollen and painful. Secondary infection of the mouth is common. There may be mucosal atrophy affecting the gastrointestinal tract.
- **Reproductive organs**: vaginitis and amenorrhoea may occur.
- **Nervous system**: in mild cases there will be weakness, tremor, anxiety, depression and irritability. In severe cases delirium is common, and dementia occurs in the chronic form. There may be paraesthesia in the feet, and loss of vibration sense and proprioception. This may lead to ataxia, spasticity and increased tendon reflexes. It is difficult to separate these symptoms from vitamin B_{12} deficiency.

Treatment
Mild cases improve upon treatment with nicotinamide or nicotinic acid or by an improved diet.

Nicotinamide, in contrast to nicotinic acid, does not cause unpleasant flushing and a burning sensation; the oral dose is 100 mg 4 hourly. The response is rapid: within 24 h the erythema is reduced, the tongue is restored to normal and diarrhoea ceases. Dementia may not respond to treatment, although depression presenting as pseudodementia will remit.

Complementary vitamin B complexes, folic acid and B_{12} should also be given. It is important to restore the individual to a diet containing an array of good-quality protein from sources compatible with his or her culture.

NIACIN EXCESS

A very high dosage of niacin, 3–6 g/day, can affect liver structure and function, with hepatotoxic consequences.

RECOMMENDED REQUIREMENTS

Recommendations for niacin are associated with tryptophan ingestion. The median intake of protein in Britain is 84 g/day for men and 62 g/day for women, containing approximately 13 mg tryptophan per gram, equivalent to 17 mg/day of niacin for men and 13 mg/day for women.

The recommendations are for niacin equivalents. The RNI is 6.6 mg/1000 kcal and the LRNI 4.4 mg/1000 kcal. These estimates are based on the intake of niacin required to prevent or cure pellagra.

Infants

The general recommendation is that infant milk should provide not less than 3.3–3.85 mg preformed niacin/1000 kcal. Because of the tryptophan present in cow's milk protein, infants would have an intake similar to adults, of niacin equivalent per 1000 kcal.

Pregnancy

Because of hormonal changes in tryptophan metabolism in late pregnancy, 30 mg of tryptophan is equivalent to 1 mg of dietary niacin. There should be simultaneously increased metabolism of tryptophan, so a need for an increased dietary intake of niacin is unlikely.

Lactation

Mature human milk provides preformed niacin (2.7 mg/l). It is assumed that maternal tryptophan metabolism would compensate for this, although some would recommend an increment of 2 mg/day.

Hyperlipidaemias

Nicotinic acid, but not nicotinamide, is sometimes used therapeutically for hyperlipidaemias at 2–6 g/day.

BODY STORE MEASUREMENTS

There are no absolute laboratory assessments of niacin status. The most sensitive measurement of niacin, nicotinamide and related compounds in serum, urine and food, is by microbiological methods. In such methods an organism that requires niacin for growth is cultured in the presence of the test material, and growth is calibrated against standard solutions of niacin. An alternative is to measure the main urinary metabolites of nicotinamide, namely *N*-methyl nicotinamide over a defined time or as a ratio of creatinine in urine. The measurement of urinary *N*-methyl-2-pyridone-5-carboxamide (2-pyridone) excretion is a more sensitive method used in marginal deficiencies of nicotinamide, and is expressed as mmol/creatinine. *N*-Methyl-nicotinamide is an excretory product of nicotinic acid and is present in the urine in reduced amounts in pellagra, e.g. below 0.2 mg/6 h.

KEY POINTS

1. Nicotinic acid occurs as a pyridine derivative and is found in the body as an amide, nicotinamide.
2. Nicotinamide is a component of the coenzymes nicotinamide adenine dinucleotide (NAD^+) and nicotinamide adenine dinucleotide phosphate ($NADP^+$). These coenzymes are electron carriers. In the reaction $NAD^+ \rightarrow NADPH$, two electrons and a proton are accepted from the substrate being oxidised.

3. Dietary nicotinic acid deficiency leads to pellagra, characterised by dementia, diarrhoea and dermatitis.

THINKING POINT

1. It is curious that the Mayans of Central America were able to avoid pellagra while eating maize by making tortillas. The unusual cooking of tortillas had profound dietary consequences. Could it be that this makes a good story, but that the tryptophan content of their diet was sufficient for the synthesis of niacin?

NEED TO UNDERSTAND

1. Niacin is a very important vitamin, a component of key coenzymes.
2. Niacin has well-defined requirements and possibilities for toxicity if eaten in excess.
3. The calculation of nicotinic acid equivalents from tryptophan, and the chemistry of this, are important.

FURTHER READING

Powers, H.J. (1999) Current knowledge concerning optimum nutritional status of riboflavin, niacin and pyridoxine. *Proceedings of the Nutrition Society*, **58**, 435–40.

PANTOTHENIC ACID

INTRODUCTION

Pantothenic acid, molecular weight 219 Da, is the dimethyl derivative of butyric acid joined by a peptide linkage to the amino acid β-alanine. The biochemically active form of the vitamin is 4′-phosphopantetheine, which is present in all tissues (Figure 16.9). Pantothenic acid is widely available

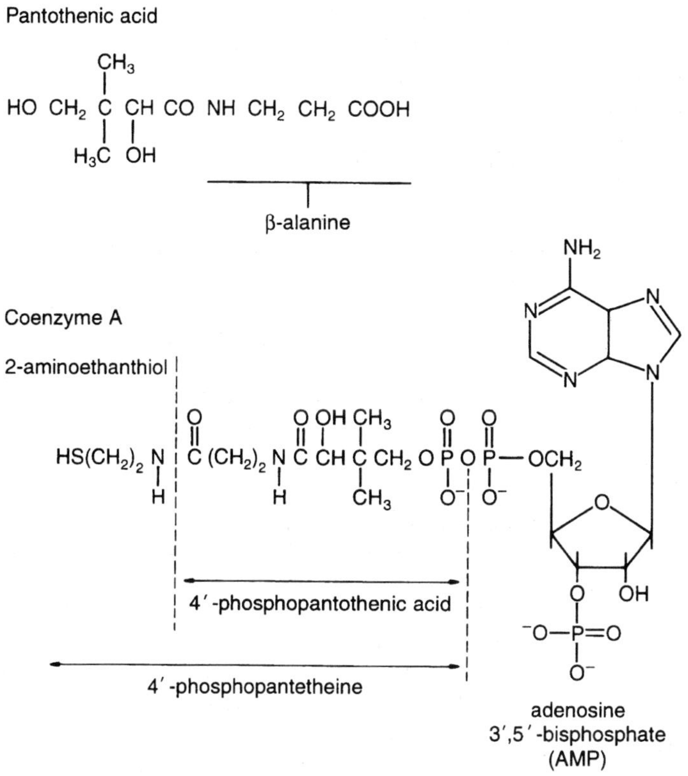

Pantothenic acid

Fig. 16.9 Structure of pantothenic acid and the active principle of coenzyme A.

in natural foods. The molecule is destroyed by heat in alkaline or acid conditions.

ACTION OF PANTOTHENIC ACID

4′-Phosphopantetheine is a constituent of co-enzymes:

- as CoA, bound covalently to an adenyl group
- as the functional part of a protein, e.g. serine hydroxyl group.

The sulfhydryl group of the 4′-phosphopant-etheine coenzyme (β-mercaptoethylene) is the functional part of the coenzyme's activity in enzymatic reactions. CoA has a central role:

- in intermediary metabolism (transfer of acyl groups to oxaloacetic acid) and in energy metabolism
- as an acyl carrier in the synthesis of lipids, fatty acids, β-oxidation of fatty acids and acylation

- in the synthesis of glycerol, glycerides, cholesterol, ketone bodies and sphingosine.

The creation of CoA esters of carboxylic acids is important in enolisation and acyl group transfer reactions.

AVAILABILITY OF PANTOTHENIC ACID

Pantothenic acid is absorbed and then excreted as the free acid in the urine. There is no storage of the vitamin.

PANTOTHENIC ACID DEFICIENCY AND EXCESS

No specific deficiency syndrome has been identified. In malnutrition there will be a general deficiency of pantothenic acid, but this will be difficult to separate from the overall problems associated with malnutrition.

No toxicity as a result of pantothenic acid excess has been identified at the dosages used.

RECOMMENDED REQUIREMENTS

Most human diets provide 3–10 mg, derived from a variety of natural foods. Estimates in the British diet give values of around 5–6 mg/day. There is no evidence of pantothenic acid deficiency at intakes of 3–7 mg; therefore, this must be an adequate intake, even during pregnancy and lactation.

The intake for children is in the order of 3 mg/1000 kcal.

BODY STORE MEASUREMENTS

No biochemical method identifies pantothenic acid status in humans. Blood levels and urinary excretion have been measured, but these are difficult to interpret in terms of dietary need.

KEY POINTS

1. Pantothenic acid is the dimethyl derivative of butyric acid joined by a peptide linkage to the amino acid β-alanine. The biochemically active form of the vitamin is 4′-phosphopantetheine.
2. Pantothenic acid is the precursor of coenzyme A.
3. No deficiency condition has been described in humans.

THINKING POINT

Considering the central place that pantothenic acid has in CoA synthesis, it is curious that dietary deficiency is so uncommon.

NEED TO UNDERSTAND

The biochemically active form of the vitamin is 4′-phosphopantetheine. Pantothenic acid is the precursor of coenzyme A.

FURTHER READING

Bender, D.A. (1999) Optimum nutrition: thiamine, biotin and pantothenate. *Proceedings of the Nutrition Society*, **58**, 427–33.

RIBOFLAVIN

INTRODUCTION

Riboflavin, molecular weight 219 Da, is a substituted alloxazine ring linked to ribotol, an alcohol derived from the pentose sugar ribose. Riboflavin is stable in boiling acid but not in boiling alkaline solution or on exposure to light.

Dietary sources are liver, milk, cheese, eggs, some green vegetables and beer. Other sources are yeast extracts, e.g. Marmite, and meat extracts, e.g. Bovril.

ACTION OF RIBOFLAVIN

In plant and animal tissues riboflavin links with phosphoric acid as flavin mononucleotide or riboflavin-5′-phosphate (FMN) which, with adenosine monophosphate, forms flavin adenine dinucleotide (FAD) (Figure 16.10). FMN and FAD are similar in their coenzyme activity. These are the prosthetic groups of the flavoprotein enzymes. The functional part of the coenzyme is the isoalloxane ring. These flavoproteins are stronger oxidising agents than NAD^+ and are versatile redox coenzymes. They are involved in one- or two-electron reactions with free radicals or metal ions. In the

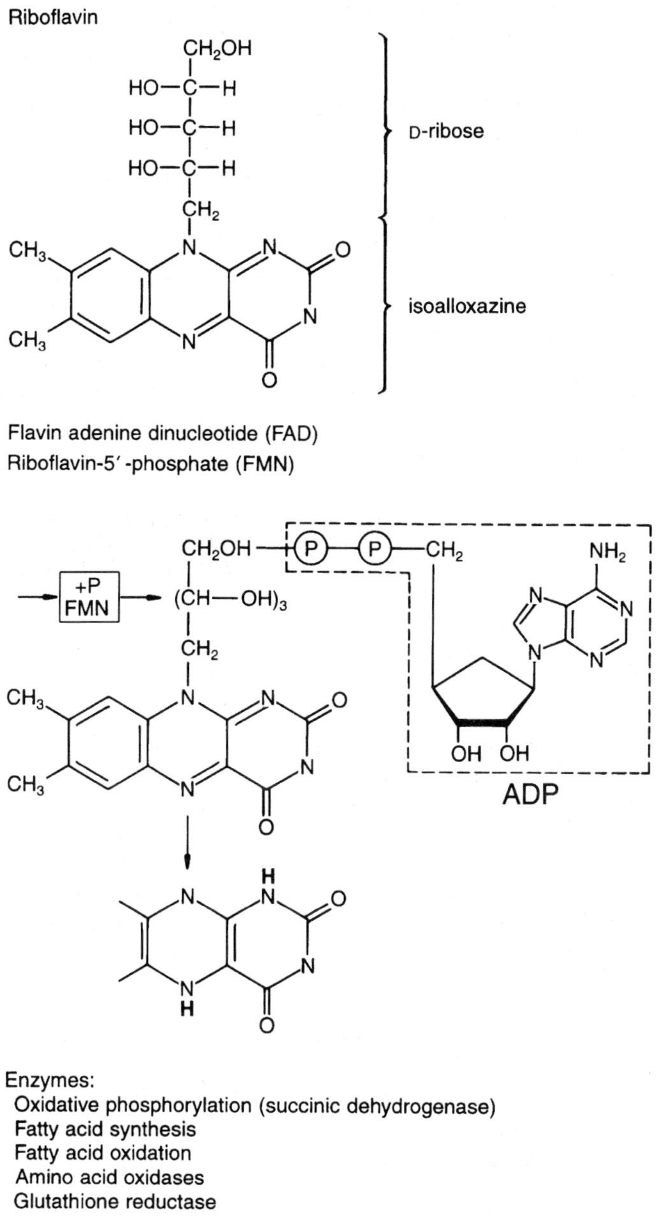

Riboflavin

D-ribose

isoalloxazine

Flavin adenine dinucleotide (FAD)
Riboflavin-5′-phosphate (FMN)

ADP

Enzymes:
Oxidative phosphorylation (succinic dehydrogenase)
Fatty acid synthesis
Fatty acid oxidation
Amino acid oxidases
Glutathione reductase

Fig. 16.10 Structure of riboflavin and role in flavin adenine dinucleotide and riboflavin-5′-phosphate.

reduced form they react with oxygen in hydroxylation reactions.

Flavoproteins are involved in metabolism, with the oxidation of glucose and fatty acids and the production of ATP, which is significant in anabolic processes. Important metabolic processes involving FAD/FMN include:

- as a coenzyme in oxidation/reduction reactions
- electron transport and oxidative phosphorylation, e.g. succinic dehydrogenases
- fatty acid synthesis and oxidation
- amino acid oxidases
- xanthine oxidase
- glutathione reductase.

AVAILABILITY OF RIBOFLAVIN

Riboflavin is absorbed in the upper gastrointestinal tract, does not appear to be stored, and is excreted unchanged in the urine. Chronic infection can affect urinary riboflavin excretion.

RIBOFLAVIN DEFICIENCY AND EXCESS

Riboflavin deficiency causes minimal morbidity, but is associated with cheilosis, angular stomatitis and superficial interstitial keratosis of the cornea. Nasolabial seborrhoea can occur.

No toxic effects have been shown for riboflavin.

RECOMMENDED REQUIREMENTS

Adults

The RNI is 1.3 mg/day for men and 1.1 mg/day for women. The LRNI in adults, male and female, is 0.8 mg/day; the EAR is 1.0 mg/day for men and 0.9 mg/day for women.

Infants

The average riboflavin content of breast milk in Britain is approximately 1.4 µmol/l. The range varies enormously, depending on the mother's intake. The RNI is 0.4 mg/day. The RNIs for children range between 0.4 mg/day for infants aged up to 3 months and 1.0 mg/day for those aged 7–10 months.

Pregnancy and lactation

Because of the extra demands for riboflavin the requirement is increased by 0.3 mg/day during pregnancy and 0.5 mg/day during lactation.

The elderly

Although the resting metabolism and riboflavin intake decrease with age, the RNI for elderly individuals should be the same as for young people.

BODY STORE MEASUREMENTS

The brilliant greenish-yellow fluorescence in ultraviolet light provides a mechanism for detecting riboflavin. Riboflavin status can be estimated by measuring:

- urinary riboflavin
- red blood cell riboflavin
- erythrocyte glutathione reductase activation coefficient (EGRAC).

The EGRAC test is a measure of tissue saturation and long-term riboflavin status. EGRAC values below 1.3 imply complete saturation of the tissue with riboflavin.

Methods used to measure tissue saturation depend on protein intake and positive nitrogen balance. A negative nitrogen balance complicates the measurement of riboflavin requirements, because riboflavin and protein are involved in the formation and storage of flavoproteins in lean tissue. A negative niacin balance and tissue breakdown increases urinary excretion of riboflavin and the saturation of red cell glutathione reductase.

Urinary riboflavin measurement was formerly the method used to assess riboflavin status. There is a linear relationship between intake and urinary excretion when there is a riboflavin intake in excess of dietary requirements. However, when riboflavin intake is less than tissue requirements there are adaptive changes in the utilisation of riboflavin coenzymes, reducing riboflavin excretion.

Glutathione reductase activity depends on riboflavin. This is used in the erythrocyte glutathione reductase stimulation test, which measures tissue saturation and long-term riboflavin status. A fingerprick blood sample is used and is not affected by the age or gender of the subject. It is sensitive only at low levels of riboflavin intake and is affected by circulating riboflavin when nutritional status is poor. An EGRAC of between 1.0 and 2.5 indicates adequate intake.

KEY POINTS

1. Riboflavin is a substituted alloxazine ring linked to ribotol, an alcohol derived from the pentose sugar ribose.

2. Riboflavin links with phosphoric acid as flavin mononucleotide or riboflavin-5′-phosphate (FMN) which, with adenosine monophosphate, forms flavin adenine dinucleotide (FAD). These are the prosthetic groups of the flavoprotein enzymes. The functional part of the coenzyme is the isoalloxane ring.
3. These flavoproteins are strong oxidising agents and versatile redox coenzymes.
4. Riboflavin deficiency is associated with cheilosis, angular stomatitis and superficial interstitial keratosis of the cornea.

THINKING POINT

Consider riboflavin as an example of a chemical with central roles in both plant and animal physiology.

NEED TO UNDERSTAND

The active role of the vitamin is as a flavin adenine dinucleotide precursor.

FURTHER READING

Bacher, A., Eberhardt, S., Fischer, M. *et al.* (2000) Biosynthesis of vitamin B$_2$ (riboflavin). *Annual Review of Nutrition*, **20**, 153–67.
Powers, H.J. (1999) Current knowledge concerning optimum nutritional status of riboflavin, niacin and pyridoxine. *Proceedings of the Nutrition Society*, **58**, 435–40.

THIAMIN

INTRODUCTION

Thiamin has a molecular weight of 337 Da. Thiamin hydrochloride consists of a substituted pyrimidine ring linked by a methylene group to a sulfur-

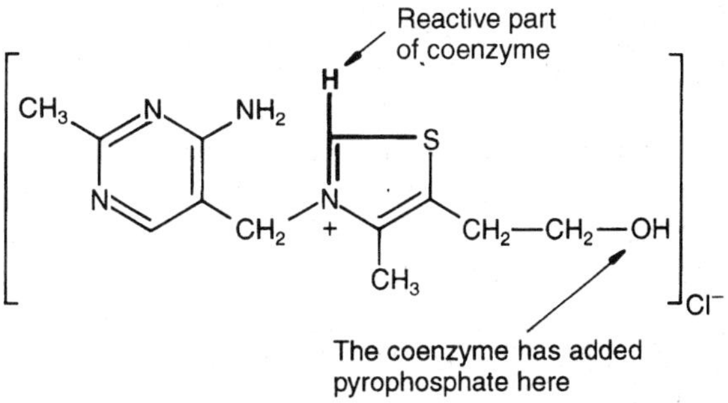

Fig. 16.11 Structure of thiamin and structure as a coenzyme. The reactive part of the coenzyme is shown in bold type.

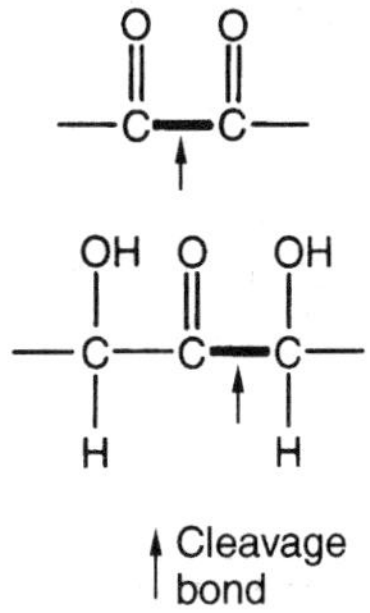

Fig. 16.12 Thiamin pyrophosphate is involved in the cleavage of ketoacids (ketoacid decarboxylation).

containing thiazole ring (Figure 16.11). Oxidation results in the inactive product thiochrome, which is strongly fluorescent in ultraviolet light; this effect can be used in the chemical estimation of the vitamin.

All animal and plant tissues contain thiamin. The important sources are plant seeds and the germ of cereals, nuts, peas, beans, pulses and yeasts. Green vegetables, roots, fruit, meat and dairy products contain modest amounts of the vitamin. Loss occurs during cooking, when rice and vegetables are boiled. Alkaline conditions result in destruction of the vitamin.

ACTION OF THIAMIN

Thiamin pyrophosphate is the coenzyme in α-ketoacid decarboxylation reactions (Figure 16.12). Thiamin pyrophosphate is the coenzyme of the carboxylase that is involved in the oxidative decarboxylation of pyruvic acid to acetyl-CoA. Thiamin pyrophosphate is also required for the decarboxylation of α-ketoglutarate in the Krebs citric acid cycle and in the transketolase reaction in the hexose monophosphate shunt.

AVAILABILITY OF THIAMIN

Absorption is by passive diffusion and active absorption from the upper gastrointestinal tract. Thiamin is not stored in the body and the only reserve is the thiamin bound functionally to enzymes. Metabolism is extensive and multiple endproducts are excreted in the urine.

THIAMIN DEFICIENCY

Thiamin deficiency results in beri-beri, which was first recognised as a widespread problem among the rice-eating peoples of the East. The widespread occurrence of the condition was a result of eating highly polished rice, the bran being sold for cattle food. The disease occurs in three forms:

- wet beri-beri (oedema and high output cardiac failure)
- dry beri-beri (polyneuropathy)
- infantile form.

Thiamin deficiencies are also found in chronic alcoholics:

- alcoholic neuropathy, which is similar to that of dry beri-beri
- thiamin-responsive cardiomyopathy
- encephalopathy (the Wernicke–Korsakoff syndrome).

In these thiamin deficiency conditions the metabolism of carbohydrates is impaired because of the role of thiamin pyrophosphate as an essential coenzyme in the decarboxylation of pyruvate to acetyl-CoA. Pyruvic acid and lactic acid accumulate in tissues and fluids, because of the lack of thiamin pyrophosphate, the coenzyme for transketolase in the hexose monophosphate pathway, and for decarboxylation of 2-ketoglutarate to suc-

cinate in the citric acid cycle. Such accumulation results in peripheral dilatation and oedema.

Clinical features

Initially, the symptoms are anorexia, malaise, a feeling of heaviness and weakness of the legs, and problems with walking. There may be a little oedema of the legs and face and precordial pain and palpitations. There may be calf tenderness, pins and needles, numbness in the legs and reduced tendon jerks. Anaesthesia of the skin over the tibiae is a feature that may persist over prolonged periods. The consequence of this mild affliction is a reduction in stamina.

Wet beri-beri
Palpitations, breathlessness, anorexia and dyspepsia are common, with exercise-related leg pain a feature. Oedema affects the legs, face, trunk, lungs and peritoneal cavity. This may be compensated for by an increased cardiac output. When the heart is unable to sustain this increased cardiac output, cardiac failure results. This is a high output failure.

There is evidence of congestive cardiac failure with increased jugular venous pressure, cardiomegaly with displacement of the apex beat and hypotension. The extremities are warm, and there is a water-hammer pulse, as in aortic regurgitation. With cardiac failure there is evidence of decompensation, coldness and cyanosis. The individual with cardiac failure may deteriorate rapidly and die suddenly.

Dry beri-beri
In the later stages the muscles become progressively wasted and weak, resulting in great difficulty in walking. The patient becomes emaciated and there may be evidence of Wernicke encephalopathy.

Infantile beri-beri
This occurs in breast-fed infants, usually between the second and fifth months. Infantile beri-beri may be acute or chronic; in the acute form cardiac failure develops rapidly, the child becomes restless, cries frequently, is oliguric, oedematous, cyanotic and dyspnoeic, and has a tachycardia. The child may develop convulsions and become comatose.

In the chronic form, symptoms of gastrointestinal upset, constipation and vomiting appear, and the child is fretful and sleeps poorly. The muscles may be soft and toneless, but not markedly wasted. The skin may show pallor with cyanosis about the mouth. Cardiac failure and sudden death are common.

Alcoholic neuropathy

This is a neuropathy affecting both sensory and motor nerves. Sensory nerve dysfunction may manifest itself by paraesthesiae and severe nerve pain, the loss of sensation, numbness of the extremities and loss of proprioception. Motor nerve lesions include foot drop, muscle wasting and impaired knee and ankle jerks. In addition to this there may be cardiomyopathy.

Wernicke–Korsakoff syndrome

This consists of a weakness of eye muscles so that the patient cannot look upwards or sideways. The patient may be disorientated and apathetic and has nystagmus and commonly is ataxic and confabulates. The anatomical lesions appear symmetrically in the brainstem, diencephalon and cerebellum. In severe cases there may be tissue necrosis with destruction of myelin.

Treatment

Treatment of wet beri-beri is by intramuscular thiamin, 25 mg twice daily for 3 days; a dose of 10 mg two or three times daily should be sufficient thereafter. Large doses of thiamin, given sufficiently early, may effect substantial, but not complete, improvement. The reversal of the clinical signs is rapid, with improvement in heart size, respiration and physical performance.

Improvement following the treatment of dry beri-beri is slow; the neurological abnormalities, in particular, reverse slowly.

In infantile beri-beri, treatment of the mother benefits the child via breast feeding. The mother should receive 10 mg thiamin twice daily and the child may be given thiamin intramuscularly 10–20 mg once a day for 3 days and thereafter 5–10 mg twice daily.

Prevention

Beri-beri can be prevented by the use of unmilled rice, by the fortification of rice with thiamin, by the use of pulses and other foods containing thiamin, or by medicinal preparations of thiamin.

THIAMIN EXCESS

Long-term intakes in excess of 50 mg/kg body weight, or more than 3 g/day are toxic, leading to headaches, irritability, insomnia, rapid pulse, weakness, contact dermatitis, pruritis and even death. At 'normal' dosages, toxicity is unknown.

RECOMMENDED REQUIREMENTS

Adults

Thiamin requirements are related to energy metabolism. The average requirement is 0.3 mg/1000 kcal. The RNI is 0.4 mg/1000 kcal. However, intakes for men and women should not be less than 0.4 mg/day.

Infants

The thiamin concentration in human milk is approximately 0.5 µmol/l, which is equivalent to 0.3 mg/1000 kcal. The RNI for infants is 0.3 mg/1000 kcal.

Children

The RNI for children is the same as for adults.

Pregnancy and lactation

There is no evidence of any increased need for thiamin during normal pregnancy. The loss of 0.14 mg thiamin per day in milk should be met by a recommended increase in energy intake. The RNI is unchanged during pregnancy and lactation.

Therapeutic use

Thiamin is used in the treatment of cardiovascular and infantile beri-beri, in Wernicke encephalopathy and some cardiomyopathies.

BODY STORE MEASUREMENTS

It is possible to estimate dietary status by measurement of urinary thiamin, although this is laborious and difficult. The thiamin:creatinine ratio has been used for random samples. Loading doses of 1–5 mg of thiamin are given orally or intramuscularly and the urinary thiamin is measured over 4–24 h. If the proportion of urinary thiamin is below 20% of the administered dose over the subsequent 24 h then thiamin deficiency is suggested.

An alternative method is the reactivation of the cofactor-depleted red cell enzyme transketolase. However, the biochemical response to a given intake varies enormously between individuals.

KEY POINTS

1. Thiamin hydrochloride is a substituted pyrimidine ring linked by a methylene group to a sulfur-containing thiazole ring.
2. Thiamin is the precursor of the coenzyme thiamin pyrophosphate. This is the essential coenzyme involved in the action of enzymes that catalyse the cleavage of C-C and C-X bonds, e.g. in many α-keto acid decarboxylations.
3. Thiamin deficiency causes beri-beri.

THINKING POINTS

1. Thiamin deficiency is at its most common with refinement of rice and dependence on too narrow a dietary base.
2. Such a restricted choice, however, has much to do with poverty and ignorance.

NEED TO UNDERSTAND

1. Thiamin is a precursor of the coenzyme thiamin pyrophosphate and the reactions involved in this coenzyme.
2. Two different syndromes result from thiamin deficiency, wet and dry beri-beri.

FURTHER READING

Bender, D.A. (1999) Optimum nutrition: thiamin, biotin and pantothenate. *Proceedings of the Nutrition Society*, **58**, 427–33.

VITAMIN B$_6$

INTRODUCTION

Vitamin B$_6$, molecular weight 168 Da, comprises a family of free and phosphorylated compounds that includes pyridoxine, pyridoxal and pyridoxamine (Figure 16.13). Vitamin B$_6$ is found in cereals, meat (particularly liver), fruit and leafy and other vegetables. The free form is most commonly found in plants; the phosphorylated form, pyridoxamine phosphate, is more commonly found in animal tissues.

ACTION OF PYRIDOXINE

Pyridoxal-5'-phosphate is a coenzyme with a major role in the intermediary metabolism of amino acids, in α-decarboxylation, aldolisation and transamination reactions (Figure 16.14). The coenzyme is also involved in the β-carboxylation of aspartic acid. The aldehyde group of pyridoxal 5'-phosphate forms a Schiff base with the α-amino acid group of amino acids. Pyridoxal-5'-phosphate catalyses several different types of bond cleavage, by stabilising the electron pairs at the α- or β-carbon atoms of α-amino acids.

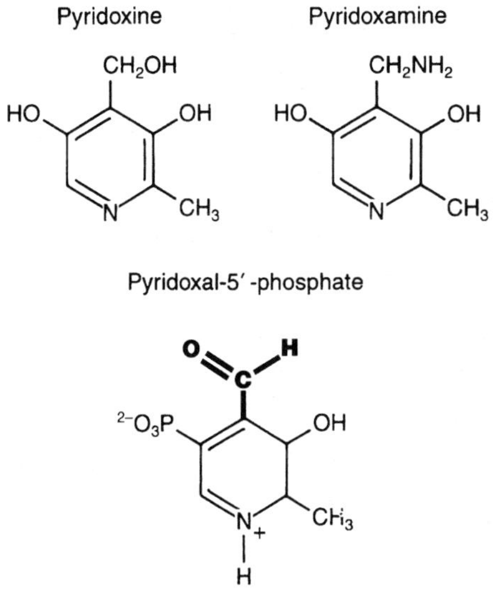

Pyridoxine   Pyridoxamine

CH_2OH CH_2NH_2

Pyridoxal-5'-phosphate

Fig. 16.13 Structure of pyridoxine, pyridoxamine and pyridoxal-5'-phosphate. The reactive part of the molecule is shown in bold type.

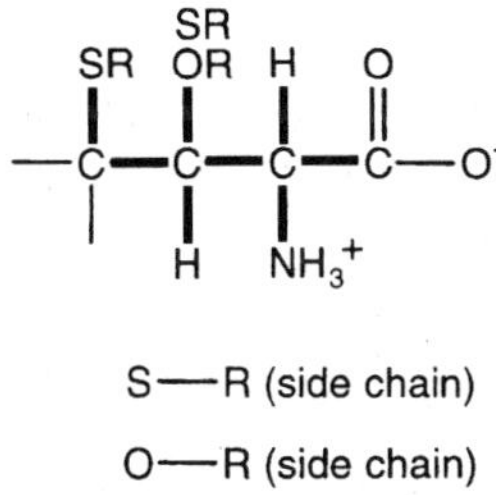

S——R (side chain)

O——R (side chain)

Fig. 16.14 Bonds (bold type) cleaved by enzymes requiring pyridoxal-5'-phosphate, including α-amino acids in transamination, α-decarboxylation and α, β-eliminations.

Metabolic roles of pyridoxine include:

- transamination enzymatic reactions: the vitamin forms pyridoxamine phosphate, which accepts the α-amino group of the amino acid, and then is released with the transfer of the amino group to a keto acid. Some of the vitamin B_6-dependent enzymes are rate limiting in metabolic processes, e.g. the degradation of tyrosine (tyrosine aminotransferase). The amount of these enzymes is modulated by corticosteroids and glucagon substrate concentration

- decarboxylation in the synthetic pathway of the neuroactive amines serotonin, tyramine, histamine and γ-aminobutyric acid. Other decarboxylation reactions include δ-aminolevulinic acid and intermediates in the synthesis of lecithin and taurine and the decarboxylation pathway, and removal of the sulfur that occurs with cysteine
- oxidative removal of the amino group from serine and threonine as ammonia to form α-keto acids
- formation of glycine and formate from serine, removal of alanine from kynurenine and 3-hydroxy-kynurenine, and the splitting of cystathione in the degradation of methionine.

AVAILABILITY OF PYRIDOXINE

The vitamin is absorbed in the free form and subsequently phosphorylated for use in enzymes. It is excreted in the urine largely as 4-pyridoxic acid.

PYRIDOXINE DEFICIENCY AND EXCESS

Primary dietary deficiency has not been reported in adults, largely because of the widespread distribution of the vitamin in foods. Nevertheless, a deficiency may occur in alcoholics and in patients taking certain drugs, e.g. p-aminosalicylic acid. This deficiency condition may result in increased urinary excretion of urea, xanthurenic acid, kynurenine, hydroxyurenine and oxalic acid. The hyperoxaluria may lead to urinary stone formation. In infants there may be hyperirritability, convulsions and anaemia.

The anti-tubercular drug isoniazid (hydrazide) inactivates pyridoxal phosphate by forming a hydrazone and results in a peripheral neuropathy, unless the pyridoxine is given with isoniazid to prevent such problems.

Few toxic effects have been observed, except in women taking pyridoxine supplements for premenstrual tension.

RECOMMENDED REQUIREMENTS

Cereals, meat, fruit, and leafy and other vegetables contain vitamin B_6 in the range of 0.1–0.3 mg/ 100 g, whereas liver contains 0.5 mg/100 g.

The total body pool of vitamin B_6 is in the order of 40–250 mg, with a half-life of 33 days. This would imply a daily intake of 0.6–3.78 mg. Deficiency develops more rapidly on high protein intakes, around 80–160 g/day, than on protein intakes of 30–50 g/day.

For adults, both men and women, the RNI is 15 µg/g dietary protein. The LRNI and EAR are 11 and 13 µg/g protein, respectively. EARs for infants vary from 6 µg/g protein at less than 3 months to 13 µg/g protein at 7–10 years. There is no evidence of an increased requirement during pregnancy or in the elderly.

BODY STORE REQUIREMENTS

Biochemical markers include plasma pyridoxal phosphate concentrations, red cell transaminase activation and urinary excretion of B_6 degradation products. No single marker is sensitive at all levels of dietary intake. The plasma pyridoxal phosphate concentration and the erythrocyte transaminase activation coefficient both have drawbacks. Two metabolic loading tests are used to measure vitamin B_6 status. In the tryptophan load test the potentially rate-limiting enzyme kynureninase is sensitive to vitamin B_6 depletion. The excretion of kynurenic and xanthurenic acid is measured before and after the loading dose of tryptophan. Another test is the methionine load test.

KEY POINTS

1. Vitamin B_6 is found in several forms: pyridoxal, pyridoxamine and pyridoxine, as the free form in plants and the phosphorylated form, pyridoxamine phosphate, in animal tissues.
2. Pyridoxal-5′-phosphate is a coenzyme with a major role in the intermediary metabolism of amino acids, in α-decarboxylation, aldolisation,

transamination reactions and the β-carboxylation of aspartic acid.
3. The aldehyde group of pyridoxal-5′-phosphate forms a Schiff base with the α-amino acid group of amino acids. Pyridoxal-5′-phosphate catalyses several different types of bond cleavage by stabilising the electron pairs at the α- or β-carbon atoms of α-amino acids.
4. Dietary pyridoxine deficiency has not been demonstrated in humans.

FURTHER READING

Powers, H.J. (1999) Current knowledge concerning optimum nutritional status of riboflavin, niacin and pyridoxine. *Proceedings of the Nutrition Society*, **58**, 435–40.

CARNITINE

INTRODUCTION

L-Carnitine [(β-hydroxy-)-γ-N-trimethylaminobutyrate], molecular weight 161 Da (Figure 16.15) is a natural constituent of the flesh of higher animals.

Acylcarnitine is found in a variety of food sources, but primarily those of animal origin. Red meat and dairy products are particularly rich sources.

AVAILABILITY OF CARNITINE

Carnitine is not an essential nutrient in the diet of adult humans. The amino acid can be synthesised in tissues, but it is not known whether synthesis is sufficient for requirements. Individuals consuming cereal-based diets, low in carnitine, can maintain similar plasma carnitine concentrations to those of populations where dietary carnitine is readily available.

Carnitine is derived from lysine, a limiting amino acid in diets, and methionine. *S*-adenosylmethionine

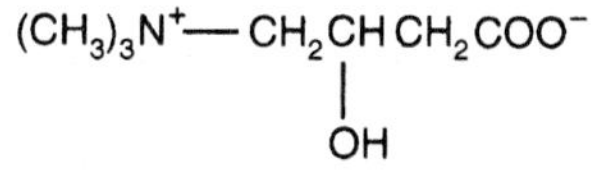

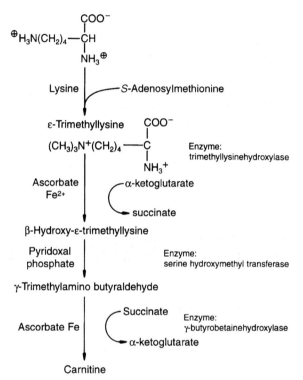

$$(CH_3)_3N^+\!\!-\!CH_2CHCH_2COO^-$$
$$|$$
$$OH$$

Fig. 16.15 Structure of carnitine.

Fig. 16.16 Carnitine synthesis from lysine. The reactions involved require ascorbate, iron, pyridoxal phosphate and S-adenosylmethionine.

provides the methyl groups for enzymatic trimethylation of peptide-linked lysine (Figure 16.16). Proteins that contain ε-N-trimethyllysine residues include histones, cytochrome C, myosin and calmodulin. An important enzyme in the synthesis of lysine to carnitine is γ-butyrobetaine hydroxylase, present in human liver, kidney and brain, but not in skeletal muscle or heart. The activity of this enzyme is dependent on age; the hepatic enzyme activity reaches adult values by the age of 15 years.

Skeletal muscle contains over 90% of total body carnitine in humans. Normal carnitine muscle levels range from 11 to 52 nmol/mg non-collagen protein, the concentration being approximately 70-fold greater than in plasma. The turnover time for carnitine in skeletal muscle and heart is approximately 8 days, in other tissues, primarily liver and kidney, 12 h, in extracellular fluid 1 h, and in the whole body 66 days. Carnitine is conserved in the human by renal reabsorption.

Glucose is a major metabolic fuel for the foetus. At birth the infant adapts to lipid as a major source of calories, when there is a rapid increase in blood free fatty acids and β-hydroxybutyrate concentrations, due to the release of free fatty acids from adipose tissue. Fatty acids become the preferred fuel for heart and skeletal muscle and so carnitine becomes an important cofactor for energy production in the neonate.

Human milk contains 28–95 nmol/ml of carnitine. Milk-based formulae also contain carnitine, although artificial formula milks manufactured from soya bean protein or casein contain little or no carnitine, with consequently reduced plasma carnitine concentration.

The rate of carnitine biosynthesis in infants may be limited by relatively reduced hepatic γ-butyrobetaine hydroxylase activity. Low plasma and tissue concentrations of carnitine may affect lipid utilisation by the infant, e.g. during parenteral nutrition and the use of infused triglycerides. Experimental studies do not show a relationship between carnitine levels and the ability to handle triglycerides by the infant.

ACTION OF CARNITINE

Carnitine plays a role in the transport of long-chain fatty acids into the mitochondrial matrix. Fatty acid acyl-CoAs are unable to cross the inner membranes of mitochondria, until they are converted into the acylcarnitine derivative (Figure 16.17). The enzymes involved are carnitine acyltransferases, each enzyme with a specific fatty acid chain length. Within the mitochondria the reaction is reversed by carnitine acyltransferase II with the restoration of the fatty acid CoA. Several mitochondrial reactions result in CoA esters of short- and medium-chain organic acids. These esters may be further metabolised to regenerate free CoA. During stress, when there is an excess production of these esters, the organic acid may be *trans*-ester-

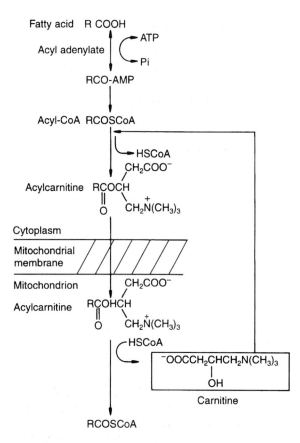

Fig. 16.17 Coenzyme A and its derivatives are unable to pass across the mitochondrial inner membrane. Acyl groups bonded to coenzyme A cross the inner membrane combined with carnitine. Acyl carnitine is exchanged at either side for acetyl-CoA.

ified to carnitine, releasing reduced CoA for involvement in other mitochondrial pathways, e.g. the tricarboxylic acid cycle. Carnitine is a mitochondrial buffer for excess organic acids; although this role is normally minor, but may become important during abnormal conditions.

Renal excretion of carnitine esters may be a mechanism for removing excess short- or medium-chain organic acids. Hyperthyroidism markedly increases urinary carnitine excretion, whereas hypothyroidism decreases urinary loss of carnitine. Prolonged fasting in normal subjects decreases renal excretion of free carnitine, but there is increased excretion of acylcarnitine esters.

CARNITINE DEFICIENCY

Carnitine deficiency syndromes in humans result from inborn errors of metabolism. Clinical symptoms of carnitine deficiency in infants are rarely seen.

Primary genetic carnitine deficiency

There are two clinical types: systemic and myopathic. Primary muscle carnitine deficiency is characterised by mild to severe muscle weakness and various excesses of lipids in skeletal muscle fibres due to defective transport of carnitine into muscle. Other symptoms are: metabolic encephalopathy, hypoglycaemia, hypoprothrombinaemia, hyperammonaemia and lipid excess in liver cells. This resembles Reye's syndrome.

Carnitine deficiency can also be associated with organic aciduria, e.g. in long- and medium-chain acyl-CoA dehydrogenase deficiency, isovaleric acidaemia, glutaric aciduria, propionic and methylmalonic acidaemia and short-chain acyl-CoA dehydrogenase deficiency.

Carnitine deficiency has been reported in ageing, diabetes and chronic heart failure.

KEY POINTS

1. L-Carnitine [(β-hydroxy-)-γ-N-trimethylaminobutyrate] is a natural constituent of higher animals.
2. Carnitine is derived from lysine, which is a limiting amino acid in diets. The precursors of carnitine are lysine and methionine. S-Adenosylmethionine provides the methyl groups for enzymatic trimethylation of peptide-linked lysine.
3. Carnitine plays a role in the transport of long-chain fatty acids into the mitochondrial matrix. Fatty acid acyl-CoAs only cross the inner membranes of mitochondria after they have been converted into the acyl carnitine derivative. The enzymes involved are carnitine acyltransferases.
4. Carnitine deficiency syndromes in humans result from inborn errors of metabolism. Clini-

cal symptoms of dietary carnitine deficiency in infants are rarely seen.

THINKING POINT

Carnitine is not an essential nutrient, but may be regarded as a 'conditionally indispensable, or even 'conditionally dispensable' contributor to nutrition.

NEED TO UNDERSTAND

The dietary sources of carnitine and the limited but very important role that carnitine plays in the transport of fatty acids across membranes.

FURTHER READING

Kerner, J. and Hoppel, C. (1998) Genetic disorders of carnitine metabolism and their nutritional management. *Annual Review of Nutrition*, **18**, 179–206.

Rebouche, C.J. and Seim, H. (1998) Carnitine metabolism and its regulation in microorganisms and mammals. *Annual Review of Nutrition*, **18**, 39–61.

INOSITOL (*myo*-inositol)

INTRODUCTION

Myo-inositol (Figure 16.18), molecular weight 180 Da, is found in the diet in the free form, as inositol containing phospholipid and as phytic acid

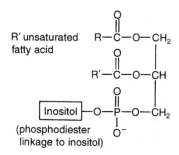

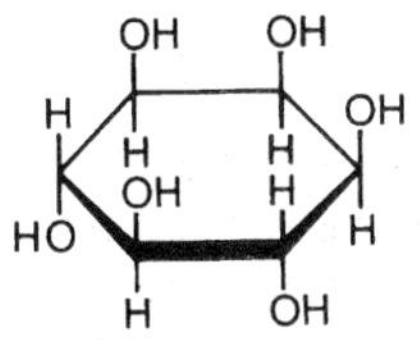

Fig. 16.18   Structure of (*myo*-)inositol.

Phosphoinositides

Phosphatidylinositol

R' unsaturated fatty acid

Inositol

(phosphodiester linkage to inositol)

Fig. 16.19   Structure of phosphoinositides and 1,4,5-phosphatidylinositol.

(inositol hexaphosphate). The cyclitols include the inositols, of which there are nine possible isomers of hexahydroxycyclohexane.

Inositol is found throughout the animal and plant kingdom. In a mixed North American diet an adult eats approximately 1 g of inositol each day from plant foodstuffs in the form of phytic acid. Inositol hexaphosphate, found in cereals, is an important contributor to the total dietary phosphorus intake. Inositol is also present in animal products such as fish, poultry, meat and dairy products in the form of free and inositol-containing phospholipids (phosphatidylinositol) (Figure 16.19). The concentration of *myo*-inositol in cow's milk is 170–440 μmol/l.

ACTION OF INOSITOL

Glucose-6-phosphate can be converted into inositol-1-phosphate (enzyme inositol 1-phosphate synthase), followed by dephosphorylation (enzyme inositol-1-phosphatase). Inositol can be incorporated into phosphoinositides. The *de novo* synthesis involves the reaction of inositol with the

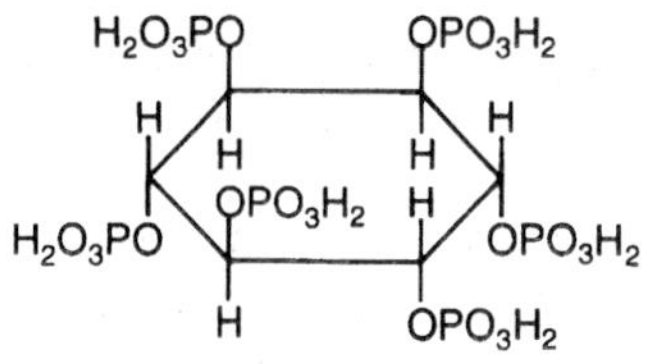

Fig. 16.20   Phytic acid (inositol hexaphosphate).

liponucleotide CDP-diacylglycerol (enzyme CDP-diacylglycerol:inositol phosphatidyltransferase), a microsomal enzyme. Free inositol can react with endogenous phospholipid to become phospho-inositide, by a microsomal manganese-stimulated exchange reaction.

The fatty acid composition and distribution in inositols is unusual in being rich in stearic and arachidonic acids. Stearate is found in the sn-1-position and arachidonate in the sn-2-position of the sn-glycerol backbone of the phosphoinositides. Phosphatidylinositol synthesis takes place in the endoplasmic reticulum of cells. Phosphatidylinositol exchange proteins are found in the cytoplasm of several tissues. Phosphatidylinositol is the precursor for the intracellular inositol lipids. The inositol head group has five free hydroxyl groups which are phosphorylated in different combinations. They are found in membranes and are substrates for kinases and lipases. They function on many aspects of cell biology, including vesicle trafficking, growth, DNA synthesis, regulation of apoptosis and cytoskeletal changes.

Myo-inositol is an essential growth factor for many cells and is important in promoting growth in children. Inositol acts as a lipotropic factor (see section on Lipotropes). The type of dietary triglyceride may influence the function of dietary inositol as a lipotrope, which is not simply related to the degree of saturation of the fat. Membrane phosphatidylinositol can regulate enzyme activity and transport processes, while providing a source of free arachidonic acid for the synthesis of eicosanoids.

Myo-inositol functions in the cell in membrane phosphoinositides, by stimulating the release of the second messengers 1,2-diacylglycerol and inositol triphosphate in stimulated cells.

Phytic acid (inositol hexaphosphate) (Figure 16.20) is found in plant foodstuffs and is hydrolysed

in the gut by an enteric enzyme phytase. This releases free inositol, orthophosphate and intermediate products, including the mono-, di-, tri-, tetra- and pentaphosphate esters of inositol. Dietary phytic acid can reduce the bioavailability and utilisation of both calcium and zinc by binding these metals and preventing their enteric absorption. Calcium phytate is excreted in the faeces, with the loss of both phytate and calcium. Inositol crosses the small intestinal brush border membrane by active transport against a concentration gradient, which is Na^+ and energy dependent and independent of the D-glucose pathway. It is possible that dietary polyphosphoinositides are hydrolysed by a pancreatic phospholipase A in the intestinal lumen. The product can be reacylated through acyltransferase activity upon entering the intestinal cell or further hydrolysed with the release of glycerylphosphorylinositol.

AVAILABILITY OF INOSITOL

The plasma concentration of free inositol in normal human subjects is approximately 30 μmol/l. The human reproductive tract is particularly rich in free inositol. Unbound inositol concentrations in the brain, cerebrospinal fluid and choroid plexus are also higher than in plasma. The concentration of inositol is about 0.6 μmol/l at 3–7 months' lactation in human breast milk. There is also a disaccharide form of inositol, 6-β-galactinol, in human breast milk, approximately 17% of the total non-lipid inositol at the 18th day of lactation.

In tissues and cells inositol occurs in the free form, bound covalently to phospholipid as phosphatidylinositol. Lower concentrations of the polyphosphoinositides (phosphatidyl-4-phosphate and phosphatidyl-4,5-biphosphate) are found.

KEY POINTS

1. *Myo*-inositol is found in the diet in the free form, as inositol-containing phospholipid and as phytic acid (inositol hexaphosphate). The cyclitols include the inositols, of which there are nine possible isomers of hexahydroxycyclohexane.

2. *Myo*-inositol functions in the cell in membrane phosphoinositides by stimulating the release of the second messengers 1,2-diacylglycerol and inositol triphosphate in stimulated cells.

THINKING POINT

Inositol is not an essential nutrient, but may be regarded as a 'conditionally indispensable' or 'conditionally dispensable' contributor to nutrition.

NEED TO UNDERSTAND

Inositol in its varied, active forms can function either as a messenger relay system or by reducing absorption in the intestine.

FURTHER READING

Holub, B.J. (1986) Metabolism and function of *myo*-inositol and inositol phospholipids. *Annual Review of Nutrition*, **6**, 563–97.

Rhee, S.G. (2001) Regulation of phosphoinostide-specific phospholipase C. *Annual Review of Biochemistry*, **70**, 281–312.

Vanhaesebroeck, B., Leevers, S.J., Khatereh, A. *et al.* (2001) Synthesis and function of 3-phosphorylated inositol lipids. *Annual Review of Biochemistry*, **70**, 535–602.

LIPOTROPES

INTRODUCTION

The lipotropes include choline, methionine, vitamin B_{12} and folic acid. Choline and folic acid are found in both animal and plant foods. Animal products and microorganisms are the sole dietary sources of methionine and vitamin B_{12}.

ACTION OF LIPOTROPES

The lipotropes are a group of biologically active compounds with a major role in cellular metabolism. They are essential to the synthesis and methylation of DNA, the metabolism of lipids and the maintenance of tissue integrity. The lipotropes interact with each other and with other nutrients (Figures 16.21 and 16.22). Folate, vitamin B_{12} and methionine are important in the transfer of one-carbon units (Figures 16.23–16.25). Methyl groups are involved in:

- purine ring formation
- pyrimidine biosynthesis
- amino acid interconversions
- formate metabolism.

Vitamin B_{12} and folate are essential for the growth and proliferation of mammalian cells. Rapid availability of nucleotide precursors is important to the lymphatic system, which depends on proliferation and cell division in response to a foreign stimulus. Folate and B_{12} deficiency, leads to a defect in thymidylate synthesis and hence DNA synthesis. Vitamin B_{12} is involved in the isomerisation of methylmalonate to succinate, which is a link between carbohydrate and lipid metabolism.

The methylation of homocysteine to methionine is the metabolic link between vitamin B_{12}, folate and methionine metabolism. The enzyme transmethylase, which requires vitamin B_{12}, is necessary for the conversion of homocysteine to methionine. By this process tetrahydrofolate (THF) is regenerated. Since methionine is available from other sources, i.e. the diet and amino acid pool, the rate-limiting step is a regeneration of THF. Folic coenzymes carrying single-carbon units in different states of reduction are involved in reactions in which methyl groups are transferred. Cellular DNA synthesis depends on the availability of the four nucleotide precursors. While thymidylate can be formed directly from thymidine, most cells convert deoxyuridine monophosphate to thymidine monophosphate, utilising the enzyme thymidylate synthetase. This is the rate-limiting step in DNA synthesis and requires 5,10-methylene-THF (Figure 16.26) as a cofactor. The cofactor is reduced to dihydrofolate, which can be further reduced

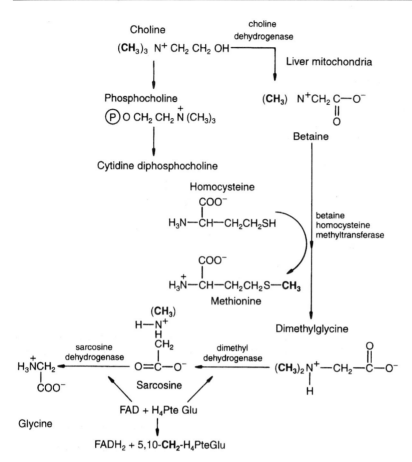

Fig. 16.21 Metabolism of dietary choline. Synthesis to cytidine diphosphocholine or, alternatively, to betaine, dimethyl glycine, sarcosine and glycine. Choline acts as a methyl donor in the biosynthesis of methionine and in the generation of 5,10-CH_2-H_4-Pte Glu.

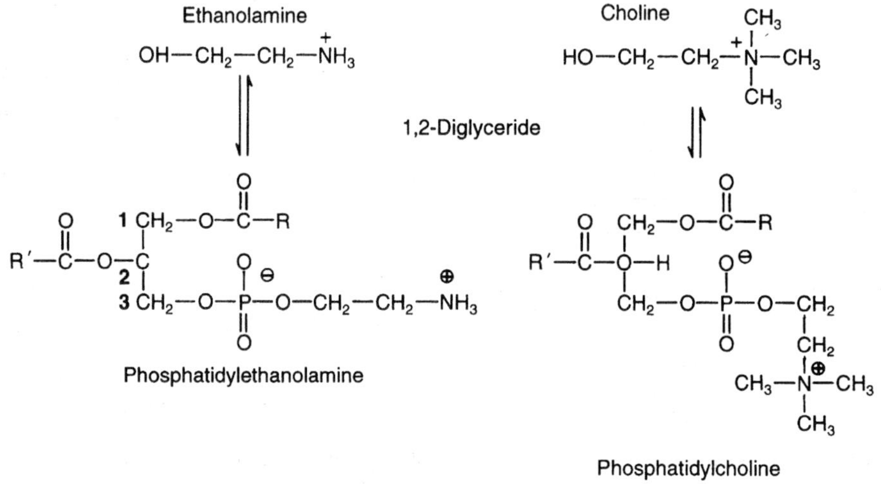

Fig. 16.22 Ethanolamine and choline are synthesised into phospholipids, namely phosphatidylethanolamine and phosphatidylcholine. R: fatty acid; R': usually unsaturated fatty acid.

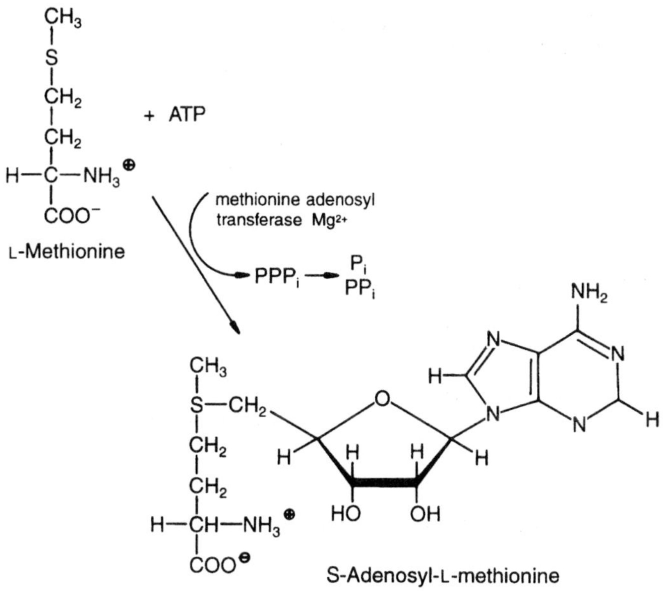

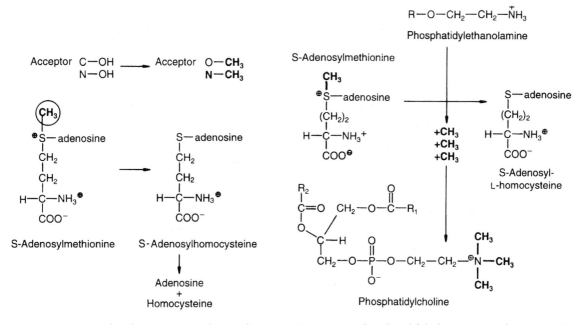

Fig. 16.23 Methionine is a methyl donor (e.g. to amines or alcohols) in the form of *S*-adenosyl-L-methionine, a reaction catalysed by methionine adenosyl transferase. *S*-Adenosyl-L-methionine is the form in which methionine is activated for methylation reactions.

Fig. 16.24 *S*-Adenosylmethione is a contributor of CH_3 to acceptor groups containing N or O. The *S*-adenosyl-methionine loses the CH_3 group to form *S*-adenosylho-mocysteine and adenosine and homocysteine.

Fig. 16.25 Phosphatidylcholine is a ready source of methylating groups and is synthesised from phos-phatidylethanolamine with three CH_3 groups (donated by *S*-adenosylmethionine) available for transfer.

through dihydrofolate reductase to THF. Alternatively, THF may be regenerated through the B_{12}-dependent methyl transferase reactions in which the methyl group is transferred from 5-methyl-THF in the synthesis of methionine. The folate-derived methyl groups go through successive stages of reduction and in so doing are converted to 5,10-methylene-THF, a cofactor for thymidylate synthetase (Figure 16.27), or may be further, irreversibly reduced to 5-methyl-THF. This folate coenzyme must be converted to THF for the methyl group to re-enter the methyl pool. In vitamin B_{12} deficiency this cannot take place and 5-methyl-THF accumulates. Patients with vitamin B12 deficiency show an increase in excretion of formiminoglutamic acid, formate and 4(5)-amino-5(4)imidazole-carboxamide. These require folate cofactors for further conversion and are restored by dietary methionine. Methionine is an essential amino acid which also serves as a methyl donor.

There is a liver enzyme for the direct methylation of homocysteine through betaine, but most cells use the vitamin B_{12}, 5-methyl-THF-dependent methyl transferase reaction to synthesise methionine. This can then be further converted to S-adenosylmethionine, an inhibitor of the 5-methyl-THF:homocysteine transmethylase reaction and of 5,10-methylene THF reductase, which reduces the amount of 5-methyl-THF formed and increases the availability of the folate cofactors. Methionine is also involved in the conversion of formate into carbon dioxide.

AVAILABILITY OF LIPOTROPES

The lipotropic nutrients methionine, choline, folic acid and vitamin B_{12} are stored in the body and turn over at different and specific rates. Vitamin B_{12} has the largest store relative to its daily requirements. Methionine is stored in tissue proteins which constantly turn over as a tRNA derivative and in an active form, S-adenosylmethionine, essential to transmethylation. Folic acid and choline stores are quite small.

Choline is stored as choline phospholipids, which are widely distributed in tissues. Phospholipids are important components of the membrane in two respects:

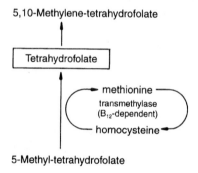

Fig. 16.26 The conversion of 5-methyl-tetrahydrofolate to tetrahydrofolate is a critical step in one-carbon metabolism. This is a transmethylase reaction in which methionine is regenerated from homocysteine; the transmethylase enzyme is vitamin B_{12} dependent. In this reaction methionine, folic acid, vitamin B_{12} and (indirectly) choline interreact.

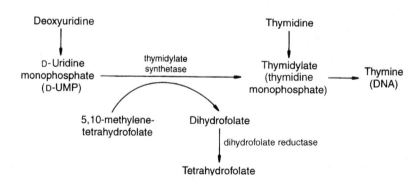

Fig. 16.27 5,10-Methylene-tetrahydrofolate is important in the methylation of D-uridine monophosphate (D-UMP) to thymidine monophosphate, which is a rate-limiting step in DNA synthesis.

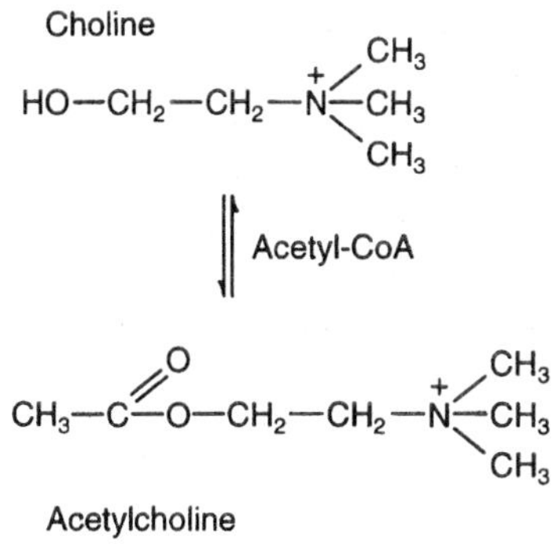

Fig. 16.28 Choline is a contributor to the synthesis of the neurotransmitter acetylcholine.

- as amphipathic compounds with both polar and non-polar groupings, making a membrane with varied charges. The cell membranes are the site of enzyme activity, e.g. for lipid synthesis
- as a source of important precursors of biologically active substance, e.g. arachidonic acid and eicosanoids, and choline and acetylcholine (Figure 16.28).

Phosphatidylcholine and phosphatidylethanolamine are important phospholipids. Their biosynthesis begins with dietary choline entering the cell. Choline is phosphorylated to phosphocholine by choline kinase. Phosphocholine and cytidine-5′-phosphate (CMP) form CDP-choline (enzyme CTP:phosphocholine cytidyltransferase), a rate-limiting enzyme. This enzyme is inactive in the cytosol and activated on the endoplasmic reticulum by phospholipids. The CDP-choline reacts with diacylglycerol, the enzyme involved being attached to the endoplasmic reticulum. Phosphatidylethanolamine is synthesised from ethanolamine in a similar series of reactions to phosphatidylcholine. In the lung the phosphatidylcholine is dipalmitoylphosphatidylcholine (palmitic acid in sn-1 and sn-2 positions) and acts as the lung surfactant.

KEY POINTS

1. The lipotropes include choline, methionine, vitamin B_{12} and folic acid.
2. These are a group of biologically active compounds with a major role in cellular metabolism.

They are essential to the synthesis and methylation of DNA, the metabolism of lipids and the maintenance of tissue integrity. The lipotropes interact with each other and with other nutrients. Folate, vitamin B_{12} and methionine are important in the transfer of one-carbon units as methyl groups.

3. The methylation of homocysteine to methionine is the metabolic link between vitamin B_{12}, folate and methionine metabolism. The enzyme transmethylase, containing vitamin B_{12}, is required for the conversion of homocysteine to methionine. By this process tetrahydrofolate (THF) is regenerated.

THINKING POINTS

1. The lipotropes are one of the great interconnecting systems in human biology.
2. Here the body has peculiar dependence on dietary constituents.

NEED TO UNDERSTAND

The chemistry of the interrelationship between vitamin B_{12}, folate and methionine, and their metabolism.

FURTHER READING

Eskes, T.K. (1998) Open or closed? A world of difference: a history of homocysteine research. *Nutrition Reviews*, **56**, 236–44.

Finkelstein, J.D. (2000) Homocysteine: a history in progress. *Nutrition Reviews*, **58**, 193–204.

McKinley, M.C. (2000) Nutritional aspects and possible pathological mechanisms of hypercysteinaemia: an independent risk factor for vascular disease. *Proceedings of the Nutritional Society*, **59**, 221–37.

Newberne, P.M. and Rogers, A.E. (1986) Labile methyl groups and promotion of cancer. *Annual Review of Nutrition*, **6**, 407–32.

Selhub, J. (1999) Homocysteine metabolism. *Annual Review of Nutrition*, **19**, 217–46.

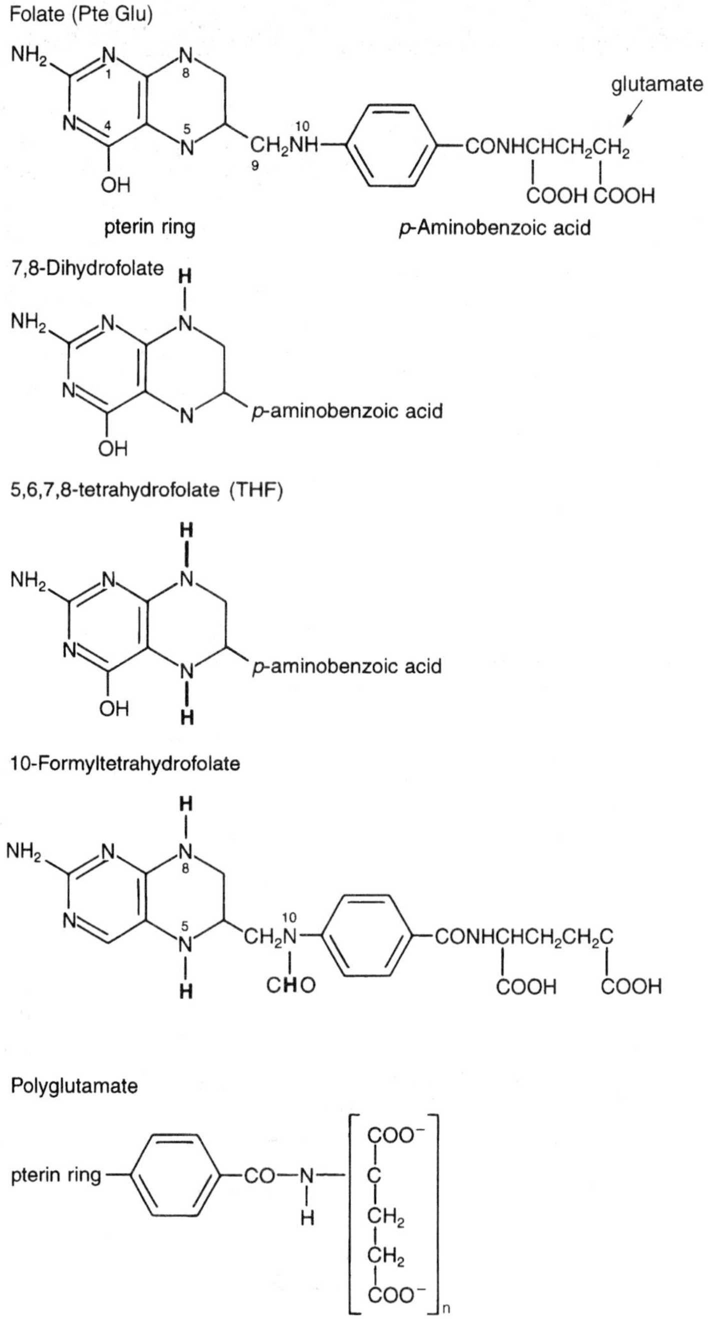

Fig. 16.29 Structure of folate: 7,8-dihydrofolate, 5,6,7,8-tetrahydrofolate (THF), 10-formyltetrahydrofolate and polyglutamate.

FOLIC ACID

INTRODUCTION

Folates, which are derivatives of folic acid, are found in many forms throughout nature. Folic acid, molecular weight 441 Da (pteroylglutamic acid), consists of a pterin ring (2-amino, 4-hydroxypteridine) attached to a *p*-aminobenzoic acid conjugated to L-glutamic acid (PteGlu). The compound is stable in acid solutions, sparingly soluble in water, but unstable in neutral or alkaline media. Variations on folic acid (Figure 16.29) include:

- di- and tetrahydro forms of the pteridine ring
- a single-carbon substitution (methyl –CH₃, formyl –CHOH, methenyl =CH–, methylene = CH₂ or formimino –CHNH) at N5 or N10)
- a chain of glutamates attached to the L-glutamate (in humans the number varies between four and six).

In human tissues and fluids, folic acid is found principally as monoglutamate derivatives, the majority as 5-methyltetrahydrofolate (methyl-THF) and some as 10-formyltetrahydrofolate (10-THF).

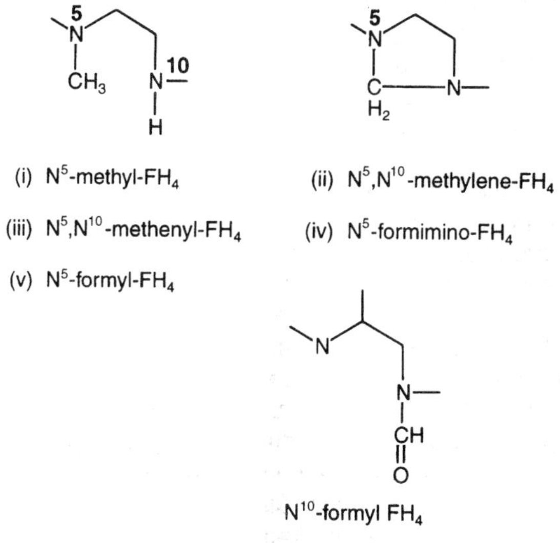

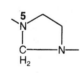

(i) N⁵-methyl-FH₄

(ii) N⁵,N¹⁰-methylene-FH₄

(iii) N⁵,N¹⁰-methenyl-FH₄

(iv) N⁵-formimino-FH₄

(v) N⁵-formyl-FH₄

N¹⁰-formyl FH₄

Fig. 16.30 Tetrahydrofolate (THF; FH₄) is an important source of one-carbon units; N-5 or N-10.

Important sources of folate include liver, yeast extract and green leafy vegetables. Folic acid is found in diets that contain other B vitamins.

ACTION OF FOLIC ACID

Folic acid undergoes a number of metabolic changes involving the transfer of one-carbon groups on the N-5 or N-10 position to other compounds (Figure 16.30) Of these, the most important folic acid one-carbon derivatives (tetrahydrofolate, THF) are 5-methyl-THF, 5,10-methylene-THF, 5,10-methenyl-THF, 5-formyl-THF and 10-formyl-THF, and 5-formimino-THF.

The folic polyglutamates may be the active coenzyme within the cell metabolic system. The reactions in which folic acid is involved include amino acid interconversions and DNA synthesis. In some reactions concerned with purine and pyrimidine synthesis, folate is oxidised to the dihydro form. The enzyme dihydrofolate reductase reduces dihydrofolate to the tetrahydo form. In the role of folic acid as a coenzyme, there is some irreversible splitting of the C9–10 bond, particularly during increased DNA turnover, which results in extra requirements for dietary folic acid.

Amino acid interconversions

- Serine → glycine: requires the transfer of a formaldehyde group from serine to the tetrafolate cofactor (enzyme serine hydroxymethyltransferase). This reaction is particularly important in the dividing cell.
- Homocysteine → methionine (enzyme 5-methyl-THF methyltransferase): also involves vitamin B₁₂ (Figure 16.31).

DNA synthesis

- purine nucleotide synthesis (5,10-formyl-THF and 10-formyl-THF), e.g. glycinamide ribotide → formyl glycinamide ribotide (enzyme glycinamide ribotide transformylase) (Figure 16.32)
- pyrimidine nucleotide synthesis (5,10-methylene-THF as coenzyme), e.g. deoxyuridine monophos-

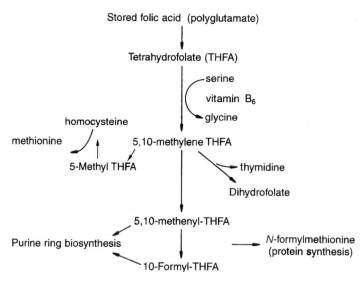

Fig. 16.31 Folic acid is available as tetrahydrofolate in reactions including homocysteine, thymidine, purine ring biosynthesis and protein synthesis.

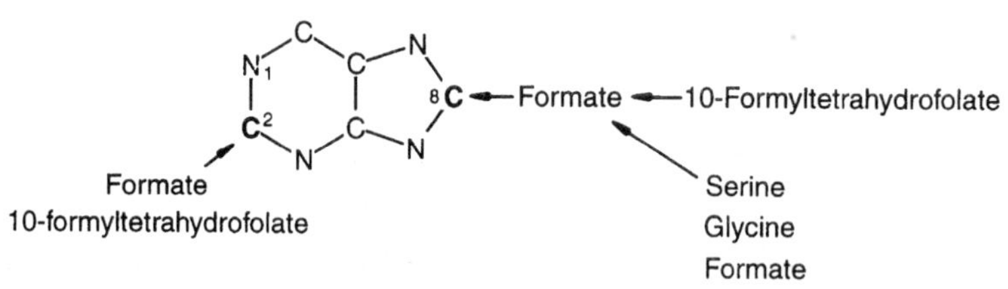

Fig. 16.32 Tetrahydropteroyl glutamate (10-formyl-H_4 Pte Glu) supplies the carbon-2 and carbon-8 in purine synthesis.

phate → thymidine monophosphate (enzyme thymidylate synthetase)
• methylation of transfer RNA.

The folates provide methyl groups for many methyltransferase reactions. This is achieved by the conversion of 5,10-methylene-THF to 5-methyl-THF, which in turn methylates homocysteine to methionine by the vitamin B_{12}-dependent enzyme methionine synthase.

Folate polyglutamates are the main intracellular forms of folic acid. Folate polyglutamates do not cross or are poorly transported across cell membranes. Therefore, the metabolism of pterolymonoglutamates to polyglutamate allows cells to concentrate folates.

AVAILABILITY OF FOLIC ACID

Most of the folate eaten in food is in the polyglutamyl form. Dietary forms of folate are typically conjugated, so that digestion to the monoglutamyl form is necessary for membrane uptake in the intestinal epithelium (Figure 16.33). Gastric and duodenal juice contents do not appear to hydrolyse the γ-glutamyl peptide chain. Absorption is most efficient in the proximal duodenum. Polyglutamates are deconjugated to the monoglutamate in the lumen, the brush border and the lysozymes of the intestinal cells by folate conjugases, γ-L-glutamyl carboxypeptidases. Each location has a

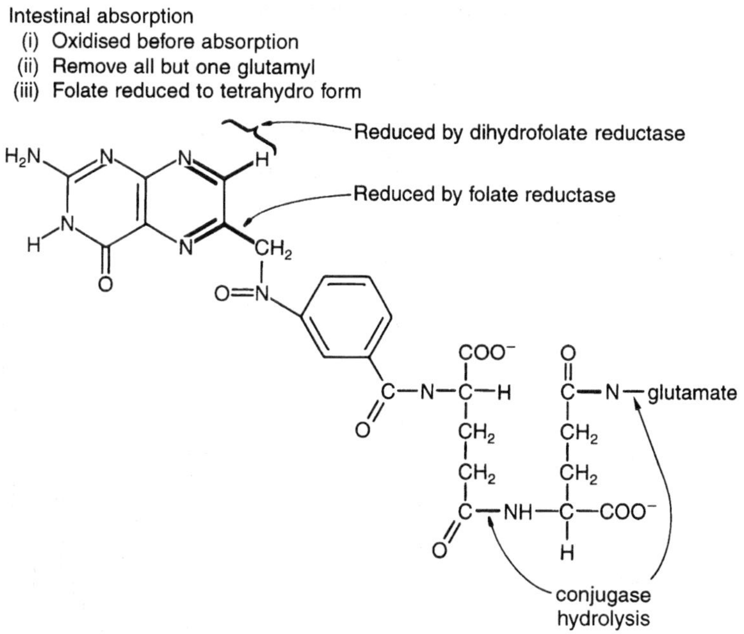

Intestinal absorption
(i) Oxidised before absorption
(ii) Remove all but one glutamyl
(iii) Folate reduced to tetrahydro form

Fig. 16.33 Dietary folate and the bonds susceptible to enzymatic cleavage.

distinct folate conjugase activity. The brush border enzyme, the most important, has an optimum pH of 6.5–7.0, is an exopeptidase and requires Zn^{2+}. This enzyme may be inhibited by alcohol, which may be important in the folic acid deficiencies that may accrue from alcohol abuse. The drug sala-zopyrine, used in the treatment of ulcerative coli-tis, may have a similar effect. The intracellular lysosomal hydrolase has a pH optimum of 4.5, is an endopeptidase and has no metal requirements.

Monoglutamyl folate is primarily absorbed by a carrier-mediated system, although there may be an element of passive absorption. Folate uptake can occur by saturable and non-saturable mechanisms. The polyglutamate being absorbed is reduced to the tetrahydro state and methylated at N_5. Methyl THF enters the portal vein for transport to the liver. Folate bound to a high-affinity folate binding protein in milk is absorbed from the ileum. This may be important in the suckling infant.

Half of the body store of folic acid is stored in the liver at a concentration of approximately 5–15 µg/g. Most cellular folate is bound to protein divided between the cell mitochondria and the cytoplasm, with minor amounts in the nucleus.

Folate is transported into the cell by three mech-anisms:

- folate binding proteins/folate receptors, which act in one direction into the cell and and utilise endocytosis
- reduced folate carriers, mobile carrier-mediated folate transport system
- passive diffusion.

The folate is transported as a single glutamate, cannot function as a cofactor and readily passes from the cell. The folylpolyglutamates are the active coenzyme forms and are held in the cell. Otherwise, the monoglutamates are removed by transport systems. There are several pools of folate, turning over at differing rates, varying from hours to days. The folate is either removed from the cell as the monoglutamate or degraded to active degradation products. The iron storage protein heavy-chain fer-ritin can catabolise folate and decrease intracellu-lar folate concentrations.

Conditions that increase folate utilisation include pregnancy and neonatal growth, oral contracep-tive use, anticonvulsant therapy, alcoholism and cancer.

FOLIC ACID DEFICIENCY

Folic acid deficiency may arise for a number of reasons:

- as a dietary defect
- from malabsorption, as in coeliac disease
- owing to excess demands, as in increased cell proliferation, e.g. in leukaemia
- owing to interference with folic acid metabolism by drugs: anticonvulsants used in the treatment of epilepsy and salazopyrine used in the treatment of colitis
- in inborn errors of folic acid metabolism (extremely rare).

Folic acid deficiency is an important cause of megaloblastic anaemia. This anaemia develops because of inhibition of DNA synthesis. The functional relationship between folic acid and vitamin B_{12} is in the tetrahydropteroylglutamate methyltransferase reaction determining intracellular folate. A cellular deficiency develops and the synthesis of purines and pyrimidines is reduced. Red cell formation is also reduced in the bone marrow and a megaloblastic anaemia results (see Lipotropes).

Pregnancy

Neural tube defects (NTDs) is a collective term for congenital deformities of the spinal cord and brain. NTDs include spina bifida (50% of cases), anencephalus (40%), encephalocoele and iniencephaly. NTDs have different prevalence rates in different populations. Folic acid deficiency has long been regarded as a cause of NTDs. It is believed that a genetic predisposition may be aggravated by environmental factors, the prevalence rising with increasing parity. Prevalence amongst populations ranges from 1 to 6 per 1000, and is increased 10-fold if there has already been a pregnancy with a baby affected by NTDs.

Epidemics of increased NTD-affected births have been recorded. Inadequate nutrition, infectious diseases, climatic factors, and seasonal usage of chemical fertilisers and pesticides are possible aetiological factors. Seasonal changes in dietary folic acid availability may alter the aetiological significance of folate in NTDs throughout the year. Excessive intake of vitamin A or zinc has frequently been suggested as a possible cause of NTDs. Most studies have also considered vitamin B_{12}, vitamin C and zinc dietary status.

Closure of the neural tube occurs early in pregnancy, before the first antenatal visit. At the first antenatal visit no differences have been noted in blood folic acid concentrations between mothers whose babies are subsequently diagnosed with NTDs and mothers of normal babies. Pregnancy, however, places a demand on folate and may deplete reserves, although this is not reflected in low blood levels early in pregnancy. However, red cell folate concentrations are more significant, those in mothers of affected babies being reduced. The biological basis of the disrupted development is a common dependence on cells that originate in the neural epithelium. The mechanism of the defect may be locally reduced concentrations of folic acid or a disturbance of methionine metabolism. Three groups of genes may be involved: folate-receptor genes, genes that regulate methionine–homocysteine metabolism and N-methyl-D-aspartate receptor genes.

In intervention studies, mothers with a previously affected baby were given an iron and multivitamin preparation with 360 µg of folic acid. The result was impressive, the rate of NTDs being 0.6% compared with 5% in an unsupplemented control group. Other larger studies have demonstrated a protective effect of folic acid containing multivitamins during the first 6 weeks of pregnancy.

RECOMMENDED REQUIREMENTS

Adults

The LRNI has been estimated to be 100 µg/day. Median folate intakes in Britain are 300 (range 145–562) µg/day for men and 209 (range 95–385) µg/day for women. An RNI of 200 µg/day has been set for adults.

Infants and children

Breast milk provides 40 µg/day and formula milk 60–70 µg/l (equivalent to 50–60 µg/day). An RNI of 50 µg/day has been suggested for formula-fed infants.

Pregnancy

The mean intake of additional folic acid required to maintain plasma and red cell folate concentrations above those of non-pregnant women is 100 µg/day. National authorities have recommended that women planning a pregnancy should increase their intake of folic acid from the usual 0.2 mg/day to 0.4 mg by capsule supplement. A dietary supplement would require eight glasses of orange juice, 10 servings of broccoli or three servings of Brussels sprouts.

Lactation

The total excretion of folic acid in breast milk averages 40 µg/day. To replace this from the diet, an intake of 60 µg/day (dietary reference value, DRV) has been suggested.

The elderly

There is little evidence that the elderly require enhanced intakes of folic acid.

BODY STORE MEASUREMENTS

Until recently the most efficient way of measuring folic acid was by microassay methods, but now high-pressure liquid chromatographic (HPLC) measurements are providing more consistent results.

The best assay of folate status is to measure folate concentration in serum and red cells. Red cell folate is a better estimate of long-term status, as it reflects body stores. If the concentration in red cells falls below 100 µg/ml then the individual may be considered to be deficient in folate. Folic acid is susceptible to oxidation and therefore if long-term storage is required suitable antioxidants should be added to the sample. To obtain a complete picture of folate status, serum and red cell folate with serum vitamin B_{12} are important measurements. Radioassay kits have replaced microbiological assays in the measurement of folate. The lower limit of normal serum folic acid is 3 µg/ml.

Urinary folate excretion is less than one-tenth of dietary intake.

KEY POINTS

1. Folates are found in many forms throughout nature. Folic acid (pteroylglutamic acid) is a pterin ring (2-amino,4-hydroxy pteridine) attached to p-aminobenzoic acid conjugated to L-glutamic acid (PteGlu). Variations on folic acid include di- and tetrahydro- forms of the pteridine ring; a single-carbon substitution (methyl –CH_2, formyl –CHOH, methylenyl =CH–, methylene =CH_2 or formimino –CHNH) at N5 or N10, and a chain of four to six glutamates attached to the L-glutamate.
2. The tetra hydrofolates function as cosubstrates for enzymes involved in one-carbon (1-C) metabolism.
3. Dietary folic acid deficiency is a cause of megaloblastic anaemia. Supplementation of dietary folic acid before conception and during pregnancy reduces the incidence of neural tube defects in the foetus.

THINKING POINTS

1. The central role that folic acid plays in DNA and other crucial metabolic paths imposes a curious reliance on a nutrient.
2. Rapidly growing tissue, neuronal in the foetus and red cells in the adult are very much at risk.
3. This also has implications for malignant tissues.

NEED TO UNDERSTAND

The chemistry of folic acid as a one-carbon donor.

FURTHER READING

Antony, A.C. (1996) Folate receptors. *Annual Review of Nutrition*, **16**, 501–21.

Butterworth, C.E. and Bendich, A. (1996) Folic acid and the prevention of birth defects. *Annual Review of Nutrition*, **16**, 73–98.

Chanarin, I. (1990) *The Megaloblastic Anaemias*, 3rd edn. Blackwell Scientific Publications, Oxford.

Gregory, J.F. III and Quinlivan, E.P. (2002) *In vivo* kinetics of folate metabolism. *Annual Review of Nutrition*, **22**, 199–220.

Rosenquist, T.H. and Finnell, R.H. (2001) Genes, folate and homocysteine in embryonic development. *Proceedings of the Nutrition Society*, **60**, 53–61.

Scott, J.M., Kirke, P.N. and Weir, D.G. (1990) The role of nutrition in neural tube defects. *Annual Review of Nutrition*, **10**, 277–95.

Scott, J.M. (1999) Folate and vitamin B_{12}. *Proceedings of the Nutrition Society*, **58**, 441–8.

Shane, B. and Stokstad, E.L.R. (1985) Vitamin B_{12}/folate inter-relationships. *Annual Review of Nutrition*, **5**, 115–41.

Sirotnak, F.M. and Tolner, B. (1999) Carrier-mediated membrane transport of folates in mammalian cells. *Annual Review of Nutrition*, **19**, 91–122.

Smits, L.J.M. and Essed, G.G.M. (2001) Short interpregnancy intervals and unfavourable pregnancy outcome: role of folate depletion. *Lancet*, **358**, 2074–7.

Suh, J.R., Herbig, A.K. and Stover, P.J. (2001) New perspectives on folate catabolism. *Annual Review of Nutrition*, **21**, 255–82.

VITAMIN B_{12}

INTRODUCTION

Vitamin B_{12} contains cobalt and has a molecular weight of approximately 1350 Da. The structure of vitamin B_{12} is complex (Figure 16.34), consisting of four linked pyrrole rings (a corrin) co-ordinating with a cobalt atom at the centre. As the corrin forms the core of the molecule, such a molecule is a corrinoid.

The prefix 'cob' implies the presence of cobalt. The term cobalamin is used for those cobinamides that play a part in human metabolism. The naturally occurring forms of the vitamin B_{12} are methylcobalamin and adenosylcobalamin. These carry a carbon–cobalt bond that is not found anywhere else in nature. The other form of cobalamin found in tissues is hydroxycobalamin, which can be converted to the methyl or adenosyl form, but only when the valency of the cobalt is reduced from 3 to 1. This hydroxy form, which may be the stored form, is the precursor and is readily converted to the coenzyme form. In plasma the predominant form is the methyl cobalamin, and in red cells the adenosyl cobalamin.

Cyanocobalamin is an artefact of the extraction process from the sources and is converted into active forms. This form, which is given therapeutically, is soluble in water, and stable in boiling water at neutral pH, but not in the presence of alkali.

SYNTHESIS OF VITAMIN B_{12}

Vitamin B_{12} is not found in any plant, cobalamin synthesis being confined to microorganisms. Colonic bacteria produce cobalamin, but it is not absorbed from the colon. Yeast is a source of cobalamin that is also found in several forms in animal food, primarily as adenosyl- and hydroxycobalamin, of which one-third and one-half, respectively, is absorbed. Methylcobalamin is found in egg yolk and cheese, and sulfitocobalamin in some foods. Little or no cyanocobalamin occurs in food, except for cow's milk, which contains 3 μg/l.

A vegetarian diet free of eggs, milk and other foods of animal origin leads to the risk of vitamin B_{12} deficiency.

ACTION OF VITAMIN B_{12}

Vitamin B_{12} itself is not active as a coenzyme but has two enzymatically active derivatives, Co-5'-deoxyadenosylcorrinoid and aquacorrinoids (methyl B_{12}). Co-5'-deoxyadenosylcorrinoid accounts for 80% of tissue cell stores, principally in the mitochondria. Only three reactions require vitamin B_{12} (Figure 16.35):

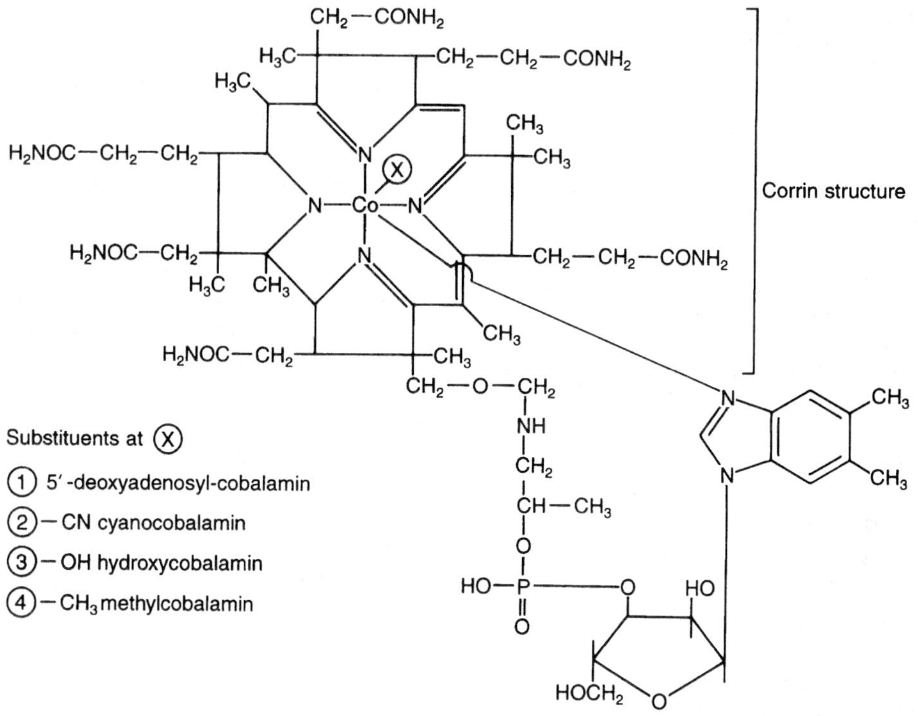

Fig. 16.34 Structure of vitamin B_{12}: 5'-deoxyadenosyl, cyanocobalamin, hydroxycobalamin and methylcobalamin.

- isomerisation of methylmalonyl-CoA to succinyl-CoA (enzyme methylmalonyl-CoA mutase; coenzyme Co-5'-deoxyadenosylcorrinoid)
- isomerisation of α-leucine to β-leucine
- methyltransferase reactions, e.g. homocysteine to methionine.

The enzyme methyltetrahydrofolate homocysteine methyltransferase requires methyl cobalamin to transfer a methyl group from N-5-methyl-THF to homocysteine, which converts homocysteine to methionine. These reactions occur in the cytoplasmic and mitochondrial fractions of mammalian cells.

In nature, vitamin B_{12} is combined with a protein. At the pH of the stomach, cobalamin is separated from the dietary protein–cobalamin complex by acid and pepsin. Vitamin B_{12} forms complexes with haptocorrin at the pH of the stomach. Haptocorrin (formerly known as R-type binder) mediates cobalamin uptake through an asialoglycoprotein receptor. The cobalamin is released from the haptocorrin by pancreatic enzymes and binds to

intrinsic factor. Intrinsic factor is a glycoprotein secreted by the parietal cells of the stomach. Secretion is stimulated by histamine, pentagastrin and cholinergic agents.

The production of intrinsic factor does not follow the same post-prandial time-course as hydrochloric acid, intrinsic factor secretion being completed earlier in the meal. Vitamin B_{12} is absorbed from the ileum as an intrinsic factor complex. There is binding to a mucosal receptor which is specific to the absorption of this complex. The receptor has a molecular weight of 75–80 kDa and requires Ca^{2+} ions. Binding of the complex is very species dependent and the intrinsic factor should preferably be from the same species in order to be absorbed. As ileal receptors are limited in number, absorption rates are low, and both dietary and biliary-excreted vitamin B_{12} are necessary. Absorption from the receptor is probably as the intrinsic factor–cobalamin complex.

Vitamin B_{12} has an important role in the maintenance of myelin in the nervous system. This may be due to a dependence of propionate catabolism

1. Intramolecular group transfers, e.g. methyl malonyl-CoA
   mutase, requires deoxyadenosyl cobalamin:

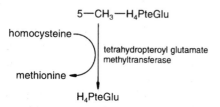

L-Methylmalonyl-CoA   Succinyl-CoA

2. Methyl transferase reactions, e.g. tetrahydropteroyl
   glutamate methyltransferase requires methyl cobalamin:

$$5-CH_3-H_4PteGlu$$

homocysteine

tetrahydropteroyl glutamate
methyltransferase

methionine

$$H_4PteGlu$$

Fig. 16.35 Two enzyme families require vitamin B_{12}: intramolecular group transfers and methyl transferase reactions.

on vitamin B_{12}. The normal sequence for propionyl-CoA reactions is through methylmalonyl-CoA to succinyl-CoA, which is metabolised in the citric acid cycle. Deoxyadenosyl vitamin B_{12} is essential for the last step.

AVAILABILITY OF VITAMIN B_{12}

Cobalamin is carried in the blood by three proteins, transcobalamins I, II and III. Of these, II is the most important and rapidly releases vitamin B_{12} to the tissues. The other two are more lasting binders of the vitamin.

Some 80% of the body storage (2–5 mg) is contained in the liver and the turnover is very slow, at 0.05–0.2% of the body pool per day. The kidneys and pituitary also contain stored cobalamin. There is efficient conservation by the kidneys and the enterohepatic circulation.

The release of protein-bound cobalamin in food may be affected by cooking, the nature of the food binding the cobalamin, and the presence of

gastric, pancreatic or ileal disease or advancing age. In pregnancy, plasma concentrations of cobalamin fall, but absorption rates are increased.

The tapeworm *Diphyllobothrium latum* can infect humans and may grow to a length of 15 m. This worm competes with the host for vitamin B_{12}, with a resultant reduction in the absorption of this vitamin. Similarly, bacteria can modify vitamin B_{12} absorption, as in enteric colonisation which occurs spontaneously in the elderly, or in conjunction with a surgical blind loop or small-bowel diverticula. Some drugs, e.g. *p*-aminosalicylic acid, biguanides, slow-release potassium and colchicine, can also interfere with the absorption of vitamin B_{12}.

Most vitamin B_{12} is excreted in the urine and some in the bile; up to 2 μg daily is excreted in the faeces, although faecal vitamin B_{12} may be of bacterial synthetic origin.

Cobalamin-binding proteins, which are found in amniotic fluid, are synthesised by the human foetus as early as 16–19 weeks of gestation.

VITAMIN B_{12} DEFICIENCY

A deficiency of vitamin B_{12} results in megaloblastic anaemia and neurological disorders, especially in the posterolateral columns of the spinal cord.

Pernicious anaemia is characterised by large red cells in insufficient numbers in the peripheral blood, a failure to produce acid in the stomach, gastritis, and antibodies in the blood to parietal cells and intrinsic factor. Intrinsic factor is not produced or secreted into the stomach, with resultant changes in release of cobalamin from the haptocorrin complex and ileal absorption. Secondary causes include the consequences of gastric surgery, pancreatic insufficiency, Zollinger–Ellison disease and ileal resection. The megaloblastic anaemia is believed to occur due to the loss of methyl availability and the consequent effect on methionine reductase (see Lipotropes).

In vitamin B_{12} deficiency, odd-number carbon (C15 and C17) fatty acids and branched-chain fatty acids accumulate in the nervous tissue. Neurological problems ensue, which are believed to result from a deficiency of mutase activity and the accumulation of methylmalonyl-CoA, which is used in fatty acid synthesis rather than acetyl-CoA, with resulting fatty acid biosynthesis impairment. The abnormal odd-numbered fatty acids incorporated into myelin result in an unstable myelin sheath. S-Adenosylmethionine (SAM)-dependent methyltransferases are involved in the methylation of arginine residues of myelin basic proteins. An inability to regenerate methionine from homocysteine in nerve tissue may lead to an inadequate supply of methionine and SAM, and hence demyelination.

Vitamin B_{12} deficiency can occasionally lead to infertility.

Deficiency in the young

Defects that affect adenosylcobalamin lead to metabolic ketoacidosis in the young, and methylmalonic acidaemia and aciduria. Methylcobalamin deficiencies result in failure to thrive, neurological problems, homocysteinuria and hypomethionaemia. Treatment is with the hydroxylated cobalamin.

VITAMIN B_{12} EXCESS

Vitamin B_{12} has extremely low toxicity and as much as 3 mg/day may be tolerated.

RECOMMENDED REQUIREMENTS

Adults

The average dietary intake requirements appear to be less than 1 μg/day. The LRNI is set at 1 μg/day. The RNI of 1.5 μg/day for adults would meet requirements over a prolonged period, e.g. up to 5 years without any supplementary vitamin B_{12} intake. There is no evidence that elderly subjects have an increased requirement, although the release of protein-bound cobalamin may be affected by age.

Pregnancy and lactation

It is not known whether additional intake is required during pregnancy, but 1.5 μg/day is probably sufficient to cover the needs of a pregnant woman. During lactation an increment of 0.5 μg/day should ensure an adequate supply for breast milk, which contains approximately 0.2–1.0 μg/l vitamin B_{12} when the lactating woman has a diet adequate in vitamin B_{12}.

Infants

In infants the LRNI is 0.1 μg/day.

BODY STORE MEASUREMENTS

Vitamin B_{12} status is estimated from serum concentrations. The relationship between dietary intake and serum concentrations is not linear because the body stores of B_{12} are largely in the liver. Thus, the serum concentration only divides individuals into broad nutritional categories.

The plasma concentration in a healthy person lies between 200 and 960 pg/ml (150–710 pmol/1). A value of under 80 pg/ml (60 pmol/l) indicates vitamin B_{12} deficiency. B_{12} absorption is measured using radioactive cobalt B_{12}, with or without intrinsic factor (Schilling test). An alternative method of measurement is to use a whole-body scanner.

KEY POINTS

1. Vitamin B_{12} is a complex consisting of four linked pyrrole rings (a corrin) co-ordinating with a cobalt atom at the centre.
2. Vitamin B_{12} has two enzymatically active derivatives, Co-5'-deoxyadenosylcorrinoid and aquacorrinoids (methyl B_{12}). Co-5'-deoxyadenosylcorrinoid accounts for 80% of tissue cell stores, principally in the mitochondria.
3. Only three reactions require vitamin B_{12}: (i) isomerisation of methylmalonyl-CoA to succinyl-CoA (enzyme methylmalonyl-CoA mutase; coenzyme Co-5'-deoxyadenosylcorrinoid); (ii) isomerisation of α-leucine to β-leucine; and (iii) methyltransferase reactions (homocysteine to methionine). The enzyme methyltetrahydrofolate homocysteine methyltransferase requires methyl cobalamin in the transfer of a methyl

group from *N*-5-methyl-THF to homocysteine, which converts homocysteine to methionine.

4. A deficiency of vitamin B_{12} results in megaloblastic anaemia and neurological disorders, especially in the posterolateral columns of the spinal cord. Vitamin B_{12} has a role in the synthesis of fatty acids in the myelin of nerve tissue.

THINKING POINT

Vitamin B_{12} is a very unusual vitamin, a cobalt-containing chemical and a large molecule that is absorbed in a most complex manner.

NEED TO UNDERSTAND

The curious mechanism of absorption of vitamin B_{12} and its limited but central role in metabolism.

FURTHER READING

Baik, H.W. and Russell, R.M. (1999) Vitamin B_{12} deficiency in the elderly. *Annual Review of Nutrition*, **19**, 357–77.

Newberne, P.M. and Rogers, A.E. (1986) Labile methyl groups and the promotion of cancer. *Annual Review of Nutrition*, **6**, 407–32.

Scott, J.M. (1992) Folate-vitamin B_{12} interrelationships in the central nervous system. *Proceedings of the Nutrition Society*, **51**, 219–24.

Scott, J.M. (1999) Folate and vitamin B_{12}. *Proceedings of the Nutrition Society*, **58**, 441–8.

Seetharam, B. (1999) Receptor-mediated endocytosis of cobalamin (vitamin B_{12}) *Annual Review of Nutrition*, **19**, 173–95.

VITAMIN D

INTRODUCTION

There is a number of compounds with vitamin D activity occurring in several forms, including vitamin D_3, molecular weight 384 Da, and vitamin D_2, molecular weight 397 Da.

Vitamin D_3 (cholecalciferol)

Most of the vitamin D_3 required by humans is produced in the skin by the ultraviolet irradiation of 7-dehydrocholesterol (provitamin D) present in animal fats (Figure 16.36). The rate of production is dependent on skin exposure to sunlight and the melanin content of the skin, which reduces the irradiation of 7-dehydrocholesterol. Increasing age is associated with a decline in the capacity to produce vitamin D_3 in the skin.

Cholecalciferol is also found in fatty fish that eat plankton that live near the surface of the sea. Oils from these fish, e.g. cod-liver oil, are an important dietary source; other sources include eggs and chicken liver.

Cholecalciferol should be regarded primarily as a hormone rather than a vitamin.

Vitamin D_2 (ergocalciferol)

The major dietary source of vitamin D in humans is ergocalciferol, from the artificial exposure of the natural sterol ergosterol to ultraviolet light. This photosynthetic process results in a number of products, some of which are toxic, but only ergocalciferol has a beneficial effect on rickets. Ergocalciferol differs from cholecalciferol by having an extra methyl group at C24 and a double bond at C22.

SYNTHESIS OF VITAMIN D

Both vitamin D_2 and vitamin D_3 are biologically inactive, lipid soluble and bound to α-globulin (transcalciferol) for transport in the blood to the liver. A proportion is converted into 25(OH)-vitamin D (calcifediol), which has modest biological activity. In the liver, calcifediol is converted to 25(OH)-vitamin D (calcitriol) or to 24,25(OH)$_2$-vitamin D. Because the hydroxylation process in the liver is a cytochrome P450-dependent process, the hydroxylating enzymes can be induced by drugs, e.g. phenobarbitone, with consequences for vitamin D status. (Figure 16.37).

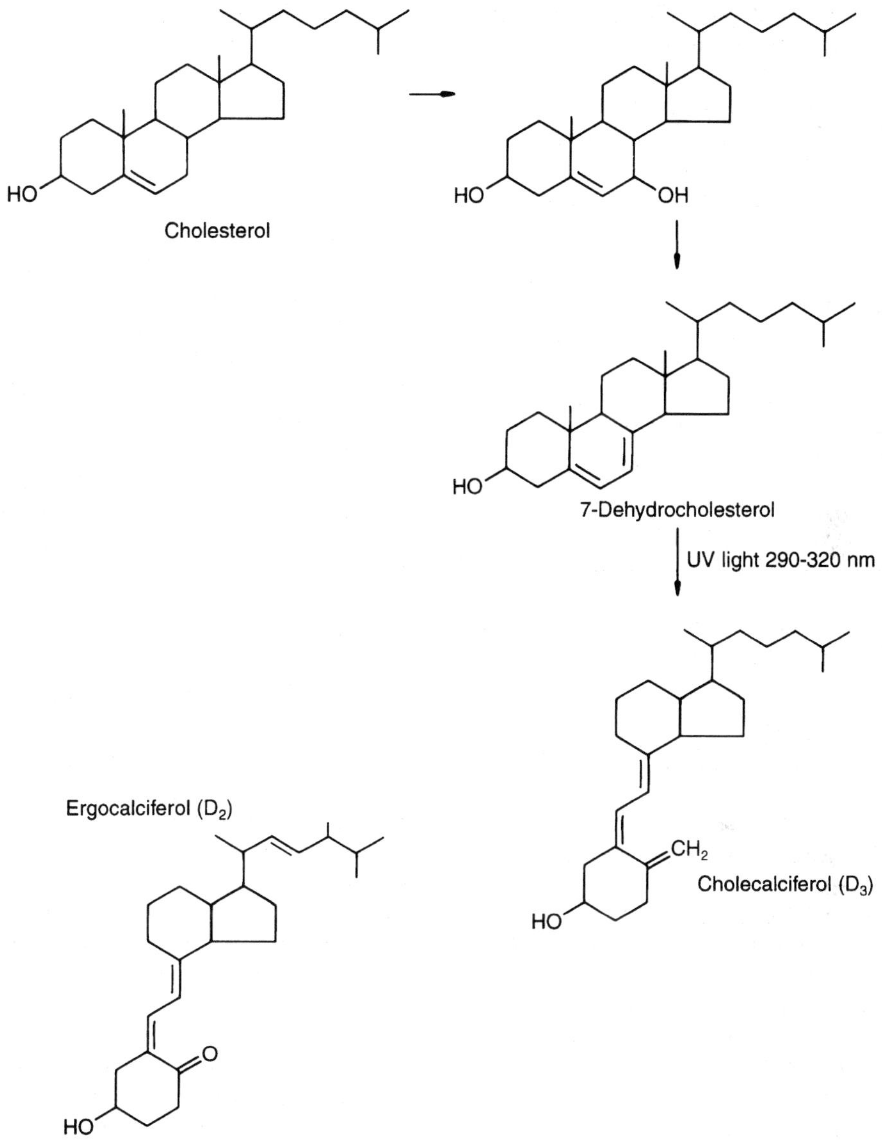

Fig. 16.36 Synthesis of vitamin D_3: structure of cholesterol; 7-dehydrocholesterol (produced from cholesterol) is converted by ultraviolet light to cholecalciferol (D_3); D_2 is ergocalciferol.

The active form of vitamin D is 1,25-dihydroxy-cholecalciferol [1,25(OH)$_2$-vitamin D], which is formed in the kidney by a specific mitochondrial hydroxylase acting on 25(OH)-vitamin D. 1,25(OH)$_2$-vitamin D is the biologically active form of vitamin D and is 100 times more potent than 25(OH)-vitamin D.

Vitamin D and its various products are stored in fat with a very long half-life: several months for vitamin D and 2–3 weeks for calcifediol. Both also circulate in the enterohepatic circulation. The half-life of 1,25(OH)$_2$-vitamin D is less than 24 h, the vitamin being converted to more polar inert products within the liver that are excreted in bile and urine.

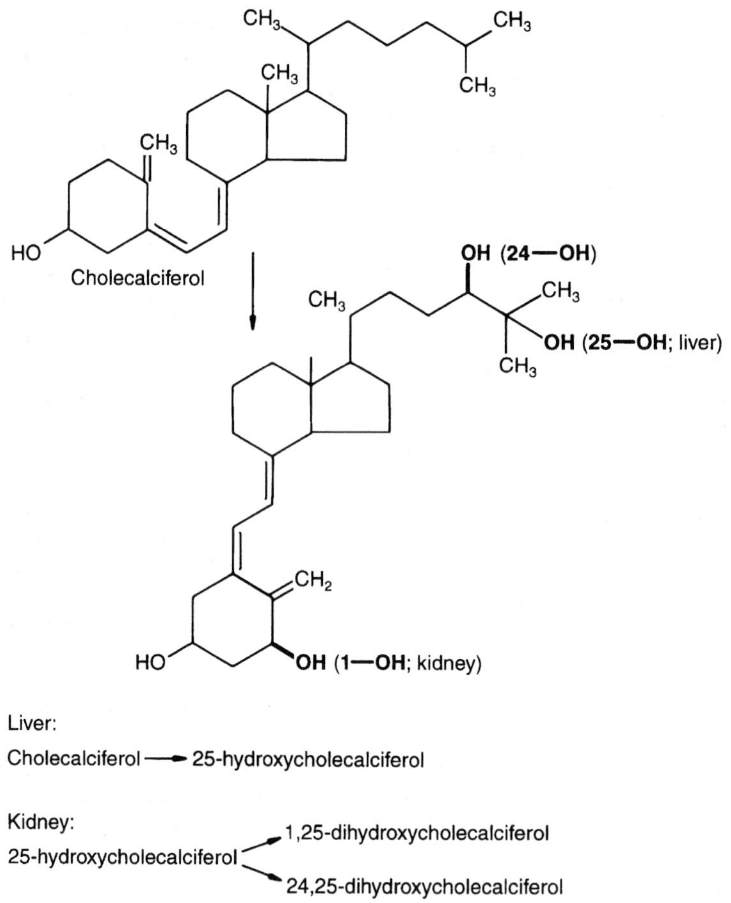

Fig. 16.37 Metabolism of cholecalciferol to 25-hydroxycholecalciferol in the liver, 1,25-dihydroxycholecalciferol in the kidney or 24,25-dihydroxycholecalciferol.

ACTIONS OF VITAMIN D

Calcium homoeostasis

The action of 1,25(OH)$_2$-vitamin D is to regulate calcium and phosphate metabolism. A reduction in plasma calcium concentration stimulates the secretion of parathyroid hormone, which stimulates 1-hydroxylation of 25(OH)-vitamin D in the renal tubule mitochondria.

1,25-Dihydroxycholecalciferol [1,25(OH)$_2$-vitamin D] is required for optimum intestinal absorption of calcium. It increases the transport of calcium across the brush border of the intestinal epithelial cell and export from the intestinal cell

into the bloodstream. A number of mechanisms may be involved.

- Through production of a specific messenger RNA and synthesis of a specific calcium-binding protein (CaBP), integral membrane calcium-binding protein (IMCAL) or alkaline phosphatase, or changes in the lipid composition and fluidity of brush border membranes, increased endocytosis of calcium and increased calmodulin binding to specific proteins in the brush border. The overall effect is possibly on the rate-limiting step in calcium absorption.
- Calcium must then move across the cytoplasm of the enteric brush border cell. This is facilitated by the action of vitamin D, the intracellular dif-

fusion of calcium or calcium binding to intracellular proteins.

- Vitamin D may also have a role in the movement of calcium into the bloodstream by either stimulating the calcium pump, stimulating Na^+/Ca^{2+} exchange, or increasing exocytosis or open voltage-dependent Ca^{2+} channels.
- In the presence of parathyroid hormone there is activation in the osteoblast of a number of functions related to bone formation. These include stimulation of the osteoblasts and osteoclasts, mobilising calcium from bone. $1,25(OH)_2$-Vitamin D acts on the osteoblast, stimulating non-matrix proteins. This allows parathyroid hormone activated mobilisation of calcium from bone and the activation of the giant osteoclast, an early step in the bone remodelling process.
- Phosphate absorption is stimulated through a separate phosphate transport mechanism in intestinal epithelial cells. Vitamin D stimulates the sodium-dependent component of phosphate absorption and movement across the basolateral membrane.
- $1,25(OH)_2$-Vitamin D acts on the distal renal tubular cells. Renal reabsorption of calcium in the distal tubule involves both parathyroid hormones and $1,25(OH)_2$-vitamin D.
- $1,25(OH)_2$-Vitamin D acts directly on the parathyroid cells to suppress parathyroid hormone production and secretion.

Vitamin D as a steroid hormone

$1,25(OH)_2$-vitamin D functions through nuclear receptors (molecular weight 55 kDa) that belong to the steroid thyroid hormone receptor family. The gene for this receptor is on chromosome 12 in humans. $1\alpha,25(OH)_2D_3$ acts as a ligand for the one vitamin D receptor (VDR) and the liganded VDR activates the gene expression at the transcriptional level. VDR forms a complex with one of the three retinoid receptors (RXRα, RXRβ, RXRγ). This complex binds to specific enhancers, the vitamin D response elements. Such binding initiates a sequence of events, including phosphorylation, which stimulates transcription of the gene, production of mRNA and synthesis of the accessory protein for vitamin D. Vitamin D may have two modes of action, acting on gene function (genomic) and

on receptors not controlling genes (non-genomic). The concentrations required for non-genomic actions are high and may not be physiological.

Vitamin D as a more general hormone

Receptors for $1,25(OH)_2$-vitamin D are also found in the parathyroid glands, the islet cells of the pancreas, the keratinocytes of skin, mammary epithelium, endocrine cells of the stomach and some cells in the brain. $1,25(OH)_2$-vitamin D may be a developmental hormone inhibiting proliferation and promoting differentiated function in cells.

The many genes and hormones influenced by $1,25(OH)_2$-vitamin D fall into four main groups:

- gene products associated with mineral metabolism
- regulators of vitamin D secosteroids
- differentiators of events in the skin and immune system
- regulators of DNA replication and cellular proliferation.

Vitamin D probably has little influence on magnesium absorption, but increases the absorption of aluminium, lead and selenium. This may be important when there is excess aluminium or lead in the diet with resultant impairment of calcium absorption.

AVAILABILITY OF VITAMIN D

Dietary vitamin D is absorbed in the small intestine, by similar mechanisms to fat digestion and absorption. There is subsequent transport to the liver in chylomicrons. In the liver all forms of vitamin D are converted by hepatic microsomes to the 25-hydroxylated form (Figure 16.37), which is carried in the plasma on a specific transport globulin. Storage is primarily in adipose tissue. Vitamin D may be excreted in bile in the form of hydroxylates and conjugates (glucuronides).

VITAMIN D DEFICIENCY

The most important consequence of vitamin D deficiency is rickets, in which there is a failure to mineralise the bony skeleton.

Rickets

Vitamin D deficiency affects bone, causing a failure of mineralisation of the osteoid matrix, which results in the formation of soft bone.

Bone exists in two major forms: cortical bone in the long bones, and trabecular solid bone at the ends of bones and in the vertebrae. Bone is a very active organ, but trabecular bone has a faster turnover than cortical bone. The formation, resorption and composition of bone are immediately controlled by bone cells, which in turn are managed by mechanical factors and hormones, calcitonin, parathyroid hormone and vitamin D.

The cells involved in bone modelling are:

- osteoblasts (bone-forming cells): collagen formation, secretion and mineralisation
- osteoclasts and osteocytes, which resorb bone.

The bone matrix is an organic matrix which is 90% type I collagen, each collagen molecule being synthesised within osteoblasts as α-chains, which then form a helix of three such chains. There are several different collagens with distinct genetic origins. The helical collagen molecules form cross-linked fibres, arranged in such a way that there are spaces in which bone mineral, a calcium phosphate complex, is laid down, giving the bone rigidity. Bone undergoes constant change, in the young as growth and in the adult as remodelling. There is a regular cycle of synthesis and calcification of the cartilage matrix, this is removed, then bone tissue is added, after which mineralisation, involves coupling factors that link bone resorption and formation. Control of calcium and phosphorous metabolism is central to bone growth and stability. The hormones involved are vitamin D, parathyroid hormone and calcitonin. Vitamin D deficiency alters this balance and failure of calcification results in soft, weak bones.

Clinical features

The bony abnormalities that accrue depend on the age of onset and the way in which gravity stresses the bone at the age of onset. The child's appearance may not indicate the development of rickets; the child may be well-built, but restless with somewhat flabby and hypotonic muscles. The limbs are able to twist into unusual positions; this is called 'acrobatic rickets'. There is excess sweating on the head and the abdomen is distended because of weak abdominal muscles. Diarrhoea, respiratory infection and delayed development of teeth are not uncommon. The most common finding is enlargement of the lower end of the radius and the costochondral junction of the ribs, 'rachitic rosary'. Later, there is bossing of the frontal and parietal bones, delayed closure of the anterior fontanelle, and 'pigeon chest', an undue prominence of the sternum with a transverse depression passing outwards from the costal margins towards the axilla. All of these features are due to pressure on the soft bones when the child is lying and standing, and are associated with breathing. This pressure deformation continues when the child is upright, so that the somewhat softened main-frame bones bend, leading to kyphosis of the spine and enlargement of the lower ends of the femur, tibia and fibula. Consequently, the legs are bowed with, for example, anterolateral bowing of the tibia at the junction of the middle and lower third. Kyphosis is often replaced by lordosis. Pelvic deformity has long-term consequences for childbirth in the fertile adult female.

Tetanic spasm

If the concentration of plasma ionised calcium falls then infantile tetany can result. This is manifested by spasm of the hands, feet and vocal chord, resulting in high-pitched cries and breathing problems.

Diagnosis

In addition to the clinical picture described above, plasma measurements of raised plasma alkaline phosphatase and particularly plasma 25(OH)-vitamin D are important.

Risk factors

- Inadequate exposure to sunlight: particularly in northern communities, resulting in reduced conversion of cholesterol to vitamin D_3. It is particularly marked in children and adolescents, who require vitamin D for growth.
- Strict vegetarianism: there is a risk of excluding vitamin D from the diet with an increased risk of osteomalacia or rickets.
- Breast feeding: if an infant is fed on milk for more than 3 months, or from a mother deficient in vitamin D for more than 3 months, the risk of infantile rickets increases.

- Skin pigmentation: there is a minor risk due to screening of the metabolically active skin sites by melanin and reduced conversion of cholesterol to vitamin D_3. Pigmented races in areas of reduced sunlight are particularly vulnerable to vitamin D deficiency.
- Secondary osteomalacia and rickets occur in conjunction with gastrointestinal disease, the malabsorption syndrome following peptic ulcer surgery where lipid absorption and hence vitamin D absorption are impaired.

Prevention
The risk of rickets can be removed by a supplement of 10 µg of vitamin D daily or regular exposure to sunlight. Protein-energy malnutrition may be associated with rickets.

Osteomalacia

This may present as pain and muscular weakness, and painful ribs, sacrum, lower lumbar vertebrae, pelvis and legs. A waddling gait may develop, as well as tetany, characterised by carpopedal and facial twitching. Spontaneous fractures may also occur.

X-ray features include rarification of the bone and translucent bands (pseudofractures, Looser's zones) characteristic of osteomalacia, which may be symmetrical and occur at points where there is compression stress, in the ribs, the scapula, the pubic rami and the cortex of the upper femur.

Osteomalacia and other bone disorders occur in individuals with chronic renal failure, with impaired hydroxylation and hence impaired synthesis of $1,25(OH)_2$-vitamin D in the kidneys. This can also occur in congenital conditions such as Fanconi's syndrome, where activation of cholecalciferol by 1,25-hydroxylation is impaired. Osteomalacia of hepatic origin results when there is a failure of 25-hydroxylation of vitamin D in the liver.

Other diseases related to vitamin D

- Renal osteodystrophy results from a renal inability to produce $1,25(OH)_2$-vitamin D. Patients on renal dialysis may have calcium replaced, but these patients can develop severe secondary

hyperparathyroidism. Treatment with $1,25(OH)_2$-vitamin D is very effective and suppresses parathyroid hormone production.
- Vitamin D-dependent rickets type 1 is an autosomal genetic disorder in which children have rickets despite normal intake of vitamin D. This defect is in the 1α-hydroxylation of 25(OH)-vitamin D. The defect is treated by physiological amounts of $1,25(OH)_2$-vitamin D or large doses of vitamin D.
- Vitamin D-dependent rickets type 2 is an end-organ-resistant defect, with autosomal recessive inheritance. This is due to a mutation of the gene for the $1,25(OH)_2$-vitamin D receptor. Mutations include changes to the two zinc fingers of the receptor that bind vitamin D response elements from target cells. A mutation in a nucleotide results in a premature stop codon, leading to a truncated receptor that does not function. This form of rickets is resistant to $1,25(OH)_2$-vitamin D.
- Osteoporosis has been suggested to be an oestrogen deficiency disorder. However, age-related osteoporosis is in part a defect in 25(OH)-vitamin D 1-α-hydroxylase.
- In X-linked hypophosphataemic vitamin D-resistant rickets, there is a renal phosphate leak and severe hypophosphataemia unrelated to defective vitamin D function. This is treated by frequent administration of oral phosphate. Such treatment results in increases in ionised calcium and secondary hyperparathyroidism; additional hydroxylated vitamin D compound

---

Vitamin D

The tissue concentrations of vitamin D may be important in cancer and infection.

Reduced intake of vitamin D is associated with an increased risk of colorectal cancer. There is evidence of regulation of the gene encoding 1α-hydroxylation of 25-hydroxycholecalciferol in colonic cancer tissue.

Resistance to infection involves several genes, including the vitamin D receptor. 25-Hydroxycholecalciferol deficiency can be found in populations with increased rates of tuberculosis, e.g. people of Asian origin living in London.

supplements are required to correct the secondary hyperparathyroidism.

VITAMIN D EXCESS

Hypervitaminosis D can occur during infant supplementation and also with replacement therapy in people who previously had osteomalacia. The consequence is an increase in plasma calcium concentration, tetany, electrocardiographic changes, convulsions and, occasionally, death.

Excess sunlight does not lead to an excess and toxic synthesis of 7-dehydrocholesterol.

Vitamin D given in milligram amounts is lethal, and vitamin D has been used as a rodent killer at 0.1 of the diet. The action may be through the blockade of receptors normally used by $1,25(OH)_2$ vitamin D by vitamin D and 25(OH)-vitamin D.

RECOMMENDED REQUIREMENTS

Adults

Plasma 25(OH)-vitamin D concentrations range from 15 to 35 ng/ml in summer and from 8 to 18 ng/ml in winter. No minimum dietary intake has been identified for individuals living predominantly exposed to the sunlight, but for those without this exposure an RNI of vitamin D of 10 µg/day is suggested. The duration of exposure is not easy to define because the degree of sunlight in various countries differs, and there are individual and racial differences in production of vitamin D. Exposure of hands, arms and face for 5–10 min, two to three times a week in good, direct sunlight in the spring, summer and autumn is adequate. Long periods of exposure require sunscreen with a sun-protecting factor of 15.

Infants and children

The vitamin D concentration in breast milk varies through the year, with winter milk containing very little vitamin D. Vitamin D intakes usually decline when the infant is weaned, as most weaning foods are modestly fortified and are low in vitamin D, as is whole cow's milk. Plasma 25(OH)-vitamin D is

therefore reduced in the second 6 months of life, a much more vulnerable period for the growing infant than the first 6 months. After this, plasma 25(OH) vitamin D concentrations are satisfactory.

Low vitamin D status is relatively common in individuals of Asian origin living in northern Europe, especially children, adolescents and women, mainly owing to vegetarian diets, low calcium intake and limited exposure to sun because of the mode of dress. Pigmented races living in northern climes with a reduced exposure to sun should therefore receive dietary supplements of vitamin D.

Pregnancy and lactation

Pregnant and lactating women should receive supplementary vitamin D to ensure an intake of 10 µg/day despite seasonal variations.

The elderly

The elderly may have reduced stores because of insufficient exposure of skin to the sun in the summer. A daily 30 min exposure of the face and legs will raise 25(OH)-vitamin D levels at a latitude of 37° N, whereas 1–2 h may be necessary in the north of Britain. To maintain winter 25(OH)-vitamin D concentrations above 8 ng/ml would require a summer plasma concentration of 16 ng/ml, which is two to three times higher than values often recorded in the elderly. Such deficiency may result in osteomalacia developing in a small proportion of this age group. It is recommended that the elderly should consume 10 µg/day of vitamin D to achieve satisfactory 25(OH)-vitamin D concentrations.

BODY STORE MEASUREMENTS

The best measure of the vitamin status in humans is the plasma 25(OH)-vitamin D concentration. This reflects the availability of vitamin D in the body and 1,25(OH)-vitamin D metabolic need. Dietary intake may be reasonably assessed from measurements of plasma 25(OH)-vitamin D concentrations in individuals minimally exposed to sunlight. The threshold of risk associated with osteomalacia is a concentration of 25(OH)-vitamin D less than 12.5 nmol/l. In contrast, where there is exposure to sunlight, the lower limit of 25(OH)-vitamin D should be 12–25 nmol/l.

KEY POINTS

1. Compounds with vitamin D activity occur in several forms, including vitamin D_2 (ergocalciferol) and vitamin D_3 (cholecalciferol).
2. Vitamin D_3 is produced in the skin from 7-dehydrocholesterol. Cholecalciferol is also found in fatty fish. Cholecalciferol may be regarded primarily as a hormone rather than a vitamin.
3. The major dietary source of vitamin D in humans is ergocalciferol. This differs from cholecalciferol in having an extra methyl group at C24 and a double bond at C22.
4. Both vitamin D_2 and vitamin D_3 are biologically inactive. The active form of vitamin D is 1,25-dihydroxycholecalciferol [1,25(OH)$_2$-vitamin D]; this is formed in the kidney by a specific mitochondrial hydroxylase acting on 25(OH)-vitamin D and is regulated by parathyroid hormone and plasma phosphate concentration.
5. The actions of the vitamin D family include calcium homoeostasis [an interaction of parathyroid hormone and 1,25(OH)$_2$-vitamin D], steroid hormone action [1,25(OH)$_2$-vitamin D functions through nuclear receptors] and a role as a more general hormone.
6. 1,25(OH)$_2$-Vitamin D may be a developmental hormone inhibiting proliferation and promoting differentiated function in cells.
7. The most important consequence of vitamin D deficiency is rickets, in which there is a failure to mineralise the bony skeleton. The site of the consequent bony deformities depends on weight bearing on the softened bones.

THINKING POINTS

1. Ensuring adequate vitamin D supplies is an unusual problem, as both sunlight and diet are important.
2. The relevance of lifestyle is important particularly for immigrants adapting to life in a new climate.

NEED TO UNDERSTAND

1. Vitamin D is essential for bone structure and a number of other receptor functions.
2. The different strands of the precursors of vitamin D are important, as are the signs of the various clinical and nutritional causes of vitamin D deficiency.

FURTHER READING

Fleet, J.C. (1999) Vitamin D receptors: not just in the nucleus anymore. *Nutrition Reviews*, **57**, 60–4.

Fraser, D.R. (1995) Vitamin D. *Lancet*, **345**, 104–7.

Gennari, C. (2001) Calcium and vitamin D nutrition and bone disease of the elderly. *Public Health Nutrition*, **4**, 547–59.

Holick, M.F. (2001) Sunlight 'D'ilemma: risk of skin cancer or bone disease and muscle weakness. *Lancet*, **357**, 4–6.

Kato, S. (2000) Molecular mechanism of transcriptional control by nuclear vitamin receptors. *British Journal of Nutrition*, **84** (Suppl. 2), S229–33.

Mawer, E.B. and Davies, M. (2001) Vitamin D nutrition and bone disease in adults. *Review of Endocrine and Metabolic Disorders*, **2**, 153–64.

Ogunkolade, B.W., Boucher, B.J., Fairclough, P.D. *et al.* (2002) Expression of 25-hydroxyvitamin D-1-α-hydroxylase mRNA in individuals with colorectal cancer. *Lancet*, **359**, 1831–2.

Omdahl, J.L., Morris, H.A. and May, B.K. (2002) Hydroxylase enzymes of the vitamin D pathway. *Annual Review of Nutrition*, **22**, 139–66.

Pfeifer, M., Begerow, B., Minne, H.W. *et al.* (2000) Effects of a short term vitamin D and calcium supplementation on body sway and secondary hyperthyroidism in elderly women. *Journal of Bone and Mineral Research*, **6**, 1113–18.

Van Leeuwen, J.P., van Driel, M., van den Bemd, G.J. and Pols, H.A. (2001) Vitamin D control of osteoblast function and bone extracellular matrix mineralization. *Critical Reviews in Eukaryotic Gene Expression*, **11**, 199–226.

Wilkinson, R.J., Llewelyn, M., Toossi, Z. *et al.* (2000) Influence of vitamin D deficiency and vitamin D receptor polymorphism on tuberculosis among Gujarati Asians in west London: a case-control study. *Lancet*, **355**, 618–21.

VITAMIN K

INTRODUCTION

Vitamin K is a naphthoquinone which occurs in two forms, vitamin K_1 and K_2 (Figure 16.38). Vitamin K_1, molecular weight 450 Da, was isolated from the plant lucerne and is a phytylmenaquinone (an alternative name is phylloquinone), but in the pharmacopoeia is called phytomanadione. The vitamin consists of 2-methyl-1,4-naphthoquinone (menadione or menaquinone) attached to a 20-carbon phytyl side-chain. This is a yellow oil and is the only form that occurs in plants. Vitamin K_2, molecular weight 649 Da, is one of the family of chemical homologues produced by bacteria with 4–13 isoprenyl units in the side-chain. These are called menaquinone-4 to menaquinone-13, depending on the number of isoprenyl units.

Vitamin K_1 is present in fresh green vegetables, e.g. broccoli, lettuce, cabbage and spinach. Beef liver is a good source, but other animal tissues, cereals and fruit are poor sources. Vitamin K_2 as menaquinones is produced by intestinal bacteria.

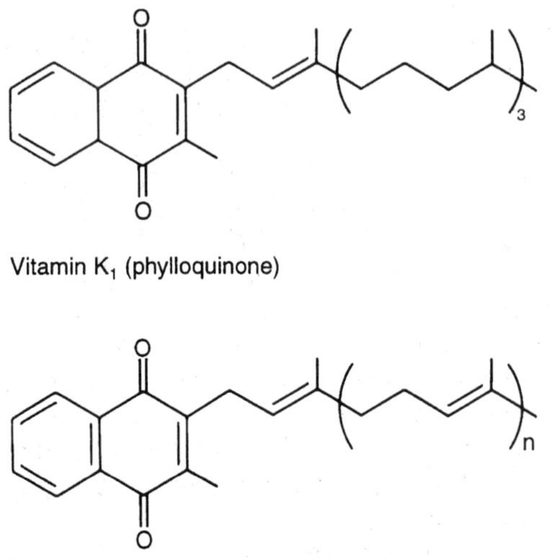

Vitamin K_1 (phylloquinone)

Vitamin K_2 (menaquinone series)

Fig. 16.38 Structure of vitamin K_1 (phylloquinone) and K_2 (menaquinone).

ACTION OF VITAMIN K

Vitamin K is involved in the synthesis of proteins central to blood coagulation, prothrombin, and factors VII, IX and X (Figure 16.39). Vitamin K is necessary for the post-translational carboxylation of glutamic acid to γ-carboxyglutamate (Figure 7.40) in the coagulation proteins, which allows the binding of calcium and phospholipids during the formation of thrombin. When warfarin, an anticoagulant, is given, the change from glutamic acid to γ-carboxyglutamate does not occur and the proteins no longer function in clotting mechanisms.

Vitamin K may have a role in the homoeostasis of bone metabolism. Two mechanisms may be involved, one of which is the γ-carboxylation of osteocalcin, a protein involved in bone mineralisation but also, directly in calcium metabolism.

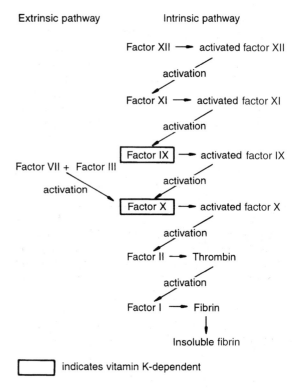

Fig. 16.39 Coagulation and fibrinolysis. There are two pathways of fibrin formation, extrinsic and intrinsic. The production of factor IX and factor X is vitamin K dependent.

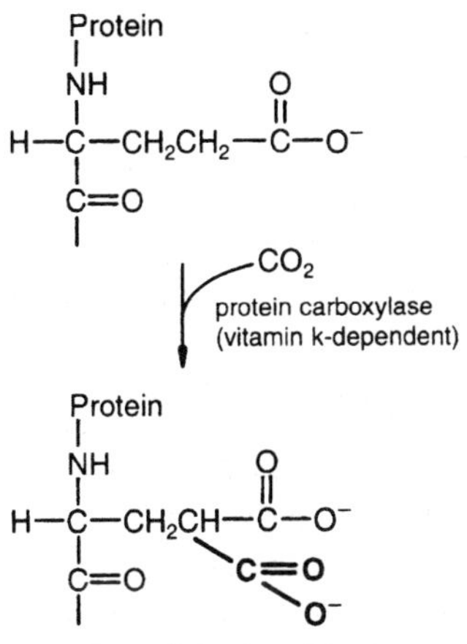

Fig. 16.40 Vitamin K is a coenzyme in the carboxylation of glutamic acid residues in proteins and forms γ-carboxyglutamic acid. This reaction is important in the clotting cascade.

AVAILABILITY OF VITAMIN K

Vitamin K_1 is absorbed in the same way as any other lipid and is transported from the intestine in the blood in chylomicrons as β-lipoproteins. Vitamin K of bacterial origin is also absorbed from the colon.

VITAMIN K DEFICIENCY

In vitamin K deficiency, the activities of factors VII, IX and X are reduced, and the blood clotting time is prolonged. Vitamin K deficiency may occur in infants but rarely in adults. Infant deficiency is the combined result of a sterile intestinal tract and a dietary deficiency due to human and cow's milk containing only small amounts of vitamin K. The problem is compounded by the immature liver of the infant being slow to synthesise prothrombin.

Acquired deficiencies of vitamin K malabsorption

These include any condition in which fats are mal-absorbed, including biliary obstruction, malabsorption, bacterial colonisation and liver disease.

VITAMIN K EXCESS

In general, natural vitamin K preparations are free from toxic effects. Synthetic preparations of menadione have little biological activity, and the high reactivity of the unsubstituted 3-position can lead to haemolysis and liver damage in the newborn.

Antagonists and anticoagulants

Spoilt sweet clover, in which a dicoumard is produced, prolongs the prothrombin time of the cow, causing a bleeding condition. This observation led to the development of dicoumarol, an analogue of vitamin K, which was used to prolong prothrombin time in clinical medicine, but has been replaced by warfarin and phenindione.

RECOMMENDED REQUIREMENTS

Adults

The accepted criterion for vitamin K requirements is the maintenance of normal plasma concentration of the vitamin K-dependent coagulation factors, assessed by prothrombin times. Most estimates of the dietary requirements of phylloquinone give figures between 0.5 and 1.0 μg/kg body weight/day.

Infants

Vitamin K in human milk is almost entirely in the form of phylloquinone, and may vary between 1 and 10 μg/litre. A reasonable DRV for an infant fed on breast milk would be approximately 8.5 μg phylloquinone.

Vitamin K is given in haemorrhagic disease of the newborn. In approximately 1 in 800 newborn babies, bleeding into the tissues occurs (including the skin, peritoneal cavity, alimentary tract and central nervous system) between the second and fifth days. In some countries, e.g. Britain, vitamin K is given routinely at delivery. Water-soluble analogues of vitamin K are not used in the newborn, particularly the premature newborn, because they may cause hyperbilirubinaemia. A dose of 1 mg of vitamin K_1 is given intramuscularly. Vitamin K preparations may be important supplements when there is lipid malabsorption in the intestine and in reversing the effects of anticoagulants.

BODY STORE MEASUREMENTS

Vitamin K deficiency can be detected by the blood prothrombin time, which measures the prolongation of clotting time.

KEY POINTS

1. Vitamin K is a naphthoquinone. There are two forms: vitamin K_1 is from the plant lucerne, a phytylmenaquinone (phylloquinone); vitamin K_2 is produced by bacteria and has 4–13 isoprenyl units in its side-chain.
2. Vitamin K is involved in the synthesis of blood coagulation proteins, prothrombin and factors VII, IX and X. Vitamin K is necessary for the post-translational carboxylation of glutamic acid to γ-carboxyglutamate in the coagulation proteins, which allows the binding of calcium and phospholipids in the formation of thrombin.
3. When warfarin, an anticoagulant, is prescribed, conversion to γ-carboxyglutamate does not occur and the coagulation proteins are ineffective in clotting mechanisms.
3. In vitamin K deficiency, the activities of factors VII, IX and X are reduced and the blood clotting time is prolonged.

THINKING POINTS

1. Blood clotting is a complex system. How does the system stop clotting?
2. Aspirin affects platelet stickiness. So here are two important plant-origin effectors on blood clotting (aspirin and vitamin K).

NEED TO UNDERSTAND

The mechanism of vitamin K's activity on the coagulation proteins.

FURTHER READING

Barton, J.S., Tripp, J.H. and McNinch, A.W. (1995) Neonatal vitamin K prophylaxis in the British Isles: current practice and trends. *British Medical Journal*, **310**, 632–3.

Berkner, K.L. (2000) The vitamin K dependent carboxylase. *Journal of Nutrition*, **130**, 1877–80.

Dowd, P., Ham, S.W., Naganathan, S. and Hershline, R. (1995) The mechanism of action of vitamin K. *Annual Review of Nutrition*, **15**, 419–40.

Ferland, G. (1998) The vitamin K-dependent proteins: an update. *Nutrition Reviews*, **56**, 223–30.

Nelsestuen, G.L., Shah, A.M. and Harvey, S.B. (2000) Vitamin K dependent proteins. *Vitamins and Hormones*, **58**, 355–89.

Suttie, J.W. (1995) The importance of menaquinones in human nutrition. *Annual Review of Nutrition*, **15**, 399–417.

Suzuki, S, Iwata, G. and Sutor, A.H. (2001) Vitamin K deficiency during the perinatal and infantile period. *Seminars in Thrombosis and Hemostasis*, **27**, 93–8.

Weber, P. (2001) Vitamin K and bone health. *Nutrition*, **17**, 880–7.

VITAMIN E

INTRODUCTION

The term vitamin E is used for any mixture of biologically active tocopherols. Eight tocopherols and tocotrienols are known that have vitamin E activity. The tocopherols are the most potent of the vitamin E compounds, while the tocotrienols are less potent, the differences being in the number and positions of the methyl groups around the ring of the molecule (Figure 16.41). While all have

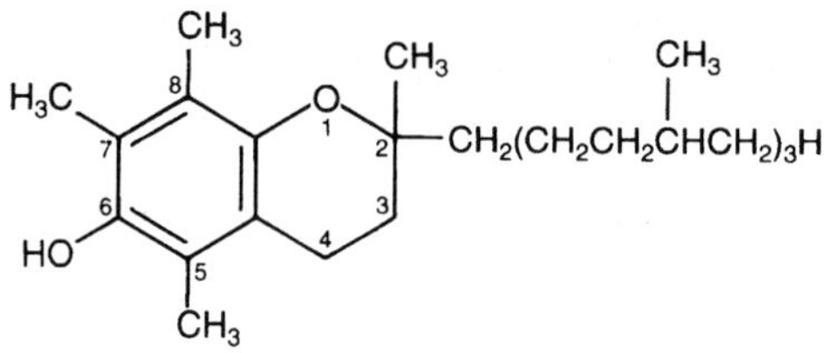

In β-tocopherol, the 7-methyl group is absent

In γ-tocopherol, the 5-methyl group is absent

In δ-tocopherol, the 5- and 7-methyl groups are absent

In tocotrienols, the side-chain is

Fig. 16.41 Structure of vitamin E (tocopherol), α-tocopherol, β-tocopherol, γ-tocopherol (no 5-methyl group), δ-tocopherol and tocotrienols.

the same physiological properties, α-tocopherol, molecular weight 430 Da, a synthetic product, is the most potent; β- and γ-tocopherol and β-tocotrienol have an activity of 48% and 20% relative to α-tocopherol. Other analogues have little vitamin type activity.

Abundant sources are vegetable oils, wheat germ, sunflower seed, cottonseed, safflower, palm, rapeseed and other oils. Vitamin E is found in all cell membranes where it inhibits the non-enzymatic oxidation of polyunsaturated fatty acids (PUFAs) by molecular oxygen.

ACTION OF VITAMIN E

The biological function of vitamin E is not specific. It acts as an antioxidant or a free radical scavenger in chemical systems. Vitamin E is the only known lipid-soluble antioxidant in plasma and red blood cell membranes.

Ascorbic acid may reduce tocopheroxyl radicals formed by the scavenging of free radicals during metabolism. This enables the single molecule of tocopherol to scavenge many radicals. Vitamin C is therefore protective against free radical damage in membranes. Vitamin C is very water soluble, but as vitamin E is buried within the membrane

Free-radical scavengers

The special radical-scavenging properties of vitamin E are found in the fused chroman ring system; the phytyl side-chain does not affect the radical-scavenging properties of this chroman. The antioxidant properties are due to the positioning of the pair of small pi-electrons of the ethereal oxygen in the ring. Vitamin E is associated with membranous organelles, largely because of its lipid solubility, being miscible with the lipids of the biological membrane. The phytyl chain allows the tocopherol molecule to enter the hydrophobic environment of the membrane.

organelles in cells, the mechanisms by which these substances may interact are not known. Glutathione may be the donor of electrons in most tissues.

Vitamin E is a protective vitamin for PUFAs. It is curious that vitamin E deficiency is not that of PUFA deficiency but rather a neurological abnormality, suggesting more specific functions of vitamin E in metabolism. Roles for vitamin E are being found in cell proliferation, protein kinase C activity and signal transduction regulation.

AVAILABILITY OF VITAMIN E

The absorption characteristics are as for all lipid-soluble nutrients. Normal lipoprotein concentrations of vitamin E as α-tocopherol range from 11 to 37 μmol/l. α-Tocopherol forms 90% of vitamin E found in tissues. Because vitamin E is not soluble in water, transport through aqueous fluids requires lipid transport systems. Vitamin E is transported in plasma by all plasma lipoproteins; there does not appear to be a specific carrier protein. This has the advantage that there is protection for PUFAs that are also being transported in the same system. Tocopherol enters the systemic circulation in chylomicrons and intestinal very low-density lipoproteins (VLDL).

Efficient removal of vitamin E from the circulation depends on lipoprotein lipase. Vitamin E is either taken up by the liver or transferred to other lipoproteins, e.g. secreted into the bloodstream within nascent VLDL. α-Tocopherol is secreted preferentially to other stereoisomers of tocopherols.

DEFICIENCY AND EXCESS OF VITAMIN E

Deficiency

Deficiency may occur as a result of gastrointestinal malabsorption and in premature infants. Deficiency may present as neurological disabilities, ataxia, lost reflexes, decreased vibration sensation and oculomotor weakness.

Excess

There appear to be no adverse effects of large doses of vitamin E, up to 3200 mg/day.

RECOMMENDED REQUIREMENTS

Adults

The average intake in Britain is 6 mg/day, of which 26% is derived from fats and oils and 9% from cereals. The required amount of vitamin E is dependent on the needs of sites in membranes, which are determined by the PUFA content of tissues; this in turn reflects the PUFA content of the diet. The relationship between PUFA intake and vitamin E requirements is neither simple nor linear; hence, identifying vitamin E requirements is very difficult.

Daily intakes of 4–10 mg and 3–8 mg of α-tocopherol equivalents for men and women, respectively, have been recommended by various committees. An alternative provision would be 0.4 mg α-tocopherol equivalents/g dietary PUFA/day. This formula could also be used for infant formulae. For a PUFA intake of 6% of the diet, the vitamin E dietary requirement would be approximately 7 mg/day.

Infants

Human milk has a varied vitamin E content, up to concentrations of 1 mg α-tocopherol equivalents/100 ml in colostrum, which may fall to 0.32 mg/100 ml at 12 days and remain constant thereafter. This would give the infant consuming 850 ml of breast milk a daily intake of 2.7 mg.

BODY STORE MEASUREMENTS

Vitamin E status can be measured by the plasma tocopherol concentration. To some extent dietary vitamin E intake is reflected in blood tocopherol concentrations. However, the value of all the biochemical indices and dietary intake calculations is modest. The absorption of the vitamin is incomplete and varies from 20 to 80%. Furthermore, because of the variable biological activity of the different tocopherols, the value of these measurements is limited. Plasma concentrations of α-tocopherol of less than 11.5 μmol/l suggest vitamin E deficiency. Vitamin E is also correlated with the total lipids in the blood, particularly the cholesterol fraction. The molar cholesterol:vitamin E ratio is approximately 200:1. An alternative ratio is vitamin E:cholesterol. A plasma tocopherol concentration of 11 mmol/l or a tocopherol:cholesterol ratio of 2.25 μmol/mmol is considered normal. A ratio of less than 2.2 μmol α-tocopherol/mmol of cholesterol is suggestive of high risk. A functional test of vitamin E status is the hydrogen peroxide haemolysis test (erythrocyte stress test).

KEY POINTS

1. Vitamin E is a term for any mixture of biologically active tocopherols. Eight tocopherols and tocotrienols with vitamin E activity are known, the differences being in the number and positions of the methyl groups around the ring of the molecule.
2. Vitamin E acts as antioxidant or a free-radical scavenger in chemical systems and is associated with membranous organelles,

miscible with lipids of the biological membrane.
3. Vitamin E is the only known lipid-soluble anti-oxidant in plasma and red cell membranes.
4. Ascorbic acid may reduce tocopheroxyl radicals formed by the scavenging of free radicals during metabolism. This enables the single molecule of tocopherol to scavenge many radicals. Vitamin C is therefore protective against free-radical damage in membranes.

NEED TO UNDERSTAND

Vitamin E is an antioxidant protective agent.

FURTHER READING

Blatt, D.H., Leonard, S.W. and Traber, M.G. (2001) Vitamin E kinetics and the functions of tocopherol regulatory proteins. *Nutrition*, **17**, 799–805.

Cohn, W., Gross, P. and Grum, H. *et al.* (1992) Tocopherol transport and absorption. *Proceedings of the Nutrition Society*, **51**, 179–88.

McCay, P.B. (1985) Vitamin E. Interaction with free radicals and ascorbate. *Annual Review of Nutrition*, **5**, 323–40.

Morrissey, P.A. and Sheehy, P.J.A. (1999) Optimum nutrition, vitamin E. *Proceedings of the Nutrition Society*, **58**, 459–68.

Ricciarelli, R., Zingg, J.M. and Azzi, A. (2001) Vitamin E: protective role of a Janus molecule. *FASEB J*, **15**, 2314–26.

17

Plant secondary metabolites and herbs

PLANT SECONDARY METABOLITES

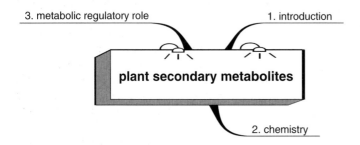

3. metabolic regulatory role

1. introduction

plant secondary metabolites

2. chemistry

Fig. 17.1 Section outline.

INTRODUCTION

Four-fifths of known natural products are of plant origin, either primary or secondary metabolites. Plant primary metabolites, e.g. amino acids, sugars, fatty acids and vitamins, are involved in plant metabolism, growth, maintenance and survival. The primary metabolites are important in nutrition and metabolism across all kingdoms.

Plants also contain a group of chemicals called secondary metabolites. These are chemically diverse natural products synthesised and stored only in plants, often peculiar to a few plant species and even parts of the plants, root, shoot, leaf or storage organ. Secondary metabolites are synthesised from a few key intermediates of primary metabolism and include non-protein amino acids, alkaloids, phenols and isoprenoids. Many have no immediately obvious function in cell growth and are produced by cells that have stopped dividing.

Secondary metabolites are regarded as being either toxins or attractants to predators or potential pollinators. They have a role in protection from animals. They also have important hormonal and other central roles in regulating physiological function. It is possible that the function of secondary metabolites also extends across the kingdoms. They have effects on the mammalian central nervous and cardiovascular systems, of which plants have no obvious equivalent. Such metabolites include opium, cannabis, digitalis and oubain.

CHEMISTRY

Alkaloids

Alkaloids are a vast family of more than 5000 different chemicals occurring naturally in plants. Structurally, they are the most diverse class of secondary metabolites ranging from simple structures such as coniine to exceedingly complex structures. The alkaloids are usually classified by the amino acid or derivatives from which they arise. The most important classes are derived from the amino acids ornithine and lysine, from the aromatic amino acids phenylalanine and tyrosine, or from tryptophan. Other alkaloids are derived from anthranilic acid, nicotinic acid, polyketides and terpenoids.

Phenolics

Phenolics are aromatic compounds with hydroxyl substitutions. The parent compound is phenol but most are polyphenolic. In addition to monomeric and dimeric phenolics there are the lignins of plant cell walls, melanin compounds and tannins. There are also substituted phenolic terpenoids, e.g. $\Delta 1$-tetrahydrocannibol. Phenols are classified according to the number of carbon atoms in the basic skeleton. Simple phenols include phenol and catechol (1,2-dihydroxybenzene). Derived classes have one, two or three side-chains, e.g. salicylic acid, p-hydroxyphenylacetic acid, hydroxycinnamic acid and caffeic acid.

Flavonoids

Flavonoids are polyphenolic glycosides that occur in edible plants, e.g. citrus fruits, berries, root vegetables, cereals, pulses, tea and coffee. They are hydrolysed by bacteria in the saliva and intestine to quercetin, kaempferol and myricetin.

Isoprenoids

The common denominator in this diverse array of compounds is their universal five-carbon building block. They are compounds with C5, C10, C15, C20 ... C40 skeletons, monoterpenes, sesquiterpenens and diterpenes. Steroids are a separate category. Mevalonic acid, a C6 acyclic compound, is the precursor of all isoprenoids. Isoprenoids that are classified as primary metabolites include sterols, carotenoids, growth regulators and the polyprenol substitutions of dolichols, quinone and proteins. These compounds are essential for plant membrane integrity, photoprotection and the orchestration of developmental programmes.

METABOLIC REGULATORY ROLE

How might these diverse chemicals be relevant to animal metabolism? The concept of shared evolutionary ancestry was introduced in Chapter 7: mammals and plants have conserved genes and proteins that are wholly or partially similar.

Ancient conserved proteins are preserved through evolution either almost intact or in the functional domains of the protein. About 900 ancient conserved regions may account for most of the similarities observed between different phyla. Although eukaryotes as divergent as yeast and humans have a total gene repertoire that differs in size by a factor in excess of 19, most proteins are likely to be members of only a few thousand gene families.

These proteins are often regulated by secondary metabolites in plants. The secondary metabolites act in physiological amounts in the plants, but are subsequently stored. They may be stored in seeds and other organs in large amounts, e.g. oxalic acid in rhubarb leaves, opium in poppy seed, nicotine in tobacco seed, salicylic acid in willow bark.

The concentration of these metabolites increases in the plant. When an animal ingests the plant, the effect will vary from physiological to pharmacological and even the toxic, depending on the amount.

Biological functions may be regulated by coarse and fine control systems. Coarse control requires changes in the regulatory genes that orchestrate transcription, structural genes coding for biosynthetic enzymes, the control of catabolic reactions or the secretion and intracellular targeting of a compound. Fine control involves post-translational mechanisms that are on/off switches for biosynthetic processes, but which also ensure that the synthetic rate is consistent with the immediate demands of a cell. These include modulation of enzyme activity through protein modification, e.g. protein phosphorylation, feedback regulation through a reaction product or pathway endproduct, and other kinetic controls that affect the catalytic efficiency of a biosynthetic enzyme. Secondary metabolites in plants can regulate gene and protein function.

Plant secondary metabolites have at least two properties:

- **type I function**: the plant uses the secondary metabolites to interact with other organisms in a protective or an attractive manner:
  - **kairomones** are members of a heterocyclic group of chemical messengers emitted by organisms of one species that benefit members of another species. These include attractants, phagostimulants and other substances that attract predators to their prey, herbivores to their food plants and parasites to their hosts
  - **allomones** are chemical substances produced by an organism to its own benefit. When the organism contacts an individual of another species, allomones evoke a behavioural or developmental reaction in the receiver that is adaptively favourable to the transmitter
- **type II function**: the secondary metabolite acts as an **ectocrine**, a metabolite that, when released from the generating organism, differentially affects other organisms of the same or a different species. It may be harmful to some members of a community and beneficial to others.

The secondary metabolites with type I properties tend to be non-protein amino acids and alkaloids; type II are phenolic and terpenoid families. Metabolites with type II properties are probably those that have nutritional and metabolic benefits to humans.

The systems affected are:

- **genes and protein regulation**: promotors of gene activity include monoterpenes, abscinic acid, methyl jasmonate, flavonoids, gibberillic acid, okadaic acid and 2,4-dichlorphenoxyacetic acid
- **mevalonic acid**: the precursor of the animal and plant sterols of all forms. 3-Hydroxy-3-methyl-glutaryl-coenzyme A (HMG-CoA) reductase is controlled by a number of chemicals, including plant secondary metabolites, e.g. brassinosteroids
- **transmembrane channel receptors**: these can be modulated by a number of chemicals, including secondary metabolites, e.g. opiates, cardiac glycosides and abscisic acid
- **kinase family of enzymes**: important control enzymes which, in turn, are controlled by phosphorylation
- **cytochrome P450 superfamily**: this central haemoprotein enzyme system in the liver has evolved from the same ancestor throughout the kingdoms. Human P450 activity can be altered by plant secondary metabolites.

KEY POINTS

1. Plants contain a wide range of secondary metabolites, non-protein amino acids, alkaloids, phenols and isoprenoids. Many of these have important biological effects when eaten by humans.
2. The benefits provided by fruit and vegetables may rely substantially on these secondary metabolites, although this is an uncharted field.

THINKING POINT

The vitamins may be but one class of important plant micronutrients. This is potentially the most exciting area for the future in our understanding of nutrition and health.

NEED TO UNDERSTAND

The basic chemistry of the secondary metabolites, non-protein amino acids, alkaloids, phenols and isoprenoids.

FURTHER READING

Aoyama, Y., Noshiro, M., Gotoh, O., *et al.* (1996) Sterol 14-demethylase P450 (P45014DM) is one of the most ancient and conserved P450 species. *Journel of Biochemistry (Tokyo)*, **119**, 926–33.

Doolittle, R.F., Feng, D.-F., Tsang, S., *et al.* (1996) Determining divergence times of the major kingdoms of living organisms with a protein clock. *Science*, **271**, 470–7.

Eastwood, M.A. (2001) A molecular biological basis for the nutritional and pharmacological benefits of dietary plants. *Quarterly Journal of Medicine*, **94**, 45–8.

Fraenkel, G.S. (1959) The raison d'être of secondary plant substances. *Science*, **129**, 1466–70.

Harborne, J.B., Baxter, H. and Moss, G.P. (1996), *Dictionary of Plant Toxins*. John Wiley, Chichester.

Herrlich, P., Blattner, C., Knebel, A., *et al.* (1997) Nuclear and nonnuclear targets of genotoxic agents in the induction of gene expression. Shared principles in yeast, rodents , man and plants. *Biological Chemistry*, **378**, 1217–29.

Lam, H.-M., Chiu, J., Hsieh M.-H. *et al.* (1998) Glutamate-receptor genes in plants. *Nature*, **396**, 125–6.

Mann, J., Davidson, R.S., Hobbs, J.B., *et al.* (1994) *Natural Products. Their Chemistry and Biological Significance*. Addison Wesley Longman, Harlow.

Powis, D.A. and Bunn, S.J. (1995) *Neurotransmitter Release and its Modulation*. Cambridge University Press, Cambridge.

Ross, J.A. and Kasum, C.M. (2002) Dietary flavonoids: bioavailability, metabolic effects and safety. *Annual Review of Nutrition*, **22**, 19–34.

Tugendreich, S., Bassett, D.E., McKusick, V.A., *et al.* (1991) Genes conserved in yeast and genes. *Human Molecular Genetics*, **3**, 1509–17,

WEBSITE

www.ars-grin.gov/duke   Duke's phytochemical ethnobase

HERBS

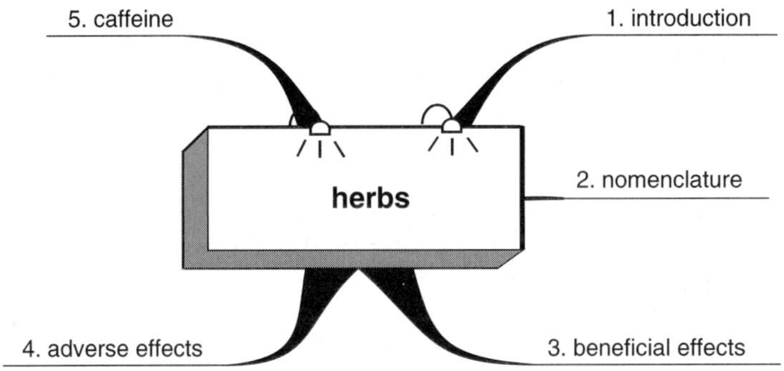

Fig. 17.2   Section outline.

INTRODUCTION

Ethnobiology is the study of the traditional lore of plants and animals. This is the wisdom of the herbal healers, shamans and medicine men. Some 25 000 plants, 10% of all species, are used medicinally throughout the world. Plant chemicals have an effect in mammals, including humans, both to promote health and to minimise disease. The mechanisms are not fully understood, for example: how can a chemical which has one function in a plant function in a quite different manner in an animal?

Herbs traditionally added to food may also have effects that are distinct from their flavour-enhancing properties, e.g. non-nutritional, physiological, pharmacological or even pathological properties.

NOMENCLATURE

Herb nomenclature may include:

- the English common name
- a transliteration of the herb name
- the Latinised pharmaceutical name
- the scientific name.

For example, corresponding names for ginseng would be:

- ginseng
- ren-shen
- radix ginseng
- *Panax ginseng*.

The naming is in practice imprecise, e.g. the term ginseng is given to oriental American as well as Siberian ginseng.

BENEFICIAL EFFECTS

There are many examples of traditional plant remedies which, following careful extraction and pharmacological studies, result in the identification of a drug with a general and accepted use in medicine. The bark of the willow was chewed to relieve fevers, pains and rheumatism; the active principle identified was salicylic acid (aspirin). The rosy periwinkle was originally thought to be useful for diabetes and eventually proved to be an effective antileukaemic agent.

Qinghaosu (*Artemisia annua* L.), also known as annual or sweet wormwood in the Western world, has a variety of medical uses, including the treatment of fevers and haemorrhoids, and as an antimalarial. The active principle is artemisinin, a sesquiterpine.

Herbal remedies contain active principles in varying amounts which are dependent on the way in which the plant is grown and stored and the specific characteristics of the individual plant. Herbs must be precisely identified and given in the correct amount to minimise the risk of toxicity. This was apparent in the development of digitalis from the foxglove, which had varying efficacy until effective biological assays and digoxin were developed.

ADVERSE EFFECTS

The traditional herbal cures are not without their complications, which may include hepatic and renal failure. Comfrey, a traditional cure for broken bones, bronchitis and ulcers, contains chemicals that may cause liver cancer. The purple pennyroyal, taken for indigestion, headaches and menstrual pain, contains substances causing irritation of the skin and urinary tract, and possibly abortion. Many people believe that garlic is protective against ischaemic heart disease, but garlic may cause allergic skin reactions. The onion has well-known effects on the tear glands, inducing crying in the cook. The

betel-nut or supari is widely used in India, chewed alone or as 'pan', which is a mixture of supari, lime and sometimes tobacco. There is a causal relationship between this habit and oral cancer. Qat, commonly chewed in Somalia and other countries in the Horn of Africa, has addictive properties. The most potent form of qat, miraa, grows on small farms alongside coffee and tea plants. Reddish-green twigs are plucked from the trees daily and placed in bundles which must be used rapidly as they wither and lose potency. The average user may chew bundles of 100 fresh twigs a day.

Table 17.1 details some hazards of traditional herbal remedies.

The secondary metabolites in plants are important in pharmacological amounts in herbal medicine. However, both in the eating of fruit and vegetables and in herbal medicine these chemicals interact with pharmaceutical drugs (Table 17.2). Beneficial or adverse interactions may also occur with less easily identified nutritional components.

Various interactions may occur:

- absorption interactions
- protein binding interactions
- metabolic interactions, including competing for the same enzyme (competitive inhibition interactions)
- induction of metabolic processes
- effects on excretion (biliary, faecal or urinary), either by altering metabolism to the excretion product, or by changing transport across membranes, e.g. kidney tubules.

CAFFEINE

Caffeine is currently the most used plant chemical that does not have a nutritional benefit. It has a variety of physiological and psychological actions that are thought to be mediated by the blockade of adenosine receptors. The direct central nervous-stimulating effect of caffeine has not been established, yet such an action is widely believed to occur. Increased alertness, and improved mood and behaviour are well-recognised and valued responses to caffeine-containing drinks. The elimination of caffeine from the body is dependent on acetylation, a process that is genetically determined to be either

Table 17.1 Traditional remedies and modern warnings

Plant	Traditional remedy	Modern warnings
Monkshood	Sedative	Poisonous in excess
Camomile	Sedative	Skin rashes
Cuckoo pint	Aphrodisiac	Poisonous in excess
Greater celandine	Treatment of liver complaints	Poisonous in excess
Broom	Laxative	Poisonous; large doses can cause abortion
Larkspur	Treatment of skin parasites	Poisonous in excess
Fox glove	Treatment of heart complaints	Poisonous in excess
Lily of the valley	Treatment of heart complaints	Poisonous in excess
Alder, buckthorn	Treatment of constipation	Poisonous in excess
Ivy	Treatment of hangovers	Poisonous in excess
St John's wort	Sedative; treatment of depression	Skin blisters
Juniper	Improved eyesight	Irritates the intestine
Colts foot	Treatment respiratory problems	Linked to liver cancer
Mistletoe	Sedative	Gastroenteritis and/or liver damage

Table 17.2 Interactions between plant chemicals and other substances

Plant chemical	Substances affected	Effects
Alcohol	Antidepressants	Increased sedation
Vitamin K in broccoli, spinach, lettuce, Brussels sprouts	Anticoagulants	Problems with anticoagulant control
Solanaceous glycoalkaloids in potatoes, tomatoes, aubergines	Slow the metabolism of muscle relaxants and anaesthetic agents, e.g. suxamethonium, mivacurium and cocaine	Alters the sensitivity to anaesthetic agents used for surgery
Grapefruit juice, unknown effector	Omeprazole	Alters omeprazole metabolism and reduces its plasma concentration
Cranberry juice, unknown effector	Not known	Beneficial effects for urinary tract infections
Glycyrrhic acid in liquorice	Interferes with 17β-hydroxysteroid dehydrogenase	Raised blood pressure

slow or fast. Slow acetylators will accumulate caffeine, with the potential for intolerance, whereas fast acetylators may never achieve such concentrations.

Vegetables in the brassica (cabbage) family are known stimulators of the cytochrome P450 enzyme system in the liver. Several consecutive helpings of cabbage will reduce the half-life of caffeine by approximately 20%, illustrating the interaction between dietary constituents and the metabolism of xenobiotic compounds.

Glucuronolactone may be used as an additive to caffeine drinks. This synthetic stimulant was first used by the US military in Vietnam by tired soldiers and causes profound central nervous system complications.

KEY POINTS

1. Ethnobiology is the study of the traditional lore of plants and animals, the wisdom of the ancients. Some 10% of all plant species are used medicinally. Herbs, traditionally added to food, have effects that are distinct from their flavour-enhancing properties. Many herbal substances have non-nutritional properties: physiological, pharmacological and pathological.
2. Herb nomenclature includes the English common name, the transliteration of the herb name, the Latinised pharmaceutical name and the scientific name.
3. Traditional plant remedies include the bark of the willow, which was chewed; its active principles include salicylic acid (aspirin). Herbal remedies contain active principles in varying amounts which are dependent on specific characteristics of the plant and how it is grown and stored.
4. Plants may have adverse effects on hepatic and renal function and may be carcinogenic.
5. Caffeine is the most ubiquitous plant chemical that has no nutritional benefit but has a variety of physiological and psychological effects.

THINKING POINT

While it is important to eat five different pieces of fruit and vegetables a day, these food sources are different and contain an array of chemicals which are developed to function in a different context than in humans. It is therefore important to vary the plant sources in the diet.

NEED TO UNDERSTAND

1. Plants are a mix of essential nutrients and other chemicals that may not be so nutritious.
2. The science of phytochemistry is very important in the contribution of vegetables to the diet.

FURTHER READING

But, P.P. (1993) Need for correct identification of herbs in herbal poisoning. *Lancet*, **341**, 637.

Depeint, F., Gee, J.M., Williamson, G. and Johnson, I.T. (2002) Evidence for consistent patterns between flavonoid structures and cellular activities. *Proceedings of the Nutrition Society*, **61**, 97–103.

D'Mello, J.P.F., Duffus, C.M. and Duffus, J.H. (eds) (1991) *Toxic Substances in Crop Plants*. Royal Society of Chemistry, Cambridge.

Izzo, A.A. and Ernst, E. (2001) Interactions between herbal medicines and prescribing drugs: a systematic review. *Drugs*, **61**, 2163–75.

James, J.E. (1991) *Caffeine and Health*. Academic Press, London.

Schenker, S. (2001) Cranberries. *British Nutrition Foundation, Nutrition Bulletin*, **26**, 115–16.

Tassaneeyakul, W., Vannaprasaht, S. and Yamazoe, Y. (2000) Formation of omeprazole sulphone but not 5-hydroxyomeprazole is inhibited by grapefruit juice. *British Journal of Clinical Pharmacology*, **49**, 139–44.

Thurnham, D. (1996) Physiologically active substances in plant food. *Proceedings of the Nutrition Society*, **55**, 371–46.

Walker, B.R. and Edwards, C.R. (1994) Licorice-induced hypertension and syndromes of apparent mineralocorticoid excess. *Endocrinology Metabolism Clinics of North America*, **23**, 359–77.

WEBSITE

www.ars-grin.gov/duke   Duke's phytochemical ethno-database

18

Water, electrolytes, minerals and trace elements

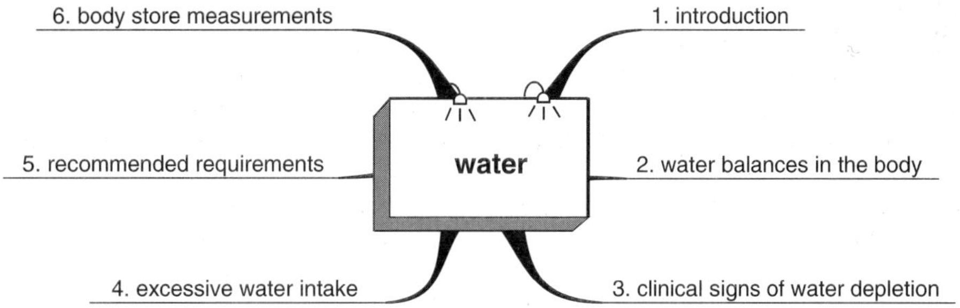

Fig. 18.1 Section outline.

INTRODUCTION

Water is the basic chemical of life, acting both as a bulk and a localised solvent for the body. Water is an angular molecule with two vertical planes of symmetry, and is an acceptor and donator of protons. Water freezes at 0°C to form ice (a stable phase), with a variety of structural formations. The chemical potential of ice is much less than that of liquid water. As water is warmed the structure becomes more open and has a maximum volume at 4°C. Water molecules are held apart by hydrogen bonds between structures.

Water readily dissolves a number of chemicals and such solubility is important in biological processes:

- cell structure
- blood

- excretory systems, e.g. urine and bile.

Equally important are water-insoluble lipid phases, which form separate and distinct functional units:

- cell membranes
- hydrophobic domains in enzymes.

The charges on the water molecule allow other atoms and molecules to be variably charged.

Solutions

A solution is a homogeneous mixture of two components. In a solution atoms of A, the solute, are surrounded by atoms of B, the solvent, and other atoms of A. A sample of the solution, however small, will be representative of the whole.

In solution, ions will be positively or negatively charged and often the water provides the complementary charge to the ion. The solution must be electrically neutral and the counter-ions move over each other, anion over cation and cation over anion, to create a neutral ionic atmosphere.

Osmolality and osmolarity

Osmolality is a measure of the number of osmoles of solute per kilogram of solvent. Osmolarity is the number of osmoles per litre of fluid. Thus, 1 mmol of a non-polar solute, e.g. sucrose, gives a 1 mosmol solution; 1 mmol of a salt, e.g. NaCl, dissociates to give two ions and therefore a 2 mosmol solution. In the body the major contributors to osmolality are sodium, and its anions chloride, bicarbonate and sulfate, and glucose and urea.

Osmolality is measured in the blood and urine by depression of freezing point measurements; 1 g molecule of any non-ionised substance in 1 kg water is equal to 1 osmol. For monovalent ions 1 equivalent weight has an osmolality of 1 osmol; for divalent ions 0.5 osmol. A mixture can be identified in terms of the total concentration of ions.

Function

Water is the major solute for the processes of metabolism and life. Water forms 50–60% of body weight. One-third is extracellular fluid, and two-thirds are intracellular (e.g. in a 65 kg man, 15 and 30 litres, respectively). These compartments are separated by cell membranes, often freely permeable to water movement, dictated by osmolality.

Water as a solvent

In any given situation the water molecule is surrounded by other molecules or atoms. In pure water, other water molecules surround each molecule at the corner of a tetrahedron, similar to the formation of ice. Other chemicals may dissolve in water to a varying extent, dependent on ions, molecular charge and hydration, which is the ability to tolerate a shell of water molecules. Water is the solvent, and the substance dissolved is the solute. Solutes will dissolve to varying degrees in water. Sucrose and salt are very soluble in water, whereas triacylglycerides are very insoluble. A large protein molecule will have regions that associate with water (hydrophilic) and other regions that are hydrophobic and are not associated with water. Phase diagrams can be constructed to portray the solubility of one or several solutes in a solvent at differing concentrations of each solute. Various thermodynamically stable boundaries will develop where the phases will exist in equilibrium, e.g. soluble, partially insoluble and totally insoluble.

The body is a complex phase diagram with differing areas defined by boundaries, osmolality and solubilities. The movement of substances between these phases, e.g. intracellular and extracellular, is important metabolically and physiologically. Water crosses plasma membranes by two mechanisms, diffusion through the lipid layer and transit through water-selective channels. Water channels, aquaporins, enable the rapid transport of water across the water-resistant cell membranes in response to osmotic gradients. These channels are important in physiological processes such as renal water conservation, neurohomoeostasis, digestion, regulation of body temperature and reproduction. In mammals there are at least ten families of water channels. The channel consists of a long hydrophobic pore and a minimal number of solute binding sites which facilitate rapid water transport.

WATER BALANCES IN THE BODY

Homoeostasis of water ensures that water intake meets metabolic requirements and losses. Humans meet their requirements for water by drinking at regular intervals. This is dictated by social habits, or by drinking water after or during meals, stimulated by thirst and regulated by water-retention mechanisms through antidiuretic hormone (ADH, vasopressin), regulated by enteroreceptors.

Water is absorbed throughout the gastrointestinal tract. Water by mouth is largely absorbed in the jejunum by a process that is passive, although glucose and sodium dependent, but is also absorbed in the colon. Water absorption occurs largely through the paracellular pathways in the jejunum. There is also transcellular water flow by lipid-mediated osmosis. Over 2 litres of intestinal fluid enters the caecum, but only small amounts, normally in the order of 10–300 ml, are excreted in the faeces.

Oral water has substantial effects in increasing blood pressure, depending on the health status of an individual. After drinking 500 ml (1 pint) of water, the response varies from 10 to 100 mm Hg, starting to rise minutes after the water is drunk, peaking at 20 min, remaining raised for 25 min and returning to normal in 80 min.

Water is lost from the body as urine, in faeces, and by evaporation from the skin and lungs. The visible water loss is readily measured as urine and faecal water, although the faecal water weight is usually very small. The sensation of thirst and the drinking of water depend on an equilibrium between fluid intake and fluid loss.

The amount lost from the skin and lungs is very temperature dependent. Sweating is an important cause of water loss, with rates as high as 2500 ml/h in hot climates. Water loss of 500 ml/h is not unusual. Expired air is saturated with water vapour and the water loss is in the order of 300 ml/day. When the air is very dry or during hyperventilation, losses may be considerably increased. The evaporative water loss is 'invisible weight loss', which is the weight of food and liquid consumed plus or minus any change in body weight, minus the weight of urine and faeces. The evaporation water loss equals the invisible water loss, minus the weight of carbon dioxide expired plus the weight of carbon dioxide absorbed.

Water is also lost through the gastrointestinal tract. In Britain the usual faecal weight is 50–300 g/day, but in diarrhoea the water loss may become considerable, as in cholera. Other causes of profound loss are intestinal fistulae and persistent vomiting. In such diarrhoeal states, body fluid volume may be lost very quickly, with fatal results.

Renal excretion of water is, in part, dependent on fluid intake, which in turn determines urine output. Urine is more concentrated than blood and there are renally induced concentration mechanisms. The blood usually has an osmolality of just under 300 mosmol/kg and urine of around 1200 mosmol/kg. The main constituents of the urine are 80% nitrogen endproducts and sodium chloride, although many other substances are present. These account for less than 50% of the osmolality.

Osmolality in the urine is also under the regulation of the posterior pituitary gland, ADH and osmoreceptors present in the hypothalamus.

Thirst

During thirst there is increased secretion of ADH from the neurohypophysis. During severe water shortage and dehydration, the person craves water. The physiological situations that arouse thirst and hypersecretion of ADH are:

- deficit of water without corresponding loss of sodium (hypovolaemic hypernatraemia)
- osmotic shift of water from the cells to the extracellular fluid, due to excess sodium intake (hypervolaemic hypernatraemia).

In both situations cellular dehydration, hyperosmolar body fluids and increased extracellular sodium concentration are evident. Dehydration causes increased osmotic pressure in the blood and in severe instances in cells, and consequent thirst and ADH secretion. Some 90% of the osmolality of the interstitial fluid and the blood plasma is provided by sodium and associated anions. Sodium is excreted continuously from cells in exchange for potassium by active enzymatic cation transport. The osmotic regulation of water intake in part controls the normal plasma sodium concentration. There is a close relationship between plasma ADH concentration and plasma osmolality.

The thirst threshold provides an effective, comprehensive mechanism or stimulus to drink water in response to the increase in plasma ADH when the renal action of the hormone can no longer prevent an undue increase in plasma sodium and

---

Diet and urine osmolality

In general, the effect of diet on urine osmolality is: 1 g of dietary nitrogen leads to approximately 2 g of urea. Therefore, when an individual eats 100 g/day of protein, this yields 30 g of urea and results in urine with an osmolality of 500 mosmol. Thus, 2 g of sodium chloride will give an osmolar load of 340 mosmol. The protein and salt in the diet will lead to a urine osmolality of 840 mosmol. To excrete this with an osmolality of 1200 mosmol, the individual must pass 830 ml of urinary water, which is the obligatory water required to dissolve the chemicals excreted by the kidney. The additional water excreted, which reflects excess fluid intake, is known as free water.

Osmolality and thirst

The average normal plasma osmolality is
287 mosmol/kg. A 2% increase in total body water
suppresses ADH secretion below detectable levels,
and induces maximal urine excretion and dilution.
The thirst threshold is reached at 2% deficit of body
water, average plasma osmolality 294 mosmol/kg,
and ADH secretion increases.

osmolality. The renal mechanism provides fine tuning.

In addition to osmotic regulation and ADH release, water intake is regulated by the volume of fluid. Volume regulators include the effective circulating blood volume, the cardiovascular reflexes and the renal renin–angiotensin system. This volume regulation is secondary to osmotic regulation during moderate fluctuations in the extracellular fluid volume. More than 20% of the blood volume needs to be lost before the thirst mechanism becomes activated. About a 10% reduction of the blood volume is required before there is an increase in plasma ADH. Afferent impulses moderate the osmotic regulation of water intake and ADH secretion. This regulation is predominantly through cerebral sensors, which are stimulated when the carotid blood osmolality is increased with sodium salts and other cell-dehydrating substances, e.g. fructose and sucrose. The sensors for thirst and ADH secretion appear to be located close to the cerebroventricular system, particularly in the anterior wall of the third ventricle of the brain. Arterial baroreceptors and left heart arterial pressure receptors create a tonic inhibition of neurohypophyseal ADH release.

Thirst is not satisfied until sufficient water has been absorbed to bring the activity of cerebral sensors to a level below that required to stimulate drinking. Drinking-induced temporary depression of the thirst drive is activated mainly in the mouth and pharangeal region, and also from the stomach, suggesting that mechanical, thermal and chemical factors are involved. It is possible that there are water taste fibres in the oropharangeal region. If too much fluid is drunk then a water diuresis follows.

A craving for water that persists in the absence of known osmotic and non-osmotic thirst is called primary polydipsia.

CLINICAL SIGNS OF WATER DEPLETION

Water depletion may result from a lack of available water, an inability to ingest water or increased losses from the skin, lungs, alimentary tract and urine. These occur in association with a hot environment, excessive exercise, hyperventilation, high altitudes, prolonged vomiting and diarrhoea, osmotic diuresis (as in diabetes mellitus) and loss from fistulae or nasogastric tube suction.

Evidence of loss of water includes: the features (particularly the eyes) are sunken, the skin and tongue are dry, and the skin becomes loose and lacks elasticity. A useful symptom and sign is a reduced urine output; this indicates the need for increased water intake. The most important sign, however, is haemoconcentration, in which there is an increase in the blood urea and possibly, but not always, increased plasma sodium and potassium.

In severe water loss, caused for example by diarrhoea in cholera and other enteric infections, oral water with glucose and sodium chloride is the basis of therapy and restoration of fluid volume.

EXCESSIVE WATER INTAKE

Excess water intake may rapidly induce hyponatraemia and cause pulmonary oedema. Alternatively, cerebral damage may lead to essential hypernatraemia, in which there is an effect on the osmotic regulation of water intake and ADH release.

Water on its own is drunk in excess only in illness (polydipsia). More frequently, fluid intake is dictated by social circumstances and the vehicle for the water, e.g. alcoholic beverages, tea or coffee. The effect of excess then becomes entwined with the congener, e.g. alcohol or caffeine. An immediate effect of increased fluid intake is increased urinary output, which is dictated by plasma osmolality, plasma ADH concentration and urinary osmolality.

If an individual drinks water in excess, symptoms do not occur until the plasma sodium concentration falls below 120 mmol/l. Confusion and headache may be followed by coma and fits in extreme instances.

Oxytocin infusions can occasionally result in severe and dangerous water intoxication in pregnant women.

Abnormal fluid intakes are usually due to abnormalities in one or several of the control mechanisms.

Conditions associated with abnormal water balance

Diabetes insipidus
- **Primary**: this condition results from an abnormality of the synthesis, storage or release of ADH in the anterior hypothalamus of the brain.
- **Secondary**: this usually follows damage to the hypothalamus, e.g. by trauma or birth injury, during some procedures, or as a result of tumour growth, abscess formation, infection or vascular thrombosis.

Psychogenic polydipsia
Drinking bouts alternate with normal intake. This results in varying plasma osmolality, unlike the constant large urine output and consistently reduced plasma osmolality of diabetes insipidus. Fluid intake may exceed 40 litres/day, with attendant low osmolalities of under 240 mosmol.

Psychoactive drugs
Drugs used in the treatment of depression and schizophrenia, e.g. thioridazine, amitriptyline and chlorpromazine, cause dryness of the mouth with resultant polydipsia.

Ecstasy (3,4-methylenedioxymethamphetamine, MDMA) has metabolic effects over and above the mood-enhancing effects of other drugs used at dance events (raves), e.g. lysergic acid diethylamide (LSD), herbal ecstasy, khat and Eve. Ecstasy has mild amphetamine stimulant actions which release brain messenger transmitters, especially serotonin (5-hydroxytryptamine). This results in increased wakefulness, euphoria, sexual activity, adrenaline release with tachycardia, raised blood pressure and metabolic hyperactivity. Exercise increases these pharmacological effects, which may result in malignant hyperthermia and severe dehydration, especially if there is little access to fluids. Death

results from hyponatraemia, convulsions and acute renal failure. Rarely there is a consequence of rapid release of ADH from the pituitary, which can lead to brain damage or death. In this variant condition, excess water is contraindicated.

Renal resistance to antidiuretic hormone
This is found in inherited nephrogenic diabetes insipidus, potassium depletion and hypercalcaemia, and may be induced by drugs, e.g. lithium carbonate (in 40% of patients), dimethylchlortetracycline, amphotericin B, methoxyfluorane anaesthesia, propoxyphene and gentamicin.

Kidney disease
Kidney disease of all types reflects an inability to concentrate urine.

Solute diuresis
This is one of the cardinal symptoms in diabetes mellitus (glucose) and uraemia (urea). In these conditions there is increased excretion of the problem chemical, e.g. glucose or urea, and a large volume of water is necessary to dissolve and remove these, with a consequential to loss of water.

RECOMMENDED REQUIREMENTS

Adults

Water intake includes fluid drunk and the water in food. In addition, metabolic water is produced by the oxidation of carbohydrates, protein and fat:

- 1 g starch produces 0.60 g water
- 1 g protein produces 0.41 g water
- 1 g fat produces 1.07 g water.

Fluid intake is usually in the order of 2–2.5 litres/day for the average adult in a temperate climate. This intake will be affected by temperature, activity, diet and health.

Babies

The renal system of newborn babies takes several days to adjust to extrauterine life. During the first 2 days, daily urine output is around 20 ml. By 2 weeks, daily output is 200 ml, with a milk intake of 500 ml. At 3 months the daily milk intake is 800–900 ml and urine output 300 ml. Loss by evaporation is high because of the high surface area:body weight ratio.

The elderly

The secretory response to ADH with water deprivation is increased in the elderly; thirst is therefore less of a feature in the elderly. Urinary incontinence may be a problem in the elderly and fluid intake may be restricted, a strategy that does not help the problem. It is important to monitor fluid intake in the elderly as fluid requirements are unchanged.

BODY STORE MEASUREMENTS

Body stores are dependent on fluid intake and urinary output. Methods to quantify water stores include:

- monitoring of body weight over a set period, with water intake/output volume measurements
- blood urea levels
- blood osmolality
- tritiated water dilution studies.

KEY POINTS

1. Water is both a bulk and a localised solvent for the body. Water is an angular molecule with two vertical planes of symmetry, and is an acceptor and donor of protons.
2. Water is the basic chemical of life and readily dissolves a number of chemicals. Such solubility is important in biological processes, cell structure, blood and excretory systems, e.g. urine, bile.
3. The body is a complex phase system with differing areas defined by boundaries of osmolality and by solubilities. The movement of substances between these phases is important metabolically and physiologically.
4. Water forms 50–60% of body weight. One-third is extracellular fluid and two-thirds are intracellular. These compartments are separated by cell membranes, often freely permeable to water movement, dictated by osmolality.

5. Humans satisfy their requirements for water by drinking habits that are not necessarily dependent on true thirst. The efficient thirst mechanism and regulation of the water retention through antidiuretic hormone (ADH, vasopressin) are important for water balance.
6. It is essential to well-being that the body contains an appropriate amount of water. Insufficient or too much water, or reduced or excessive loss, results in well-characterised clinical conditions. Such imbalances can result from both natural and pathological causes.

THINKING POINTS

1. Fluid balance, i.e. fluid intake and loss, is an important measurement in health and disease.
2. The prime sources of loss will vary.

NEED TO UNDERSTAND

1. Water is central to life and the body pool of water is very defined.
2. The control mechanisms for water homoeostasis are important.

FURTHER READING

Anderson, B., Leksell, L.G. and Rundgren, M. (1982) Regulation of water intake. *Annual Review of Nutrition*, **2**, 73–89.

Atkin, P.W. (1990) *Physical Chemistry*, 4th edn. Oxford University Press, Oxford.

Borgnia, M., Nielsen, S., Engel, A. and Agre, P. (1999) Cellular and molecular biology of the aquaporin water channels. *Annual Review of Biochemistry*, **68**, 425–58.

Bourque, C.W. and Oliet, S.H.R. (1997) Osmoreceptors in the central nervous system. *Annual Review of Physiology*, **59**, 601–19.

Desjeux, J.F., Nath, S.K. and Taminiau, J. (1994) Organic substrate and electrolyte solutions for oral rehydration in diarrhoea. *Annual Review of Nutrition*, **14**, 321–42.

Errington, J.R. and Debenedetti, P.G. (2001) relationship between structural order and the anomalies of liquid water. *Nature*, **409**, 318–21.

Kirk, K. and Strange, K. (1998) Functional properties and physiological roles of organic solute channels. *Annual Review of Physiology*, **60**, 719–39.

Lichtenberger, L.M. (1995) The hydrophobic barrier properties of gastrointestinal mucus. *Annual Review of Physiology*, **57**, 565–83.

Mathias, C.J. (2000) A 21st century water cure. *Lancet*, **356**, 1046–7.

Spring, K.R. (1998) Routes and mechanism of fluid transport by epithelia. *Annual Review of Physiology*, **60**, 105–19.

Sui, H., Han, B.-G., Lee, J.K. and Jap, B.K. (2001) Structural basis of water-specific transport through the AQP1 water channel. *Nature*, **414**, 872–8.

Ward, D.T., Hammond, T.G. and Harris, H.W. (1999) Modulation of vasopressin-elicited water transport by trafficking of aquaporin2-containing vesicles. *Annual Review of Physiology*, **61**, 683–97.

Weatherall, D.J., Ledingham, J.G.G. and Warren, D.A. (eds) (1996) *Oxford Textbook of Medicine*, 3rd edn. Oxford Medical Publications, Oxford.

ELECTROLYTES AND MINERALS

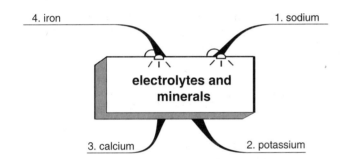

Fig. 18.2 Section outline.

SODIUM

Introduction

The distribution of sodium in the body is quite distinct from that of potassium, despite their total body pools being similar.

- Atomic weight, 23; valency 1
- natural isotope, 23
- relative abundance in Earth's crust, 2.64%.

A common source of sodium in the diet is salt, added to food at the table, in cooking, and in processed foods. Salt is an important food preservative that has always been used for preserving meat and fish, to provide food during long winters and periods of hardship.

The sodium content of natural food varies between 0.1 and 3.3 mmol/100 g. In contrast, processed foods have a sodium content of 11–48 mmol/100 g, partly for taste and partly because sodium nitrate is used as a preservative.

Function

Sodium is a major cation and contributor to the osmolality of the extracellular fluid of the body, which is one-third of the body water in adults.

Because the body is a multiphasic system divided into distinct separate compartments, controlled transport between these compartments is important.

Molecules may pass down a concentration gradient by diffusion, or move by active transport against a concentration gradient, i.e. active energy-requiring transport. Sodium is concentrated in the extracellular fluid, giving osmolarity and charge properties to the sodium. Therefore, when sodium

Group	1	2	3	4	5	6	7	8	9	10	11	12	13	14	15	16	17	18
Period																		
1	1 H																	2 He
2	3 Li	4 Be											5 B	6 C	7 N	8 O	9 F	10 Ne
3	11 Na	12 Mg											13 Al	14 Si	15 P	16 S	17 Cl	18 Ar
4	19 K	20 Ca	21 Sc	22 Ti	23 V	24 Cr	25 Mn	26 Fe	27 Co	28 Ni	29 Cu	30 Zn	31 Ga	32 Ge	33 As	34 Se	35 Br	36 Kr
5	37 Rb	38 Sr	39 Y	40 Zr	41 Nb	42 Mo	43 Tc	44 Ru	45 Rh	46 Pd	47 Ag	48 Cd	49 In	50 Sn	51 Sb	52 Te	53 I	54 Xe
6	55 Cs	56 Ba	71 Lu	72 Hf	73 Ta	74 W	75 Re	76 Os	77 Ir	78 Pt	79 Au	80 Hg	81 Ti	82 Pb	83 Bi	84 Po	85 At	86 Rn
7	87 Fr	88 Ra	103 Lr	104 Rf	105 Db	106 Sg	107 Bh	108 Hs	109 Mt	110 Uun	111 Uuu	112 Uub	113 Uut	114 Uuq	115 Uup	116 Uuh	117 Uus	118 Uuo
–																		
Lanthanides			57 La	58 Ce	59 Pr	60 Nd	61 Pm	62 Sm	63 Eu	64 Gd	65 Tb	66 Dy	67 Ho	68 Er	69 Tm	70 Yb		
Actinides			89 Ac	90 Th	91 Pa	92 U	93 Np	94 Pu	95 Am	96 Cm	97 Bk	98 Cf	99 Es	100 Fm	101 Md	102 No		

Fig. 18.3 Periodic table. Elements with biological roles are highlighted.

moves from the extracellular fluid into cells there is a change in charge and concentration. This becomes important in the following mechanisms.

- **Direct active transport**: sodium is important in the transport of chemicals across selectively permeable cell membranes. The cell cytosol contains a high concentration of potassium and the extracellular fluid a high concentration of sodium. These concentration differences are due to the active transport of both ions by the Na^+/K^+-ATPase transporter. With adenosine triphosphate (ATP) providing the energy, three Na^+ ions are pumped out of the cell and two K^+ are pumped in. This leaves a charge and concentration differential. The resting potential prepares nerve and muscle cells for the propagation of action potentials necessary for nerve impulses and muscle contraction. One-third of the energy generated by mitochondria is used to drive the ATPase pump.
- **Voltage-gated ion channels**: in the excitable cells, e.g. neurones and muscle, channels open and close in response to changes in the charge across

the cell membrane. When a nerve impulse passes down a neurone or a cardiac muscle strand, the voltage opens sodium channels in the adjacent portion of the membrane. Sodium (Na^+) influxes into the cell and the change in charge allows the impulse to travel. Sodium penetrates more rapidly than potassium, which increases the electrical charge. The sodium is then pumped out. This channel remains open for 1 ms.
- **Active transport**: the increase in concentration of sodium outside the cell is accompanied by water.
- **Indirect active transport**: This utilises the downhill flow of an ion, often sodium, to pump other molecules or ions against its gradient. The sodium is then returned by the Na^+/K^+-ATPase exchange pump system. The concentration gradient of Na^+ releases energy to run indirect pumps.

Glucose and amino acids cross the cell membrane by a process of facilitated diffusion in response to this concentration gradient. This is dependent on carrier molecules, against a concentration gradient, achieved by the sodium co-transport system.

Na$^+$/K$^+$-ATPase exchange pump system

There is an influx of two potassium ions as three sodium ions are pumped out. In this way, the negative potential within the cell is maintained. The presence of Mg-ATP is essential for this transport system. Energy for the carrier is provided by ATP hydrolysis and a sodium/potassium-ATPase enzyme. The Na$^+$/K$^+$-ATPase exchange pump system consists of two subunits. The α-subunit ($\sim$113 kDa) binds ATP, Na$^+$ and K$^+$, and is controlled by a phosphorylation kinase system which, in turn, is controlled by hormone action, thyroid, aldosterone, catecholamines and insulin. The β-unit ($\sim$35 kDa) activates and places the α-subunit. Both subunits exist in different isoforms.

The α-subunit is a receptor for digitalis and ouabain, and the binding affinities are different for different isoforms.

Oral rehydration solutions

A solution of 90 mmol/l of sodium and sugar, or rice powder of 30 g/l for adults; and 30 mmol/l of sodium for infants and the very ill has been recommended by some authorities. Potassium at 20 mmol/l is important. Bicarbonate at 30 mmol/l is helpful in correcting the metabolic acidosis in severe dehydration.

The binding of glucose to the cell membrane carrier is increased in the presence of sodium. Sodium is present in high concentrations at the luminal border of the membrane, but concentrations at the inner cell surface are kept low by the Na$^+$/K$^+$ exchange pump. When the carrier–sugar–sodium complex reaches the inside of the cell the glucose leaves the carrier, the affinity of the receptor for glucose falls, the sugar is released and the sodium is pumped back outside (by the sodium-dependent hexose transporter, SGLUT-1).

Treatment of sodium and water loss
The glucose absorption system is important in the intestine, and is exploited in the readily available and cheap resuscitation of dehydrated infant with cholera and other diarrhoeal states.

In the severe loss of water and sodium through infectious diarrhoea of a secretory nature, e.g. *Vibrio cholerae* or enterotoxigenic coliforms, the initial treatment is with oral replacement solution (ORS, water, sodium and glucose) to replace the water volume. Following the absorption of the glucose and sodium from the intestinal lumen, water is absorbed by a passive process. Sucrose and rice powder are useful sources of carbohydrate. The additional benefit of rice powder, other than its

availability in poor areas of the world, is its constituent amino acids. Glycine (at 30 mg/100 g) stimulates sodium and water absorption. There is still debate over the correct concentration of sodium in ORS for adults and the young. In children there is the risk of engendering hypernatraemic dehydration.

Millions of babies have been saved by ORS, although the very ill may need to be admitted to hospital, where it is often necessary to give intravenous fluids that are isotonic with blood.

The products of the Krebs (tricarboxylic acid) cycle are moved about the cell using the Na$^+$/K$^+$ ATPase exchange pump system. All of the amino acids are transported using this system and iodide ions are pumped into the cells of the thyroid in a similar manner.

Absorption and availability of sodium

Intestinal sodium absorption is very efficient in both the small intestine and colon. Sodium is absorbed by a variety of processes. In the proximal intestine sodium is absorbed, in part by a solute-dependent cotransport system, and is involved in nutrient absorption. In the more distal intestine and colon, sodium absorption is by a sodium/hydrogen interchange; in the colon this process is coupled to chloride/bicarbonate exchange. In the distal intestine and colon the process is electroneutral and involves protein carriers. In the distal colon active sodium transport occurs against an electrochemical gradient.

Water absorption is a passive process that requires active transport of sodium and chloride. The optimum absorption of water occurs when the concentration of glucose in the intestinal lumen is around 110 mmol/l. This finding has been of great importance in the development of ORS.

Sodium content of the body

A male adult weighing 65–70 kg has a total body sodium content of 4 mol (100 g):

- 500 mmol (11.5 g) in intercellular fluid (concentration 2 mmol/l)
- 1500 mmol (34.5 g) in bone
- 2000 mmol (46 g) in extracellular fluid (concentration 130–145 mmol/l)
- daily dietary intake is 50–200 mmol (1.15–4.6 g).

Thirst

The requirement for salt, expressed as thirst sensation, is controlled by the adrenocorticotropic hormone (ACTH)-renal response to changes in plasma sodium concentration. Hyponatraemia reduces ADH secretion, which is followed by renal loss of water and correction. Hypernatraemia results in thirst and a desire to drink water. Changes in sodium concentration result from changes in water intake, rather than the converse.

Body sodium content is affected by renal regulation of urinary loss of sodium over a range of 1–500 mmol daily.

Sodium regulation

Most of the body's sodium pool is contained in the extracellular fluid compartment. Sodium is found in significant amounts in bone, but this pool is not readily available at times of rapid loss of sodium.

The extracellular fluid sodium content is regulated in parallel with the extracellular fluid volume control. The control of the latter is monitored by changes in pressure and distension in the cardiac atria and right ventricle, the pulmonary vasculature, the carotid arteries and the aortic arch. These activate centres in the medulla and hypothalamus of the brain. When the extracellular fluid or blood volume falls, neural sympathetic activity increases, and the response comprises vasoconstriction, a redistribution of renal blood flow, reduced glomerular filtration, and increased sodium and water retention. In addition, there are increases in renin production, circulating angiotensin II, noradrenaline, adrenaline, ACTH and ADH.

Sodium excretion

Sodium is filtered from the plasma in the kidneys, the reabsorption of sodium occurring as an osmotic phenomenon in the proximal tubule, loop of Henle and distal tubule. Distal tubular absorption is very important, and is under the control of atrial natriuretic factor. Renal sodium excretion is also controlled by angiotensin II, prostaglandins and the kallikrein–kinin system.

Sodium depletion

Sodium is lost largely via the urine, with only minimal loss occurring via the faeces or skin, unless there are abnormal situations such as diarrhoea or excessive sweating. A reduced body sodium pool results in reduced extracellular fluid volume.

Increased sodium loss in urine can occur in diseases, e.g. diabetes mellitus and Addison's disease (adrenal cortical insufficiency), following excessive doses of diuretic drugs, and in cases of renal tubular damage, as in chronic renal failure.

Sweating

Significant amounts of water and electrolytes may be lost during sweating. Up to 3 litres/h may be lost during continuous hard physical exercise. The sodium content of sweat is in the order of 20–80 mmol/l. Consequently, exercising hard in a hot climate may result in the loss of a significant amount of water and sodium. In situations where there is increased loss of sweat and exercise, e.g. marathon running, daily losses of sodium in the sweat may be up to 350 mmol.

Alimentary tract losses

It is possible to lose substantial amounts of water, sodium and potassium in diarrhoea. These losses may be rapid during infections such as cholera.

Clinical signs of sodium depletion

The signs of sodium depletion are often non-specific psychological and behavioural changes. The rate of decrease in body sodium is may be closely associated with the onset of these symptoms. A slow change is often more tolerable than a rapid loss.

In true sodium depletion there is an avid retention of sodium in the plasma, even if the concentration is reduced. This conservation is reflected by a urinary sodium of less than 10 mmol/24 h.

A low blood sodium is not always due to sodium depletion. In inappropriate ADH excess there is a normal body sodium but a retention of water; this leads to an apparent decrease in plasma sodium. The phenomenon is recognised by the plasma osmolality being reduced or the urinary sodium being more than 50 mmol over 24 h. Inappropriate ADH syndrome may be caused by malignancy, e.g. carcinoma of the lung, intakes of fluid in excess of urinary excretion or use of the drug ecstasy (see Psychoactive drugs, earlier in this chapter).

The normal excretion of water is 10–20 ml/min. Consistently more than this may be achieved by individuals with emotional problems and by high-consumption beer drinkers (beer drinker's potomania). Excessive intravenous administration of water with glucose, cardiac failure, cirrhosis and renal failure may produce a dilutional hyponatraemia.

Excess sodium intake

An excess of sodium leads to an increase in body extracellular volume, unless the excess sodium is cleared by the kidneys and urine. The most common cause is, however, secondary to water loss, or iatrogenic sodium excess. Insufficient water intake relative to sodium is also an important cause.

Infants can develop this problem if they are taking formula milk and the milk powder is made up with insufficient water, as the infant's ability to excrete sodium is slow to develop. With a high plasma sodium there is even a risk of infantile convulsions.

In adults, especially the elderly, congestive cardiac failure may occur with sodium and hence water retention.

Salt intake and blood pressure

There is a strong correlation between the average salt intake of a population and the incidence of high blood pressure and cardiovascular complications of high blood pressure, such as stroke. Other variables such as body weight, nutrition, cultural factors and smoking complicate this finding. An individual's blood pressure is not related to salt intake. Studies of spouses' salt intake and blood pressure do not support the salt and blood pressure theory. Reduction in salt intake does not reduce blood pressure except at very low intake, of under 10 mmol/day. However, conventional dietary wisdom is to reduce the intake of sodium to assist blood pressure control.

Recommended requirements

The dietary intake of sodium varies between populations (100–200 mmol/day in Britain). The recommended dietary intake is not universally agreed; suggested figures include a lower reference nutrient intake (LRNI) of sodium for adults of 25 mmol/day with a reference nutrient intake (RNI) of 70 mmol/day. The LRNI in infants up to 6 months, based on calculations for breast-fed infants, should be approximately 6 mmol/day, and the RNI 9–12 mmol/day.

Measurement of sodium status

The 24 h urinary excretion of sodium is generally a good indicator of dietary intake. Normal faecal excretion of sodium is approximately 2–4 mmol/day, and of little physiological consequence, although in diarrhoeal states the faecal sodium becomes significant and must be measured. The 24 h urinary excretion of sodium reflects 95–98% of dietary sodium intake. The within-person variability in sodium excretion is 30%; 24 h urine collections may be incomplete and hence there will be poor correlation between individual estimates of diet and urinary sodium excretion. For good correlations at least 7 days of urine collections and diet history or measurements are required.

KEY POINTS

1. The distribution of sodium and that of potassium in the body are quite distinct, while the total body pools are similar. Sodium is a major cation and contributor to the osmolality of the extracellular fluid of the body. Sodium is important in the transport of chemicals across cell mem-

branes. Sodium and potassium are exchanged across nerve membranes during nerve conduction.

2. The requirement for salt, or rather thirst sensation, is controlled by the adrenocorticotropic hormone–renal response to changes in plasma sodium concentration. Hyponatraemia reduces the secretion of antidiuretic hormone (ADH) which is followed by renal loss of water and correction. Hypernatraemia results in thirst and there is an increased water intake. Changes in sodium concentration result from changes in water intake, rather than the converse.

3. Sodium is lost in urine, sweat and minimally in faeces under a variety of physiological and pathological circumstances.

4. In severe secretory diarrhoea, oral replacement solutions (ORS), i.e. water with glucose, sucrose or rice powder (30 g/l) and sodium 90 mmol/l, or 30 mmol/l in infants, should be used to replenish sodium levels.

THINKING POINT

Salt is one of the proscribed elements in the diet. How strong is the evidence at a personal level, as opposed to a general statistical trend?

NEED TO UNDERSTAND

The central role that sodium and the Na^+/K^+-ATPase exchange pump system play in the maintenance of the compartments of the body. Such compartmentalisation is a prerequisite for a multicellular organism.

FURTHER READING

Catterall, W.A. (2001) A 3D view of sodium channels. *Nature*, **409**, 988–91.

Crill, W.E. (1996) Persistent sodium current in mammalian central neurons. *Annual Review of Physiology*, **58**, 349–62.

Dietary Reference Values for Food Energy and Nutrients for the United Kingdom (1991) Report on Health and Social Subjects, No. 41. HMSO, London.

Freedman, D.A. and Petitti, D.B. (2001) Salt and blood pressure. Conventional wisdom reconsidered. *Eval Review*, **25**, 267–87.

Kaplan, M.R., Mount, D.B., Delphire, E. *et al.* (1996) Molecular mechanisms of NaCl cotransport. *Annual Review of Physiology*, **58**, 649–68.

Kromhout, D. (2001) Epidemiology of cardiovascular diseases in Europe. *Public Health Nutrition*, **4**, 441–57.

Matalon, S. and O'Brodovich, H.(1999) Sodium channels in alveolar epithelial cells. *Annual Review Physiology*, **61**, 627–61.

Pajor, A.M. (1999) Sodium coupled transporters for Krebs cycle intermediates. *Annual Review of Physiology*, **61**, 663–82.

Swales, J. (2001) Salt, blood pressure and health. *Nutrition Bulletin*, **26**, 133–9.

Weatherall, D.J., Ledingham, J.G.G. and Warrell, D.A. (eds) (1996) *Oxford Textbook of Medicine*, 3rd edn. Oxford Medical Publications, Oxford.

POTASSIUM

Introduction

- atomic weight, 39; valency 1
- abundance in Earth's crust, 2.4%
- natural isotopes, 39, 40.

Availability

In natural and processed foods the potassium content varies from 2.8 to 10 mmol/kg. Dietary potassium tends to be derived from fresh vegetables and meat.

Function

The transport of potassium into cells is under the control of the Na/K-ATPase enzyme, and allows transport of potassium against a concentration gradient. The ratio of extracellular to intracellular potassium concentration is important in the membrane potential difference in neurone and muscle cells (see Na^+/K^+-ATPase exchange pump system, in the Sodium section).

Transport and absorption of potassium

Over 90% of dietary potassium is absorbed in the proximal small intestine. In the small intestine potassium absorption is passive, but in the colon it is an active process. In the sigmoid colon absorption is mediated by a K/H^+ mechanism.

Body stores of potassium

Most of the potassium is intracellular, i.e. in the cell fluid compartment. An adult male weighing approximately 70 kg contains 2800–3500 mmol (110–137 g), of which 95% is intracellular (150 mmol/l). Cellular potassium concentrations are affected by pH, aldosterone, insulin and the adrenergic nervous system.

The plasma concentration of 3.5–4.5 mmol/l is dependent on intake, excretion, and the balance between extracellular and intracellular compartments. There is a direct, reciprocal relationship between plasma potassium and aldosterone production. Control is mainly through urinary loss, with some additional colonic loss. Insulin excretion is increased when the plasma potassium increases, possibly provoking cellular uptake of potassium.

Potassium homoeostasis

The homoeostasis of potassium in the body is controlled by renal glomerular filtration and tubular secretion.

Chronic increased dietary potassium intake increases potassium secretion via the kidneys. There is an associated degree of hyperaldosteronism. Increased sodium entering the distal nephron results in an increased, simultaneous urinary loss of potassium.

Renal conservation of potassium

Proximal tubular reabsorption is partially an active process and is complete by the end of the proximal segment. There is potassium excretion in the pars recta and descending limb of the loop of Henle, with further control through absorption in the ascending limb.

Excretion

Potassium is largely lost in the urine, although 10% of the daily loss occurs through the distal ileum and colon. Small amounts are lost in sweat and vomit.

Potassium deficiency and excess

Deficiency

This can occur as a result of vomiting, diarrhoea and chronic usage of purgatives. It may also occur as a result of urine loss in wasting disease and starvation, overdosage with drugs (e.g. diuretics and corticosteroids), endocrine disturbances, aldosterone excess, Cushing's syndrome and hypertension. Deficiency may also occur in hepatic cirrhosis and renal disease.

During the breakdown of tissue, there is an important loss of potassium, e.g. in underfeeding, in diabetes and after injury. The loss of 1 kg muscle mass results in the loss of 105 mmol of potassium and 210 g of protein (equivalent to 34 g of nitrogen).

Potassium depletion results in muscular weakness and mental confusion, and is reflected in electrocardiographic changes and loss of smooth muscle motility, e.g. in the intestine.

Rarely, potassium deficiency is due to familial periodic paralysis, in which there is episodic oversecretion of aldosterone by the adrenal cortex. Such a non-specific diagnosis may be sought when there is excess vomiting or at any time when the patient's health appears compromised.

Excess

Plasma potassium concentrations in excess of normal may occur in total parenteral nutrition, on renal failure dialysis and in liver failure. If not corrected, cardiac arrhythmias and even cardiac arrest may result.

Recommended requirements

Habitual daily potassium intakes are maintained at suitable levels to ensure optimal metabolism of potassium. Reported potassium intakes by Western populations are in the range of 40–150 mmol/day. Potassium replacement, if necessary, should be gradual; a 4 g tablet of potassium chloride provides 53 mmol potassium.

Measurement of potassium status

The urinary excretion of potassium is generally a good indicator of dietary intake. Faecal losses vary from 5 to 13 mmol/day, which is approximately 11–15 % of the dietary intake. The within-person variation in potassium excretion is 24% for each 24 h collection. In populations where diarrhoea is endemic, potassium loss in the faeces may be 30% of the dietary intake.

Sources of inaccurate results in balance studies include losses through sweating and breast feeding.

KEY POINTS

1. The distribution of potassium in the body differs from that of sodium; body pools are, however, similar.
2. The extracellular:intracellular potassium ratio is important in the membrane potential difference in cells. Most of the potassium is in the cell fluid compartment.
3. The homoeostasis of potassium in the body is controlled by renal glomerular filtration and tubular secretion. Proximal tubular reabsorption is partially an active process and is complete by the end of the proximal segment.
4. Potassium is lost in urine or faeces under a variety of physiological and pathological circumstances.

THINKING POINT

Potassium is an intracellular ion and is dangerous in increased amounts in the extracellular fluid.

NEED TO UNDERSTAND

The role that potassium plays in the Na^+/K^+-ATPase exchange pump system.

FURTHER READING

Aldrich, R.W. (2001) Fifty years of inactivation. *Nature*, **411**, 643–4.

Barry, D.M. and Nerbonne, J.M. (1996) Myocardial potassium channels: electrophysiological and molecular diversity. *Annual Review of Physiology*, **58**, 363–94.

Benatar, M. (2000) Neurological potassium channelopathies. *Quarterly Journal of Medicine*, **93**, 787–97.

Dietary Reference Values for Food Energy and Nutrients for the United Kingdom (1991) Report on Health and Social Subjects, No. 41. HMSO, London.

Haddad, G.G. and Jiang, C. (1997) O_2-Sensing mechanisms in excitable cells: role of plasma membrane K^+ cells. *Annual Review of Physiology*, **59**, 23–43.

Lin, S.-H., Lin, Y.-F. and Halperin, M.L. (2001) Hypokalaemia and paralysis. *Quarterly Journal of Medicine*, **94**, 133–9.

Miller, C. (2001) See potassium run. *Nature*, **414**, 23–4.

Nichols, C.G. and Lopatin, A.N. (1997) Inward rectifier potassium channels. *Annual Review of Physiology*, **59**, 171–91.

Seino, S. (1999) ATP-sensitive potassium channels: a model of heteromultimeric potassium channel/receptor assembles. *Annual Review of Physiology*, **61**, 337–62.

Weatherall, D.J., Ledingham, J.G.G. and Warrell, D.A. (eds) (1996) *Oxford Textbook of Medicine*, 3rd edn. Oxford Medical Publications, Oxford.

CALCIUM

Introduction

- Atomic weight, 40; valency, 2
- natural isotopes, 40, 42, 43, 44, 46
- abundance in Earth's crust, 3.39%.

Availability

The most important source of dietary calcium is milk, which may provide over half of the required intake. The calcium content of milk is 35 mg/100 ml for human milk and 120 mg/100 ml for cow's milk. Other important sources of calcium include cheese (hard 400–1200 mg/100 g, soft 60–75 mg/100 g), nuts (13–250 mg/100 g), herring, vegetables, eggs, cereals and fruit (20–70 mg/100 g). Meat and rice are very modest sources.

Function

Calcium is concentrated in the organelles and blood, and is very important in the structure of the skeleton and maintenance of the extracellular fluid calcium concentration.

Skeletal calcium

A positive calcium balance is required before bone growth can occur. Calcium intake and skeletal modelling and turnover determine calcium balance during growth. The majority of the total calcium pool is contained in the bony skeleton, which contains some 1 kg of calcium (see Chapter 41).

Non-skeletal calcium function

Half of the plasma calcium (2.25–2.6 mmol/l) is ionised, the remainder being bound to albumin (40%) and globulin (10%). This ionised fraction affects humoral controls, which are important in dictating intestinal absorption, renal loss and calcium bone metabolism. A small (approximately 25 mmol) but very important part of the total calcium pool is that of calcium in soft tissues and extracellular fluid.

Intracellular concentrations of calcium are 100 times lower than those in the extracellular fluid. There is a substantial concentration of calcium in mitochondria. Hormonal and pharmacological activation of cells, membrane function and enzyme activity may all be affected by the local concentrations of calcium. Calcium is bound within the cell to enzyme proteins; this binding alters the protein configuration and hence enzyme activity. Calcium has a wide range of activity, being involved in muscle contraction, endocytosis, exocytosis, cell mobility, the movement of chromosomes and the release of neurotransmitters. Calcium acts as an intracellular messenger. A Ca^{2+} release messenger system involves the activation of phospholipase by acetylcholine and cholecystokinin, producing the messenger inositol 1,4,5-triphosphate (IP_3). Diacylglycerol is also produced in this hydrolysis reaction and activates protein kinase. This is a typical hormone and neurotransmitter system resulting in calcium release. Plasma membrane Na^+/Ca^{2+} exchange is an essential feature of Ca^{2+} signalling pathways, especially in the heart, where the exchange is important in cardiac contractility, and also in the kidney, smooth muscle and brain.

Activity is low in the liver. The Na^+/Ca^{2+} exchanger rapidly removes calcium from the cardiac myocytes, an effect determined by the Na^+/Ca^{2+} exchange gradient. In this, three Na^+ are exchanged for one Ca^{2+} resulting in one positive charge. The calcium entering the calcium channels is the prime trigger for cardiac contraction. The Na^+/Ca^{2+} exchanger is a member of a calcium exchanger superfamily.

Calcium-regulating hormones

The major regulating hormones for calcium are parathyroid hormone (PTH), calcitonin, vitamin D and, to a lesser extent, growth hormone, thyroid hormone, adrenal steroids, sex hormones and some gastrointestinal hormones.

Parathyroid hormone

PTH is secreted as a single peptide chain of 84 amino acids (molecular weight 5500 Da), of which only the first 32–34 amino acids have biological activity. Extra amino acids are attached for the pro-hormone format, and cleavage of these extra amino acids in the liver generates biological activity. The separated polypeptide fragments are degraded in the liver, kidney and skeleton. A reduction in the ionised calcium activates PTH excretion. Several hormones also influence PTH secretion. PTH directly affects body calcium through bone resorption, and kidney proximal and distal tubular calcium reabsorption.

PTH stimulates the 1-α-hydroxylase enzyme, which is involved in the hydroxylation of 25(OH)-vitamin D3 to 1,25(OH)$_2$-vitamin D$_3$, resulting in increased calcium absorption from the intestine.

Calcitonin

This consists of 32 amino acid residues with a disulfide bond between cystine residues in positions 1 and 7. Increased secretion from the parafollicular cells of the thyroid results from increases in blood calcium concentrations and from the actions of glucagon, gastrin and β-adrenergic hormones. Bone resorption is inhibited, and tubular resorption of calcium, sodium, phosphate, magnesium and potassium is decreased.

Calcitriol

Calcitriol [1,25(OH)$_2$-vitamin D] increases the

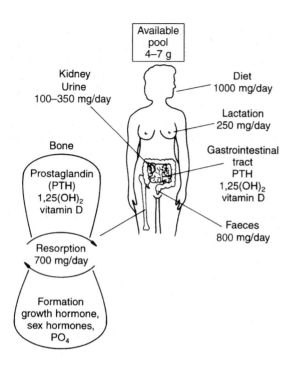

Fig. 18.4 Calcium fluxes in the body through the gastrointestinal tract, lactation, bones and urine. PTH: parathyroid hormone.

availability of calcium and phosphorus by increasing bone resorption.

Calcium absorption and balance

Calcium absorption is largely from the jejunum, but may also occur in the ileum and colon. The predominant absorptive process is by active transport and there is also some simple passive diffusion in the ileum. Calcium absorption is by paracellular and transcellular pathways. The transcellular pathway consists of:

- crossing the brush border
- transport through the cytoplasm complexed with specific calcium-binding proteins; these calcium-binding proteins are synthesised following the binding of a vitamin D metabolite to a nuclear receptor in the enterocyte
- active extrusion of calcium from the basolateral membrane into the bloodstream.

Calcium and phosphate may well be absorbed independently. Phosphorus has no effect on calcium absorption and retention. The average dietary intake of calcium is 25 mmol (1000 mg), of which 10 mmol is absorbed (Figure 18.4). The amount absorbed is highly dependent on age, skeletal and metabolic requirements. The amount absorbed and retained will be regulated by $1,25(OH)_2$-vitamin D_3, hormone and PTH activity. During infancy and adolescence, the time of maximum skeletal and overall growth, a greater proportion of the dietary calcium in the diet is absorbed than at other times of life. Intestinal absorption of calcium decreases with advancing age.

Phytate binds calcium to form insoluble salts within the intestinal lumen, and reduces calcium absorption. Phytic acid, a constituent of wholemeal flour, is the hexaphosphoric acid ester of inositol [(1,2,3,4,5)-(6-hexakis) (dihydrogen phosphate, *myo*-inositol)]. Calcium absorption is compromised when there is heavy dependence on wholemeal flour.

Fatty acids form insoluble soaps with calcium, although the effect on absorption of calcium is unknown.

Approximately 60% of the total plasma calcium is filtered in the kidney glomeruli, and in health 97% of this calcium is reabsorbed. Urine contains 100–350 mg of calcium per day (Figure 18.4). There is effective conservation and reabsorption of calcium by the proximal and distal renal tubules. Several hormones are involved, including PTH, with increased absorption of calcium and decreased tubular absorption of phosphate. This is achieved by cyclic adenosine monophosphate (cAMP) and activation of adenylate cyclase in the renal cortex. The proximal renal reabsorption of bicarbonate is decreased. All of these adjustments are determined by the dietary calcium, protein and sodium intake. Urinary calcium excretion figures are variable. If intestinal absorption is low, 70% of calcium is retained at low calcium intakes and 30% at high intake. Urinary excretion of calcium varies proportionally with dietary protein. With age there is a reduction in calcium glomerular filtration rate. This is dependent on the individual and may be increased during summer, presumably because of sunlight and vitamin D status. There is some increase in urinary calcium in women after the menopause.

Intestinal biliary, pancreatic and intestinal secretions account for a daily enteric loss of 5 mmol calcium. Calcium is excreted in urine, but there are also losses in faeces, sweat, skin, hair and nails. The loss to the gastrointestinal tract of approximately 400 mg of calcium per day is through bile, pancreatic secretions and desquamated cells from the mucosal lining.

There is some colonic absorption of calcium, dependent on poorly understood factors.

Calcium deficiency and excess

Deficiency
PTH deficiency leads to hypocalcaemia. A reduction in plasma calcium results in tetany, a hyperactivity of the motor muscles, facial spasm, and spasm in the wrist and metacarpophalangeal joints.

Excess
Hypercalcaemia may occur in infants who have been given an excess of vitamin D, as with cod-liver oil fortification of infant foods. The infant loses appetite, vomits, loses weight, is constipated and has a characteristic facial appearance. The calcium, urea and cholesterol concentrations in the plasma are increased. The blood pressure may increase. Prolonged increased plasma concentrations result in calcification of the heart and kidneys, and even cerebral damage and death.

In adults, hypercalcaemia can occur in hyperparathyroidism or excessive dosage of vitamin D. This used to happen in individuals who had peptic ulcer surgery and to whom calcium and high-dosage vitamin D were given on an empirical basis.

Recommended requirements

It is difficult to define requirements for calcium because of its long-term accumulation; hence, the study of calcium metabolism is extremely complex.

The skeleton of a newborn infant contains 25 g of calcium and, during the first years of life, the calcium content of the body increases quickly. Vitamin D and dietary calcium are important dictates of calcium balance.

Calcium absorption in early infancy is approximately 150 mg/day and this declines to approximately 100 mg/day by the age of 3 years. There is

a steady increase to a maximum at puberty, during the adolescent growth spurt, an effect that occurs to a greater extent, and later, in boys than in girls. Thereafter, there is a fall in calcium absorption, plateauing in adults at between 250 and 400 mg/day. In children, approximately 20–30% of dietary calcium is absorbed, compared with the infant where the absorption rate is 40–60%. Calcium uptake increases in pre-adolescence and puberty, during which time 45% of the adult skeleton is formed. Bone mineral content increases at approximately 9% a year. There is also substantial urinary loss of calcium, so that an enhanced absorption rate is necessary. The majority of individuals reach the peak bone mass by the age of 30 years.

Between the ages of 18 and 30 years, bone density increases by a further 10% and 120 g of calcium (about 25 mg/day) is added to the skeleton during this period (see Chapter 41).

Another period of enhanced calcium requirement is during pregnancy, which requires increased absorption by the mother of up to 30 g of calcium, for utilisation by the foetus.

The average daily calcium intake for British adults is 940 mg (24 mmol) for men and 730 mg (18 mmol) for women. The average intake varies from country to country (range 350–1200 mg; 9–30 mmol), the range being influenced by milk intake and food fortification policies.

The bioavailability of calcium for absorption in the intestine is important in establishing the dietary reference value (DRV). It has been estimated that the dietary intake necessary to achieve calcium absorption of 4 mmol (160 mg/day) is 20 mmol/day (800 mg) to achieve 20% absorption, and 5.8 mmol/day (230 mg) to achieve 70% absorption. It has proved exceedingly difficult to calculate the estimated average requirement (EAR), and

---

Calcium intakes

Dietary calcium average intake in the UK is approximately 20 mmol (800 mg) per person per day, although this varies geographically. Typically, calcium is obtained from:

- milk and milk products: 12.8 mmol (512 mg)
- vegetables: 1.2 mmol (46 mg)
- fortified cereals: 4.5 mmol (181 mg)
- hard water: 3.9 mmol (154 mg)

figures are based on the retention of calcium. These vary considerably with age and gender.

Infants

In early infancy calcium balance may be negative. The daily rate of calcium retention is approximately 4 mmol (160 mg). Breast-milk calcium is absorbed at about 66% efficiency, so that in the first year 6 mmol/day (240 mg) would be adequate. In contrast, absorption from infant formulae is about 40%, so the EAR is 10 mmol/day (400 mg). The RNI would be 13 mmol/day (520 mg).

Children

Calcium retention for skeletal growth increases from 1.8 to 3.8 mmol/day (70 to 150 mg) between the ages of 1 and 10 years. Absorption is approximately 35%; therefore, this degree of calcium retention requires 7 mmol/day (280 mg) and 10.6 mmol/day (425 mg) at 1 and 10 years, respectively. Corresponding RNIs are 8.8 and 13.8 mmol/day.

Adolescence

During adolescence 6.3 mmol/day (250 mg) for girls and 7.5 mmol (300 mg) for boys is retained. Absorption effectiveness is approximately 40%. The EARs are 15.6 mmol/day (625 mg) and 18.8 mmol/day (750 mg), respectively.

Adults

The EAR has been recommended as 3.8 mmol/day (150 mg) plus an estimated 0.25 mmol/day (10 mg) for losses through skin, sweat, hair and nails. Absorption is estimated to be 30%. Therefore, the EAR is 13.1 mmol/day (525 mg), the RNI is 17.5 mmol/day (700 mg) and the LRNI is 10 mmol/day (400 mg).

Pregnancy

There is some mobilisation of maternal calcium depots rather than a dietary absorption increment during foetal growth. Maternal bone density may diminish in the first 3 months of both pregnancy and lactation to provide an internal calcium reservoir which is replenished by 6 months. A deficiency of absorbed calcium arises in pregnant compared with non-pregnant women. However, if pregnancy occurs in adolescence, then the growth requirements of the mother and foetus require a doubling of calcium provision.

Lactation

Food intake is increased during lactation, with consequent benefits to calcium intake. A lactating mother will secrete some 150–300 mg (48 mmol) of calcium. Approximately an additional 14 mmol/day (550 mg) of calcium may be required during lactation.

Post-menopause

Osteoporosis results from the loss of all components of bone, not just of calcium. Therefore, the post-menopausal increase in bone loss, the main cause of osteoporosis, is not due to calcium loss. Oestrogen and other hormone deficiencies may be important. Oestrogen replacement can prevent and possibly reverse bone loss.

The elderly

It is not clear that there is any need for an increase in calcium intake by individuals aged 60 years or over.

Body store measurements

Plasma calcium, especially the ionised form, is the most consistent value in calcium metabolism. The maintenance of a positive calcium balance is required to preserve the skeleton. However, study of the conservation of the skeleton is not easy in other than short-term studies. It has not proved easy to generate meaningful data in studies of calcium loss. Urinary calcium excretion reflects dietary intake and, if increased, may lead to the formation of kidney stones.

KEY POINTS

1. Calcium is concentrated in the body in organelles and blood. Calcium is very important in the structure of the skeleton and to ensure an adequate extracellular fluid calcium concentration. A positive calcium balance is required before growth can proceed. Calcium intake and skeletal modelling and turnover determine calcium balance during growth.

2. Hormonal and pharmacological activation of cells, membrane function and enzyme activity

may all be affected by the local concentrations of calcium. Calcium is bound within the cell to enzyme proteins; this binding alters the protein configuration and hence enzyme activity. Calcium has many roles, including that of an intracellular messenger.

3. The major regulating hormones for calcium are parathyroid hormone, calcitonin and vitamin D. Growth hormone, thyroid hormone, adrenal steroids, sex hormones and some gastrointestinal hormones are involved to a lesser extent.

4. A reduction in plasma calcium results in tetany, which is due to hyperactivity of the motor muscles. This results in spasms in the face, wrist, hands and feet.

5. A sustained deficiency of dietary calcium can result in osteomalacia, a loss of calcium in the bone.

THINKING POINTS

1. Calcium dynamics are very complex, within a compartmented system of varied size and turnover.

2. On the one hand there is the fast movement of calcium across the muscle membrane during heart contractility, and on the other hand the massive and slow turnover of the bone calcium.

3. There are large changes in requirements during different stages of life: foetus, childhood growth, pregnancy and lactation, and in the ageing process.

NEED TO UNDERSTAND

1. Calcium is a divalent ion with significant functions in cell signalling, contractility and bone structure.

2. Bone also acts as a store of calcium, although too much drainage from the store has effects on bone structure.

3. Calcium's poor solubility in water means that it is better to restrict absorption rather than to rely on renal excretion, and such control is important in calcium homoeostasis.

FURTHER READING

Abrams, S.A. (2001) Calcium turnover and nutrition through the life cycle. *Proceedings of the Nutrition Society*, **60**, 283–9.

Cashman, K.D. and Flynn, A. (1999) Optimal nutrition: calcium, magnesium and phosphorous. *Proceedings of the Nutrition Society*, **58**, 477–87.

Dietary Reference Values for Food, Energy and Nutrients for the United Kingdom (1991) Department of Health Report on Health and Social Subjects, No. 41. HMSO, London.

Farrugia, G., Holm, A.N., Rich, A. *et al.* (1999) A mechanosensitive calcium channel in human intestinal smooth muscle cells. *Gastroenterology*, **117**, 900–5.

Matkovic, V. (1991) Calcium metabolism and calcium requirements during skeletal modelling and consolidation of bone mass. *American Journal of Clinical Nutrition*, **54**, S245–60.

Philipson, K.D. and Nicoll, D.A. (2000) Sodium–calcium exchange: a molecular perspective. *Annual Review of Physiology*, **62**, 111–33.

Prentice, A. (2000) Calcium in pregnancy and lactation. *Annual Review of Nutrition*, **20**, 249–72.

Putney, J.W., Jr (2001) Channelling calcium. *Nature*, **410**, 648–9.

Weatherall, D.J., Ledingham, J.G.G. and Warrell, D.A. (1996) *Oxford Textbook of Medicine*, 3rd edn. Oxford Medical Publications, Oxford.

IRON

Introduction

- Atomic weight, 56
- found in two forms, ferrous and ferric, which interchange: $Fe^{2+} \longleftrightarrow Fe^{3+} + e^-$
- natural isotopes, 54, 56, 57, 58
- abundance in Earth's crust, 4.7%.

There are many important sources of iron, including meat, meat products, cereals, vegetables and fruit. A prime source is black pudding (20 mg/100 g), and most foods contain 1–10 mg/100 g. There are regional variations in the iron content of plant foods, depending on the soil in which the plants are grown. Milk is a poor source of iron.

Iron is present in all cells of the body and plays a key role in many biochemical reactions. The iron must be readily available for the synthesis of essential iron proteins, e.g. haemoglobin and myoglobin, and enzymes, e.g. catalase. In the normal adult there is 4–5 g of iron, 75% of which is in the form of haemoglobin (2.5 g), myoglobin (0.15 g), haem enzymes and non-haem enzymes. The remainder is stored as ferritin and haemosiderin in the hepatic reticuloendothelial system, spleen, bone marrow and hepatic parenchymal cells. Women have a reduced iron pool due to menstrual loss.

Function

Haemoglobin

The haemoglobin molecule is central to oxygen transport. It has a molecular weight of 64.5 kDa and is formed from four haem groups linked to four polypeptide chains. Haemoglobin can bind four molecules of oxygen. Divalent iron (Fe^{2+}) in haem reversibly binds oxygen for transport to tissues, while oxidation of iron to the ferric (Fe^{3+}) in methaemoglobin causes haemoglobin to lose its capacity to carry oxygen. The average plasma haemoglobin concentration is 11 g/100 ml, and is higher in healthy males than in healthy females.

Cytochromes

The cytochromes transport electrons to molecular oxygen through the reversible valency changes of iron atoms present in these molecules. There is a stepwise release of energy by the haem-containing proteins of the mitochondrial electron transport apparatus.

Iron complexes are all octahedral, and paramagnetic because of unpaired electrons in the 3d orbital. Haem coenzymes contain Fe^{2+} and are directly involved in catalysis. Many redox enzymes, including electron–transferring protein NADH dehydrogenase, contain iron–sulfur complexes that catalyse one-electron transfer reactions. The complex is usually two or four iron and sulfur ions bound as an equal complex to the cysteinyl–sulfur group of the protein. The cytochrome P450 system involves haem, iron–sulfur complexes, flavin coenzymes and nicotinamide coenzymes in a multienzyme system (see Chapter 31).

Myoglobin

This is important in the storage of oxygen in muscle. It has a molecular weight of 17 kDa and is formed from one polypeptide chain and one haem molecule. Myoglobin is a reservoir of oxygen for muscle metabolism, with a higher affinity for oxygen than haemoglobin. Oxygen is released to cytochrome oxidase, which has a greater affinity for oxygen than myoglobin. Iron is an integral part of haem protein cytochromes, catalase, and peroxidases, and as a cofactor.

All of these are reversible acceptors or donors of electrons. There is a controlled interaction between molecular oxygen and haem iron proteins, iron–sulfur proteins and non-haem iron-containing oxygenases. Ribose is converted to DNA by the iron-containing ribonucleotide reductase.

Absorption and transport of iron

Absorption

Although 10–15 mg/day of iron is ingested, only 1–2 mg (between 10 and 15% of dietary iron) is absorbed in a steady state to compensate for daily losses, and is taken up either by the bone marrow for haemoglobin formation or by the reticular endothelial tissue stores. There is increased iron absorption during growth, blood loss and pregnancy. Absorption takes place in the upper small intestine and is controlled by the mucosal cells, mediated by specific receptors on the intestinal mucosal surface. Dietary iron absorption is dependent on overall iron stores.

Iron absorption from food depends on the form of the iron and other constituents in the diet. Iron is absorbed as both haem and non-haem iron. Most iron is present as haem iron in animal foods, in the Fe^{2+} form. Haem iron is absorbed more readily than inorganic iron from vegetable foods and is little affected by other constituents in the diet. Haem iron is absorbed from the intestine by a different process to that for non-haem iron. Within the intestine, haem is released from haemoglobin, myoglobin or cytochromes by proteolytic degradation of the protein fraction. Haem is then transported through the brush border of epithelial cells bound to a receptor. Once absorbed within the cell the iron is liberated enzymatically from haem by a haem oxygenase.

Iron in vegetable food is present as non-haem complexes as Fe^{3+} bound to protein, phytates, oxalates, phosphates and carbonates. Most of the non-haem iron is in a high molecular weight form and is less well absorbed than soluble iron. Binding to low molecular weight chelators, sugars, amino acids, ascorbic acid and glycoproteins forms soluble iron complexes and increases absorption. Non-haem iron is taken from the gut lumen through border membranes at receptor sites, which may be glycoproteins. The absorbed iron passes into the plasma and is bound to the transferrin protein. Inorganic iron uptake is facilitated by ascorbic acid; the reducing ability of ascorbic acid expedites the conversion of Fe^{3+} to the more water-soluble Fe^{2+}. Gastric hydrochloric acid facilitates the absorption of non-haem iron by converting ferric to ferrous iron; achlorhydria is a cause of iron-deficiency anaemia. Prolonged iron deficiency may lead to gastric atrophy. Partial gastrectomy and malabsorption can cause iron-deficiency anaemia.

Phytic acid in cereals, phosphate, carbonates, oxalate and pancreatic bicarbonate bind iron and decrease iron absorption.

Enhancers of iron absorption

Physiological
Iron deficiency, an anaemic state, fasting, pregnancy.

Dietary
Ascorbic acid, citric acid, lactic acid, malic acid, tartaric acid, fructose, sorbitol, alcohol, amino acids, e.g. cystine, lysine, histidine.

Inhibitors of iron absorption

Physiological
Iron overload, achlorhydria, copper deficiency.

Dietary
Tannins, polyphenols, phosphates, phytate, wheat bran, lignin, proteins, egg albumin and yolk, legumes, protein, inorganic elements, calcium, manganese, copper, cadmium, cobalt.

Transferrin

Transferrin is a glycoprotein, molecular weight 80 kDa. Two Fe atoms are carried on each molecule, on two high-affinity sites. Transferrin is the major supplier of iron for most cells. The diferric transferrin binds to a transferrin receptor present on the cell membrane, and the diferric transferrin complex is taken into the cell by receptor-mediated endocytosis. The apoferritin remains bound to the receptor until the Fe is released and then recycles. There are specific receptors for transferrin and the transferrin iron complex on reticulocytes.

Iron absorption is greatly increased when there is increased red blood cell production, and may double in iron-deficient individuals. The control of iron uptake depends on both bone marrow activity and iron stores. Iron stores fall during pregnancy owing to the needs of the foetus, which is a stimulus to increase iron absorption.

Transport
Iron is transported into the bloodstream bound to a globular protein transferrin, which is synthesised in the liver. The transferrin concentration in the plasma is 2–2.5 g/l. The concentration of iron in the plasma is 16–18 µmol/l.

There are wide diurnal variations (the range varying by 100% over 24 h) in plasma iron concentrations. The iron is carried to the marrow (80% of the total), where new red blood cells are formed. The life of a red cell is 120 days, so each day 1/120th of body haemoglobin is degraded and resynthesised. Each day 20 mg of iron passes from the spleen, liver and other lymphoreticular tissue, the site of red cell breakdown. The total amount of intracellular iron is approximately 500 mg.

Storage of iron

The typical pool of iron increases from 300 mg in infants to 4000 mg in adults, an increase of 0.5 mg/day. Both ferric and ferrous iron form complexes with organic and inorganic ions. Ionic iron is very toxic, so iron is held throughout the body in a bound form. The distribution of iron in the body is shown in Table 18.1.

Table 18.1 Distribution of iron in the body of an adult male

Organ	Compound	Amount (g)
Liver, spleen, bone marrow stores	Ferritin	0.70
	Haemosiderin	1.00
Tissues	Myoglobin	0.30
	Haem enzymes	0.10
	Non-haem enzymes	0.40
Blood	Haemoglobin	2.50
Total		5.00

Iron storage compounds

Haemosiderin and ferritin each contain approximately 1 g of iron, the majority in ferritin. Ferritin is present in all cells, but particularly in the liver, spleen and bone marrow. Normal iron stores range over 0.75–1 g in men and 0.3–0.5 g in women, largely in the liver as ferritin. Iron is stored in the reticuloendothelial cells of the liver, spleen and bone marrow.

A balance between the synthesis of ferritin and the plasma membrane receptor for transferrin regulates iron availability. The transferrin receptor is required for the uptake of iron, and ferritin is necessary for the storage of any iron in excess of requirements.

Iron in the infant

During pregnancy some 700 mg of iron passes through the placenta from mother to foetus, this transfer being most marked in the second half of pregnancy. This poses problems for the premature infant, as less time is available and maternal milk is not rich in iron. At delivery late clamping of the umbilical cord can increase the infant's transferred haemoglobin and therefore iron store. The baby's iron stores are related to body weight. During the first 6 weeks of life there are major shifts of iron stores from haemoglobin to other iron protein complexes.

Iron loss, deficiency and excess

Iron loss

Daily losses of endogenous iron include: desquamated gastrointestinal cells (0.14 mg), haemoglobin (0.38 mg), bile (0.24 mg) and urine (0.1 mg).

Ferritin

Ferritin has a molecular weight of 450 kDa, which increases to 900 kDa when loaded with iron. Ferritin is a soluble complex, with Fe^{3+} in the core as insoluble ferric hydroxyphosphate surrounded by a coat of apoferritin proteins. This prevents excessive iron from damaging cells and allows the storage of up to 4500 ferric atoms. The removal of free iron from the cytoplasm protects against the peroxidation of cell lipids, DNA and some proteins. Ferritin consists of 24 protein subunits of two types, heavy (H) and light (L). These are formed as truncated molecular pyramids. The shell is formed of subunit proteins, four long and one short helical segments making a rigid structure. The rest of the subunit proteins consist of non-helical segments connecting the helices. The amounts of these proteins are controlled by their mRNA activity. There is probably only one expressed copy of the L-gene and one of the H-gene in human genomes. The expressed H- and L-genes of the human have three introns separating four exons. Gene translation from mRNA to amino acids is modified to provide protection for cell molecules against peroxidation by accumulated iron. This is achieved by dormant ferritin mRNA, which is activated by iron when present in excessive amounts. This occurs through an iron-dependent protein (IRE-BP), which binds to regions of the mRNA for each regulatory protein. Iron removes a specific protein that blocks the translation of ferritin mRNA. Iron causes the cytoplasmic pool of dormant ferritin mRNA to become active by association with polysomes. The L-subunit of ferritin is transcribed preferentially in response to increased iron intake, whereas the H-subunit responds to cell differentiation. This affinity decreases as iron availability increases. This is a simple control mechanism.

Normally, the amount of iron absorbed equals the amount of iron lost by dead cells desquamated from surfaces, skin and intestine. Iron is also lost by bleeding and, in the female, through menstruation. Iron-deficiency anaemia in the male and post-menopausal female is uncommon, and when this does occur a pathological cause must be sought, since it usually results from a source of bleeding in the gastrointestinal tract. In some parts of the world hookworm infestations (*Ancylostoma duodenale* and *Nector americanus*) cause loss of blood from the gastrointestinal tract. Urinary loss of iron is small in the normal person, less than 100 µg/day. The loss of iron in sweat is small and is in the order of 250–500 µg/day.

Iron deficiency
Iron deficiency is associated with a low serum iron and results from dietary insufficiency, an excess loss of blood through menstruation, pregnancy, insufficient iron stores (as in the premature baby), or loss from lesions in the gastrointestinal tract.

Iron deficiency results in anaemia. In the young and during growth iron deficiency results in impaired psychomotor development, with reduced attention span and cognitive function. Iron deficiency also reduces work performance, particularly endurance work. In pregnancy, iron deficiency is associated with low birth-weight babies and perinatal mortality. In the older population, anaemia resulting from iron deficiency can cause tiredness and increased risk of complications associated with atherosclerosis, e.g. angina, myocardial infarction and stroke.

Iron excess
An excess of iron in the body is known as siderosis. The body store of iron is reflected in and measured by the plasma ferritin.

Haemochromatosis is a failure to control iron absorption from the small intestine, with a progressive inappropriate increase in total body iron

---

Haemochromatosis

Idiopathic haemochromatosis is an autosomal recessive genetic condition. Individuals who are heterozygous may show some phenotypic expression of the disease by an increased serum transferrin saturation. The abnormal gene lies close to the histocompatibility locus antigen complex (HLA) on chromosome 6. The haemochromatosis-associated gene is called HFE; this is present throughout the intestine but is particularly expressed in the small intestine. The encoded protein forms a complex with the transferrin receptor and decreases the affinity of this receptor for transferrin. Mutations in the HFE disrupt the control of iron absorption in association with other host and environmental factors.

---

stores, which may be aggravated by parenteral iron loading. Excess deposition of iron may result in cellular and organ damage. The causes of haemochromatosis are:

- **genetic**: primary idiopathic haemochromatosis, a very common genetic disorder affecting 1 in 300 in populations of northern European stock, with a carrier frequency of 1 in 20 individuals
- **acquired**: secondary haemochromatosis. This can be secondary to: (i) anaemia and ineffective erythropoiesis, thalassaemia and major sideroblastic anaemia; (ii) high oral iron intake, prolonged ingestion of medicinal iron or intake of iron with alcohol; or (iii) liver disease, including porphyria cutanea tarda and alcoholic cirrhosis, or following portacaval anastomosis.

Pathology
Iron accumulates over time, and plasma iron and percentage saturation of transferrin increase. The tissues may contain over 20 g of iron. This may result in tissue injury from disruption of iron-laden lysosomes or mitochondrial lipid peroxidation. The excess iron is deposited in the lysosomes of the parenchymal cells of the liver, and in hepatic fibrosis and cirrhosis. Such iron loading results in diabetes mellitus, heart problems and excess skin pigmentation.

In the early stages of haemochromatosis haemosiderin is deposited in the periportal hepatocytes, particularly in the pericanalicular cytoplasm within lysosomes. This progresses to deposition of iron and perilobular fibrosis in bile duct epithelium, Kupffer cells and fibroceptor cells. An irregular macronodular cirrhosis develops later.

A nutritional iron overload can occur when the dietary iron intake exceeds 40 mg/day. This can occur from absorption from iron vessels used for cooking and making alcoholic drinks.

Recommended requirements

Infants and children
Breast-fed infants are capable of absorbing 50% of the iron present in mother's milk, whereas iron absorption from formulated milks may be only

10%. The LRNI for infants aged 0–3 months is 0.9 mg/day; the EAR is 1.3 mg/day and the RNI 1.7 mg/day. This should treble during the next 6 months of life to an EAR of 3.3 mg/day.

By the age of puberty the intake of iron should be 1 mg/day.

Menstruation

Median and mean losses of blood in menstruation are 30 and 44 ml, respectively. The calculated loss of iron is therefore approximately 20 mg, averaging 0.7 mg/day. In Britain the average iron intake among fertile women is in the order of 12 mg/day. To allow for the varied amounts of menstrual blood loss, an EAR of 11 mg/day, an LRNI of 8 mg/day and an RNI of 15 mg/day have been suggested.

Pregnancy

It has been estimated that the toll of pregnancy on the mother's iron stores is approximately 700 mg. This should come from pre-existing body stores. In part, this will be met by the cessation of menstrual losses, increased intestinal absorption and the mobilisation of maternal stores. Therefore, additional iron is not necessary unless the iron stores are insufficient at the beginning of pregnancy.

Lactation

Breast milk contains 7 µmol/l at 6–8 weeks postpartum, decreasing to 5 µmol/l during weeks 17–22. The total loss is around 5–6 µmol/day. This secretion will be balanced by the amenorrhoea generally associated with lactation.

Blood donors

A pint of blood given every 6 months is more than compensated for by increased iron absorption. However, more frequent donations, especially by women of child-bearing years, can upset iron stores.

Adults

Iron intakes in Britain average 14 mg/day for men and 12 mg/day for women.

Body store measurements

Haemoglobin in part reflects iron status. Normal values for plasma iron range from 12 to 30 µmol/l and the total plasma iron-binding capacity 45–70 µmol/l. In healthy people, plasma ferritin closely reflects body iron stores (normal range 12–250 µg/l).

There is a large amount of ferritin in storage tissues but little in serum. A plasma ferritin level of 1 µg/l corresponds to 8–10 mg storage iron in the average adult. Serum ferritin is relatively increased in the newborn and falls rapidly in the first few months as iron is required for the increasing red cell mass. The concentration increases slowly during childhood until late adolescence, males having values three times those of females. The female ferritin level is low during the child-bearing years and increases thereafter. A plasma ferritin of less than 12 µg/l is not useful in assessing iron deficiency, especially in infants and during pregnancy.

KEY POINTS

1. Iron is found in two forms, ferrous and ferric, which interchange: $Fe^{2+} \longleftrightarrow Fe^{3+} + e^{-}$.
2. The iron must be readily available for the synthesis of essential iron proteins, e.g. haemoglobin and myoglobin, and enzymes, e.g. catalase.
3. Iron is central to oxygen metabolism: 2.5 g circulates in haemoglobin and 0.3 g is present in myoglobin. Haemoglobin has a molecular weight of 64.5 kDa and is formed from four haem groups linked to four polypeptide chains. Divalent iron (Fe^{2+}) in haem reversibly binds oxygen for transport to tissues, while oxidation of iron to the ferric (Fe^{3+}) state in methaemoglobin causes haemoglobin to lose its capacity to carry oxygen. Iron is present in all cells of the body and plays a key role in many biochemical reactions.
4. Iron deficiency occurs with loss of blood in menstruation, insufficient iron stores (as in the premature baby) or loss from lesions in the gastrointestinal tract. In pregnancy, iron deficiency is associated with low birth-weight babies and perinatal mortality. Iron deficiency results in anaemia, impaired psychomotor development and reduced cognitive function in the young and during growth. Iron deficiency also reduces work performance (particularly endurance work).

THINKING POINT

The ferric/ferrous interplay is critical to oxygen transfer and also to metabolism in the body.

NEED TO UNDERSTAND

1. Iron stores and conversion to haemoglobin and myoglobin are sensitively allied to intestinal absorption of iron.
2. Increased loss may be physiological in the female, but is of concern in the post-menopausal female and in the male.

FURTHER READING

Andrews, N.C., Fleming, M.D. and Gunshin, H. (1999) Iron transport across biologic membranes. *Nutrition Reviews*, **57**, 114–23.

Burke, W., Impertore, G. and Reyes, M. (2001) Iron deficiency and iron overload: effects of diet and genes. *Proceedings of the Nutrition Society*, **60**, 73–80.

Chesters, J.K. (1992) Trace element/gene interactions. *Nutrition Reviews*, **50**, 217–23.

Cook, J.D. (1999) Defining optimal body iron. *Proceedings of the Nutrition Society*, **58**, 489–95.

Cook, J.D., Baynes, R.D. and Skikne, B.S. (1992) Iron deficiency and the measurement of iron status. *Nutrition Research Reviews*, **5**, 189–202.

Crawford, D.H.G., Powell, L.W. and Halliday, J.W. (1996) Factors influencing disease expression in hemochromatosis. *Annual Review of Nutrition*, **16**, 139–60.

Griffiths, W.J.H., Kelly, A.L., Smith, T.M. and Cox, T.M. (2000) localization of iron transport and regulatory proteins in human cells. *Quarterly Journal of Medicine*, **93**, 575–87.

Hallberg, L. (2001) Perspectives on nutritional iron deficiency. *Annual Review of Nutrition*, **21**, 1–21.

Halliday, J.W. (1998) Hemochromatosis and iron needs. *Nutrition Reviews*, **56**, S30–7.

Kuhn, L.C. (1998) Iron and gene expression: molecular mechanisms regulating cellular iron homeostasis. *Nutrition Reviews*, **56**, S11–19.

Lonnerdal, B. and Iyer, S. (1995) Lactoferrin: molecular structure and biological function. *Annual Review of Nutrition*, **15**, 93–110.

Mascotti, D.P., Rup, D. and Thach, R.E. (1995) Regulation of iron metabolism. *Annual Review of Nutrition*, **15**, 239–62.

Munro, H. (1993) The ferritin genes – their response to iron status. *Nutrition Reviews*, **51**, 65–73.

Rosmurdoc, O., Poupon, R., Nion, I. *et al.* (2000) Differential HFE expression in hemochromatosis heterozygotes. *Gastroenterology*, **119**, 1075–86.

Wessling-Resnick, M. (2000) Iron transport. *Annual Review of Nutrition*, **20**, 129–51.

Winzerling, J.Y. and Law, J.H. (1997) Comparative nutrition of iron and copper. *Annual Review of Nutrition*, **17**, 501–26.

TRACE ELEMENTS

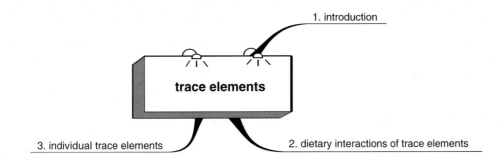

Fig. 18.5 Section outline.

INTRODUCTION

Trace elements are important in the body by virtue of:

- establishing potential differences across membranes; such differences have to be maintained by energy-requiring reactions, e.g. Na^+, K^+, Ca^{2+}
- allowing oxidation–reduction (redox) enzymatic reactions to take place, e.g. iron, copper
- acting as cofactors in enzymatic reactions, e.g. zinc
- maintaining the structure (conformation) of proteins, e.g magnesium
- maintaining the structure of hormones, e.g. iodine in thyroxine.

Trace elements are required in small amounts, although their concentrations in the diet will vary. In communities totally dependent on locally grown food the trace element content of the local soil and drinking water is relevant. In communities buying from sources from all over the world such restrictions may not apply.

Trace elements and protein structure

The trace elements adsorb to protein in specific configurations. Such ligands may act as cofactors or structural elements by virtue of high concentrations of positive charges, directed valences that interact with two or more ligands, acting as bridges in two or more valency states. Alkali metals, Na^+ and K^+, which have a single positive charge and no d-electronic orbital for sharing, rarely form complexes with proteins. Occasionally the divalent alkaline metals Mg^{2+} and Ca^{2+} complex with proteins. The other elements in biological systems come from the first transition series of the periodic table, have partially filled 3d orbitals and exist in more than one oxidative state, which is important in oxidation–reduction reactions. Zinc, unusual in having a full 3d orbital, chelates with nitrogen, in histidine side-chains or sulfur-containing amino acid chains, e.g. cysteine, and makes the structure of a protein rigid.

Zinc–phytate interactions

Dietary phytate:zinc ratios exceeding 25:1 can inhibit zinc utilisation, provided that dietary calcium is maintained at or above the currently accepted RDA. There is a synergistic effect of dietary calcium on the phytate:zinc relationship. The action of phytate is dependent on the available free phytate, which is not already bound to some other element, e.g. calcium. Phytate is degraded by bacterial hydrolysis by phytases in the intestinal mucosa. Free amino acids (histidine, cysteine, methionine) can desorb zinc from an insoluble complex (ZnCu–phytate). The yield of soluble copper or zinc from such complexes is directly proportional to the amino-nitrogen content of the intestinal soluble phase.

DIETARY INTERACTIONS OF TRACE ELEMENTS

The amount and chemistry of dietary inorganic constituents affect the efficiency of absorption of the essential elements. An example is the inhibition of calcium and trace metal absorption, e.g. zinc by dietary phytate. The ease of release of metals from their complexes with phytate is in the order: copper > cadmium > manganese > zinc > lead.

Copper absorption is affected by interactions acting on its intraluminal solubility and competitive interactions determining its transport through the mucosa.

A mild degree of iron depletion increases the uptake of other metals. Dietary iron in such depletion states increases not only the efficacy of iron absorption, but also that of lead, zinc, cadmium, cobalt and manganese. A clue possibly lies with apolactoferrin, which also has affinity for zinc and other metals, and this may influence absorption.

Measurement

Serum zinc, copper, manganese, chromium, molybdenum and vanadium are not good indicators of nutritional status and dietary intake. Measurement of trace elements in hair or nail clippings is of little value in determining dietary intake or body status.

FURTHER READING

Bates, C.J., Thurnham, D.I., Bingham, S.A. *et al.* (1991) Biochemical markers of nutrient intake. In *Design Concepts in Nutritional Epidemiology* (eds B.M. Margetts and M. Nelson). Oxford Medical Publications, Oxford, pp. 192–265.

Chesters, J.K. (1992) Trace elements and gene interactions. *Nutrition Reviews*, **50**, 217–23.

Cousins, R.J. (1994) Metal elements and gene expression. *Annual Review of Nutrition*, **14**, 449–69.

Diem, K. (ed.) (1962) *Documenta Geigy Scientific Tables*, 6th edn. Geigy Pharmaceutical Company, Manchester.

Dietary Reference Values for Food, Energy and Nutrients for the United Kingdom (1991) Report on Health and Social Subjects, No. 41. HMSO, London.

Fairweather-Tait, S.J. and Hurrell, R.F. (1996) Bioavailability of minerals and trace elements. *Nutrition Research Reviews*, **9**, 295–324.

Johnson, L.R., Alpelpers, D.H., Christensen, J. *et al.* (1994) *Physiology of the Gastrointestinal Tract*. Raven Press, New York.

Mill, C.F. (1985) Dietary interactions involving the trace elements. *Annual Review of Nutrition*, **5**, 173–93.

INDIVIDUAL TRACE ELEMENTS

Aluminium

- Atomic weight, 27; valency, 3
- natural isotope, 27
- natural abundance in Earth's crust, 7.51%.

Aluminium is found in all biological materials and the amount depends on the local soil and environmental conditions. High concentrations of aluminium are found in tea and orange juice. The tea plant absorbs aluminium from acid soil, concentrating 500–1500 mg/kg in its leaves. Brewed black tea contains 2–6 mg/l of aluminium. The bioavailability of aluminium in tea is low because it binds with organic compounds. Aluminium is also found in herbs, processed cheeses, baking powder and pickles.

Aluminium hydroxide was formerly used therapeutically as an antacid in the treatment of duodenal ulcers. Daily intake is approximately 20 mg/kg

of food and 0.5 mg/1500 ml fluid. Fluoride and silicon reduce bioavailability. Aluminium is excreted in urine.

The only know biological role for aluminium is as part of the succinic dehydrogenase–cytochrome C system.

Aluminium may be involved in the development of Alzheimer's disease and is present in increased amounts in the brains of sufferers. If renal dialysis fluids contain aluminium, dementia can occur in patients receiving such treatment. Such dialysis dementia is an acute condition that is often reversible with treatment. The pathology is quite different to that of Alzheimer's. There are no geographical or temporal variations in dementia relating to aluminium concentrations.

Antimony

- Atomic weight, 122; valencies, 3, 5
- natural isotopes, 121, 123
- abundance in Earth's crust, $2.3 \times 10^{-5}\%$.

Antimony does not appear to be an essential element. The intake in the North American diet is in the range of 2–10 µmol/day. The efficiency of absorption is about 15% and antimony is stored in the liver, kidneys, skin and adrenals.

Toxic effects include gastrointestinal and respiratory symptoms. Antimony poisoning can occur from drinking soft drinks that have been stored in enamel containers.

Arsenic

- Atomic weight, 75; valencies, 3, 5
- natural isotope, 75
- abundance in Earth's crust, $5.5 \times 10^{-4}\%$.

There is widespread arsenic contamination of water wells in Bangladesh and parts of India. These wells were dug to improve the life of the local inhabitants, but proved to be a source of arsenic. Arsenic is present in many plant and animal foods, but has yet to be established as an essential element in the diet. Shellfish are particularly rich in arsenic. Excessive amounts of arsenic have contaminated poultry and pig feed, and may be found in muscle and liver in amounts of 6.5 and 26 µmol/kg, respectively. In seafood, the arsenic is present as arsenobetaine.

Arsenic is rapidly absorbed and excreted in urine and bile. Inorganic forms of penta valent and trivalent arsenic are rapidly methylated in the digestive tract. Intakes are usually 0.1–0.4 µmol/day.

Tolerable daily intake
Arsenic is extremely toxic and an upper limit of tolerable daily intake is 2 µg/kg body weight.

Boron

- Atomic weight, 11; valency, 3
- natural isotopes, 10, 11
- abundance in Earth's crust, 0.0014%.

Boron is a ligand and forms complexes with organic compounds such as sugars, polysaccharides, adenosine phosphate, pyridoxine, riboflavin, dehydroascorbic acid, pyridine nucleotides and steroid hormones. Boron is an essential nutrient, found in plant foods, which is excreted in the urine. There is no evidence of a role in animal metabolism.

Recommended requirements
Human diets provide 2 mg/day. Toxic effects are experienced with intakes 50 times this amount.

Bromine

- Atomic weight, 80; valencies, 1, 3
- natural isotopes, 80, 81
- abundance in Earth's crust, $6 \times 10^{-4}\%$.

Bromine does not have an evident physiological function, but may be substituted for chlorine in some reactions. It has been reported that bromine may concentrate in the thyroid gland. Bromine is found widely in the environment and it is unlikely that deficiency will occur.

Excess
It was used clinically as a sedative and it was rumoured by British Army Infantry recruits that bromide was added to tea to reduce sexual drive.

Cadmium

- atomic weight, 112; valency, 2

- natural isotopes, 106, 108, 110, 111, 112, 113, 114, 116
- abundance in Earth's crust, $1.1 \times 10^{-5}\%$.

Cadmium is not an essential nutrient. Cadmium exposure results from industrial waste contaminating water, so that small amounts are absorbed and accumulate in tissues. Levels may reach 200–300 µmol total body deposit, with a biological half-life of 15–30 years and the highest concentration in the kidneys. Another source is from inhaling cigarette smoke containing cadmium. During pregnancy smoking increases cadmium uptake, which could affect the foetus. Cadmium may react with the intestinal mucosa and interact with zinc, copper, manganese and iron.

Caesium

- Atomic weight, 133; valency, 1
- natural isotope, 133
- abundance in Earth's crust, $7 \times 10^{-5}\%$.

Caesium is available predominantly as the radioisotope caesium 137. It is metabolised in the same way as potassium, being concentrated in the muscle. Following radioactive fallout after a nuclear explosion, radioactive caesium may concentrate in cattle and sheep feeding on contaminated grass.

Chromium

- Atomic weight, 52; valencies, 2, 3
- natural isotopes, 50, 52, 53, 54
- abundance in Earth's crust, 0.033%.

Chromium is present in all organic matter. Wheat (1.8 µg/g) and wheat germ (1.3 µg/g) are especially good sources of chromium, as is molasses (1.2 µg/g). There is little chromium in milk.

Dietary intakes range from 5 to 100 µg/day, but absorption is poor, at 1% of available chromium in the diet. Plasma concentration is 0.15 µg/ml, bound to transferrin. There is an accumulation of chromium in the spleen and heart. Chromium is excreted in urine.

The trivalent (Cr III) form is biologically active, but cannot be oxidised in tissues to the hexavalent (Cr VI) form. The role of chromium in human nutrition is uncertain, but it may act in an organic complex that influences and extends the action of insulin. There may also be a role in lipoprotein metabolism, in stabilising the structure of nucleic acids and in gene expression.

Recommended requirements

The recommended requirements for chromium are debatable. It has been suggested that a reasonable intake would be 0.5 µmol/day for adults and between 2 and 19 nmol/kg/day for children and adolescents. The usual body content in adults is 100–200 µmol. A reasonable requirement is 0.4 µmol/day. The chromium content of breast milk has a range of 0.06–1.56 ng/ml; this gives the infant an intake of 15–1300 ng/day.

Cobalt

- Atomic weight, 59; valencies, 2, 3
- natural isotope, 59
- abundance in Earth's crust, 0.0018%.

Wheat, especially wholemeal flour (0.5–0.7 µg/g), and seafoods (1.6 µg/g) are good sources of cobalt.

Cobalt is a constituent of vitamin B_{12}. This appears to be the only biological function of the element.

Absorption of cobalt is facilitated by incorporation into vitamin B_{12}. The intestinal absorption of the cobalt salt is high, at 63–97% efficiency. The plasma concentration ranges from 0.007 to 6 µg/100 ml, bound to albumin.

The main organs and tissues of storage are the liver and fat; cobalt is excreted in the urine.

Recommended requirements

Average intakes of cobalt are approximately 0.3 mg/day and the total body content is about 1.5 mg.

Cobalt can have serious toxic effects, including causing goitre, hypothyroidism and heart failure. In Quebec, cobalt was added to beer to improve the head. This led to cobalt concentrations of 15 µmol/l, which was toxic to men with heavy alcohol consumption. They developed severe cardiomyopathy from which some died.

Copper

- Atomic weight, 64; valencies, 1, 2
- natural isotopes, 63, 64
- abundance in Earth's crust, 0.010%.

Sources of copper include green vegetables, fish, oysters and liver; these foods provide copper at approximately 4 µmol/kcal. Milk, meat and bread provide less than 0.5 µmol/kcal.

Function

Copper is an important component of enzymes, including cytochrome oxidase and superoxide dismutase. Copper may also have a role in iron metabolism, when Fe^{2+} released from ferritin is oxidised to Fe^{3+} for binding to transferrin. Copper is excreted in bile and eliminated in the faeces.

Absorption

The absorption efficiency of copper appears to be 35–70% and may well diminish with age. The bioavailability of copper from milk-based formulae is approximately 50%. Absorption is facilitated by a complicated, specific transport system, which is energy dependent. Factors involved in absorption include the intestinal luminal concentration of amino acids, chelating agents, e.g. gluconate, citrate or phosphate, and the effect of other minerals, e.g. zinc. Cupric copper is more soluble than cuprous, so reducing agents such as ascorbic acid inhibit absorption.

Availability

Copper is bound to a specific blood copper-binding protein, caeruloplasmin, and to a lesser extent to albumin. Caeruloplasmin is present in serum at a concentration of 25–45 mg/100 ml. Each molecule of the protein contains six atoms of copper. The copper is not exchangeable, so the protein is not a transporter protein. The transport and cellular metabolism of copper depend on a series of membrane proteins and a smaller soluble peptide, which form an integrated system to shuttle copper to its site of action. The protein has an *in vitro* oxidase activity to aromatic amines, cysteine, ferrous ions and ascorbic acid.

The total copper in an adult is approximately 50–80 mg, mainly concentrated in muscle and liver. In pregnancy, copper is transferred from the maternal to the foetal liver, where there is storage before birth in the infant's liver (8 mg) for early extrauterine life.

Deficiency

Copper deficiency has not been reported in humans, as there is a wide variety of dietary sources. Premature birth may result in low copper stores. Menke's syndrome is is a rare congenital failure of copper absorption, with poor mental development, failure to keratinise hair, skeletal problems and degenerative changes in the aorta.

Excess

Copper can accumulate excessively in the body in rare, genetically determined conditions. Wilson's disease is a hepatolenticular condition resulting from an accumulation of copper in the body due to a failure to excrete copper in bile. Efficient synthesis of caeruloplasmin leads to copper being transported in the plasma and into albumin. Excess copper is deposited in tissues, particularly the liver and the basal nuclei of the brain, leading to sclerosis, and kidney, corneal and brain abnormalities. This is now treated with D-penicillamine, a chelating agent that facilitates copper excretion.

Acute poisoning and toxicity may present with haemolysis, and brain and hepatic cellular damage. In chronic excess there is interference in the absorption of zinc and iron.

Recommended requirements

The normal adult diet provides 1.5 mg/day. The RNI for an infant is 0.3 mg/day. For children, the RNI is 0.7–1.0 mg/day and for adults an RNI of 1.2 mg/day is required.

Increasing requirements during the first, second and third trimesters of pregnancy necessitate 0.033, 0.063 and 0.15 mg/day, respectively. This increasing need is met by improved absorption through adaptation of enteric absorption rates.

Milk has a copper content of 3.5 μmol/l and the absorption efficiency is said to be 50%. Therefore, the maternal increment required during lactation is approximately 0.4 mg/day.

Body store measurements

Copper binds to two main plasma proteins, albumin and caeruloplasmin. The major copper transport protein may be albumin. Concentrations of caeruloplasmin and a second major copper protein, copper–zinc superoxide dismutase, are unrelated to dietary copper.

Fluorine

- Atomic weight, 19; valency, 1
- natural isotope, 19
- abundance in Earth's crust, 0.027%.

Fluoride forms crystalline calcium fluorapatite in the structure of teeth and bone. There is a general overall acceptance of a role for fluoride in the care of the teeth. When drinking water contains 1 mg/l (1 ppm) there is a coincidental 50% reduction in tooth decay in children.

Absorption and metabolism

Fluoride is absorbed passively from the stomach, but protein-bound organic fluoride is less readily absorbed. Fluoride appears to be soluble and rapidly absorbed, and is distributed throughout the extracellular fluid similarly to chloride.

Concentrations in blood, where fluorine is bound to albumin and tissues, are small. Fluoride is rapidly taken up by bones but equally rapidly excreted in the urine.

Excess

High intake of fluoride, in excess of 1 mg/l, results in mottling of the teeth; the enamel is no longer lustrous and becomes rough, an effect particularly marked on the upper incisors. In concentrations well in excess of 10 parts per million, fluoride poisoning can occur, with a loss of appetite and sclerosis of the bones of the spine, pelvis and limbs. There may be ossification of the tendon insertion of muscles.

Doubts over the fluoridation of water have been raised by many groups. One argument other than teeth mottling is an increased incidence of osteoporosis and hip fractures. This is an immensely complicated area, complicated by previous use of the contraceptive pill, exercise, walking and smoking.

Recommended requirements

There is no known requirement for fluoride and no RNI is recommended.

It has been suggested that adults should have a mean dietary intake of 95 μmol/day or 150 μmol from fluoridated water. Tea is an important source of fluoride.

Body store measurements
A high proportion of the dietary intake of fluoride appears in the urine. Urinary output in general reflects the dietary intake.

Germanium

- Atomic weight, 73; valencies, 2, 4
- natural isotopes, 70, 72, 73, 74, 76
- abundance in Earth's crust, $1 \times 10^{-4}\%$.

Germanium is present in the diet at trace levels, and is consumed at the rate of 1 mg/day and rapidly excreted in urine.

Excess
Consumption of germanium in the order of 50–250 mg/day (0.7–3.4 mmol) over a prolonged period may result in morbidity and even death.

Iodine

- Atomic weight, 127; valencies, 2, 4
- natural isotope, 127
- abundance in Earth's crust, $6 \times 10^{-6}\%$.

Most foodstuffs except for seafood are poor sources of iodine. Fruit, vegetables, cereals, meat and meat products may contain up to 100 μg/kg depending on the soil content where they are grown. Water is not an important source of iodide and contains only small amounts (1–50 μg/l), although the iodine content of the soil water in which plants and cereals are grown is important. Milk is a major source of iodine, with a content in the order of 0.2–23 μmol/kg. Iodine-supplemented cattle feed, iodinated casein, is a lactation promoter in cows. Contamination of milk by iodophors, used as sterilising agents, is an important source of iodine.

Function
Iodine is required for the thyroid hormones, thyroxine 3,5,3',5'-tetraiodothyronine (T_4) and 3,5,3'-triiodothyronine (T_3). Iodide is oxidised to iodine and bound to tyrosine, forming mono- and diiodotyrosines. Subsequent metabolism produces T_3 (triiodothyronine) and T_4 (thyroxine).

Thyroid hormones

Thyroxine is bound to thyroglobulin, which may be stored in the vesicles of the thyroid gland. Thyroid hormone release is dependent on thyrotropic hormone activity from the pituitary gland. Thyroxine is important in cellular metabolism by inducing an increase in the number, size and activity of mitochondria and constituent enzymes. Cellular protein synthesis is increased by thyroid hormones by increased mRNA transcription. Thyroid hormones increase the utilisation of ATP through increased transmembrane transport. Fatty acids are released from adipose tissue under the action of thyroid hormones. Selenium is important in thyroid hormone production, particularly in the conversion of T_4 to the active T_3. It is possible that zinc is also involved. All T_4 is synthesised in the thyroid, whereas 80% of plasma T_3 is derived from 5'-monoiodination of T_4 in liver, kidney and possibly muscle. The enzyme involved in the peripheral conversion of T_4 to T_3 in liver and kidney is type 1 iodothyronine deiodinase (idi), the activity of which is reduced in selenium deficiency. The enzyme is a selenoenzyme.

Absorption
Dietary iodine from food and water is absorbed as inorganic iodide. Some of this is transported to the thyroid gland, depending on the activity and requirements of the gland.

The body content of iodine is 20–50 mg (160–400 μmol). About 8 mg is found in the thyroid gland.

Deficiency
Iodine deficiency is of great importance in thyroid enlargement, namely goitre, in areas where iodine is deficient in the soil. Iodine deficiency disorders have consequences for normal growth and development.

Iodine deficiency results in reduced thyroid iodine stores and production of T_4, There is increased production of pituitary thyroid-stimulating hormone, ineffective hyperplasia of the thyroid and the development of goitre. Iodine deficiency can be demonstrated by urinary iodine excretion measuring 24 h samples (normal range 100–150 μg/day). Goitre may arise through eating plant inhibitors of iodine uptake (goitrogens), e.g. thiocyanate. Staple

Iodine-deficient food crops are found in areas where the iodine has been leached from the soil by glaciers, high rainfall or flooding, such as the Himalayas, the Andes and the vast mountain ranges of China, the Ganges valley and Bangladesh. All the food grown in such soil is iodine deficient and the iodine deficiency will persist in the local population until there is dietary diversification and an increased provision of iodine in the diet. There are 800 million people in the world at risk from iodine deficiency, of whom 190 million may develop goitre and more than 3 million are cretinous. In some populations apathy has been found even among domestic animals as a result of iodine deficiency.

foods in developing countries, e.g. cassava, maize, bamboo shoots, sweet potatoes, lima beans and millet, contain cyanogenic glucosides that produce cyanide that may, in turn, give rise to thiocyanate. In general, this not a problem as they are found in the inedible portions of the plant.

Iodine deficiency in the foetus results from iodine deficiency in the mother and can be reversed by thyroid hormone replacement. Maternal deficiency is associated with a high incidence of stillbirths, spontaneous abortions and congenital abnormalities. The perinatal death rate is also increased.

A consequence of foetal iodine deficiency is endemic cretinism, found in mountainous regions of India, Indonesia and China. This occurs in populations where the iodine intake is less than 25 μg/day, the requirement being 80–150 μg/day. Thyroid hormone is essential for brain development. The human brain has reached only one-third of its full size at birth and continues to grow rapidly until the second year. Severe iodine deficiency adversely affects neonatal thyroid function and hence brain development, with resultant learning disabilities, deaf–mutism and spastic diplegia. This is the nervous or neurological type, in contrast to the myxoedematous type found with hypothyroidism and dwarfism. This community problem can be reversible with replacement of iodine.

Iodine deficiency in children causes goitre. The incidence of goitre increases with age and is maximal in adolescence and particularly marked in girls. The results are poor school performance and reduced intelligence quotients (IQs). However, assessment of IQ is often difficult as the iodine-deficient areas are likely to be remote and to suffer from social deprivation, resulting in poorer school facilities, poverty and poorer general nutrition.

The problems of iodine deficiency may be reversed by using iodised oil.

Excess
A modest increase in the incidence of hyperthyroidism has been described following iodised salt programmes. This condition is found in individuals over 40 years of age, who form a small proportion of the population of a developing country. The condition is readily controlled with anti-thyroid drugs.

Correction of deficiency
People in deficient areas can receive iodine as an additive to food or water, or by direct administration of iodised oil, potassium iodide or iodine in Lugol's solution.

Iodinated salt: salt is usually produced from the evaporation of seawater or brine using the sun's heat, or rock deposits. The crude salt is refined by recrystallisation or milling. Iodine can be added by dry mixing the iodine compound with salt or by dripping a solution of iodine onto the salt on a conveyor belt. Potassium iodide and iodate are the most common additives. The drip-feed system is the simplest and cheapest, but a spray-mix method allows more uniform distribution of iodine with very fine salt. Iodide is cheaper, but iodate is more stable in warm, humid climates. Iodine is usually added at a ratio to salt of 1:10 000 to 1:50 000; this gives an iodine intake of 50–150 μg with a salt intake of 3–15 g/day.

Iodised oil: iodine covalently bound to vegetable oils is given intramuscularly or orally. A single dose of iodised oil is sufficient iodine for at least 3 years, e.g. iodinated poppy seed oil (lipiodol) contains 38% iodine by weight. Iodinated walnut or soya bean oil contains 25% iodine. A single oral administration is effective for at least 1 year. There is the added advantage that injections are not required removing the risk of spreading diseases such as hepatitis and AIDS with non-sterile syringes. Iodised oil is used as an emergency stop-gap measure to control iodine deficiency in severely affected areas until there is an effective programme for iodinated salt. High intakes do not appear to be harmful.

Recommended requirements
Adults have an intake of 70 µg/day. The RNI has been suggested as 140 µg. In infants and children the LRNI is around 40–50 µg/day and the RNI 50–100 µg/day.

Body store measurements
Thyroid hormone measurements reflect iodine status. A high proportion of the dietary intake of iodine appears in the urine, so urinary output in general reflects the dietary intake.

Lead

- Atomic weight, 207; valencies, 2, 4
- natural isotopes 204, 206, 207, 210, 211, 212, 214
- natural abundance in Earth's crust, 0.002%.

There is no evidence that lead is of any importance physiologically. In an industrialised society, 1–2 µmol is ingested in the food daily, and 90% of this is not absorbed. Plasma concentrations are in the range of 15–40 µg/100 ml, bound to protein. Lead is deposited in bone and excreted in bile.

Toxicity
Lead has been widely used in cooking utensils and water pipes. Consequently, it has been an important, albeit toxic, element in the diet. Lead poisoning may lead to anaemia, peripheral neuropathy and encephalopathy. This has been a problem in lead workers, e.g. plumbers, in the past. Water, especially when slightly acidic, that has been held overnight in the pipes, is particularly dangerous. Other lead hazards are pewter vessels, lead toys, paints and leaded petrol, from which a substantial concentration of lead may develop in the atmosphere. Undue exposure to lead may affect the IQ of children growing in this environment. Lead is used in the manufacture of crystal decanters and can be leached from the glass by alcoholic beverages over a long period, e.g. by sherry kept in a decanter.

A blood concentration of more than 1.4 µmol/l is undesirable.

Lithium

- Atomic weight, 7; valency, 1
- natural isotopes, 6, 7
- abundance in Earth's crust, 0.005%.

There is no known role for lithium in normal physiology. The main interest in lithium is in its important role in the prophylactic management of manic–depressive psychosis. Lithium is absorbed efficiently by the intestine and excreted in the urine. The blood therapeutic concentration is 0.6–1.0 mmol/l and side-effects are seen at higher concentrations. Toxicity is associated with abnormalities of glucose metabolism, teratogenicity, hypothyroidism and renal problems.

Magnesium

- Atomic weight, 24; valency, 2
- natural isotopes, 24, 25, 26
- natural abundance in Earth's crust, 1.94%.

Magnesium is present in most foods, particularly those of vegetable origin containing chlorophyll, e.g. green leaves and stalks. Typically, a diet contains 200–400 mg/day. Magnesium is a component of magnesium–porphyrin complexes in chlorophyll in some plant sources.

Function
Magnesium is complexed with ATP in ATP-dependent enzyme reactions, e.g. glycolysis and the Krebs cycle, adenyl cyclase in cAMP formation, phosphatases, and in protein and nucleic acid synthesis.

Magnesium is an important cofactor for cocarboxylase and is involved in the replication of DNA and synthesis of RNA.

Availability
The whole body content of magnesium is about 1 mol (25 g). Almost two-thirds of body magnesium is found in bone in association with phosphate and bicarbonate. The remaining 30% is found intracellularly in soft tissues, bound to protein.

The homoeostasis of magnesium is controlled by a system that involves parathyroid hormones. Excretion is by the kidneys and is related to dietary intake.

Absorption
Magnesium is absorbed from the distal intestine by active transport, although there is also some additional passive diffusion. The maintenance of magnesium homoeostasis includes the reabsorption of endogenous magnesium in enteric secretions. The influence of vitamin D in the absorption process appears to be minimal.

The plasma concentration is 0.6–1.0 mmol/ l; the intracellular concentration is about 10 mmol/l.

Deficiency
Magnesium deficiency is manifested by progressive muscle weakness, failure to thrive, neuromuscular dysfunction, tachycardia, ventricular fibrillation, coma and death. Alcohol abuse and diuretics are important causes of a low serum magnesium.

Recommended requirements
In adults, magnesium balance is achieved with an intake of 50 mg/day. The effectiveness of absorption increases from 25% on a high magnesium diet to 75% on a magnesium-restricted diet. The LRNI for magnesium is 190 mg/day for adult men and 150 mg/day for women. The EAR is 250 mg for men and 200 mg/day for women. The RNI is 300 mg for men and 270 mg/day for women.

Human milk contains approximately 0.12 mmol per 100 ml, so infant intake is approximately 1 mmol/day (25 mg). By 3 months the intake is 0.25 mmol (6mg)/kg/day.

The foetus requires approximately 8.0 mg/day over 40 weeks, so the maternal requirement during pregnancy is around 16 mg/day. Increased effectiveness of absorption and the use of maternal stores ensure adequate provision for the foetus.

The magnesium content of breast milk is approximately 1.2 mmol/l, producing about 25 mg/day. It is suggested that the lactational increment should be 50 mg/day.

Body store measurements
Urinary magnesium is the best method available of assessing dietary intake, but is not very accurate. Urinary output in general reflects dietary intake.

Manganese

- Atomic weight, 55; valencies, 2, 3, 4
- natural isotope, 55

- natural abundance in Earth's crust, 0.085%.

Good sources of manganese are various forms of wheat: wholemeal 50 µg/g, wheat germ 130 µg/g and nuts 17 µg/g. Tea is another source of dietary manganese, as well as unrefined vegetarian diets, e.g. it is found in cereals, legumes and leafy vegetables. Meat, milk and refined cereals are poor sources.

Function
Manganese is important in enzyme activity, e.g. pyruvate carboxylase, mitochondrial superoxide dismutase and arginase. It may also activate other enzymes, e.g. glycosyl transferases, hydrolases, kinases, prolinase and phosphotransferases.

Absorption
Manganese absorption occurs along the entire intestine but overall is only 3–4%. The absorption efficiency in the small intestine is low. High concentrations of calcium, phosphorus, fibre and phytate reduce manganese absorption through interactions. Plasma concentrations are 1–2 µg/g, bound to transferrin.

Manganese is stored in liver and bone. The body pool is largely intracellular and is 0.2–0.4 mmol. The pancreas and liver have the highest concentration and about 25% is in the skeleton. Manganese is excreted in bile and intestinal secretions.

Deficiency
Manganese deficiency has not been reported in humans.

Recommended requirements
The average daily intake in Britain is said to be approximately 4.6 mg/person, half of which is derived from tea. The content of manganese in breast milk in the first 3 months postpartum is 1.9 µg/day and 1.6 µg/day thereafter. Healthy infants fed cow's milk will have an intake of 28–42 µg/kg/day.

Mercury

- Atomic weight, 200; valencies, 1, 2
- natural isotopes, 196, 198, 199, 200, 201, 202, 204
- natural abundance in Earth's crust 2.7×10^{-6}%.

Mercury is present in food in trace amounts, possibly because it has important uses in industry and therefore is a widespread contaminant. It is not an essential element.

Toxicity
Mercuric poisoning may occur with contamination of food in excess of 145 µmol/kg. The toxic forms of mercury are the alkyl derivatives, methyl mercury and ethyl mercury, which can produce an encephalopathy. This was a problem for workers who made top hats in which mercury was used; hence the 'Mad Hatter' in *Alice in Wonderland*. Grain that has been sprayed with alkyl mercury compounds, to prevent fungal disease, has on occasions been eaten by unsuspecting peasant families. This may lead to ataxia and visual disturbances, and even paralysis and death. Alkyl mercury derivatives may be a hazard when eaten with carnivorous fish from polluted waters. Lakes may contain up to 25 µmol of mercury/litre of water, which then passes into the food chain. Microorganisms may be contaminated with inorganic mercury from this water. This is converted into methyl mercury, which may then pass into the food chain via plant-eating small fish to carnivorous large fish, e.g. tuna, swordfish and pike. Most deep-sea fish contain small amounts of mercury, e.g. cod may contain 400 nmol/kg, while fish living in coastal waters near estuaries may contain 2.5 µmol/kg. These may then be eaten by humans or other predators. This may not be a real hazard but it is noteworthy.

Molybdenum

- Atomic weight, 96; valencies, 2, 3, 4
- natural isotopes, 92, 94, 95, 96, 97, 98, 100
- natural abundance in Earth's crust, $7 \times 10^{-4}\%$.

The amount of molybdenum in plants is dependent on where they are grown and on the soil content. Vegetables grown in neutral and alkaline soils with a high content of organic matter have a higher content of molybdenum. Important dietary sources are wheat flour and wheat germ (0.7 and 0.6 µg/g, respectively), legumes (1.7 µg/g) and meat (2 µg/g).

Function
Molybdenum is essential for the enzymes xanthine oxidase/dehydrogenase, aldehyde oxidase and sulfite oxidase, important in the metabolism of DNA and sulfites.

Absorption
Intestinal absorption efficiency is high, at 40–100%; there is a carrier-dependent active process in the stomach and proximal intestine.

Availability
Plasma concentration is 1 µg/100 ml, bound to protein. Storage is in the liver and excretion in urine.

Deficiency and excess
As yet, there have been no reports of molybdenum deficiency in humans.

Gout may be attributed to high intakes of molybdenum (10–15 mg/day). Molybdenum intake at this level may also be associated with altered metabolism of nucleotides and impaired copper bioavailability.

Recommended requirements
These are 50–400 µg/day for adults. For breast-fed infants a requirement of 0.5–1.5 µg/kg/day has been suggested.

Nickel

- Atomic weight, 59; valencies, 2, 3
- natural isotopes, 58, 60, 61, 62, 64
- natural abundance in Earth's crust, 0.018%.

Nickel may be essential in some animals and birds, but deficiency in humans has never been proven.

Absorption
Intestinal absorption from the diet is meagre, at 3–6%. Plasma concentrations are 2–4 µg/100 ml, some bound to albumin, the remainder in free solution. Nickel is excreted in urine.

Deficiency
Nickel deficiency may result in depressed growth and haemopoiesis, but there is uncertainty as to whether nickel is essential.

Phosphorus

- Atomic weight, 31; valencies, 3, 5
- natural isotope, 31
- natural abundance in Earth's crust, 0.12%.

Phosphorus is present in all natural foods. The usual diet in Britain provides 1.5 g of phosphorus daily. Approximately 10% of dietary phosphorus is present as food additives. An excessive intake of aluminium hydroxide antacids may bind dietary phosphate and result in secondary phosphate depletion. This results in muscle weakness and bone pains.

Function
Phosphorus is an important component of the crystalline structure of the bony skeleton with calcium (see Chapter 41). Phosphorus is important in oxidative phosphorylation as part of ATP. Under normal physiological conditions, electron transport is tightly coupled with phosphorylation. ATP generation depends on electron flow, which only occurs when ATP can be synthesised.

Other critical roles are in nucleic acids through the phosphorylation of sugars as a base–sugar–phosphate nucleotide, the phosphate group being a connector between nucleotides in the polynucleotide chain. Phosphorus is important in the control of enzyme activity through phosphorylation. The activity of an enzyme may be changed through alteration in its covalent structure. One way is by phosphorylation of hydroxyl groups in the enzyme, usually the side-chain of serine, threonine or tyrosine residues by a protein kinase and reversed by a phosphoprotein phosphatase. The enzyme is therefore in either an active or inactive conformation. Glycogen phosphorylase is controlled in this manner. The control becomes complex, as in addition to substrate availability there are two control enzymes.

Absorption
Phosphorus absorption is as the dietary free inorganic phosphorus with an efficiency of 50–70%, reaching 90% at low dietary intakes. Phosphorus in the form of phytate may not be hydrolysed or absorbed. Other sources of phosphorus in the intestine include salivary and intestinal secretions. Absorption is by active transport controlled by 1,25(OH)$_2$-vitamin D, at both the brush border and basolateral membrane. The process is active, sodium independent and non-saturable. The jejunum absorbs better than sites further along the intestine. The plasma concentration is 0.8–1.4 mmol/l and is dependent on excretion.

Availability
About 80% of the phosphorus in the human body (19–29 mol; 600–900 g) is found in the skeleton as the calcium salt. The remainder is present as inorganic phosphate and forms part of essential metabolic components such as ATP.

Intracellular are higher than extracellular concentrations; the former are about 5–20 mmol/l and act as an intracellular buffer.

Plasma phosphate concentrations are controlled by renal excretion, although there is some excretion in faeces. Urinary phosphate secretion undergoes diurnal variation governed by adrenocortical hormones through phosphate reabsorption in the renal tubules. Vitamin D metabolites, glucocorticosteroids and growth hormones increase urinary phosphorus excretion. Oestrogens, thyroid and parathyroid hormones, increased plasma calcium concentrations and exercise increase renal reabsorption and hence conservation.

Phosphate metabolism may be disturbed in a number of conditions, particularly those affecting the kidneys and bone.

Recommended requirements
In general, phosphorus requirements are estimated as equimolar to calcium.

Selenium

- Atomic weight, 79; valencies, 2, 4
- natural isotopes, 74, 76, 77, 78, 80, 82
- abundance in Earth's crust, 8×10^{-5}%.

Selenium is found in a number of forms in food, as selenoamino acids, e.g. selenocysteine and selenomethionine, in selenoproteins, and as selenide, selenite or selenate.

The main sources of selenium are cereal, meat and fish: meat 2 µg/g, seafood 0.5 µg/g, nuts 0.7 µg/g and wheat flour 0.3 µg/g. Milk, vegetables and fruit contain little selenium.

Function

Selenium is an essential nutrient. Selenoenzymes, i.e. selenium-dependent enzymes such as iodothyronine, deiodinase and glutathione peroxidases, protect the cell from peroxidative damage. Selenium is part of the active site of these enzymes as selocystine. Selenoprotein activity includes the hepatic microsomal deiodination of thyroxine.

Metallothioneins are small, cysteine-rich proteins that bind divalent metal ions. They act as a store for metals such as zinc. Their concentration in tissues is dependent on metal ion availability. They also act as RNA transcriptional enhancers. Proteins (metal-responsive transcription factors) interact with one of the inducing metal ions and facilitate the transcription of the metallothionein gene.

> Selenocysteine is recognised as the 21st amino acid in ribosome–mediated protein synthesis. Genetic control of the conversion of selenocysteine into selenoproteins involves the codon U(T)GA. This is normally a stop codon, but marks a site of insertion of a selenocysteine residue in each selenoprotein. Insertion of selenocysteine is through an unusual transfer tRNA, which is charged with a serine residue and then converted to selenocysteine. The concentration of the mRNA responsible for glutathione peroxidase is linked to the dietary selenium intake.

Absorption

Absorption is efficient at 35–85%. Selenium absorption may be through a wide variety of mechanisms, e.g. amino acid pathways as selenoamino acids.

Plasma concentration is 7–30 µg/100 ml, bound to protein. Excretion is via the urine and possibly bile.

Deficiency

There is an overlap between selenium deficiency and vitamin E deficiency in a number of animals. This is because selenium is involved in glutathione peroxidase, which destroys lipid hydroperoxides and is important in stabilising lipid membranes by inhibiting oxidative damage. In New Zealand, Venezuela and China the soil is poor in selenium and deficiency problems are reported. In China,

selenium deficiency has been associated with a cardiomyopathy in children (Keshan's disease). Selenium deficiency results in a decrease in glutathione peroxidase activity.

Recommended requirements

The adult RNI has been suggested at 1 µg/kg, which is approximately 70 µg/day in a British adult; 40 µg/day is a suitable LNRI.

Fertility is dependent on an adequate selenium intake. There are adaptive changes in metabolism during pregnancy. In lactation, the concentration of selenium in colostrum varies from 50 to 80 ng/ml. The concentration in breast milk during the first month of lactation is between 18 and 30 ng/ml. This demands an increase in dietary intake of about 15 µg/day.

Breast-fed infants receive approximately 5–13 µg/day. Intakes from formula feeds are generally lower, around 2–4 µg/day. The non-breast-fed infant's RNI is in the order of 1.5 µg/kg/day at 4–6 months.

The RNI for children has been estimated to be equivalent to that for the adult per kg body weight.

Body store measurements

Urine is the major route of excretion and is a reasonable marker of intake. Plasma concentrations reflect intake to an extent, although there is a wide range of variation. Red cell selenium and glutathione peroxidase activity are markers of medium-term status. Hair and toenail concentrations reflect long-term status, but these measurements may be invalidated by the use of shampoos.

Silicon

- Atomic weight, 28; valency, 4
- natural isotopes, 28, 29, 30
- natural abundance in Earth's crust, 25.8%.

Silicon occurs as a silicate, which is very insoluble in water. Cereal grains, other forms of dietary fibre and drinking water (2–12 µg/ml) are important sources of silicon.

Function

The role of silicon in human nutrition is unclear, although it is an essential nutrient for the growing chick and rat. Silicon may be important in the proteoglycans of cartilage and of the ground substance of connective tissue. The human aorta, trachea, lungs and tendon are rich in silicon. The aortic silicon content may decline with age, particularly in the presence of atherosclerosis.

Absorption and storage
Silicic acid in foods and drink is absorbed quickly. The body storage pool is approximately 3 g in a 60 kg man. Maximal levels occur in skin and are found as the free monosilicic acid in plasma (500 μg/100 ml). Only trace amounts are found in tissues, especially skin, cartilage and tissues containing glycosoaminoglycans (glycans, i.e. polysaccharide polymer, containing a substantial proportion of aminomonosaccharide units).

Recommended requirements
The dietary requirements of silicon are not known.

Silver

- Atomic weight, 108; valency, 1
- natural isotopes, 107, 109
- natural abundance in Earth's crust, $4 \times 10^{-6}\%$.

Silver occurs in low concentration in soil, plants and animal tissues. It may interact with copper and selenium, but has no known essential function in humans.

Strontium

- Atomic weight, 88; valency, 2
- natural isotopes, 84, 86, 87, 88 89
- natural abundance in Earth's crust, 0.017%.

Strontium is widely distributed in the environment and in plants, particularly in wheat bran, rather than the endosperm of grains, and in the peel of root vegetables. The strontium content of drinking water varies from 0.02 to 0.06 mg/l, although higher values have been recorded.

Strontium is present in foods that are rich in calcium, e.g. milk and fresh vegetables, and is stored in bone. The concentration is approximately 1000 times lower than that of calcium. Cow's milk has a higher content of strontium than human milk;

therefore, bottle-fed babies have a greater intake of strontium than breast-fed infants. The amount of strontium retained in the body is dependent on urinary loss. Strontium is lost in urine, sweat, other fluids and hair.

Absorption and storage
The body store is in the order of 3.5–4 mmol, of which 99% is present in bones. The efficiency of absorption of strontium is approximately 20%.

Dietary intake
The dietary intake is of the order of 1–3 mg/day. When strontium-90, resulting from atomic explosions is a contaminant, bony malignant lesions, e.g. sarcoma may result. Strontium has no known function and hence is not essential in humans.

Sulfur

- Atomic weight, 32; valencies, 2, 4
- natural isotopes, 32, 33, 34, 36
- abundance in Earth's crust, 0.048%.

Function
Sulfur occurs in tissues as the sulfate, SO_4^{2-}, a component of the proteoglycans that are important in extracellular matrices, cartilage, vascular and reproductive systems, as dermatan sulfate, chondroitin sulfate and keratin sulfate. Disulfide cross-linkages are also important in the specific three-dimensional folding of proteins.

Sulfate is involved in the hepatic enzymatic detoxification of phenols, alcohols and thiols, in part by increasing water solubility and facilitating excretion. Sulfate is involved in an active form of phosphoadenosine and phosphosulfate, and is derived from cysteine and methionine using the molybdenum-dependent sulfite oxidase system. Sulfur is part of glutathione and some coenzymes, including coenzyme A. Sulfur is also present in sulfur-containing amino acids. L-Methionine is metabolised by transmethylation and transsulfuration.

Absorption
Sulfur is largely absorbed as amino acid conjugates, which are subsequently desulfated. It is excreted as free sulfate or as organic and inorganic sulfates.

S-Adenosylmethionine

In methionine metabolism the high-energy sulfonium, S-adenosyl-L-methionine, is formed. This is both a methyl donor for transmethylation reactions and the precursor of decarboxylated S-adenosyl-L-methionine, which is the aminopropyl donor for the synthesis of polyamines. S-Adenosyl-L-methionine is the methyl donor for all known biological methylation reactions, with the possible exception of those involved in methylation of L-homocysteine. S-Adenosyl-L-homocysteine is hydrolysed to l-homocysteine, which can be remethylated to methionine or condensed with serine to form cystathionine. S-Adenosyl-L-methionine may be decarboxylated, to be the donor of aminopropyl groups for the synthesis of spermidine and spermine. The methyl group of adenosyl methionine is transferred to a nitrogen, oxygen or sulfur group of a wide range of compounds in reactions catalysed by numerous methyltransferases.

There is an important reduction of sulfate to sulfide in the colon, which influences the production of hydrogen sulfide or methane gas in the colon.

Recommended requirements
Dietary intake is in the order of 0.7 mg/day.

Body store measurements
Free sulfate in the diet is freely absorbed and freely excreted in the urine.

Tin

- Atomic weight, 119; valencies, 2, 4
- natural isotopes, 112, 114, 115, 116, 117, 118, 119, 120, 122, 124
- natural abundance in Earth's crust, $6 \times 10^{-4}\%$.

Absorption
Human diets may contain 150–200 µg/day, although how much tin is from food and how much from tin cans is not clear. The lacquering of the interior of cans reduces the amount of tin available for absorption. It is not known whether tin is an essential nutrient.

Ingested tin is poorly absorbed and mainly excreted in the faeces. Tin (Sn II) is four times more easily absorbed than the (Sn IV) form. Tin accumulates in the skeleton, liver, spleen and lung, and is excreted in urine.

Deficiency and excess
No naturally occurring tin deficiency has been reported.

High intakes of inorganic tin lead to gastrointestinal symptoms.

Recommended requirements
The upper limit permissible in a canned food is 2.1 mmol/kg. Average intakes in Britain have been estimated at 190 µg/day for an adult, but 99% of the tin is excreted in faeces.

Vanadium

- Atomic weight, 51; valencies, 2, 3, 4
- natural isotopes, 50, 51
- natural abundance in Earth's crust, 0.016%.

Vanadium is present in most human foods, particularly shellfish, mushrooms and peppers. The daily intake in the American diet may be 25 µg.

Function
The biological function and nutritional requirements of vanadium have yet to be identified.

Absorption
Absorption efficiency is meagre, at 0.1–1.5%. This is in part because of the number of non-absorbable complexes that vanadium forms. Vanadium may occur in oxidation states from –1 to +5. Tetravalent and pentavalent ions are the most common form in foods. The reduced vanadyl ion (VO_2^{2+}) binds to ferritin and is transported in the blood in that form. Plasma concentrations are in the order 0.5–2 µg/100 ml, with some binding to transferrin. Excretion is in the urine.

Recommended requirements
These are in the order of 1–2 µg/day, but this is only a rough estimate.

Zinc-finger 'proteins'

There are a several generic classes of gene transcriptional regulators, including those based on helix-turn-helix, leucine-zipper and zinc-finger transcription motifs. The number of different zinc-finger proteins may exceed 100.

Most zinc-finger proteins relate to genes transcribed by RNA polymerase II and bind to a promoter lying outside the coding region. Zinc-finger proteins include at least two distinctly different groups of transcription factors, the C2-H2 and C2-C2 series and GAL4. Polypeptide loops are stabilised by being held together by a zinc ion, tetrahedrally co-ordinated to a cysteine residue. The C2-C2 zinc-finger proteins are important as nuclear receptors for the steroid and thyroid hormones and for retinoids. All of the zinc-finger proteins have been shown to be transcriptional control factors. The zinc ions are essential for their function.

Zinc

- Atomic weight, 65; valency, 2
- natural isotopes, 64, 66, 67, 68, 70
- natural abundance in Earth's crust, 0.02%.

Dietary sources of zinc are meat (3–5 mg/100 g), whole grains and legumes (2–3 mg/100 g) and oysters (70 mg/100 g). White bread, fats and sugars are not very good sources.

Zinc is essential in the human diet.

Function

Zinc is required for many enzymatic functions, DNA synthesis, cell division and protein synthesis. Zinc is involved in enzyme activity, including carbonic anhydrase, alcohol dehydrogenase, alkaline phosphatase, lactate dehydrogenase, superoxides, dismutases and pancreatic carboxypeptidase. The role of the zinc ion is to stabilise a highly reactive hydroxide ion, so that an activated nucleophile is available for catalysis.

It has long been believed that zinc is important for wound healing.

Absorption

Approximately 20% of dietary zinc is absorbed. During digestion free zinc is complexed with ligands such as amino acids, phosphates and organic acids. Phytates and oxalates may form insoluble complexes that inhibit absorption. The coincidental presence of copper and iron may inhibit absorption.

Normal plasma concentration is 11–22 µmol/l, bound to albumin.

The adult body content of zinc is over 2 g (30 mmol). The prostate gland, choroid of the eye and semen have high concentrations of zinc, but the greatest amount is in bones (about 200 µg/g). Red blood cells contain 13 µg/ml and hair contains 120–250 µg/g, both in newborns and adults.

Urinary loss is in the order of 6–9 µmol (average male 0.63 mg; female 0.44 mg)/day. Most zinc is lost in the faeces, and the control of zinc homoeostasis is by colonic absorption. Other routes of loss of zinc are kidney, integument (0.4–5 mg/day, male and female), semen (0.1 mg/ejaculation), and menses.

Deficiency

Zinc deficiency is rare, as zinc is so widely available in foods, but where it has been described it has been associated with increased zinc losses from the body. The clinical syndrome of growth retardation, male hypogonadism, skin changes, mental lethargy, hepatosplenomegaly, iron-deficiency anaemia and geophagia has been reported from studies of male dwarfs in Iran, which are said to be due to true zinc deficiency. This secondary sexual retardation is in part due to reduced serum testosterone, dihydrotestosterone and androstenedione concentrations. These deficiencies are treatable with zinc supplementation (15 mg, three times a day as zinc acetate) for at least 12 months. The mechanism by which zinc affects testosterone concentration in zinc-deficient subjects is not known, but a zinc-dependent enzyme may be important in sex hormone synthesis.

The dermatological signs of severe zinc deficiency include progressive bullous-pustular dermatitis at the extremities and the oral, anal and genital areas, combined with paronychia and generalised alopeciae. These respond to dietary supplementation of zinc sulfate.

Zinc deficiency has been reported in alcoholics who have low serum zinc concentrations. Similarly, hepatic cirrhosis is associated with low serum and hepatic zinc, and increased urinary zinc excretion. Zinc deficiency has been reported in patients with steatorrhoea and, presumably, zinc malabsorption, or when there is loss of zinc protein complexes into the intestinal lumen in malignancies. Extensive burns may also result in reduced plasma zinc concentration, due to a loss of zinc through the skin. In renal disease excess zinc may be lost in the urine, with a consequent reduction in plasma and tissue concentrations.

Iatrogenic causes of zinc deficiency include the use of antimetabolites and diuretics.

Genetic disorders: acrodermatitis enteropathica is a potentially lethal autosomal recessive trait that manifests itself in infancy after weaning, and consists of pustular and bullous dermatitis, alopecia and diarrhoea. Zinc supplementation is necessary. The condition is due to zinc malabsorption. Sickle-cell anaemia may be associated with zinc deficiency. Zinc supplementation for sickle-cell anaemia promotes weight gain, growth of pubic hair, serum testosterone concentrations, plasma zinc, tissue zinc and neutrophil alkaline phosphatase activity.

Excess
Excessive zinc can lead to nausea, vomiting and fever.

Recommended requirements
The recommended intake varies between 7 and 15 mg/day, although only 20–30% of this is absorbed.

Adult requirements of zinc are approximately 2–3 mg/day (30–40 µmol). Minimal losses are in the order of 30 and 20 µmol/day in men and women, respectively. Since absorption is only 20–30% efficient, this suggests RNIs of 145 and 110 µmol/day for men and women, and LRNIs of 85 and 60 µmol, respectively.

Human milk is not a rich source of zinc, and the infant is highly dependent on the stores accumulated in the last 3 months of intrauterine life. Assuming a daily requirement of 1 mg/day and an absorption efficiency of 30%, an EAR of 3 mg/day has been suggested, and an RNI of 4 mg/day.

The EAR in children is around 3.8–5.4 mg/day, with an RNI of 5–7 mg/day.

Extra zinc is required during pregnancy. Zinc in the order of 8 mg is needed by the foetus during the last 3 months of gestation, requiring an additional maternal intake of 2 mg/day, assuming an

Summary of activity of trace elements

Enzyme co-factors	Aluminium, copper, magnesium, manganese, molybdenum selenium, zinc
General Ligand	boron
Protein ligand	sulfur, phosphorous
Coenzyme	phosphorous
Hormones	iodine
Vitamin	cobalt
Conjugation reactions	sulfur
Gene transcription	selenium, zinc
Skeletal structure	fluorine, magnesium, phosphorus, silicon, sulfur
No evident nutritional function	bromine, cadmium, caesium, chromium, germanium, lead, lithium, mercury, nickel, silver, strontium, tin, vanadium

absorption efficiency of 20–30%. This means that the dietary requirement is 6–14 mg/day. It is not known whether there is an increased dietary need during lactation.

Supplementary zinc may be given as zinc sulfate.

Body store measurements
The concentration of plasma zinc that is neither haemolysed nor contaminated is a measure of zinc status. An alternative is the plasma copper:zinc ratio. An increase in this ratio of greater than 2 is suggested to be related to zinc deficiency. Zinc in the red blood cells and hair gives a long-term assessment of zinc status, as the zinc turnover in red cells and hair is slow.

Neutrophil alkaline phosphatase activity has been used to assess zinc status. Urinary excretion of zinc is decreased during zinc deficiency.

KEY POINTS

1. Trace elements are present in the diet in milligram amounts.
2. They are important in that they establish potential differences across membranes; such

differences have to be maintained by energy requiring reactions.

3. They are also co-factors for enzyme oxidation-reduction reactions; the active principle may be copper, iron, magnesium, manganese or sulfur; in addition, phosphorus has a role in controlling the enzyme active sites.

4. They are important in maintaining the structure of proteins and nucleic acids; trace elements, e.g. zinc, may adsorb to proteins in specific configurations. Such trace elements act as cofactors or structural elements by high local concentrations of positive charges, in two or more valency states, e.g. copper, molybdenum and selenium.

5. Trace elements are also important in the structure of hormones and vitamins, e.g. iodine in thyroxine and cobalt in vitamin B_{12}.

6. Trace elements are involved in skeletal structure, e.g. fluorine, magnesium and phosphorus in bone and teeth, and silicon in cartilage.

7. Na^+ and K^+, with single positive charges, rarely form complexes with proteins. Occasionally, the divalent alkaline metals Mg^{2+} and Ca^{2+} complex with proteins. The other elements in biological systems are from the first transition series and exist in more than one oxidative state, which is important in oxidation-reduction reactions.

8. Some trace elements are toxic, e.g. lead, aluminium, mercury and arsenic. These may reduce intellect in the young and elderly. The function of some trace elements, e.g. vanadium, has still to be established.

THINKING POINT

Elements in the free form are toxic, but bound to molecules they are essential.

NEED TO UNDERSTAND

The role of trace elements in metabolism and the differentiation of the essential from the toxic.

FURTHER READING

Ahmad, K. (2001) Report highlights widespread arsenic contamination in Bangladesh. *Lancet*, **358**, 133.

Anon. (1992) Aluminium, a dementing ion. *Lancet*, **339**, 713–14.

Anon. (1992) Essential trace elements and thyroid hormones. *Lancet*, **339**, 1575–6.

Aposhian, H.V. (1997) Enzymatic methylation of arsenic species and other new approaches to arsenic toxicity. *Annual Review of Pharmacology and Toxicology*, **37**, 397–419.

Cashman, K.D. and Flynn, A. (1999) Optimum nutrition: calcium, magnesium and phosphorus. *Proceedings of the Nutrition Society*, **58**, 477–87.

Combs, G.F. Jr (2001) Selenium in global food systems. *British Journal of Nutrition*, **85**, 517–47.

Cousins, R.J. (1998) The role of zinc in the regulation of gene expression. *Proceedings of the Nutrition Society*, **57**, 307–11.

Duffield, A.J. and Thomson, C.D. (1999) A comparison of methods of assessment of dietary selenium in Otago, New Zealand. *British Journal of Nutrition*, **82**, 131–8.

Failla, M.L. (1999) Considerations for determining 'optimum nutrition' for copper, zinc, manganese and molybdenum. *Proceedings of the Nutrition Society*, **58**, 497–505.

Fairweather-Tait, S. and Hurrell, R.F. (1996) Bioavailability of minerals and trace elements. *Nutrition Research Reviews*, **9**, 295–324.

Gibson, R.S. (2000) Zinc supplementation for infants. *Lancet*, **366**, 2008–9.

Hambridge, M. and Krebs, N.F. (2001) Interrelationships of key variables of human zinc homeostasis: relevance to dietary zinc requirements. *Annual Review of Nutrition*, **21**, 429–52.

Harris, E.D. (2000) Cellular copper transport and metabolism. *Annual Review of Nutrition*, **20**, 291–310.

Hausen, H.W. (2000) Fluoridation, fractures and teeth. *Lancet*, **321**, 844–5.

Hetzel, B.S. and Dunn, J.T. (1989) The iodine deficiency disorders. Their nature and prevention. *Annual Review of Nutrition*, **9**, 21–38.

Huffman, D.L. and O'Halloran, T.V. (2001) Function, structure and mechanism of intracellular copper trafficking proteins. *Annual Review of Biochemistry*, **70**, 677–701.

Jeejeebhoy, K.N. (1999) The role of chromium in nutrition and therapeutics and as a potential toxin. *Nutrition Reviews*, **57**, 329–35.

Lightowler, H.J. and Davies, G.J. (1998) Iodine intake and iodine deficiency in vegans as assessed by the duplicated-portion technique and urinary iodine excretion. *British Journal of Nutrition*, **80**, 529–35.

McDonagh, M.S., Whiting, P.F., Wilson, P.M. *et al.* (2000) Systematic review of water fluoridation. *British Medical Journal*, **321**, 855–9.

Neves, J. (2000) New approaches to assess selenium status and requirements. *Nutrition Review*, **58**, 363–9.

Osendarp, S.J.M., van Raaij, J.M.A., Darmstadt, G.L. *et al.* (2001) Zinc supplementation during pregnancy and effects on growth and morbidity in low birth weight infants: a randomised placebo controlled trial. *Lancet*, **357**, 1080–5.

Phiel, C.J. and Klein, P.S. (2001) Molecular targets of lithium action. *Annual Review of Pharmacology and Toxicology*, **41**, 789–813.

Prasad, A.S. (1985) Clinical manifestations of zinc deficiency. *Annual Review of Nutrition*, **5**, 341–63.

Rayman, M.P. (2000) The importance of selenium to human health. *Lancet*, **356**, 233–41.

Rosen, C.J. (2000) Fluoride and fractures: an ecological fallacy. *Lancet*, **355**, 247–8.

Satarug, S., Haswell-Elkins, M.R. and Moore, M.R. (2000) Safe levels of cadmium intake to prevent renal toxicity in human subjects. *British Journal of Nutrition*, **84**, 791–802.

Stadtman, T.C. (1996) Selenocysteine. *Annual Review of Biochemistry*, **65**, 83–100.

Umeta, M., West, C.E., Haidar, J. *et al.* (2000) Zinc supplementation and stunted infants in Ethiopia: a randomised controlled trial. *Lancet*, **355**, 2021–6.

Vincent, J.B. (2000) Quest for the molecular mechanism of chromium action and its relationship to diabetes. *Nutrition Reviews*, **58**, 67–72.

Vulpe, C.D. and Packman, S. (1995) Cellular copper transport. *Annual Review of Nutrition*, **15**, 293–322.

Watts, J. (2001) Mercury poisoning victims could increase by 20,000. *Lancet*, **358**, 1349.

Winzerling, J.Y. and Law, J.H. (1997) Comparative nutrition of iron and copper. *Annual Review of Nutrition*, **17**, 501–26.

19

Non-nutritive components of food

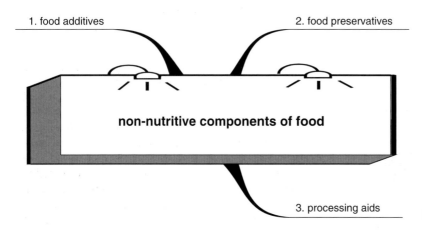

1. food additives

2. food preservatives

non-nutritive components of food

3. processing aids

Fig. 19.1　Chapter outline.

FOOD ADDITIVES

A food additive (Table 19.1) may be regarded as a substance, either synthetic or natural, that is normally not consumed as food itself, but is deliberately added, usually in small amounts. The substance is intended to remain in food for some desirable function or effect during manufacturing, production, processing, storage or packaging, or in the finished product. Food additives enhance the appearance, quality, consumer acceptability and flavour of foods, extend shelf-life and allow mass production, mass distribution and ready availability. They may facilitate and standardise preparation, enhance nutritional value or provide for specific dietary requirements. Azo dyes are colour fast and are commonly used as colouring agents.

Food additives, e.g. salts and spices, have been used throughout recorded food history. Nutrients of various types have been added to food to minimise the incidence of conditions known to be due to deficiency in the community diet. Iodine, calcium and, more controversially, fluoride have been added to food.

The functions of nutritional additives include enrichment and fortification. Enrichment replaces nutrients lost during processing through oxidation or reaction with food components, e.g. ascorbic acid and thiamin, which are lost through chemical and enzymatic degradation. Fortification is the addition during manufacture of substances to improve dietary intake, e.g. vitamins in margarine.

A distinction has to be made between toxic substances and a toxic effect. All substances have the potential to be toxic, but only at a concentration at which the substance produces that toxic effect. The use of food additives free from toxic effects is controlled by regulatory and advisory committees within the European Union, the United States Food

Table 19.1 'E' numbers

Colourings and additives	E number
Yellow	E100–E110
Red	E120–E129
Blue	E131–E133
Green	E140–E142
Brown and black	E150–E155
Plant extracts	E160–E163
Other colourings	E170–E180
Preservatives	E200–E297
Antioxidants	E300
Emulsifiers, stabilisers and auxiliary compounds	E322–E495
Acids, bases and related materials	E500–E529
Anticaking agents and auxiliary additives	E530–E585
Flavour enhancers and sweeteners	E620–E640
Glazing agents and auxiliary additives	E900–E914
Flour treatments, improvers and bleaching agents	E920–E928
Packing gases	E941–E948
Sweeteners	E950–E967

and Drugs Administration and the World Health Organisation. The decisions of these policy-making bodies are based on scientific studies (e.g. toxicity studies), which include evidence of safety to the foetus and absence of the potential to cause cancerous changes in cells. There are, however, inevitable tensions between regulations and the need to produce food economically. Nonetheless, all additive manufacturers must follow the stipulated guidelines and demonstrate both the safety of and need for their product.

The guidelines also identify a acceptable daily intake (ADI), which is an estimate of the amount of the food additive expressed on a body weight basis that can be ingested daily over a lifetime without appreciable health risk, and is expressed on a milligram/kilogram body weight basis (mg/kg BW/day). This is a widely used measurement and is applicable to people of all ages. Some additives come into the category of generally regarded as safe (GRAS), e.g. ascorbic acid.

Food additive may also have negative effects. Antioxidants, spices, gums and waxes may result in dermatitis. Tartrazine, the antioxidants BHA and BHT, and sacramen may cause urticaria. There is an increased risk of tartrazine sensitivity in aspirin-intolerant patients. Benzoic acid and sodium benzoate, which are used to suppress the growth of yeast and bacteria in food, can cause skin and asthmatic reactions, particularly in patients already suffering from asthma. Sodium monoglutamate can produce the 'Chinese restaurant syndrome': bronchospasm, flushing and headache.

FOOD PRESERVATIVES

Preservatives are added to foods that readily perish and deteriorate owing to bacterial colonisation. Perhaps the most significant example is the prevention of botulism, using vinegar (and hence low pH) and salt 15% w/v, or by heating to 121°C for at least 3 min.

PROCESSING AIDS

Despite seasonal variations in the availability of natural products, the food industry strives to ensure that products are uniform in appearance and availability. Butter naturally varies in yellow colour throughout the year and its composition, e.g. milk with variable milk sugar, protein and fat content, may have to be adjusted to achieve a consistent product.

KEY POINTS

1. Food additives are a wide range of chemicals intended to preserve and enhance the appearance of food.
2. It is useful to be familiar with the concepts, not the detail.

THINKING POINTS

1. Food additives are a controversial topic in nutrition.
2. Consider and contrast food additives, which are well-studied chemicals, with the plant secondary metabolites, which are less well characterised.

20

Agricultural chemicals in the food chain

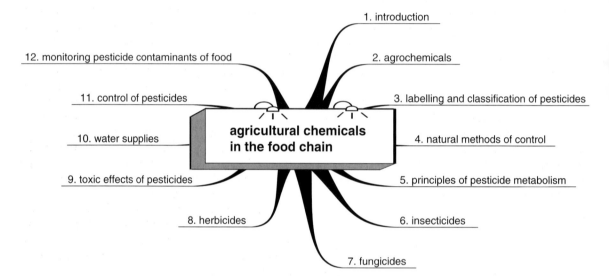

Fig. 20.1 Chapter outline.

INTRODUCTION

Why should a student of nutrition be exposed to the chemistry of agricultural chemicals? These substances are extensively applied to growing crops and are present in many sources of food, and it is therefore important to know what they are and their biology.

The agricultural industry is the source of the urban society's food. The industry looks for a predictable harvest, which requires good weather, adequate equipment, fertile soil and freedom from infestation and disease in the plants.

Food price competition places pressure on farmers to produce cheap food. Such pressure requires more intensive use of better land. Such efficiency is seen as being sustainable only with the use of fertilisers and the elimination of pests and weeds, often by chemical methods. Humans, as hunter-gatherers, had to wander over large areas to find randomly distributed sources of food, in competition with other forms of life living off these particular plant and animal foods. Intensive farming released people from hunter-gathering, but such large areas of food did not pass unnoticed by the predators, which would also enjoy the concentration of food in one area. The use of chemicals is intended to redress the balance in our favour. This has introduced other unexpected imbalances that appear to benefit no one. There is a basic need in agricultural practice for nitrogen, potassium and phosphate. The crop yield becomes more abundant as the amount of nitrogen applied increases. Inorganic nitrogen is usually applied as ammonium nitrate. Organic nitrogen in the form of manure and blood, etc., is effective, but is both smelly and bulky and is required in vast amounts to produce an equivalent amount of nitrogen.

The control of insects that are parasitic on plants used for food has a very long history. Sulfur was used to control pests by the Egyptians, the Ancient Greeks and the Romans. In the nineteenth century, the French developed the use of copper sulfate and lime as fungicides. For generations farmers in the USA have combated the Colorado beetle using the arsenical poison Paris green.

Large volumes of pesticide liquid are sprayed onto plants throughout the world, and have entered every food chain. In the USA in 1984, the value of pesticides sold by the top 16 USA manufacturers was approximately $6500 million. For a major international pesticide producer the relative amounts sold in US world-wide are:

- selective herbicides 32%
- non-selective herbicides 13%
- fungicides and insecticides 18%.

In Great Britain in 1999, the total amount applied was 22 643 tonnes, of which 18 301 tonnes was in commercial agriculture and horticulture. This outlay may be lessened in the future by the introduction of genetically modified crops, for which there is less or no need for pesticide spraying. The increasing commitment to organic farming may also have its effects. Organic agriculture is defined by the World Health Organisation (WHO) and Food and Agriculture Organisation (FAO) as a 'holistic production management system which promotes and enhances agro-ecosystem health, including biodiversity, biological cycles, and soil biological activity. This is accomplished by using, where possible, cultural, biological and mechanical methods; as opposed to using synthetic materials to fulfil any specific function within the system'.

Herbicides have had a profound effect on crop yields, allowing direct drilling, early harvesting and proven product quality. Local authorities use pesticides for weed control on footpaths and road margins, to control grass moss in sports grounds and to control slugs.

Intensive animal production is heavily dependent on disinfectants and other measures against infection such as formaldehyde, phenolics, iodine-containing sheep dips, vaccines and organophosphates, given in bolus form to ruminants.

The world-wide spread of the mite *Varroa jacobsoni* has had profound effects on bee colonies. This mite is associated with viral attacks on the enervated bees. The varroa infestation can be reduced by oxalic acid spraying or by specific chemicals.

Therapeutic antibiotics are permitted for prophylactic use when prescribed by veterinary practitioners. Nevertheless, the number of strains of bacteria resistant to these antibiotics is increasing. Feeds containing preservatives, propionic acid, minerals, vitamins and urea will supplement the requirements of the ruminal flora for nitrogen. Gut flora is manipulated by copper and zinc bacitracin.

The use of pesticides is important in limiting outbreaks of infectious diseases that may be spread by food. The use of insecticide sprays during the fly season can reduce the incidence of childhood diarrhoea, a potentially lethal condition.

The battle is not being won by the agrochemical industry. Insects and weeds are developing resistance to pesticides and herbicides, while opportunist weeds grow in the spaces left by the disappearance of other weeds.

AGROCHEMICALS

Agrochemical pesticides can be divided into four main groups:

- traditionally compromising inorganics, e.g. arsenate, sulfur and copper
- biologically selective agents: plant extracts such as nicotine and pyrethroids. More recent developments include synthetic pyrethroids that are stable when exposed to light and water
- organochlorine compounds, e.g. DDT, dieldrin and aldrin
- organophosphorus products.

A classified list in terms of usage is presented in the box below.

Pesticides

Acaricides	Insecticides
Algicides	Insect repellents
Antifeedants	Mammal repellents
Avicides	Mating disrupters
Bactericides	Molluscicides
Bird repellents	Nematicides
Chemosterilants	Plant activators
Fungicides	Plant growth regulators
Herbicide safeners	Rodenticides
Herbicides	Synergists
Insect attractants	Virucides

Each major group may be divided into chemical or other classes:

Insecticides

- Botanical and other biological products
- carbamate-insecticides
- chlorinated hydrocarbons
- organophosphates
- pyrethroids.

Fungicides

- Benzimidazoles
- diazoles
- dithiocarbamates
- diazines
- inorganics
- morpholines
- triazoles.

Herbicides

- Amides
- bipiridils
- carbamate-herbicides
- dinitroanilines
- phenoxyhormone products
- sulfonyl ureas
- triazines
- uracil
- urea derivatives.

The frequency, amount and type of agrochemicals applied vary from year to year.

LABELLING AND CLASSIFICATION OF PESTICIDES

In the UK, pesticide labels must conform to the *Data Requirements for the Control of Pesticide Regulations*, (1984) which covers the classification, packaging and labelling of dangerous substances and includes various European Union (EU) directives. A label must include:

- the trade name
- the common name with concentration
- restrictions for use
- manufacturer's recommendations on the method of usage, e.g. rate of application.

The law also requires further instructions to be followed, for example:

- precautions
- name and address of holder of approval
- registration number approval.

Dangerous pesticides are classified as those that are:

- very toxic, with an oral median lethal dose (LD_{50}) in rats of 5 mg/kg or less
- toxic, i.e. LD_{50} of 5–50 mg/kg
- harmful, i.e. LD_{50} of 50–500 mg/kg.

Other classifications are inflammable, flammable, oxidising or corrosive. It is also important that the public are aware of the presence of residues in food, including the labelling of post-harvest application.

NATURAL METHODS OF CONTROL

Pesticides

Pesticides which are acceptable to organic organisations such as the Soil Association include pyrethrum, derris, soft soap and aluminium sulfate. Derris and pyrethrum, natural products extracted from plants, may also contain piperonyl butoxide, which adds to the effectiveness of the pyrethrum. Both of these compounds are short-lived but kill a wide range of creatures, including ladybirds, bees, butterflies, fish, toads and tortoises. Soft soap kills soft-bodied insects by removing the protective wax covering of their skins.

Fungi

There are no natural organic fungicides, but there are some naturally occurring mineral fungicides, e.g. copper salts and sulfur. It is possible to minimise the spread of some fungal diseases by growing resistant, less vulnerable varieties, growing young plants in good light and well-ventilated sites and removing infected plants. Good growing conditions are important; however, the breeding of new fungus-resistant plants may also result in unexpected, unwanted modifications of the overall characteristics or specific chemistry of the plant.

PRINCIPLES OF PESTICIDE METABOLISM

Metabolism has an important role in dictating the selective action of pesticides and protects some species, including humans. Most pesticides are poorly soluble in water. Oxidation and hydrolysis are primary metabolic reactions, with the insertion or uncovering of polar groups. Sometimes the products of primary actions undergo further secondary changes, e.g. conjugation, before biliary and urinary excretion. The secondary reactions are very species dependent. There is therefore different metabolism of foreign compounds in organisms as remote as fungal mould and humans. A substance accumulates in a living organism until a toxic concentration is reached. Pesticides, therefore, are metabolised to compounds that accumulate in the target organism and either do not accumulate or are safely excreted by humans and other animals.

Enzymes that metabolise foreign compounds catalyse reactions that:

- alter the molecular structure, to a less toxic product
- increase the polarity and water solubility, and facilitate urinary and biliary excretion.

The majority of the enzymes responsible for the primary metabolism of foreign compounds are hydrolases and oxygenases (Figure 20.2).

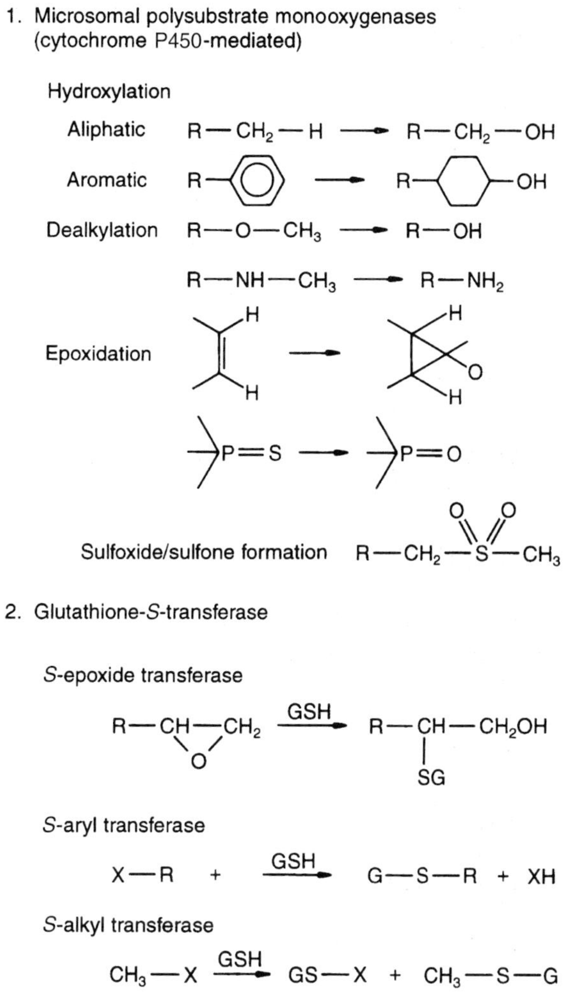

1. Microsomal polysubstrate monooxygenases (cytochrome P450-mediated)

2. Glutathione-S-transferase

Fig. 20.2 Metabolism of pesticides: microsomal polysubstrate monooxygenases and glutathione-S-transferases. GSH: glutathione.

The extent to which a chemical is metabolised dictates the persistence of pesticides in soil, plants and animals. Resistance to pesticides results from pests' developing or possessing metabolic processes that reduce the biological reaction and metabolism or increase the rate of urinary or biliary excretion.

Hydrolases

Hydrolytic enzymes are widespread in plants, animals and various parts of individual cells, including

Hydrolase actions

Many pesticides have ester, amide or phosphate linkages that are split by hydrolases:

- organophosphorus, pyrethroid, carbamate (insecticide)
- dithiocarbamate, dinitrophenol (fungicide)
- urea, carbamate (herbicide).

Substrate specificities:

- R-O-P linkage: phosphatase
- R-COOR' linkage: carboxylesterase, carboxyesterase
- R-CONHR' linkage: carboxyamide.

Esterases are of two types:

- A-esterase: involved in a hydrolytic reaction increased by organophosphates, e.g. paraoxan
- B-esterase: involved in a hydrolytic reaction inhibited by organophosphates, differing in the post-reaction dephosphorylation rate.

Malathion is detoxified by a carboxylesterase:

$$R–COO–C_2H_5 \rightarrow RCOOH + C_2H_5OH$$

Hydrolysis of esters of 2,4-dichlorophenoxyacetic acid (2,4-D) in plants leads to the development of an active metabolite within the plant cell.

vertebrate cytoplasm, microsomal membranes and the endoplasmic reticulum of liver cells.

Hydrolytic enzymes are found as membrane-bound hydrolases in microsomes. There is considerable species variation between the microsomal polysubstrate mono-oxygenases responsible for the oxidation of a number of drugs and pesticides across both the plant and the animal kingdoms, but the primary metabolites are remarkably constant from phylum to phylum.

Hydrolysis plays an important part in the metabolism of the oxime subgroup of carbamates after an initial oxidative step. Carbamates have a high affinity for esterases.

Many pesticides contain $–O–CH_3$ or $–O–C_2H_5$ groupings. These alkyl groups are removed by a glutathione transferase system (Figure 20.2). Amide groups are removed by an amidase, e.g. with dimethoate.

Propanil is a selective herbicide used to control weeds in rice fields. Rice plants are unaffected as they reduce the herbicidal activity of propanil

using an aryl carboxylamidase enzyme. Some carboxyamidases act as carboxylesterases and are able to select amides as substrates. This is important in cross-resistance over a wide range of effects of different pesticides, e.g. the ester malathion and the amide dimethoate. Resistance by insects to some insecticides results from their possessing or developing high concentrations of the enzyme carboxylesterase.

Epoxides are transient intermediates in the metabolism of unsaturated compounds. The epoxide of the organochlorine aldrin is stable, persists in fat tissues and is more toxic than the parent compound. The reaction involves a hepatic epoxide hydrolase enzyme which generates highly active epoxides that bind to DNA. Cyclic compounds with one or two double bonds readily form labile epoxides. Some organic pesticides form epoxides, e.g. dieldrin and endrin.

Oxidation reactions

The oxidation of drugs and pesticides requires microsomal polysubstrate mono-oxygenases and cytochrome P450. Such enzyme systems are found in plants, vertebrates and invertebrates. Oxidation reactions that require mono-oxygenase are:

- aliphatic and aromatic hydroxylation
- O- and N-dealkylation
- epoxidation
- substitution of oxygen for sulfur: formation of sulfoxides and sulfones, and formation of amino oxides.

Microsomal polysubstrate oxygenases are found in the smooth endoplasmic reticulum of liver cells:

$$R–H + O_2 \rightarrow R–OH.$$

These mixed-function oxidases require cytochrome P450, producing O^-, which is then hydrolysed to water.

Flavine adenine dinucleotide (FAD) oxygenases require the reduced form of nicotinamide-adenine dinucleotide (NADH) and are of limited relevance to pesticide metabolism. There are three fractions: cytochrome P450, a flavoprotein NADPH–cytochrome P450 oxidoreductase and a phospholipid. These enzymes form a group of isoenzymes that vary in different organs, are found in all species and phyla, and are under hormonal control.

Cytochrome P450 mono-oxygenases are inhibited by methylene dioxyphenols, e.g. piperonyl butoxide. These delay the metabolism of pesticides, e.g. carbamates, which then accumulate to toxic concentrations in the organism.

Aliphatic hydroxylations are a common metabolic route for aromatic or heterocyclic pesticides, e.g. a methyl group in the acid moiety of pyrethrin can be converted to a hydroxymethyl group.

Oxidative desulfuration is important in the metabolism of thiophosphate insecticides, which are NADPH dependent. The S atom is replaced to yield a substance with more potent choline esterase inhibitor efficacy than the original. This phenomenon is lethal metabolism, e.g. parathion is converted to the more lethal paraoxon.

Sulfoxidation: an FADH-containing mono-oxygenase system oxidises sulfide sulfur to sulfoxide

demeton-*S*-methyl $\rightarrow$ sulfoxide
aldicarb $\rightarrow$ aldicarb sulfoxide $\rightarrow$ aldicarb sulfone.

O-Dealkylation is a common metabolic pathway for pesticides, involving at least three mechanisms.

N-Dealkylation is common in pesticide metabolism as many pesticides are substituted amines or amides, e.g. carbamate, carbufuran or diuron, as well as the herbicide atrazine. Resistance to atrazine occurs if this metabolic pathway is well developed in the plant.

Glutathione is important in glutathione-*S*-transferase involvement in pesticide degradation.

- **Reaction 1** (catalysed by glutathione-*S*-epoxide transferase) opens epoxide rings and as an additive reaction inserts a glutathione; this is important in the metabolism of potentially carcinogenic oxides, e.g. dieldrin, endrin and heptachlor epoxide.
- **Reaction 2** (catalysed by glutathione-*S*-aryl transferase) occurs in the animal liver and also in plants, varying in activity from species to species. The reaction involves the transfer of active thiol groups, and the elimination of a hydrogen halide, e.g. dichloronitrobenzene, atrazine and other chlorinated triazine herbicides. Maize, which is resistant to atrazine, contains an abundance of this enzyme.
- **Reaction 3** (catalysed by glutathione-*S*-alkyl transferase) involves alkyl halides and the removal of methyl groups from those organophosphorus insecticides containing CH_3–O–P.

Conjugation

Conjugation and acetylation reactions involve glucuronic acid, glucose, arginine, glutamic acid, glycine and sulfate by membrane-bound enzymes and cofactors in the cytosol.

Glucuronide formation is important and occurs in terrestrial vertebrates possessing a microsomal glucuronyl transferase. The fungicide ferbam is converted to *S*-glucuronide in some animals.

INSECTICIDES

Classification of insecticides

Neurological
Acetylcholine esterase inhibitors:

- carbamates, act on synapses

Channel and receptor inhibitors and blockers:

- GABA-gated chloride antagonists, e.g. cyclodienes
- sodium channel modulators, e.g. organochlorines, pyrethroids
- acetylcholine receptor antagonists, e.g. nicotine
- acetylcholine receptor modulators, e.g. spinosyns
- chloride channel activators, e.g. benzoate

Metabolic inhibitors:

- oxidative phosphorylation disrupters, e.g. organotin miticides
- oxidative phosphorylation uncouplers, e.g. chlofenapyr
- ATPase inhibitors, e.g. propargite

Endocrine effectors:

- juvenile hormone mimics, e.g. methoprene

Selective feeding blockers, e.g. pymetrozine

Chitin synthesis inhibitors, e.g. acyl ureas

Microbial disrupters of midgut, e.g. *Bacillus thuringiensis* tenebrionis

Water balance, e.g. boric acid

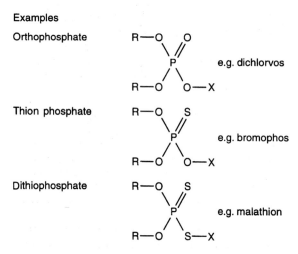

R is usually a methyl or ethyl group
X is the leaving group
These are joined by ester or thioester
They are usually complex, either aliphatic, homocyclic or
heterocyclic in nature

Fig. 20.3 Organophosphorus insecticides: general structure.

Organophosphorus insecticides

These compounds have a wide range of physico-chemical and biological properties and are used widely in agriculture to control insects and their activity. They have a common basic structure called the leaving group (Figure 20.3).

Organophosphates inhibit acetylcholine esterases either by phosphorylating the enzyme or by competing with acetylcholine for the enzyme surface. Either way, the enzyme is inactivated, inhibiting the degradation of the neurotransmitter acetylcholine, which then accumulates, resulting in the overexcitement of the nervous system. This is a slow poison, unlike the instant action of the pyrethroids.

Organophosphorus compounds have now replaced organochlorine compounds as the most common insecticides for the control of aphids and other soft-bodied insects. These compounds are less persistent and need to be sprayed at more frequent intervals. Examples are demeton-S-methyl, malathion, parathion and phorate.

The toxicity to insects of the organophosphorus compounds varies from the instantly fatal to negligible. In addition to acute and prolonged, toxic, anticholinergic effects, the organophosphorus compounds have other effects, including teratogenic activity. Chromosomal abnormalities may be found more frequently than expected in humans poisoned by malathion. The problem of safety is complicated by contaminating impurities, e.g. iso-malathion potentiates the toxicity of malathion. The impurity strongly inhibits the β-esterases that detoxify malathion and hence potentiate its action. Resistance in insects results from the development of increased carboxyesterase activity, in addition to the substrate specific activity of the various carboxyesterases.

The diet of insects may alter hepatic cytochrome P450 activity and hence the rate of metabolism of the pesticide and the potency of the insecticide.

The efficacy of insecticides depends in part on differences in the metabolic enzymes found in plants, mammals and insects.

- **Glucose** can be conjugated to an alcoholic thiol amino acid, the metabolic fate of the herbicide propanil in rice plants
- **Sulfate esters**: a sulfotransferase is found in mammalian livers and kidneys, sometimes in insects but rarely in plants.

Enzymatic hydrolysis is often rapid and depends on two types of esterase and amidase enzymes (Figure 20.4). Esterases attack the bond on the side of the carbonyl group attached to the oxygen atom, whereas amidases attack the bond on the side attached to the nitrogen atom. In most animals the primary attack on most carbamates involves oxidative N-demethylation, ring hydroxylation and epoxide formation. This weakens the molecular structure and allows more rapid enzymatic hydrolytic change. In the insect the initial reaction may involve a mono-oxygenase reaction, so the rate of detoxification may be inhibited by a methylene dioxyphenol synergist. The carbamate insecticide *carbaryl* (Figure 20.5) may inhibit cellulase activity by soil bacteria. Carbaryl is leached from the soil to deeper water layers following chemical or bac-

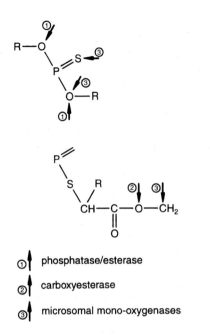

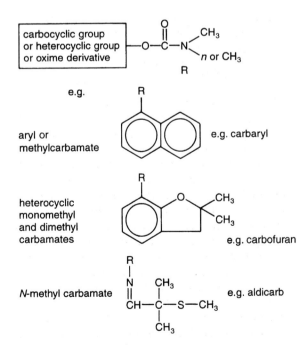

① phosphatase/esterase

② carboxyesterase

③ microsomal mono-oxygenases

Fig. 20.4 Some enzymes cleaving organophosphorus compounds: phosphatase/esterase, carboxyesterase and microsomal monooxygenases.

Fig. 20.5 Structure of carbamates.

terial chemical decomposition. Soil microbiological metabolism of the carbamates may increase over the years with prolonged exposure. In soils and animals some carbamates are degraded to sulfoxides. In anaerobic soils containing ferrous ions degradation is rapid. Soil moisture content may also affect the degradation rate. In anaerobic soil the degradation products are a nitrate and an aldehyde.

The parathion family of organophosphorus insecticides is toxic to mammals. The compounds are readily oxidised by mono-oxygenases in animals, insects and plants, and are converted to derivatives containing the P=O group, which are even more powerful cholinesterase inhibitors than the parent compound. Degradation of parathion is by an oxidative NADPH-dependent oxidase reaction. Different mechanisms are involved in methyl parathion and fenitrothion metabolism, in which there is a rupture of a P–O–CH$_3$. In general, this reaction is faster in the mammalian liver than in insects.

Oxidation of the insecticide may precede conjugation. If the oxidation product is more toxic than the parent compound, e.g. carbofuran, retention in the mammalian enterohepatic circulation is potentially harmful. The *N*-methyl carbamate derivatives of oximes, e.g. aldicarb, methomyl and oxamyl, are toxic to higher animals. Excretion in humans may be facilitated by conjugation to endogenous compounds. In the animal liver the principal primary metabolite is a sulfoxide. Some carbamates are excreted in bile to the intestine and subsequently retained in the mammalian enterohepatic circulation. The toxic aldicarb has further value in controlling phytophagous nematodes, hence its wide usage. The half-life of aldicarb in soil is variable and depends upon how much is applied and the nature of the soil.

Organochlorine insecticides

These include the potent, cheap and widely used dichlorodiphenyltrichloroethane (DDT) and gamma-hexachlorocyclohexane (γ-HCH), and have been widely and somewhat indiscriminately used, especially during World War II, for the eradication

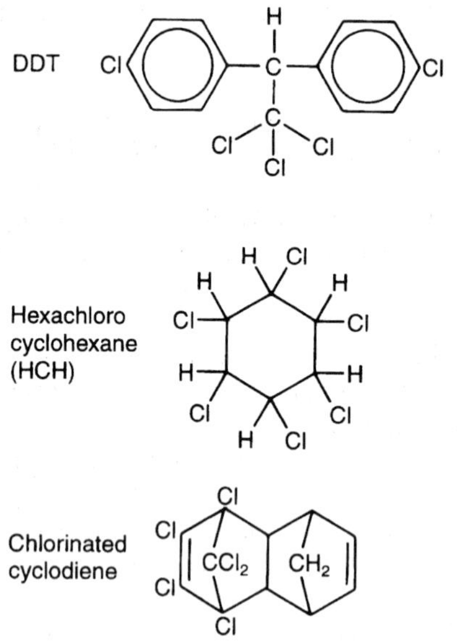

Fig. 20.6 Structure of organochlorine insecticides.

of vectors harbouring malaria, typhus, river blindness and yellow fever.

The organochlorine insecticides belong to three major groups (Figure 20.6):

- DDT related
- Gamma-HCH
- Compounds related to aldrin.

The chemical stability of these compounds results from the C–C, C–H and C–Cl bonds, which makes for slow dissimilation and hence accumulation in the environment.

DDT

DDT is effective against a wide variety of pests, although it is relatively ineffective against aphids and spider mites. The initial effect of DDT, on the peripheral nervous system, is temperature dependent; hence, efficacy is reduced in regions with a warmer climate.

DDT is very insoluble in water. In higher animals DDT accumulates in the central nervous system. The most damaging neurotoxic effects of DDT appear to be close to post-synaptic membranes of neurone–neurone or neurone–muscle contacts, by opening the Na^+ gate in nerve membranes, affecting the sodium ion channel, which interferes with

---

DDT metabolism

The major pathway for the degradation of DDT is dehydrochlorination to DDE. Removal of one chlorine from the trichloromethyl group results in p,p'-DDD [tetrachlorodiphenylethane (TDE)], a metabolic breakdown product of DDT. DDE, which is less toxic to insects, is the major DDT residue found in animal tissue. The reaction is dependent on a glutathione-S-transferase reaction. A second route is reductive dechlorination to DDD, and a third is oxidative and leads to dicofol. In many species a further metabolite is water-soluble DDA, in which $–CCl_3$ in DDT is replaced by $–COOH$. In mammals this is excreted as a free compound or conjugated in bile and faeces.

---

ion transfer in the nerve. The nerve keeps firing and the insect is stimulated to death; this is called metabolic exhaustion.

An alternative role for DDT may be on the mitochondrial membranes responsible for transmembrane conduction. Such a lipophilic substance may well distort the activities of photosynthesis, oxidative phosphorylation, active transport and nuclear division. Specifically, DDT inhibits adenosine triphosphate (ATP) synthase.

From acute experiments, the LD_{50} for DDT given in one dose to a 70 kg man would be 14 g. DDT is being phased out, but its use is still permitted in less environmentally aware countries.

Hexachlorocyclohexane (gamma-HCH, formerly BHC)

The γ-isomer (lindane) is more toxic to insets than the α- or δ- forms. γ-HCH is odourless, whereas the other isomers are smelly and taint food. The mechanism whereby this one isomer is more potent than the others is not known. The toxic action on the insect is on the central nervous system, and may well be involved in γ-aminobutyric acid (GABA), dopamine and N-acetyldopamine brain receptors. The complicated metabolism of γ-HCH requires mono-oxygenases and glutathione-S-transferases, and is species dependent. In humans, γ-HCH acts on the central nervous system.

Chlorinated cyclodiene family

These include the stereochemically related dieldrin and aldrin. Aldrin is a soil fumigant that kills wire-

Aldrin and dieldrin metabolism

The olefinic cyclodienes aldrin, isodrin and heptachlor are oxidised by microsomal oxidases to the corresponding stable epoxide. Other reactions include secondary alcohol substitution or mono-oxygenase reactions in mammalian liver. Hydrolysis of the oxirane ring by epoxide hydrolase leads to the formation of a *trans*-diol. These substances induce liver enzymes and hence hepatic excretion of the organochlorines. Another metabolite is 2-ketodieldrin. Dieldrin can be degraded in mud and soil by anaerobic organisms. These epoxide cyclodienes are toxic, especially to birds, and are particularly persistent in animal fats.

Pyrethroids

The four active principles in pyrethrium flowers are pyrethrin I and II and cinerin I and II, and small amounts of jasmolins I and II. All four are esters with an acid containing a three-carbon ring joined to an alcohol containing a five-carbon ring. Compounds designated I contain chrysanthemic acid and II pyrethric acid. The naturally occurring acids are in the *trans* form, and its esters are more toxic than the synthetic stereoisomers. The natural alcohols are in the *cis* form. The esters are unstable; storage results in 20% loss of activity, but antioxidants and dry and dark conditions can maintain potency. Water and insect tissue activity lead to hydrolysis. The esters are insoluble in water and are soluble in lipid solvents. Some methylene dioxyphenyl compounds are powerful synergens of pyrethroids. The metabolism of the pyrethroids is by liver microsome activity. Metabolism occurs not by hydrolysis of the ester linkage but by oxidation of the methyl group in the isobutenyl side-chain of the acid moiety, to a hydroxymethyl group and then to a carboxyl group in an NADPH-dependent reaction.

worms and larvae of root flies, whereas dieldrin is used for root dip and seed dressing. Aldrin is metabolised to dieldrin by an NADPH-dependent reaction in hepatic microsomes. The slowness of the reactions is important in retaining a lethal concentration.

The chlorinated cyclodiene insecticides are the most toxic and persistent of all pesticides. Many similarities exist between the central nervous system neurotoxic properties of cyclodiene and lindane.

Natural and synthetic pyrethroids

These are based on naturally occurring compounds found in the dried inflorescences of *Chrysanthemum cinerariaefolium* (Figure 20.7). These are 'knock-down' substances that stun insects in their track, without toxic effects to warm-blooded animals. A second lethal compound is required to kill the disabled insect.

Pyrethroids are attractive insecticides as they are minimally toxic to humans and mammals, and are readily destroyed by cooking and digestive juices. They are, however, expensive, readily decomposed by light and toxic to fish.

Synthetic pyrethroids, e.g. allethrin, bioresmethrin, permethrin, cypermethrin and deltamethrin are more stable in light, with varying knock-down properties and relative toxicity to flies and vertebrates, and are more expensive than natural pyrethroids. It may be that different types of pyrethroid act at different sites in the nervous system.

Permethrin
This is a non-systemic, moderately persistent insecticide, useful in domestic and veterinary medicine and effective against a wide range of phytophagous insects and for the control of mosquitos. It consists of a mixture of isomers, related *cis* and *trans* with respect to the spatial arrangement of the ester linkage and the dichlorovinyl linkage. The isomeric mixture gives rise to a large number of metabolites. Most of the initial metabolic changes involve hydrolysis or oxidation.

trans-Permethrin is usually metabolised more rapidly than is *cis*-permethrin. The initial reaction is specific, but it is difficult to follow the oxidative and hydrolytic reactions in sequence. Many metabolites are conjugates formed by secondary metabolism. There are differences in the hepatic microsomal metabolism of the *trans*-permethrin compared with the *cis*-permethrin, as the *trans*-isomer is hydrolysed by an esterase, whereas the *cis*-isomer is cleaved by an oxidase. The metabolism of permethrin by pseudoplusia is inhibited by low concentrations of organophosphorus compounds,

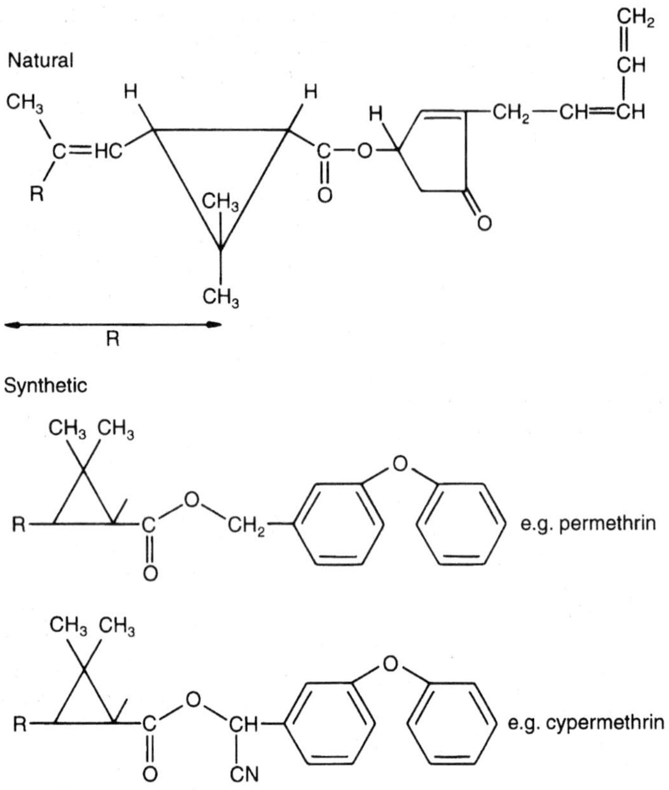

Fig. 20.7 Structure of natural and synthetic pyrethroids.

particularly the relatively non-polar ones. Such combinations are important in the potency of pesticide formulations.

Cypermethrin
This is a similar compound to permethrin, but has an α-cyano group that improves photostability, with a powerful and rapid debilitating effect on insects and an increased number of metabolic products. The degradation of cypermethrin is initiated by bond cleavage or by hydroxylation. Many birds are tolerant to cypermethrin, partly because the compound passes rapidly through the intestine to be quickly metabolised if absorbed. The nervous system of birds is relatively insensitive to this compound, which has a wide biological spectrum and is applied to numerous crops against biting and sucking insects. However, when tolerance develops in certain strains of flies, effectiveness can be restored by applying organophosphorus compounds.

Juvenile hormone mimics
These insect growth regulators act on the insect endocrine system, an action specific to insects and not toxic to mammals. Physiological juvenile hormone is produced in the insect brain and the synthetic juvenile hormone mimics keep the insect in an immature larval/pupal or larval/adult form. Normal reproductive physiology is disturbed.

Cuticle production inhibitors
These block a cell membrane transport step involving uridine disphosphate (UDP)-*N*-acetyl-glucosamine in the synthesis of chitin, an *N*-acetylglucosamine polysaccharide and the major component of the insect exoskeleton.

Alimentary toxins from Bacillus thuringiensis
During sporing, *Bacillus thuringiensis* develops a number of insecticidal protein toxins, which when eaten by insects are dissolved in the midgut and release endotoxins several hundred amino acids

long. The insect's intestinal proteases remove part of the main acid chain to create an active form that binds to the intestinal membrane and alters ionic permeability. The intestine lyses and the insect dies. This biological system is used in some genetically modified plants.

FUNGICIDES

Fungi may attack plants through the soil or through the seeds. Fungal mycelia have an almost unlimited ability to regenerate from a few surviving hyphal strands, making an established fungus very difficult to eradicate. Fungicides that kill on contact can check the growth of mycelium, limit the production of reproductive structure and delay spread from infected plants to healthy ones. Non-systemic fungicides are usually insoluble in water.

The site-specific fungicidal systemic agents affect single receptors or enzymes. Fungicides with multiple sites of action have low systemic and eradicant properties, affect non-specific targets, and may react with thiol groups and disorganise lipoprotein membranes (Table 20.1).

Copper fungicides

Copper fungicides are used against a wide variety of fungi but are toxic to many organisms. Bordeaux mixture is a concentrated solution of copper sulfate added to a slight excess of lime suspended in water. It is insoluble in water and gelatinous, and the copper binds to the leaf surface. The fungicidal efficiency of Bordeaux precipitate decreases on storage, probably owing to the changes in the extent and type of crystalline aggregation. The activity of copper may be through the chelation of amino acids, e.g. glycine and keto acids, that have exuded through the leaf surface. However, the observed leakage of amino and keto acids may also be a consequence of the toxic effect of the copper.

Mercuric compounds

Inorganic mercury compounds are still occasionally, although decreasingly used in some countries. Mercury is toxic to higher animals, and the accumulation of mercury in soil and animals represents a serious environmental hazard. Microorganisms, under aerobic and even anaerobic conditions, can interconvert different forms of mercury, organic to inorganic, inorganic to organic, and inorganic to elemental mercury. Various forms of mercury are used for sealing pruning cuts and for seed treatments, used to protect cereal seeds from a variety of diseases. All mercury-treated grain must be sown and never used as food for humans or livestock. To reduce the risk of such treated grain being accidentally eaten it is usual to colour the seed dress-

Table 20.1 Groups of fungicides

Possible multiple sites of action	Site-specific	Site(s) of action uncertain
Copper and tin compounds	Dinitrocompounds (e.g. dinocap)*	Dicarboximides (e.g.
Mercurials	Benzimidazoles (e.g. benomyl)	vinclozolin)
Sulfur	Oxathins (e.g. carboxin)	
Dithiocarbamates (e.g. thiram, maneb)	Steroid synthesis blockers	
Phthalimides (e.g. captan)	(a) Morpholines (e.g. tridemorph)*	
Phthalonitriles (e.g. chlorothalonil)	(b) C14 demethylation inhibitors	
	(e.g. prochloraz, triforine, triarimol)	
	Hydroxyaminopyrimidines (e.g. ethirimol)	
	Antibiotics (e.g. kasugamycin)	
	Phenylamides (e.g. metalaxyl)	
	Organophosphorus compounds	
	(e.g. pyrazophos, fosetyl)	
	Others (e.g. guazatine, cymoxanil, prothiocarb)	

Based on MAFF (1984), with additions.
*Systemic activity may be low or absent.

Dimethyldithiocarbamate

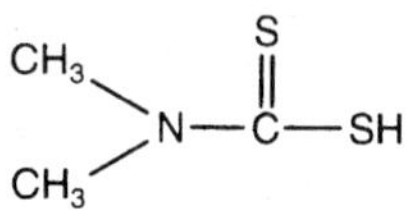

bis-Dithiocarbamate

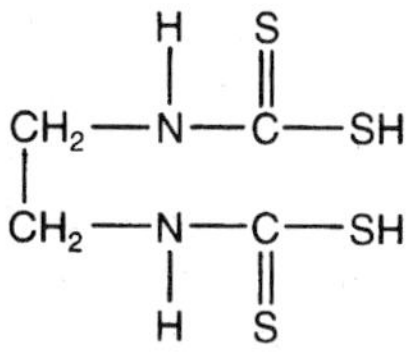

Fig. 20.8 Dithiocarbamate fungicides. There are two major groups: dimethyldithiocarbamate and bis-dithiocarbamate.

ing as a warning, and the colour code indicates the nature of the fungicide or insecticide in the dressing. Sometimes, however, starving communities wash the treated grain, wrongly assuming that the removal of colour indicates that the poison had been removed. Alkyl, but not aryl and alkoxyalkyl mercury-treated grain is a major threat to grain-eating birds.

Sulfur and lime sulfur

Sulfur was widely used by farmers in the USA in considerable amounts as a fungicide. The quantity used was partly because of the low potency of the preparation, in the order of kilograms per hectare, whereas most organic fungicides are used at a dosage of less than one-hundredth of this amount. It is not known how sulfur works; it may be that sulfur oxides are the active principle, that the sulfur is hydrolysed by water to active polysulfides, or that hydrogen sulfide is the agent.

Non-systemic organic fungicides

Fungicides can be classified into two types:

• Those that are focused at the point of delivery
• Systemics that enter the plant through the roots or leaves and are transported within the plant in xylem or phloem.

The correct and efficacious use of fungicides is much more exacting than that of insecticides or herbicides, especially in the developing world. Most organic fungicides, both non-systemic and systemic, tend to be selective. Consequently, success or failure depends on accurate identification of the fungal infection, which is not a universal farming skill. The effectiveness of a fungicidal application may also depend on timing, and an understanding of the life cycle of the particular fungus.

Dithiocarbamates
There are two fungicide dithiocarbamates, dimethyldithiocarbamate and bis-dithiocarbamate (Figure 20.8). Thiram, a disulfide oxide, is used as a fungicide; its diethyl analogue is used medically to treat alcoholism. The dithiocarbamates enter fungi either as un-ionised molecules, a weak acid or disulfide derivative, or a covalent complex. Mixtures of diethyl carbamates with other fungicides with different chemical action are often more effective than the individual components used alone. The dimethyldithiocarbamates may form toxic complexes with copper or, alternatively, may sequestrate essential trace elements.

The dimethyldithiocarbamates have a bimodal action when applied to moulds. An initial effect that declines is followed by a second phase of activity, owing to the sustained action of the varied products of dithiocarbamate generated during metabolism.

Bis-dithiocarbamate acts on the thiol group of an enzyme's coenzyme or biological carriers, with resultant breakdown to isothiocyanates and thiourea derivatives, and probably inhibits fungal respiration and growth. The active species is not known, but may be an isothiocyanate disulfide or an ethylenethiuram disulfide.

All dithiocarbamate fungicides are unstable and can be broken down chemically and photochemically, as well as by enzymes in plants and fungi. Significant amounts of ethylene thiourea are formed during the cooking of food treated by the dithiocarbamate spray maneb.

Phthalimide group
This group, which includes captan (Figure 20.9), folpet, captafol and dichlofluanid, reacts with thiol groups. The breakdown of phthalimides is accelerated by the endogenous thiol and

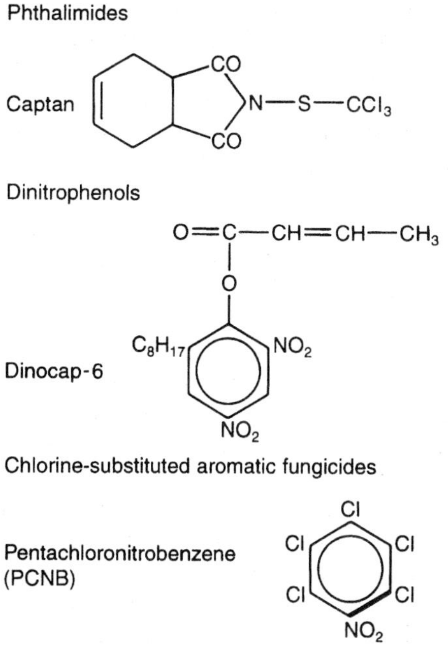

Phthalimides

Captan

Dinitrophenols

Dinocap-6

Chlorine-substituted aromatic fungicides

Pentachloronitrobenzene
(PCNB)

Fig. 20.9 Non-systemic organic fungicides: structure of phthalimides, dinitrophenols and chlorine-substituted aromatic fungicides, e.g. captan, dinocap-6 and pentachloronitrobenzene (PCNB).

glutathione. The captan group of fungicides is toxic to fish, but not to mammals. Some of these compounds indicate mutagenic properties on the Ames' test. Captan and related compounds have an unusual residual problem, in accelerating the corrosion of tin cans. This problem for the food industry is prevented if the captan is destroyed by heat processing.

Dinitrophenol derivatives
Dinocap (Figure 20.9) and binapacryl have been used as insecticides, fungicides and herbicides and for mothproofing since 1892, as a herbicide since 1932, and as fungicides since 1949. Simple dinitrophenates uncouple mitochondrial oxidation from phosphorylation. It is possible that this is an example of lethal metabolism and these fungicides are hydrolysed by fungal enzymes to liberate free dinitrophenols, which are then fungitoxic.

Chlorine-substituted aromatic fungicides
Cationic detergents have both bactericidal properties and defined but useful antifungal properties.

They are safe and are chemically related to domestic detergents. They attack lipoprotein membranes and disrupt vital membrane-dependent processes such as selective permeability and oxidative phosphorylation.

Imazalil and prochloraz
These imadazoles inhibit steroid synthesis and have a weakly systemic action, especially against seed- and air-borne pathogens. When prochloraz is fed in high doses to rats it induces the cytochrome P450 mono-oxygenase system and glutathione-*S*-transferases in the endoplasmic reticulum. Such induction leads to an accelerated metabolism of foreign compounds, including pesticides.

Systemic fungicides

A systemic fungicide attacks internal mycelium and penetrating haustria, and thereby prevents the regeneration of even small pieces of surviving mycelium.

Benzimidazole (Figure 20.10) is the parent compound of a large family of systemic fungicides including benamyl, thiophanate-methyl and thiabendazole. There are three groups, carbamates, non-carbamates and the thiophanate family, which after application are converted to benzimidazoles. The systemic fungicide families affect very specific processes. Such site-specific activities are usually mediated through single gene selection amplification or modification, and include interference with nucleotide base synthesis, protein formation, and the synthesis of steroids and components of lipoprotein membranes. The main action of the benzimidazoles is to interfere with the division of the cell nuclei and to disrupt the assembly of tubilin into microtubules. Resistance readily develops and persists.

After application, some of these compounds break down quite readily in soil, where the half-life of detectable benzimidazole derivatives is 6 months or more. Some 30% of the original benomyl can be found as breakdown products after 2 years. These degradation products are adsorbed to soil constituents, the amount being dependent on the organic matter content and the soil pH. The acute toxicity of most benzimidazoles, when eaten by humans, is low. In the mammalian gastrointestinal

tract, break down of benomyl occurs rapidly following oral ingestion. Within 24 h 40% appears in
the urine, partially conjugated to glucuronic acid,
cysteine or acetylcysteine.

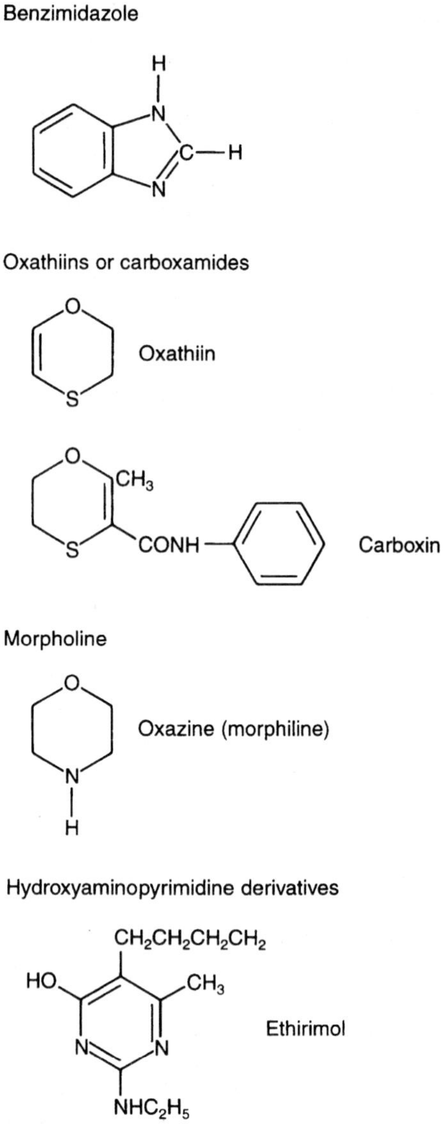

Oxathiins or carboxamides
Carboxin (Figure 20.10) is used in Britain exclusively as a cereal seed treatment against rusts, smuts
and bunts. Carboxin is fungitoxic because it
inhibits the respiration of sensitive fungi, possibly
acting on the enzyme succinate dehydrogenase and
causing mitochondrial damage. The *cis*-croto-
nanilide grouping is believed to be the active group.
In some plants, particularly peanuts, the metabolism of carboxin consists of *p*-hydroxylation of the
phenyl moiety. In barley, there is oxidation of the
sulfide sulfur to sulfoxide, which has slow fungitoxic
activity. Adding a further atom of oxygen yields the
sulfone, which reacts with lignin to produce insoluble complexes and aniline derivatives. In animals,
oral doses of carboxin are excreted largely
unchanged. In soil, carboxin loses its activity over
3 weeks.

Morpholine inhibitors of sterol synthesis
The most common of these nitrogen-containing
heterocyclic fungicides are based on the triazole
ring, pyrimidine, pyridine, piperazine or imidazole
(Figure 20.10). These control powdery mildew
infections, but some are also effective against rusts.
The mode of action of morpholines is to inhibit the
normal growth of fungal hyphae. This results from
inhibition of one or both steps in the complex
process of biosynthesis of sterol, by the inhibition
of C4-demethylation of the sterol lanosterol by the
cytochrome P450 system. This leads to an accumulation of unwanted intermediate sterols.

Hydroxyaminopyrimidine derivatives
These compounds, e.g. ethirimol (Figure 20.10),
are effective only against powdery mildews. Their
use is restricted as resistance develops very readily. The primary metabolism of ethirimol is similar
in plants and animals, with N-de-ethylation to a primary amine of low biological activity. The butyl
group can be hydroxylated, although this route is
less important in plants than in animals. Conjugation (with glucuronic acid in animals, glucoside in
plants) can occur on the C4 hydroxyl. Ethirimol has
a half-life of less than 4 weeks in barley plants,

Fig. 20.10 Systemic fungicides: benzimidazole, oxathiins (carboxamides), morpholine and hydroxyaminopyrimidine derivatives.

where uptake is through the roots. Ethirimol interferes with the enzyme adenosine deaminase,
which catalyses the conversion of the amino
groups of adenine, in the form of adenosine, to the
amino groups of hypoxanthine, in the form of
inosine.

HERBICIDES

The global weed-control programme is somewhat different from the control of insects and pathogens. Weeds only seriously reduce crop yield or quality when they compete with a crop for available moisture, nutrient and light. In general, weeds may be controlled by farmers by hand and hoe, or in more extensive farming chemicals may be used. Crop rotation is another method for weed and pest control.

Herbicides are used in agriculture to remove weeds that would otherwise compete with a crop. This can be achieved in a number of ways, not all of which require the weed killer to possess an intrinsic selectivity between the weed species and crop plants. The selective action of herbicides depends on differences in plant life cycles and morphology, so that the crop is exposed to a lower effective dose than the weed receives. Biochemical differences between crops and common weeds are exploited; for example, there is no β-oxidase in some legumes, allowing these plants to be tolerant of the herbicide 2,4-DB; maize is tolerant of atrazine.

Herbicide uptake

The physical and chemical properties of herbicides applied to foliage are very different to those of compounds normally applied through the soil. A toxic substance that is lipid soluble will penetrate the waxy cuticle when applied to leaves.

The factors influencing herbicide uptake are numerous, as are the interactions in the total metabolic process, and in consequence their action is not fully understood. Some herbicides may persist in the soil, particularly those with low solubility in water. The effectiveness of many herbicides may depend on the level of rainfall following soil application. Volatile materials such as diclobenil, certain thiolcarbamates and nitronilines have relatively short half-lives in many soils. A problem inherent in the use of soil-acting herbicides is that they accumulate over the years.

Following continuous use of a herbicide, the herbicide-degrading enzymes in the soil microorganisms increase, with an attendant increase in the rate of degradation of these herbicides. Most herbicides are readily degraded by the oxidative, reductive and hydrolytic enzymes of microorganisms. The type of soil also influences the persistence and effectiveness of any one herbicide. Some substances are strongly adsorbed onto soil organic matter, e.g. urea derivatives, triazines, carbamates and nitrophenyl ethers, while others are strongly adsorbed onto soil gritty particles, e.g. diquat. Thus, the type of soil affects the level of toxicity of a given dose of the herbicide and the retention of the herbicide within the soil.

It is therefore necessary carefully to select a herbicide for a particular purpose, especially when using soil-acting compounds. The rate of application, rainfall, soil type, temperature and microbial population all affect persistence in the soil. Some crops are relatively tolerant of some herbicides and can be sown or planted soon after application.

There is considerable specificity of herbicidal function (Table 20.2). Some are applied to the foliage of well-established plants, while others attack germinating weed seeds. Others preferentially attack dicotyledonous weeds in the presence

Table 20.2 Classification of foliage herbicides

Mode of action	Type of herbicide
Auxin growth regulators	Phenoxyaliphatic acid herbicides
	Picolinic acids
Aromatic amino acid inhibitors	Glyphosate
	Sulfosate
Branched chain amino acid inhibitors	Imidazolinones
	Sulfonylureas
	Sulfonalides
Chlorophyll/carotenoid pigment inhibitors	Amitrole
Lipid biosynthesis inhibitors	Aryloxyphenoxypropionates
	Cyclohexanediones
Cell membrane destroyers	Bipyridyliums
	Diphenyl ethers
Photosynthetic inhibitors	Triazines
	Uracils
	Phenylureas
Root inhibitors	Dinitroanilines
Shoot inhibitors	Thiocarbamates
	Chloroacetamides

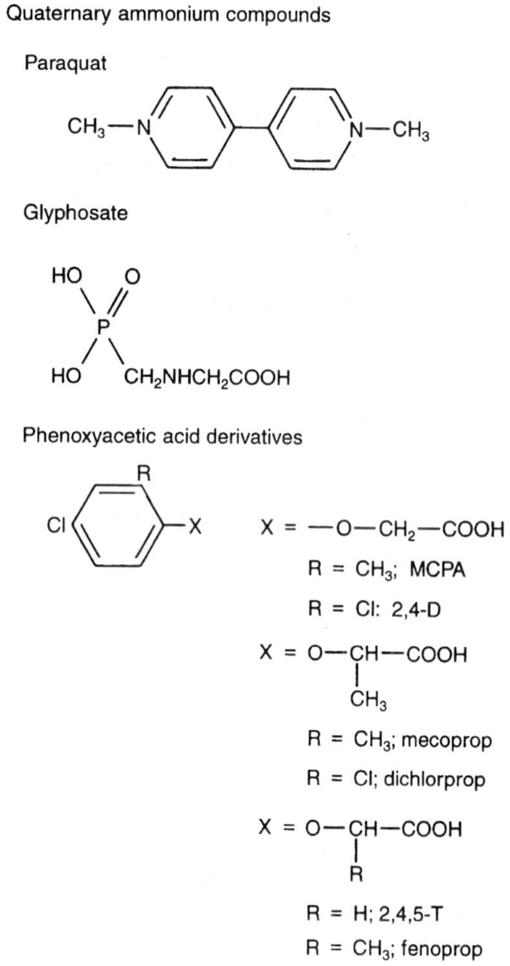

Quaternary ammonium compounds

Paraquat

$CH_3—N$ [pyridine ring structure] $N—CH_3$

Glyphosate

[phosphonate structure]
HO O
P
HO CH_2NHCH_2COOH

Phenoxyacetic acid derivatives

[benzene ring with Cl and R substituents] —X

$X = —O—CH_2—COOH$

  $R = CH_3$; MCPA

  $R = Cl$: 2,4-D

$X = O—CH—COOH$
         |
         CH_3

  $R = CH_3$; mecoprop

  $R = Cl$; dichlorprop

$X = O—CH—COOH$
         |
         R

  $R = H$; 2,4,5-T

  $R = CH_3$; fenoprop

Fig. 20.11 Herbicides: quaternary ammonium, e.g. paraquat, glyphosate and phenoxyacetic acid derivatives.

Paraquat

Paraquat inhibits the reduction of $NADP^+$ and thereby prevents reduction of carbon dioxide in the photosynthetic carbon cycle by replacing ferredoxin as an electron receptor in the photosystem. Light energy is rerouted, with paraquat being reduced by a single-electron transfer and automatically reoxidised by atmospheric oxygen to form superoxides. These attack unsaturated fatty acids in membrane lipids.

---

of monocotyledon foliage. A few selectively kill seeding cotyledons.

Foliage contact herbicides

Herbicides that kill all foliage include quaternary ammonium compounds (Figure 20.11); in addition, two such herbicides, paraquat and diquat, are bipyridylium compounds and kill exclusively by foliage contact.

Glyphosphate

Glyphosphate (Figure 20.11) is an aromatic amino acid inhibitor containing phosphonate and derived from glycine. This quaternary ammonium compound is inactivated by soil.

Glyphosphate has little selectivity of action and kills all foliage on contact. The main action appears to be on the biosynthetic pathway by which aromatic amino acids are synthesised, the shikimic acid route of synthesis (phenylalanine, tyrosine and tryptophan) in plants. Decomposition of glyphosphate, mainly to aminomethylphosphonic acid in plants, appears to occur rather slowly. Chemical decomposition in soil is also slow, but there is rapid degradation by microorganisms with the release of carbon dioxide.

Aminotriazoles are foliage herbicides that rapidly disappear after killing the weeds, but are not inactivated by soil. The major use is to control weeds in uncultivated land intended for planting in the near future. Aminotriazole blocks carotenoid synthesis, in which dehydrogenase enzymes remove hydrogen atoms to form double bonds.

In the plant, detoxification involves conjugation, producing higher molecular weight products that are poorly excreted.

Selective herbicides for broad-leaved weeds

Phenoxyacetic acid derivatives
These are used to control broad-leaved weeds in cereal crops from grasslands (Figure 20.11). Phenoxyacid herbicides, 2,4-D and 4-chloro-2-methyl phenoxyl acetic acid (MCPA), have persistent auxin-like characteristics, affect auxin growth regulation and react with the plasma membrane.

Phenoxyacetic acid derivatives readily pass through cuticular lipids at a rate dictated by their molecular polarity.

Whatever receptor or enzyme for auxin-like activity is the target of phenoxyacetic acid herbicides, activity is very structurally specific. The metabolism of phenoxyacetic acid involves side-chain degradation with a substituted phenol as a final product. Ring hydroxylation is usually the main metabolic route. Aromatic compounds chlorinated on C4 are often hydroxylated in this position and thereafter the chlorine group may migrate to the C3 or C5 position. Conjugation with glucose can occur; such glucosides form a reservoir for active phenoxyacetic acids.

The primary effect of these phenoxyacetic acid herbicides is to cause aberrant growth of young, rapidly growing tissues near the meristem. There is evidence that auxins stimulate cell-wall development, and phenoxyalkanoic acid herbicides may interfere with the metabolism of pectin, methyl esters or some other components of young cell walls.

If applied to soils, salts of MCPA and 2,4-D are readily washed away or decomposed by micro-organisms. Consequently, low levels of herbicide usually disappear 1–4 weeks after application, but may persist much longer when the soil is cold or dry. Enhanced degradation occurs with multiple application.

Auxin-like herbicides derived from benzoic acid
The most important of these are dicamba and 2,3,6-TBA (Figure 20.12). These are growth regulators and affect growth in broad-leaved weeds. They are applied to the soil and persist over long periods. Their main function is to add range and versatility to the herbicidal spectrum of phenoxyalkanoic compounds. The main metabolism of dicamba involves hydroxylation at C–S in the benzene ring and conjugation with glucose.

Bromoxynil and ioxynil
These herbicides (Figure 20.12) attack the seedlings of several of the broad-leaved weeds that are not readily controlled by phenoxyacetic acid-derivative herbicides. The herbicidal action is to interfere in a wide range of biochemical processes in plant organelles. They destabilise lipoprotein membranes, and thus affect mitochondrial electron transport and inhibit protein synthesis. These

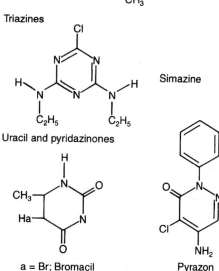

Fig. 20.12 Herbicides. Dioxin, auxin-like herbicides, bromoxynil and ioxynil, urea herbicides, triazines, uracil and pyridazinones.

herbicidal nitriles affect the light reaction of photosynthesis, possibly through the electron transport system. They prevent the incorporation of carbon dioxide into acetyl-coenzyme A (CoA) and the formation of the malonyl-CoA for fatty acid biosynthesis. They also inhibit the reduction of $NADP^+$, thereby interfering with the photosynthetic reduction of carbon dioxide. Microorganisms present in some soils appear to be able to degrade bromoxymil to carbon dioxide.

Herbicides to control grassy weeds

There are two chlorinated aliphatic acids, dalapon and trichloroacetic acid (TCA). Dalapon is internally translocated after application to the foliage; TCA is usually applied before planting in the soil to control couch and other grasses. Little is known about the mode of action of dalapon, but it may act by non-specific binding and precipitation of proteins, and also by inhibiting RNA synthesis.

Some herbicides selectively kill grasses after the emergence of the crop, e.g. phenoxybutyric acid and derivatives such as MCPB and 2,4-DB. These are of low toxicity until converted into the acetic acid member of the species by a specific β-oxidase. The degradation involves an acyl-CoA derivative found in plants and animals during fatty acid oxidation.

Dinitrophenol derivatives, e.g. dinoseb, are extremely toxic and should not be used. This group uncouples oxidation from phosphorylation in the mitochondrial electron transport system. Grasses can flourish in the absence of competitors, therefore causing considerable crop losses. Post-emergence herbicides selectively control grass growth. Herbicides in these families have names that end in -fop, e.g. fluazifop. A second family have names ending in -dim, of which sethoxydim is the best known example. Diclofop is metabolised by microorganisms and has a half-life of 10–30 days in a normal range of soils. Sethoxydim has been shown to have a half-life similar to diclofop in prairie soils, but in air-dried soils 94% of an applied dose was recovered unchanged 28 days later. The primary mode of action seems to be on chloroplast fatty acid biosynthesis in susceptible plants, the membranes of which are strikingly different to those in other plants and animals.

Soil-acting herbicides against seedlings

These herbicides are inhibitors of photosynthesis.

Urea herbicides
This family of substituted ureas, e.g. diuron and fluometuron (Figure 20.12), is trisubstituted to form ureides. One of the amino groups carries either two methyl groups or one methyl group and one methoxy group. The other amino group is substituted with a benzene ring, which may contain halogen atoms. The main action of ureides, triazines and ureciles is to disrupt the photosynthetic light reaction. Ureides are adsorbed onto soil organic matter. Microbial action is largely limited to the herbicide, which is dissolved in soil water. Degradation rates are determined by the concentration of herbicide in water and therefore by adsorption on, or desorption from, soil particles. Two major routes of degradation occur: N-demethylation and ring hydroxylation. Differences in metabolism with or without differences in uptake and translocation by the plant are major factors contributing towards a selective response and sensitivity between various crops and weeds for a particular ureide.

Triazines
Triazine herbicides, e.g. atrazine, simazine and ametryne (Figure 20.12), persist in soils for months depending on the soil type. Their mode of action resembles that of the ureides, in that they block photosynthetic processes. Metabolism of triazines is through one or more major routes. Chlorinated triedes undergo non-enzymatic but catalysed hydrolysis. Some plants contain one or more glutathione-S-transferases, which allow glutathione to conjugate directly with herbicidal triazines, of the chlorotriazine family, to form inactive products. This enzyme system and reaction may explain why the herbicidal triazine is safe for mammals. The secondary amine groups on C4 or C6 allow triazines to undergo N-dealkylation with some retention of activity.

Uracil pyridazinones
The selective action of these compounds, e.g. bromacil and pyrazon (Figure 20.12), is through metabolic reactions that act at or before cell divi-

sion. They include phenyl carbamate esters, in which a phenyl group has replaced an amino hydrogen group in aminoformic acid.

Uracil pyridazinones are metabolised by similar microsomal mono-oxygenase enzyme systems in plants and animals. Metabolic studies in rats show that 30% of the normal dose of chlorpropham is hydrolysed to chloroaniline and its N-acetylated derivative. There is subsequent hydroxylation and then acetylation. Glucuronide and sulfation conjugates are excreted.

TOXIC EFFECTS OF PESTICIDES

The fruit and vegetable marketing system insists on standards of perfect appearance in the produce, with no surface blemishes and perfect ripeness, size and colour. Those farmers who use a minimum of synthetic chemicals or organic farmers cannot completely eradicate pests, so there is some cosmetic damage. If the produce is sent to the food processing industry then blemishes are less important. The potential biological and pathological hazards to humans of the infections that cause the blemishes do not appear to be a cause for concern. However, it is possible that many consumers would accept less attractive fruit and vegetables containing a lower pesticide residue content. In a survey in the USA the majority of interviewees felt that the health benefits of fruit and vegetables outweighed the risks accruing from possible pesticide residues.

While there is a general deep concern for the environment and for children, the reappearance of ergot in Germany from untreated rye indicates the need for a balance between pests and pesticide control and residue content of crops.

Pollution and risk to health

Considerable and continued thought and monitoring are now necessary in this area. Organochlorines accumulate for months, even years in clay and manure-rich soils, with little effect on soil bacteria. However, the phenomenon of biomagnification means that there is a concentration effect in some plant species. In plants that transpire rapidly there

is substantial uptake through the roots. Contamination of water is universal and soil organochlorine residues drain off in water into the sea, rivers, reservoirs and lakes.

Some of the more toxic chemicals, including dioxin and the polychlorinated biphenyls (PCBs), are appearing in the Arctic environment. The north-east Atlantic is the largest reservoir for PCBs, evaporating from soils, waste dumps and polluted lakes, and condensing on the snow and ice.

The size of the problem is indicated by the huge amount of DDT produced and used. At least 1301 million kg was produced in the USA during 1944–1970. It is estimated that the total DDT production when sprayed would have covered the Earth's surface at a concentration of about 2.5 mg of DDT/m^2 of the Earth's surface (not allowing for degradation, binding, etc.). Residues have been detected throughout the world, including Antarctica. The most important hazards of these compounds lie with their analogues containing three chlorine carbons (CCl_3). This is largely because of the highly toxic contaminating dioxin (Figure 20.12) which is formed as a side-reaction in the chemical preparation of 2,4,5-trichlorophenol (2,4,5-T). There have been fears for individuals working in or near factories making such agrochemicals or their precursors.

In 1970, it was calculated that rain water contained 2×10^{-4} ppm, air 4×10^{-6} ppm and seawater 1×10^{-6} ppm of organochlorines (see also Biomagnification). By 1972, concentrations of DDT and their derivatives were reported as 3×10^{-4} ppm in plankton, 1×10^{-3} ppm in aqueous invertebrates and 5×10^{-1} ppm in marine fish. Vegetables contained 2×10^{-2} ppm, meat 2×10^{-1} ppm and human adipose tissue 6 ppm. Many components of the food chain are contaminated.

It is claimed that some crops may safely be harvested the same day as spraying, but concentrations double the maximum residue level (MRL, UK), i.e. 5 g/kg (UK Consumers' Association, July 1991), have been found on the same day as spraying occurred. The residue concentrations should be less than the legal MRL permitted in the UK or within the limit set by the Codex.

Pesticides may undergo chemical changes during food processing and hence may change the degree of toxic potential. The measurement of these by-products at various stages of cooking and processing

> Agricultural chemicals are present in every aspect of life.
>
> Lindane, carbaryl, permethrin, malathion and phenothrin are used for head-lice control in schools.
>
> Pesticides are used in the control of wood rot and mould. Pentachlorophenol is a hazardous wood preservative. Following the spraying of affected wood in a confined space, pentachlorophenol residue concentrations may be three times higher than recommended safe levels. The clothing of operatives who have been spraying chemicals may be contaminated by pesticides.
>
> Large volumes of pesticides are transported around the world. There is always a concern that there might be leakage of chemicals into the environment during the clearance and cleaning of the tankers. The dumping of surplus pesticides is also a problem for both industry and individuals with ecological interests.

is a difficult logistic and analytical problem. Residues may be concentrated in particular tissues, e.g. organochlorines in oils, meat, milk and fatty tissues.

Short-term toxic effects

The primary hazards with exposure to pesticides are acute toxic reactions from skin contact and inhalation over relatively brief periods. Such exposure can lead to acute eye and upper respiratory tract irritation, contact dermatitis and even serious poisoning. Individuals who work regularly with pesticides are most at risk. Many of the confirmed poisoning accidents are the result of drift from nearby spraying operations. Domestic timber treatment is another potential problem.

Small amounts of paraquat can irritate the skin or if inhaled may cause nose bleeding. When larger amounts are ingested, a non-cancerous multiplication of lung cells occurs, accompanied by proliferation of mitochondria, which continues long after all traces of the herbicide have disappeared, and leads to respiratory failure and death.

Paraquat and diquat undergo little metabolism in plants or animals. These quaternary ammonium compounds accumulate in water plants and hence

are a danger to aquatic animals. Mammals may die after running through treated areas and ingesting paraquat by licking contaminated fur.

Long-term toxic effects

Polychlorinated biphenyls (PCBs) accumulate in the environment, especially in fatty tissues. Some 450 million kg have been released into the environment. These have definite consequences for birds and humans, in whom behavioural and nervous abnormalities have been observed. The organochlorines are readily stored in fat and the animals in frozen conditions rely on an abundance of fat to survive. These fat-soluble pesticides are also found in fish oils and even fish oil supplements.

Pesticide residues have been detected in a wide range of foods, 10% of bran-based breakfast cereals, 55% of wheat germ, 93% of pure bran, 16% of processed oats, 24% of rice, one-third of sausages and nearly half of sampled burgers, cheeses and apples. Meat, eggs and milk can be contaminated, with consequences to the food chain. When cows are exposed to grass containing DDT, within 2 weeks the milk contains DDT at a steady concentration. Concentrations in human milk are even higher than in cow's milk. Despite the reduced usage of these chemicals they persist in all depots, e.g. in human fat tissue (12 ppm in 1951 in the USA).

Until recently some 40 million sheep in Britain were dipped each year. The pesticide residue presents formidable disposal problems, including concerns over seepage into deep waters. In 1985, when 1500 samples of sheep's kidney fat were analysed for pesticide residues, 71% contained residues of lindane.

Farm workers are readily contaminated during crop spraying and it has been claimed that diminution in sexual potency can result from contact with some sprays. It is now clear that there are neuropsychological risks from accumulated contact with sheep dips. Many farmers exposed to organophosphates feel unwell. The organophosphate diazinonoxon is hydrolysed by the enzyme paraoxanase (PON1), which occurs as isoforms. The PON1 192 (glutamine for arginine) polymorphism is more common in people reporting ill health. It is possible that the organophosphate could be more toxic in susceptible individuals. Phenoxyacetic acid derivatives may persist and can, for example, alter the quality of fodder. At high dosage, animals lose the ability to maintain their body temperature when moved into either a hot or cold environment, although the reason for this loss of homoeostasis is not known.

In humans, mild side-effects have been claimed; a mild neural disorder, peripheral neuropathy, has been reported.

There are possible long-term effects of insecticides, e.g. the insecticide dibromochloropropane (DBCP), on reproduction. As the organochlorines are genotoxic, the effect is to reduce the fertility of many animal breeds. Significant pesticide residues of DDT have been measured in the blood and placentas of Indian women who have had spontaneous abortions, although not in women with full-term deliveries. A survey in the USA showed a reduction in sperm density that is related to pesticide concentrations in semen. A further complication associated with dioxin residues is that the sex ratio is skewed, with a reduction in the number of males born.

Pesticides have both chronic and acute neurotoxic effects. Immune response may also be modified by these substances.

A phenomenon called the Gulf War syndrome has been reported in USA and British soldiers who went to the Gulf War in 1990–1991. They felt impairment of physical functioning, psychological upsets and poor well-being. The significance of such ill-defined symptoms has been variably accepted by governments. They are certainly more common in these soldiers than in others not active in that conflict. While there may be many causes, one strong possibility is the use of organophosphates and other chemicals .

Such organophosphate poisoning can occur when food is contaminated by organophosphates, emphasising the problems raised by the indiscriminate use of such pesticides, the insecticide function of which is dependent upon a neurotoxic effect.

DDT and PCB use has been associated with poor prenatal and, to a greater extent, postnatal development. This may be due to the substance being carried in the mother's milk. Preterm births are increased, with attendant effects on infant mortality and health.

Cancer

The International Agency for Research on Cancer (IARC) classifies chemicals by their carcinogenic potential. The IARC describes evidence for carcinogenesis under a series of categories: sufficient, inadequate, or limited.

A carcinogenic potential in animals does not necessarily apply to carcinogenesis in the human situation and vice versa. Risks to humans are categorised under:

- group I, proven to be carcinogenic in humans
- group IIA, probably carcinogenic
- group IIB, possibly carcinogenic
- group III, not classifiable
- group IV, probably not carcinogenic in humans.

Examples of group I are arsenical pesticides and vinyl chloride. One probably carcinogenic pesticide is ethylene dibromide. There are 17 possible carcinogenic pesticides and 26 not classifiable.

Various studies have tried to link exposure to pesticides to increasing prevalence of cancer of varying types. These include organochlorine and nitrates. It has been suggested that soft-tissue carcinomas are more common in workers who spray 2,4,5-T than in uncontaminated groups. Proving the case for the differing amounts of nitrate, nitrite and N-nitroso compounds in water and food is difficult as the levels vary, making a simple cause and effect relationship difficult to establish.

The United States Environmental Protection Agency has calculated that if a million people were to eat apples that had been sprayed with daminozide, which 'plumps up' apples, over a lifetime, 45 would develop cancer. This carcinogenic action is mediated through a metabolite, UDMH.

WATER SUPPLIES

The agricultural industry can contaminate water both at point source and over a wide area. Point source contamination arises in heavily farmed areas, e.g. farm slurries. Diffuse pollution from organic fertilisers, nitrates and pesticides is a problem. The pollution of river water by fertilisers is highly seasonal; it is greatest in autumn from leaching of land run-off water following heavy rain with resulting pollution of water supplies, resulting in high ammonia concentrations. In summer, concentrations are relatively low and the applied nitrate is immediately taken up by the crop. Nitrates may contaminate underground water stores as a consequence of increased fertiliser use. Long-term storage of nitrate-containing water in reservoirs leads to a 50% decrease of nitrates to nitrogen gas by bacterial reduction. Nevertheless, nitrate pollution of rivers and aquifers, which supply half of the water, is a growing problem, and more complicated in aquifers where some water takes up to 30 years to percolate from the surface soil to the water table. This means that the pollution of these underground water sources may take years to establish and even longer to reduce. The most certain health risk from high nitrate levels in water is methaemoglobinaemia. Maximum safe concentrations of nitrate in drinking water were established at 100 ppm in 1974 by the WHO.

Water-soluble pesticides and herbicides such as atrazine and simazine contaminate drinking water. A survey of British tap water found that two-thirds of samples contained pesticide levels in excess of European and British Government guidelines. In the USA aldicarb (an insecticide), triazines (a herbicide) and EDB, DCP and DBCP (soil fumigants) have been detected in drinking water.

CONTROL OF PESTICIDES

International trade in pesticides is covered by two United Nation conventions. The FAO publishes the International Code of Conduct on the use of and distribution of pesticides ('the Code'). The UN Environmental Programme has produced guidelines for the exchange of information on chemicals in international trade, known as the London Guideline.

The FAO Code covers the management and use of pesticides, their availability, distribution and trade, and recommendations for labelling, packaging, storage, disposal and advertising. The Code is intended for the guidance of governments and industry and other interested organisations.

The European Commission has increasing control over pesticide use in Europe. Under the Single European Act, Article 100A gives a strong commitment

to establish high standards of environmental, consumer and public health protection. European Union (EU) directives identify residue limits for a number of pesticides and prohibit some products.

Under the UK 1986 Control of Pesticide Regulations, when a chemical is submitted for approval it must:

- be effective against the designated pests
- be safe against plants and wildlife in general
- have no undesirable effects on the environment
- be safe to humans.

Pesticide residues

Government agencies publish details of the pesticides used, pesticide residue analysis and the quantities found in foods.

MONITORING PESTICIDE CONTAMINANTS OF FOOD

In the UK two organisations test for pesticides and pesticide residues. The Association of Public Analysts test products on behalf of local authorities. The Government's Working Party on Pesticide Residues (WPPR) publishes figures every year.

The estimated intake of pesticide residues is measured in micrograms per day, whereas acute toxic doses are many orders of magnitude greater. Such testing has shown that 2% of overall foods, 6% of cereal and cereal products and 6% of fruit and vegetables contain more than the maximum residue levels. Some 99% of apples receive pesticide treatment, the residual pesticide declining with time. Peeling apples removes 90% of the pesticide residues. Meat is not analysed. There may be more than one residue present in any one food.

Classification of pesticide concentration

Chemicals may cause either no toxic effect or an acute toxic effect after a single dose, or may have a chronic effect after repeated small and non-lethal doses. Acute toxicity is measured as LD_{50}, the dose at which 50% of the organisms die from a randomly chosen group of a batch of a species. The dosage is described in mg/kg.

- **Acceptable daily intake (ADI)**: All pesticides are tested on animals before application to crops eaten by humans. Such tests establish an ADI, which is calculated to be a safe intake over a lifetime. ADI is defined as the amount of chemical on a body-weight basis, that can be consumed daily in the diet over a whole lifetime in the practical certainty, on the basis of all the known facts, that no harm will result.
- **Acceptable operative exposure level (AOEL)**: the maximum amount of the active substance to which the operator may be exposed without any adverse health effect, measured as mg substance /kg body weight of the operator.
- **Maximum residue level (MRL)**: the maximum concentration of pesticide residues (expressed as mg/kg) expected in a product if the pesticide is applied properly. These are not safety limits. They are the maximum residue concentrations allowed for any particular pesticide in the food when leaving the farm. MRLs are calculated as the maximum quantity of the given product that anyone could eat to ensure that the ADI is not exceeded. The European Commission has made the MRL into a legal limit to be used for each pesticide. As yet, only a limited number of available pesticides has a defined MRL.
- **No observed adverse effect level (NOAEL)**: the highest exposure level in a toxicity study free from toxicity.
- **No observed effect level (NOEL)**: the maximum dose that is safe and at which specific treatment-related effects do not occur. The NOEL is used to calculate the ADI. The safety factor is set at a figure of 100-fold; this is based on a figure of 10 times to allow for variation between animals and humans, and 10 times for the possible variation among individuals. Different safety factors are given for different foods or chemicals.

  The ADI is usually set by the WHO through an international committee, the Codex Alimentarius Commission of the United Nations, which also sets MRLs.
- **Maximum admissible concentrations (MACs)**: applied to pesticides in drinking water at 0.1 parts per billion (ppb) for individual pesticides and 0.5 ppb for total pesticide content.

Occupational exposure

Occupational exposure limits (OELs), based on the long-established US threshold limit value (TLV), are not maximum exposure limits (MELs). The TLU was established by the American Conference of Government Industrialist Hygienists (ACGIH) and refers to airborne concentrations to which workers may be repeatedly exposed without adverse effects. This does not allow for the wide range of individual susceptibility or for the effects of metabolites over a prolonged period. The ACGIH committee now recommends the use of a short-term exposure limit while awaiting definitive information that would enable sensible comment on long-term effects. In the USA there is also another set of values called the integrated risk information system (IRIS), which is used to calculate long-term risks. IRIS uses maximum time-weighted air concentrations (WAC), which should cause no adverse effects in humans over a 40 year exposure. Carcinogens are considered not to be safe at any concentration. The risk factor is the amount by which the OEL exceeds the level obtained for IRIS.

During spraying, particularly with aerial pesticides, pesticides may contaminate the air and be dispersed from the sprayed area into the surrounding area. This is known as spray drift, in which tiny drops of pesticide float away from the intended crop. Only certain pesticides are approved for aerial spray and these include captan, benomyl, chlorpyrifos, 2,4-D, dichlorvos, malathion, metaldehyde and 2,4,5-T.

KEY POINTS

1. The use of agricultural chemicals has contributed to a plentiful and inexpensive food supply for many people. The real cost may be environmental.
2. Large volumes of pesticide liquid are sprayed and applied throughout the world, and have entered every food chain.
3. In the UK pesticide labels must conform to the Data Requirements for the Control of Pesticide Regulations, which cover the classification, packaging and labelling of dangerous substances.

4. Agricultural chemicals are designed to act on the intended target and be innocuous to other creatures. Following metabolism or passage into the food chain this may not be the case. Side-effects may be acute, cumulative and chronic. A toxic substance can accumulate in a living organism until a concentration is reached at which toxicity is manifest. For example, the organochlorines are toxic are readily stored in fat and reduce the fertility of many species.

5. Metabolism has an important role in dictating the selectivity of action of agricultural chemicals and protects some species, e.g. animals and humans. Enzymes that metabolise foreign compounds catalyse reactions that: (i) alter molecular structure to produce a less toxic product; and (ii) increase the polarity and water solubility to facilitate urinary and biliary excretion. Most enzymes responsible for the primary metabolism of foreign compounds are hydrolases and oxygenases. The extent of metabolism dictates the persistence of pesticides in soil, plants and animals.

6. Oxidation and hydrolysis are the primary metabolic reactions in pesticides, with the insertion or exposure of polar groups. Occasionally, products of primary actions undergo secondary changes that are species dependent.

THINKING POINTS

1. The value of clean food and water is self-evident. How this is achieved is a matter for discussion.

2. Some argue the organic approach, others would have us use genetically modified plants and sources, still others chemical control of the environment. What do you think? The decision affects everyone from the unborn child through to those individuals who live into old age.

NEED TO UNDERSTAND

1. The variety of pesticides, their general metabolism and potential for good, harm and safety.

2. Many of the pesticides influence metabolic systems that are common to plants, humans, other mammals and other animals.

FURTHER READING

Bingham, S.A. (1989) Agricultural chemicals in the food chain. *Journal of the Royal Society of Medicine*, **82**, 311–15.

Chaudhry, R., Lall., S.B., Mishra, B., and Dhawan, B. (1998) A food borne outbreak of organophosphate poisoning. *British Medical Journal*, **317**, 268–9.

Chavasse, D.C., Shier, R.P., Murphy, O.A. *et al.* (1999) Impact of fly control on childhood diarrhoea in Pakistan: community-randomised trial. *Lancet*, **353**, 22–5.

Cherry, N., Mackness, M., Durrington, P. *et al.* (2002) Paraoxonase (PON1) polymorphism in farmers attributing ill health to sheep dip. *Lancet*, **359**, 763–4.

Eichholzer, M. and Gutzwiller, F. (1998) Dietary nitrates, nitrites, and N-nitroso compounds and cancer risk. A review of the epidemiological evidence. *Nutrition Reviews*, **56**, 95–1105.

Hassall, K.A. (1990) *Biochemistry and Uses of Pesticides*, 2nd edn. Macmillan Press, New York.

Hoyer, A.P., Grandjean, .P, Jorgensen, T. *et al.* (1998) Organochlorine exposure and risk of breast cancer. *Lancet*, **352**, 1816–20.

Ismail, K., Everitt, B., Blatchley, N. *et al.* (1999) Is there a Gulf War syndrome? *Lancet*, **353**, 179–82.

Lang, T. and Clutterbuck, C. (1991) *Pesticides*. Ebury Press, London.

Longnecker, M.P., Klebanoff, M.A., Zhou, H. and Brock, J.W. (2001) Association between maternal serum concentration of the DDT metabolite DDE and small-for-gestation babies at birth. *Lancet*, **358**, 110–14.

Mocarelli, P., Gerthoux, P.M., Ferrari, E. *et al.* (2000) Paternal concentration of dioxin and sex ratio of off-spring. *Lancet*, **355**, 1858–63.

Ott, W.R. and Roberts, J.W. (1998) Everyday exposure to toxic pollutants. *Scientific American*, Feb. 72–7.

Pesticides 2001. Your Guide to Approved Pesticides. Pesticides Safety Directorate UK and Health and Safety Executive.

Pesticides Usage Survey Report 159: *Arable Farm Crops in Great Britain*. MAFF and Scottish Executive Rural Affairs Department, 1998.

Stephens, R, Spurgeon, A., Calvert, I.A. *et al.* (1995) Neuropsychological effects of long-term exposure to organophosphates in sheep dip. *Lancet*, **345**, 1135–9.

WEBSITES

www.pesticides.gov.uk Website of the Pesticides Register UK

www.foe.co.uk Friends of the Earth

www.panna.org Pesticide appraisal site

www.epa.gov/pesticides USA government site for pesticide information

www.pan-uk.org

http://ipmworld.umn.edu Integrated pest management

www.agcom.purdue.edu/AgCom/Pubs/WS/WS-23.html herbicide mode of action summary

21

Drugs and nutrition

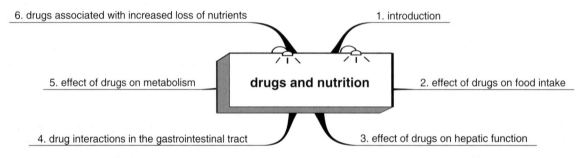

6. drugs associated with increased loss of nutrients   1. introduction

5. effect of drugs on metabolism   **drugs and nutrition**   2. effect of drugs on food intake

4. drug interactions in the gastrointestinal tract   3. effect of drugs on hepatic function

Fig. 21.1 Chapter outline.

INTRODUCTION

The long-term use of some drugs may alter appetite, dietary intake, biosynthesis, absorption, transport, storage, metabolism or excretion of nutrients. Susceptibility to such drug-induced effects may be enhanced during growth, pregnancy and lactation. The concentration of drugs and the genetic heterogeneity of drug metabolic activity may also affect the metabolism of other drugs and hence their effect on nutrients.

EFFECT OF DRUGS ON FOOD INTAKE

Digoxin and non-steroidal anti-inflammatory agents may reduce appetite, either systemically through high blood concentrations or locally through gastritis. High plasma concentrations of sulfonamides may also reduce appetite. Sialadenitis (inflammation of salivary glands) has been reported in patients taking phenylbutazone.

EFFECTS OF DRUGS ON HEPATIC FUNCTION

Drugs are known to affect hepatic function, either by altering enzyme activity or through more direct effects. Many drugs are known to induce hepatic hydroxylating enzymes. The liver microsomal hydroxylating system is concentrated in the cytochrome P450 system. The P450-dependent system includes enzymes involved in oxidation, dealkylation, deamination and sulfoxidation. Vitamin D metabolism is affected by cytochrome P450 activity in the presence of long-term anticonvulsant therapy. Alcohol can induce increases in the metabolic turnover rates of drugs, e.g. blood concentrations of the anticonvulsant drug phenytoin. A constituent of cigarette smoke, 3,4-benzpyrene, influences its subsequent hydroxylation to non-carcinogenic products. Thiazide diuretics can induce a diabetes-like state, and hyperglycaemia and glycosuria can develop in patients taking such drugs.

DRUG INTERACTIONS IN THE GASTROINTESTINAL TRACT

Many drugs interact within the lumen of the gastrointestinal tract. Some drugs are known to affect intestinal absorption by:

- a direct toxic effect causing morphological changes in the mucosa of the small intestine
- inhibition of mucosal enzymes, with or without morphological evidence of mucosal change
- binding and precipitation of micellar components, e.g. bile acids and phospholipids
- altering the physicochemical state of other drugs.

Neomycin may cause rapid and extensive microscopic damage to the intestinal mucosa. Neomycin can produce a sprue-like malabsorption syndrome, with a malabsorption of fat, cholesterol, carotene, iron, vitamin B_{12}, xylose, glucose and nitrogen. The cationic amino groups in neomycin bind to the anions of detergents that are necessary for formation of micelles in the intestinal lumen, e.g. bile acids. This precipitation results in lipids coming out of solution and being malabsorbed. A treatment for gout, colchicine, which is now less commonly used, can induce malabsorption, causing atrophy of small intestinal villi. Biguanides may reduce or slow the absorption of glucose, in part owing to the loss of matrix granules from the mitochondria of epithelial cells. This may be a sign of reduced energy metabolism. The anti-tuberculous drug p-aminosalicyclic acid can cause profound diarrhoea, steatorrhoea and malabsorption of xylose, folic acid and vitamin B_{12}. Methyldopa may cause partial villous atrophy in the small intestine, with consequent malabsorption of both xylose and vitamin B_{12}.

Drugs that alter gastrointestinal motility alter the rate at which other chemicals, nutrients or drugs are absorbed. This is particularly important when tablet dissolution is a rate-limiting step, e.g. metoclopramide in digoxin, pethidine or diamorphine absorption. Malabsorption secondary to the inges-

tion of aluminium and magnesium-based antacids is well known. The polyvalent cations, e.g. Al^{3+} and Mg^{2+}, form non-absorbable chelates with certain organic groupings, e.g. aluminium hydroxide, and may reduce the absorption of tetracyclines. Iron and tetracycline inhibit the absorption of one another. Liquid paraffin and magnesium sulfate can alter lipid absorption, but the effects are only apparent after long usage.

The anion-binding resin cholestyramine has been shown to influence fat-soluble vitamin absorption, e.g. vitamins, A and E.

Folic acid metabolism may be disturbed by anticonvulsants. The mechanism is altered hepatic microsomal enzyme activity with enhanced degradation of folic acid.

Pellagra is a rare complication of the anti-tuberculosis drug isoniazid, which may be due to impaired niacin synthesis secondary to pyridoxine deficiency. Pyridoxine deficiency is common with isoniazid therapy, leading to peripheral neuropathy. Cycloserine is another pyridoxine antagonist. The mechanism of this pyridoxine deficiency is increased urinary excretion of pyridoxine complexed with the drug or competitive inhibition of pyridoxal phosphate.

Mefenamic acid, a non-steroidal anti-inflammatory drug, is an inhibitor of prostaglandin synthetase and may also cause diarrhoea and malabsorption. The consequence of this may be profound malnutrition, which may occur even after years of trouble-free exposure.

The effects of opiates on the intestine are well known. The use of opium and morphine in the treatment of diarrhoea and dysentery has been a long-standing therapy. In the 1970s several endogenous peptides (endorphins) were discovered, with a similar action to that of opiates. These include:

- the pentapeptides methionine enkephalin and leucine enkephalin
- the 31-amino acid peptide β-endorphins
- the dynorphins and β-neoendorphins.

These are synthesised on three separate multicomponent protein precursors, the products of three separate genes. They can be found throughout the central and peripheral nervous systems, in the pituitary and adrenal glands and in the enteric nervous system. The enkephalins are found in the intestine in extremely high concentrations, particularly in neurones of the myenteric plexus. The enkephalins act as neurotransmitters and possibly as circulating hormones. Similar receptors for these opiates exist in the intestine for acetylcholine, catecholamines and histamine. It has been suggested that there are four subtypes of opiate receptor (μ, δ, ϵ or κ). Drugs such as morphine act preferentially at μ-receptors. The enkephalins act preferentially at δ-receptors, β-endorphin at ϵ-receptors, and dynorphin at κ-receptors. Opiates affect many sections of the gastrointestinal tract, including the enteric neurones, smooth muscle and epithelium. In all studied species morphine has a constipating effect, with a marked increase in the segmenting or non-propulsive contraction of the small and large intestines. Part of the action of morphine in the intestine may be mediated through the central nervous system.

Opiates such as morphine have profound effects on intestinal fluid and electrolyte transport. Morphine increases the absorption of fluids as well as sodium and chloride ions. It is possible that the antisecretory actions of the opioids act through the enkephalin-selective δ-opiate receptors in the mucosa. In contrast, receptors in the longitudinal muscle–myenteric plexus appear to be μ- or κ-receptors.

EFFECT OF DRUGS ON METABOLISM

Dihydrofolate reductase is inhibited by methotrexate, pyrimethamine, trimethamine, trimethoprim, pentamidine and triamterene. The anaesthetic nitrous oxide, may affect vitamin B_{12} metabolism by affecting methylcobalamin synthesis.

DRUGS ASSOCIATED WITH INCREASED LOSS OF NUTRIENTS

A number of drugs may result in increased loss of nutrients. Oral diuretics, including frusemide and ethacrynic acid, can cause hypercalcuria, magnesium or potassium deficiency. The psychotropic drug chlorpromazine may influence riboflavin requirements. These chemicals have a similar structure. Chlorpromazine may inhibit the incorporation of riboflavin into flavin adenine dinucleotide through an inhibition of hepatic flavokinase.

KEY POINTS

1. Drugs may alter:
    (i) appetite and dietary intake, e.g. digoxin, which is plasma concentration dependent
    (ii) biosynthesis and absorption, by affecting liver metabolism, e.g. of cytochrome P450 activity or of phenytoin and folic acid function; intestinal absorption, e.g. of neomycin; and transport, e.g. of biguanides
    (iii) intestinal motility, e.g. of codeine phosphate
    (iv) faecal and urinary excretion of nutrients, e.g. of cholestyramine and ethacrynic acid.
2. Susceptibility to such drug-induced changes may be enhanced during growth, pregnancy and lactation.

THINKING POINT

In considering a person's diet, their drug intake is an important consideration.

NEED TO UNDERSTAND

1. The manner in which drugs alter nutrient intake, absorption and metabolism is variably understood from their drug action.
2. Each interaction has to be looked at as a new problem.

FURTHER READING

Grahame-Smith, D.G. and Aronson, J.K. (2002) *Oxford Textbook of Clinical Pharmacology and Drug Therapy*, 4th edn. Oxford University Press, Oxford.
Welling, P.G. (1996) Effects of food on drug absorption. *Annual Review of Nutrition*, **16**, 383–416.

Part VI

Eating, digestion and metabolism

- Smell and taste
- Intake and satiety
- The gastrointestinal tract and food availability
- Carbohydrate digestion and absorption
- Protein absorption
- Lipid absorption
- Foetal and placental nutrition
- Thermodynamics and metabolism
- Mitochondria
- Cytochrome P450
- Free radicals
- Carbohydrate metabolism
- Liquid metabolism
- Eicosanoids
- Cholesterol and lipoproteins
- Amino acid metabolism
- Amino acid neurotransmitters
- Organ metabolic fuel selection
- Growth
- Bone

22

Smell and taste

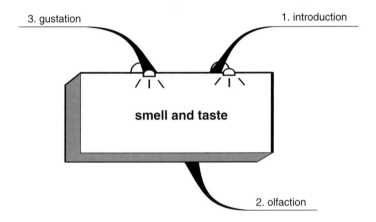

Fig. 22.1 Chapter outline.

INTRODUCTION

Gustation is the term for the sense of taste and olfaction for the sense of smell. Together, they make for the sensation of flavour. There are numerous tastes and smells that add to the joy of eating. Good nutrition must include an enjoyment of food, which is enhanced by good company and food with an appetising appearance and taste. Different animals have different sensitivities to smells, e.g. dogs can be trained to detect explosives, drugs and people. Some smells are said to affect behaviour; certainly this is the case for insects with the smells of flowers, but it may also apply to mammals. Such chemicals are pheromones which may, among other properties, have sexual attractant properties.

Taste qualities are divided into four or five sensations: salt, sour, sweet, bitter and umami. The latter is described as an amino acid type of taste, e.g. sodium glutamate. Each of these tastes is immediately recognised. Intensity only becomes relevant when a taste sensation is too strong or too weak.

Each of these tastes involves a single transducive nerve sequence and is associated with recognition of specific chemical structures. The appreciation of the flavour of food involves several sensory systems, mechanoreceptive, thermoreceptive and chemoreceptive. Many of the non-taste and non-olfactory sensations are carried to the brain by the trigeminal nerve (V). Taste is largely dependent on multiple sensations, predominantly gustation and olfaction. Taste is appreciated by specialised receptor cells in the mouth and palate that recognise chemical stimuli. The recognition of a chemical involves altering the firing rate of the sensory nerve.

OLFACTION

The olfactory system is capable of recognising thousands of different smells. The system is therefore very complex and it is not clear whether recognition takes place peripherally or centrally in the brain.

The olfactory system is a three-compartment sensory system specialised for the detection and processing of molecules called odorants. There are also three anatomical areas involved: the olfactory epithelium, the olfactory bulb and the periform epithelium. The olfactory epithelium in humans is found predominantly on the dorsal aspect of the nasal cavity, the septum and part of the superior turbinates. There are approximately 6 million ciliated olfactory receptor neurones in the 2 cm^2 area of the human olfactory tissue.

There are three layers of human olfactory mucosa:

- the superficial acellular layer, composed of mucous and cilia
- the olfactory epithelium with three morphologically defined cell types: olfactory receptor neurons, sustentacular cells and basal cells
- the lamina propria, consisting of olfactory and trigeminal nerves.

Smell is perceived by bipolar neurons of the olfactory cranial (I) nerve (Figure 22.2). The receptors are located on the ciliary processes that arise from the olfactory receptor neurones.

For a substance to be smelt it must be volatile. The detection of odours depends on their solubility in mucus. Some substances are detected in µg/l concentrations, others in mg/l amounts. The axons of the receptor cells pass through the cribriform plate to innervate the secondary projection neurones found in the olfactory bulb. Information is carried to higher cortical regions, including the periform cortex. Odour information is subsequently distributed to both cortical and subcortical structures throughout the nervous system.

Smell in prenatal infants

The ability to detect odour may be present before birth. The olfactory bulb and receptors have an

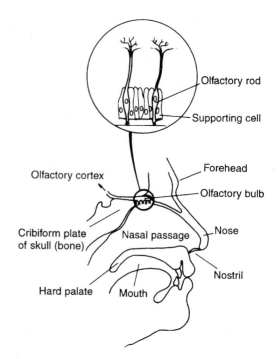

Fig. 22.2 Olfaction: anatomy of cranial nerve I and olfaction.

adult pattern by the middle of the eleventh week of interuterine life. At around 28 weeks the olfactory system is capable of detecting chemical stimuli. It would appear that infants can detect and discriminate between a variety of quite distinct smells or odorants. The breast-fed baby is able to distinguish the mother's smell from that of another lactating female. Bottle-fed infants do not make such discriminations. Breast-feeding infants cannot discriminate the axillary smells from their own father from another father. At 7 weeks, breast-fed infants will turn towards a perfume that has been worn on the mother's breast during feeding in preference to perfume worn by any other mother.

Odour classification

The classification of odours into discrete qualitative characters has tantalised scientists from the Ancient Greeks to the modern olfactory chemists. Aristotle divided flavours and smells into pungent, succulent, acid and astringent. In the modern era

Amor, by physicochemical measurements, classified odour qualities on the basis of a set of primary odours: ethereal, camphoraceus, muscae, floral, antipungent and putrid.

Many factors influence the capability to smell, including prior exposure to the test stimulus or related compound, the subject's age, gender, smoking habits, exposure to environmental toxins, drug usage and state of health. Exposure to an odorant, if recent and relatively continuous, can result in a temporary reduction in the ability to smell that odorant. This is called *olfactory fatigue*. Little is known about the degree to which the ability to smell can be improved by training. Repeated testing with an odorant results in increased sensitivity for detecting that odour. Repeated exposure to odorants makes unpleasant odours less unpleasant and pleasant odours less pleasant. Practising with feedback increases the ability to name odours. This has been used to a high degree in training food and beverage tasters, and also in testers in the perfume industry.

The intake of volatile smells (odorants) to the chemoreceptive membrane of the mouth and palate occurs in two different physical phases. Initially, the air-borne odorants pass in the air stream to the nasal chambers and the olfactory mucosa. In the second phase, fluid-borne odorants are transported through the olfactory mucus to the receptor membranes. The response is dependent on a partitioning between the air and mucus, which is dependent on water solubility. The olfactory mucus can concentrate relatively water-insoluble odorants by a factor of ten.

The physicochemical properties of the olfactory mucus regulate the access of odorants to, and their clearance from, olfactory cells, where the stimulus occurs. The viscosity of olfactory mucus varies enormously, being related primarily to the glycoprotein and water content. The olfactory mucus consists of a shallow (5 μm), superficial watery layer and a deeper (30 μm), more viscous mucoid layer. Viscosity microstructure and depth of the olfactory mucus determine the diffusion times for odorants and therefore regulate the speed with which stimulants reach the olfactory cilia. The physical properties of mucus and its chemical composition of electrolytes, glycoconjugates, proteins and enzymes are regulated by a complex interplay of odorants, cellular and neural factors.

Odorants, in general, are organic molecules with a molecular weight of less than 350 Da. They range in water solubility from infinitely soluble to poorly soluble. 'Musks', which are of higher molecular weight, are nearly always insoluble in water, with a low partition coefficient, and are classified as hydrophobic. Most organic odorants have molecular weights of less than 150 Da and are moderately water soluble. There are two complementary hypotheses to describe how odorants cross the mucus layer. The first suggests a free diffusion and the other a facilitated diffusion of odorants by transport proteins.

Olfactory receptor neurones have four primary functions:

- to detect odorants as a chemical stimulus
- to transmit the information about the chemical identity of the odorant, as well as its concentration and duration of stimulation
- to couple this information to the electrical properties of the neurone
- to transmit this information to the brain.

Odorant receptor molecules and odorant-regulated channels are found in the distal ciliary region where sensory transduction occurs. Three categories of membrane mechanism have been proposed for olfactory transduction. The first includes the odorant receptor-specific stimulation of the adenylate cyclase cyclic adenosine monophosphate (cAMP) second messenger and the phosphoinositide-derived messenger systems that activate ion-gated channels. G proteins are also involved.

Nerve fibres sensitive to noxious chemical stimuli on exposed or semi-exposed mucosal membranes respond to pungent spices, lacrimators and chemicals; the result is sneezing and skin irritation.

Another classification of chemical stimuli is based on a proposed mechanism of interaction with the nerve endings:

- those with an affinity for reaction with –SH groups on proteins
- molecules such as sulfur dioxide that do not react with –SH groups and may cleave S–S bonds in proteins
- sensory irritants belonging to neither of the above categories, e.g. ethanol.

The olfactory receptor nerve fibres for pungent chemicals serve as effectors, relaying chemically induced stimuli to the trigeminal nuclei and the brainstem. This sensory input triggers several sensory-mediated reflexes and peripheral action reflexes to protect the animal from further exposure to the irritant and remove the irritating stimulus from the nose, eye or mouth, by sneezing, withdrawing or spitting out the chemical.

Pungent-tasting vegetables contain compounds, e.g. isothiocyanate in horseradish and 1-propanyl-sulfenic acid in onion and garlic. Spices such as mustard, cloves, chilli pepper, black pepper and ginger contain active irritant principles, allyl and 3-butenyl isothiocyanate, eugenol, capsaicin, piperine, and 6-gingerol and 6-shogaol, respectively. Piperine and 6-gingerol and 6-shogaol, include an aromatic ring and an alkyl side-chain with a carbonal function. Changes in the alkyl side-group or in the amide function near the polar aromatic end abolish or reduce the pungent taste. Side-chains of nine carbon atoms' length for capsaicin and piperine and ten carbon atoms for gingerol result in more potent irritants.

Olfactory system measurements

The measurement of olfactory sensitivity is difficult because there is no simple physical measurement analogous to colour or sound pitch. Mixtures of odorants do not give predictable psychological and physiological effects in the same way as mixtures of light and sounds. The problem is not made easier when compounds with different chemical structure can all smell the same to humans. Valid measures of smell and olfactory sensitivity require reliable and reproducible procedures for presenting stimuli to the subjects. Such methods include the draw tube olfactometer of Zwardemaker, glass sniff bottles, plastic squeeze bottles, air dilution olfactometers, glass rods, wooden sticks or strips of blotting paper dipped in odorants. The results obtained include threshold measurements, the method of constant stimuli, methods of determining the limits of detection and a staircase or up/down method. Various techniques have been developed that use threshold stimuli to assess olfactory function. These can be divided into three general classes:

- those that require subjects to judge the relative amount of one or more attributes with a set of stimuli such as intensity or pleasantness (supra-threshold attributes scaling)
- those in which different thresholds are determined, e.g. the minimum increase in concentration required to make concentration A perceptibly more intense than concentration B (difference threshold measurement)
- those that specifically test the ability of subjects to detect, recognise, identify, clarify and remember after supra-threshold stimuli.

Electronic 'noses' that can detect chemicals are being developed. When a vapour binds to a polymer there is a change in the electrical characteristics of the polymer that can be recorded electronically. These can be used in food manufacturing systems and detecting malodours in foods. These machines are quite limited in the number of chemicals that they can identify.

GUSTATION

The chemoreceptor cells that experience taste are arranged into buds in the mouth. Most taste buds are found on the upper surface of the tongue, although there are some in the soft palate, larynx, pharynx and epiglottis. Taste buds are found in the lingual epithelium with connective tissue called papillae.

Fungiform papillae are found on the anterior two-thirds of the tongue and are concentrated near the anterior tip. Each fungiform papilla may contain up to 36 taste buds. A typical taste bud contains 50–150 individual taste cells, which are innervated by sensory nerve fibres from the facial glossopharyngal and vagal cranial nerves (Figure 22.3). More than half of the fungiform papillae contain no taste buds. Circumvallate papillae (large mushroom-shaped structures) are found on the posterior tongue and contain more taste buds than individual fungiform papillae. Gustatory stimulation of a single fungiform papilla is sufficient to identify correctly any of the four basic tastes, although this accuracy varies with the function and number of intact taste buds in that papilla. Taste sensitivity varies according to both regional taste

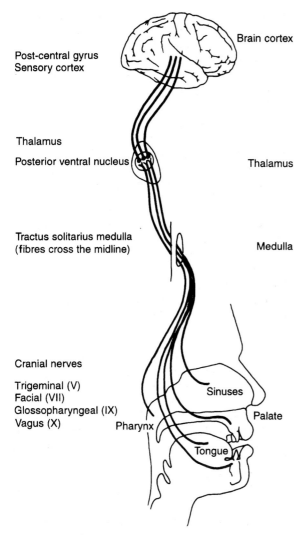

Post-central gyrus
Sensory cortex

Brain cortex

Thalamus

Posterior ventral nucleus

Thalamus

Tractus solitarius medulla
(fibres cross the midline)

Medulla

Cranial nerves

Trigeminal (V)
Facial (VII)
Glossopharyngeal (IX)
Vagus (X)

Sinuses

Palate

Pharynx

Tongue

Fig. 22.3 Sensory fibres from the taste buds transmit sensation to the trigeminal (V), facial (VII), glossopharyngeal (IX) and vagus (X) cranial nerves. These innervate the tongue, palate and pharynx, pass to the tractus solitarius in the medulla, cross the midline to the thalamus in the posterior ventral nucleus and then pass to the post-central gyrus in the sensory cortex.

bud density and the number of taste buds per papilla. There is enormous variation in taste bud density between individuals (from 3 to 514 taste buds/cm^2), which is not affected by age or gender. This is why some people may become expert tasters and gourmets, while others cannot differentiate between apparent delicacies. The anterior tongue is covered not only by the fungiform and folate papillae, but also by many coarse conical filiform papillae that may respond to mechanical stimuli.

Taste receptors are innervated by the VII, IX and X cranial nerves. The anterior two-thirds of the tongue is innervated by the VII cranial nerve, the posterior third including vallate and foliate papillae by the IX, and the soft palate, glottis and epiglottis by the X nerve (Figure 22.3). Taste cells respond to more than one taste quality. Gustatory information is carried by the VII, IX and X cranial nerves to the haustral half of the medulla. Axons from the gustatory region of the medulla enter the central tegmental tract and finish in the ventrobasal thalamus. There is a close linkage between the gustatory, somatosensory and trigeminal systems. In the olfactory cortex, inputs from an odorant receptor separate into thousands of neurones which are clustered in many olfactory areas. Information from many odorant receptors are in the same area. These inputs are then integrated and refined to give an overall smell experience.

Some textbooks on taste show a picture of the tongue with sweet receptors concentrated at the tip, salt receptors at the front, sour at the rear edges and bitter at the back of the tongue. Such tongue 'maps' are incorrect. The original work by Hanig showed that the thresholds for each of the four basic tastes are not constant over the entire tongue. The threshold for sweet is slightly lower at the front of the tongue, the threshold for bitter is slightly lower at the rear of the tongue, etc. The differences in sensitivity across each site are actually very small. All tastes are perceived well on all sites with taste receptors.

Development of taste

Taste cells are developed in the human foetus by 7–8 weeks of gestation and morphologically mature cells are found at 14 weeks. Foetal taste receptors may be stimulated by chemicals present in the amniotic fluids. The foetus begins to swallow from 12 weeks of gestation and may swallow 100–300 ml/kg/day by 9 months. Amniotic fluid contains glucose, fructose, lactic acid, pyruvic acid, citric acid, fatty acids, phospholipids, creatinine, uric acid, amino acids, polypeptides, proteins and salts. The chemical composition of the amniotic fluid varies over the course of gestation and may be abruptly altered by foetal urine. It is possible that foetuses show a preference for sweet tastes and reject bitter tastes. Swallowing amniotic fluid appears to be necessary for the proper development of the gut.

Newborn infants

The response of newborn babies to taste stimulation is judged by facial expression suggestive of contentment and liking or discomfort and rejection. Other response measurements used to measure neonatal taste perception include lateral tongue movements, autonomic reactivity, differential ingestion and sucking patterns.

The newly born baby enjoys sweet, sour and bitter tastes, and can discriminate sweet from non-sweet solutions and sour from bitter tastes, but does not appear to differentiate salt.

Older infants and young children

There have been few studies in infants aged 1–24 months. This is probably because children of this age are unwilling to co-operate or indulge scientists by eating unfamiliar food items. Children of this age are unwilling to accept unfamiliar bottles or food items from strangers or sometimes even from their mother.

Familiarity with specific foods and taste in the correct environment plays an important role in the preferences of pre-school children. Young children tend to show stronger preferences for concentrated sugar and salt than do adults.

Ageing and the taste system

The number of taste buds in the gustatory papillae does not decrease with age, and taste remains intact in old age.

Saliva

Saliva is produced by three large paired salivary glands, the parotid, submaxillary and sublingual glands. Mechanical stimulation during chewing of both food and inert substances promotes a flow of saliva, with 500–750 ml being produced each day; most is swallowed and absorbed from the gut.

Saliva performs a variety of functions.

Table 22.1   Composition of saliva

Electrolyte	Resting (mEq/l)	Stimulated (mEq/l)
Sodium	2.7	63
Potassium	46	18
Chloride	31	36
Bicarbonate	0.6	30
Magnesium	4.5*	0.4*
Calcium	42*	38*

Organic components

Proteins of acinar cell origin:
  amylase, lipase, mucus, glycoproteins, proline-rich glycoproteins, basic glycoproteins, acidic glycoproteins, peroxidase

Proteins of non-acinar cell origin:
  lysozyme, secreted immunoglobulin A growth factors, regulatory peptides

*mg/l.

- Saliva is essential for normal taste function (it is difficult to taste food with a dry mouth). It acts as a solvent for chemical stimuli in food and carries these stimuli to the taste receptors. At rest, gustatory receptors are covered with a layer of fluid that extends into the taste pores and bathes the receptors of the microvilli. Because gustatory stimulation alters salivary flow and composition, the fluid environment may alter during the activation of sensations of taste.
- Saliva has a role in the taste process. Drugs injected intravenously can be tasted as they circulate as they are secreted into saliva on the tongue. Such drugs include the intensely bitter sodium dehydrocholate and saccharine. It is not possible to taste drugs unless they are secreted in saliva.
- Saliva has a cleaning and antimicrobial action and also a buffering action that protects the teeth. Salivary glands secrete a large number of physiologically active substances, growth factor, vasoactive peptides and regulatory peptides.

Composition of saliva

Saliva is a dilute aqueous solution containing inorganic and organic constituents (Table 22.1). Its composition varies with the type of glands, species, time of day and degree and type of stimulation. Salivary flow virtually stops during sleep. With an increase in flow rate, the composition and concentration of saliva change. Sodium concentrations increase with increasing flow rate, while potassium decreases. Protein secretion by salivary glands is preceded by an initial uptake of amino acids and peptide synthesis in the gland.

High flow rates of saliva result from parasympathetic stimulation, and increased amylase secretion results from sympathetic nerve activation. The parasympathetic secretomotor neurones controlling the salivary glands arise from the salivatory nucleus of the vagus nerve. The sympathetic nerve supply to the salivary glands originates from the superior cervical ganglion.

There is an increase in salivary secretion even before (anticipatory) and certainly after food enters the mouth. Reflex secretion follows stimulation of the oral mechanoreceptors, especially periodontal ligament mechanoreceptors as well as taste buds. Not all taste stimuli by food are equally effective in promoting salivary flow. Citric acid produces a copious flow of saliva. Ingestion of sucrose is followed by significant production of salivary amylase, whereas salt stimulus produces secretion of saliva with a much higher protein content.

Taste papillae contents may control access and removal of stimuli and hence the sense of taste. During feeding and drinking, muscles controlling the jaws, tongue and face move food and fluid around the mouth and expose the solubilised tastes to the whole population of taste receptors. This is particularly important for taste receptors in the clefts of the circumvalate and foliate papillae. Muscle movements determine the rate and direction of delivery of stimuli to the receptors. Since saliva contains various ions, e.g. salt, which are themselves gustatory stimuli, taste receptors are continuously stimulated by salivary components. Thus to detect dietary salt, the concentration must exceed the concentration in saliva. Detection thresholds are reduced when the mouth is rinsed with distilled water and increased with higher concentrations of sodium chloride.

Of the many organic constituents of saliva, proline-rich proteins increase the ability to taste bitter compounds, quinine, raffinose and cyclohexamide.

Most tastes increase salivary flow in a concentration-dependent manner. Salivary proteins serve as carrier proteins for trophic substances.

Zinc has long been recognised as having an important role in taste perception as well as in taste bud maintenance.

Taste partitioning

Most tastes are water soluble and non-volatile, weak acid (sour), salts (salty and bitter), sugars (sweet), amino acids (sweet, bitter and umami) and protein (sweet and bitter). These dissolve during chewing and pass through saliva and the mucus layer covering the taste pore to reach the microvilli processes of taste receptor cells. Some tastes are lipophilic molecules, such as alkaloids, caffeine and quinine. Most hydrophobic molecules are extremely bitter-tasting and their taste detection thresholds tend to be lower than their hydrophilic counterparts.

Taste sensation begins when chemicals interact with specific sites on the apical membranes of taste receptor cells. Some tastes bind directly to receptors in ligand channels, while others stimulate signal transduction pathways for guanosine triphosphate (GTP)-binding proteins and second messengers. Salty, sour and some bitter tastes do not require specific membrane receptor proteins for stimulation. These tastes interact directly with specific ion channels located on the atypical membrane. The receptors for sweet stimuli, amino acids and bitter compounds contain a G protein, gustducin, which is cleaved when a taste chemical binds to the receptor. The T2R/TRB receptors are a family of some 40–80 receptors for bitter taste. The number of odorant receptors may be in the millions and they have been shown, in the mouse, to be encoded by up to 1000 genes. Each odorant receptor recognises several smells, but different smells are recognised by different combinations of odorant receptor.

When substances with different tastes are mixed there is often suppression of one or several tastes. Mixture interactions with food and beverages are the sum of interactions at different sites in the taste system. Each of these interactions probably depends on more than just the qualities of the mixtures. The area of tongue stimulated, the temperature of the stimuli and the way in which they are tasted, e.g. the rate of flow over the tongue, determine the taste effect.

Taste perception

Salty taste

Salty taste is experienced with sodium chloride; other alkali halides have less marked salty tastes. Larger cations have a salty but also a bitter taste. Thus, no salt substitute has been found that does not taste bitter. There is only one cation that is smaller than sodium, namely lithium, but, while lithium has a pleasantly salty taste, it can be toxic. Salts can enhance other flavours; this may be due to filtering of flavours with suppression of unpleasant flavours and enhancement of agreeable flavours.

Salty taste appreciation is mediated through an epithelial ion channel, where the influx of Na into the cell depolarises the cell membrane. This leads to alterations in voltage-sensitive ion channels, which modulate intracellular calcium activity with resulting neurotransmitter secretion. Sodium ions are removed from these cells through a Na^+/K^+-ATPase pump.

Sour taste

Sourness, while being a major taste sensation, has been poorly studied. The primary event in sourness is stimulation through an ion channel involving potassium ions and cellular depolarisation.

Sweet taste

Sweet taste has traditionally been seen as good and bitter as dangerous. This difference is because many beneficial foods are sweet and some poisonous compounds are very bitter.

Sweet and bitter tastes are typical of organic compounds. As the anion size is increased there is a change in the balance of bitter and sweet taste dependent on structure.

Many attempts have been made to develop a general theory relating chemical structure to sweetness, although such theories have not been generally successful. The sweet receptor gene is now identified as *T1R3*, which is selectively expressed in the taste cells of the tongue and mouth.

Some bulk sweeteners give body and viscosity to foods, e.g. glucose, sucrose and isomalt. A second group comprises intense sweeteners used at low concentration, e.g. saccharine, aspartame and thaumatin.

Most sugars taste sweet at a concentration of 10^{-1} M, aspartame at 10^{-3} M, aspartic derivatives at 10^{-6} M and thaumatin at 10^{-7} M. The problem in identifying sweet taste receptors is that the diversity of the chemical structure of sweet compounds is so wide. However, the sweet receptor has been identified. Sugars stimulate adenylate cyclase in a concentration-dependent manner, indicating a role for G proteins.

There is no perfect sweetener that is without additional tastes, e.g. bitterness or sourness, or differences due to surface tension and viscosity. A real problem is persistence, which is a prolonged sweet taste.

Many of the very sweet, naturally occurring compounds are at least 50–100 times sweeter than sucrose and are mainly terpinoids, flavinoids and proteins. Many are constituents of green plants, from quite different taxonomic groups, that synthesise similar classes of biochemical sweet compounds. However, if there are sweet-tasting constituents in one plant it does not follow that such sweetness will occur in other species of the same genus. As with attempts to define sweetness chemically, there is no logic that predicts the discovery of sweet compounds using plant taxonomy.

Sweet tastes

Sweet-tasting compounds from natural sources include:

- low molecular weight sugars (sucrose, fructose, glucose)
- amino acids (alanine, glycine)
- terpenoid glycosides (glycyrrhizin acid), osladin, sevioside, baiyunoside
- proteins, thaumatin, monellin, mabinilin, pentadin.

Other sweet tasting compounds include:

- amino acyl sugars, methyl-2,3-di-*O*-(1-alanyl)-α-D-glucopyranoside
- alanine D-amino sugars
- peptides, aspartame
- chlorinated hydrocarbons, chloroform, halogenated sugars, sucralose
- *N*-sulfonyl amide, saccharine
- sulfamates (cyclamate)
- polyketides, neogasperidin, anilines and ureas.

Interactions of molecules and taste

Shallemberger and Acre proposed that the sensation of sweetness was appreciated by a sweet receptor. This was called the AH,B system (Figure 22.4). A and B are electronegative atoms (usually oxygen) and AH is a hydrogen bond, which functions through intermolecular hydrogen bonds. The hydrogen donor AH and hydrogen bond acceptor are separated by about 0.3 nm, which is critical for sweetness. The entire molecular geometry as well as the AH,B system affect the hydrogen-bonded complex, the quality and the intensity of the sweet response. The bipolar system is an electrophilic–nucleophilic (e-n) system. There is an additional important role in the sweet receptor site for the hydrophobic region of the molecule at another portion of the sweet receptor. The quality and intensity of a given molecule's taste depend strongly on the e-n system, the size and shape of the hydrophobic moiety and its position relative to the e-n system.

Kier proposed a third complementary binding site involving dispersion forces. Sweetness was induced in co-operation with the AH,B receptor site. It is now thought that an ideal sweetener contains up to eight optional and co-operative binding sites.

Bitterness may well have a similar receptor shape, but of different dimensions. This may account for bitter–sweet overlap in molecules that have similar dimensions fitting roughly into both sites.

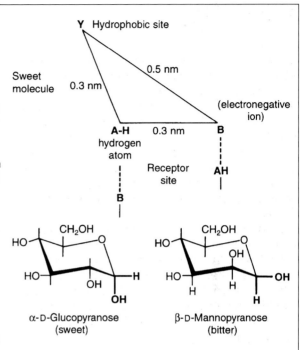

Fig. 22.4 Sweetness perception: Shallenberger's saporous unit. For a molecule to taste sweet there must be A and B electronegative atoms; AH acts as an acid while B acts as a base. The AH,B unit forms a double hydrogen bonded complex with a similar AH,B system on the taste receptor.

Field investigations and literature sources have been used to identify sweet compounds. For example, agranandulcin, a novel sesquiterpene sweetener, was rediscovered from a monograph entitled *Natural History of New Spain (Central America)*, written between 1570 and 1576 by Francisco Hernandez.

Two proteins, monellin and thaumatin, found in African berries are very sweet (100 000 times sweeter than sucrose) at concentrations of 10^{-8} M. Thaumatin is a single-chain protein of 207 residues and monellin two peptide chains of 45 and 50 amino acid residues each. Native conformation of the protein is essential for the sweet taste; although both proteins are intensely sweet they are somewhat different chemically. Antibodies raised against thaumatin cross-react with and compete with monellin and other sweet compounds, but not with chemically modified non-sweet monellin. This suggests a common chemical domain or portion of structure that confers sweetness. These proteins have little calorific content, are safe and natural, and neither introduces non-natural metabolites into the body to distort the balance of the amino acid pool. The disadvantage is that the taste profiles of these proteins differ from sugars and therefore they have limited applicability. Monellin loses its sweet taste on heating, as the two peptide chains separate. Thaumin has eight disulfide bonds and is more heat stable than monellin, but once denatured does not regain potency.

Structurally different sweeteners, amino acids, sweet peptides, aspartame and nitroaniline derivatives all bind at the sweet taste receptor. The sweet taste of sugars, amino acids, saccharine, chloroform, olefin alcohols and metanitroanilans is attributed to their ability to form two hydrogen bonds with a complementary B,AH entity at the receptor. A structure–activity relationship is based on a three-dimensional molecular theory rather than one-dimensional structural approaches. The problem is the peculiar relationship between sweet- and bitter-tasting molecules. Simple amino acids and peptides can change their taste from sweet to bitter when the chirality of the carbon adjacent to the amino and carboxyl groups is changed. This seems to point to a two-mirror-image receptor active site. A large number of synthetic sweeteners are flat rigid molecules. It might be possible to account for a change in taste of amino acids with chirality simply by inverting the AH,B entities of the twin receptors for sweet and bitter tastes. Saccharine substituted in position 6 of the aromatic ring remains sweet when the hydrogen is substituted with a methyl group, an amino group, a fluorine or a chlorine, but loses its sweet taste when hydrogen is substituted with an iodine or a methoxy group.

Amino acids and peptides: some amino acids taste very sweet. The short-chain neutral amino acids (both L- and D-configuration) are sweet, e.g. glycine. Aspartyl dipeptide is very sweet. Such sweetness does not depend on the L- or D-configuration of the second amino acid ester, but rather on the size and shape of the amino acid ester and side-chain substitutions. When R1 and R2 amino acid side-chains are sufficiently dissimilar in size the potency of the sweetener is very high. If space remains in the dipeptide ester receptor binding site at the C- or N-terminus of the sweet aspartyl dipeptide, then peptides extended at the C- or N-terminus of the sweet peptides may taste sweet. A dipeptide N-terminus is required for significant sweetness. Both sterically small and large hydrophobic moieties are required on the second amino acid for the specific sweet taste spatial orientation. It would appear that amine branching is important for a successful sweet taste. The increased steric bulk from either trimethyl or cyclopropyl substitution of the (α-carbon is required for high sweetness taste in the aliphatic series. L-Aspartyl-L-phenylalanine, methyl ester (aspartame) is 200 times sweeter than sucrose. The sweet region lies with the phenylalanine portion of the molecule.

Sugar: a simple conformational change in an asymmetrical carbon can convert a sweet to a bitter taste. β-D-Glucopyranose is sweet and β-D-

Mannopyranose is bitter. The sweet taste of sucrose can be increased by selective halogenation. The halogenation of hydroxyl groups results in an increase in sweetness of up to several thousand times. This is very stereo-specific, with many compounds being entirely tasteless. Other chlorinated carbohydrates, including derivatives of maltose and lactose, are extremely bitter.

Substitution at the carbon 6 position results in compounds 400 times sweeter than sucrose. The 6-O-methyl derivative is 500 times sweeter, whereas the 6-O-isopropyl derivative has no sweetness. Chlorination of the C2 position produces an extremely bitter compound, suggesting that the presence of a hydroxyl group at the 2 position is essential for sweetness. Increasing the size of substitution at the 4' position has a positive effect on sweetness. Sucralose, the 4,1',6-trichloro derivative of sucrose, is 650 times sweeter than sucrose and is very stable.

It is possible that the intense sweetness of some of these sugar derivatives is a consequence of the molecules that occupy multiple binding sites.

Bitter taste

Bitter taste receptors involve a G protein that activates the production of inositol triphosphate which, in turn, releases calcium from internal stores.

Many chemicals taste bitter, some of which are chemically related, e.g. quaternary amines, acetylated sugars, alkaloids, amino sugars, L-isomers and some inorganic acids.

β-D-Mannose and gentiobiose have a bitter taste, whereas their α-isomers, e.g. α-D-mannose and isomaltose, are sweet tasting. The lipophilicity of the aglycone glycosides is associated with bitterness. The methyl glycosides of glucose, galactose, mannose, fructose, arabinose and benzyl glycosides are all bitter. The bitterness increases with chain length, with the methyl glucoside being sweet, ethyl glucoside bitter–sweet and propyl glucoside bitter. D-Isomers of amino acids taste sweet, whereas the L-isomers taste bitter. The overall hydrophobicity of amino acid side-chains affects their sweet or bitter taste. Increasing the steric bulk of the amino acid with lipophilic moieties in the side-chain increases the bitter taste. Substitution of the α-carbon abolishes taste. Aromatic side-chains increase the bitter taste, e.g. phenylalanine and tryptophan are very bitter. Bitterness decreases with polar substitutions in the side-chain, i.e. hydroxy, amino and carboxylic.

Peptides may taste bitter in both L- and D-isomer forms. The taste, however, of a peptide does not appear to be related to the constituent amino acids. The sequence in which the amino acids are paired in dipeptides, in some unknown manner, dictates the taste potential. This is regardless of the taste of the constituent amino acids.

There is some genetically determined variation in ability to taste substances, e.g. some people can taste thiourea.

Phenylthiocarbamide (PTC) tastes bitter to some but is without taste for others. Such non-tasting is a simple Mendelian trait. Substances with genetically based taste thresholds similar to PTC contain an N–C=S group, e.g. 6-N-propylthiouracil. In the USA and Europe, non-tasters account for one-third of the population, whereas among other ethnic groups the taste threshold frequency is higher.

Umami

This modality of taste, which may or may not be a reality, is derived from the Japanese word for delicious or savoury. An example is monosodium glutamate.

Taste interactions

A variety of unusual taste interactions has been reported. The berries produced by *S. dulcificum* plant (miracle fruit) have the ability to make sour substances taste sweet. A glycoprotein in the berry adds a sweet taste to acidic substances. This may occur through a conformational change in the miracle fruit glycoprotein. Acids change the conformation of the glycoprotein so that the sugars bind to it and stimulate the sweet receptor sites.

The leaves of the plant *G. sylvestre* contain substances that temporarily reduce the ability to taste sweet substances. Artichokes for some, but not all, individuals cause other substances to taste sweet for up to 15 min.

KEY POINTS

1. Gustation is the term for the sensation of taste and olfaction for smell. In addition to the basic tastes of sweet, sour, bitter and salty, there is a large number of other tastes. The recognition of the flavour of food involves several sensory systems, mechanoreceptive, thermoreceptive and chemoreceptive.

2. The olfactory system is capable of recognising thousands of smells. The system is very complex and it is not clear whether recognition takes place peripherally or centrally, in the brain. The olfactory epithelium in humans is found predominantly on the dorsal aspect of the nasal cavity, the septum and part of the superior turbinates. The physical and chemical properties of olfactory mucus regulate the access of odorants to, and their clearance from, olfactory cells.

3. The olfactory bulb and receptors have an adult pattern by the middle of the 11th week of gestation. At about 28 weeks the olfactory system is capable of detecting chemical stimuli.

4. The chemoreceptor cells that experience taste, sweet, sour, bitter and salty are arranged into buds in the oral cavity. Most taste buds are found on the upper surface of the tongue, although there are some in the soft palate, larynx, pharynx and epiglottis.

5. Taste cells are developed in the human foetus at 7–8 weeks of gestation and morphologically mature cells are to be found at 14 weeks. The newborn baby enjoys sweet, sour and bitter tastes, and can discriminate tastes. The number of taste buds in the gustatory papillae does not decrease with age, and taste response remains into old age.

6. Saliva is produced by three large, paired salivary glands: the parotid, submaxillary and sublingual glands. It is a dilute aqueous solution that contains inorganic and organic constituents and has a cleaning, antimicrobial and buffering action that protects the teeth. The composition of saliva varies with time of day and degree and type of stimulation.

7. The sensation of sweetness is said to be appreciated by a sweet receptor called the AH,B system. There is a role in the sweet receptor site

for the hydrophobic region of the molecule on the sweet receptor.

8. The taste sensation is identified by receptors and the information carried to the cerebral cortex by the VII and IX cranial nerve and processed into the sensation of taste.

THINKING POINT

What, for the average person, are the relative significances of the smell and taste and nutritional value of a meal?

NEED TO UNDERSTAND

The underlying mechanisms behind the basic sensations of taste, salt, sour, sweet and bitter, and the experience of smell.

FURTHER READING

Beets, M.G.J. (1978) *Structure Activity Relationships in Human Chemoreception*. Applied Science Publishers, London.

Drewnosski, A. (1997) Taste preference and food intake. *Annual Review of Nutrition*, **17**, 237–54.

Getchell, T.V., Batoshuk, L.M., Doty, R.L. and Snow, J.B. (1991) *Smell and Taste in Health and Disease*, Raven Press, New York.

Gilbertson, T.A., Damak, S. and Margolskee, R.F. (2000) The molecular physiology of taste transduction. *Current opinion in neurobiology*. **10**, 519–27.

Mennella, J.A. and Beauchamp, G.K. (1998) Early flavor experiences: research update. *Nutrition Reviews*, **56**, 205–11.

Patterson, R.L.S., Charlwood, B.V., MacLeod, G. and Williams, A.A. (1992) *Bioformation of Tastes*. Royal Society of Chemistry, Cambridge.

Shallemberger, R.S. and Acre, T.E. (1967) Molecular theory of sweet tastes. *Nature*, **216**, 480–2.

Walters, D.E., Orthoefer, F.T. and DuBois, G.E. (eds) (1991) *Sweeteners, Molecular Design and Chemoreception*. ACS Symposium Series 450. American Chemical Society, Washington, DC.

Woods, M.P. (1998) Taste and flavour perception. *Proceedings of the Nutrition Society*, **57**, 603–7.

Zou, Z., Horowitz, L.F., Montmayeur, J.-P. *et al.* (2001) Genetic tracing reveals a stereotyped sensory map in the olfactory cortex. *Nature*, **414**, 173–9.

WEBSITE

http://dmoz.org/health/senses/smell_and_taste

23

Intake and satiety

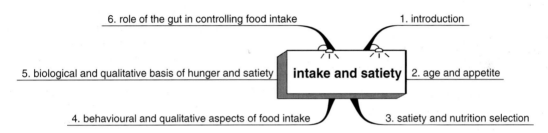

6. role of the gut in controlling food intake

5. biological and qualitative basis of hunger and satiety

4. behavioural and qualitative aspects of food intake

intake and satiety

1. introduction

2. age and appetite

3. satiety and nutrition selection

Fig. 23.1 Chapter outline.

INTRODUCTION

The sense of appetite begins with hunger and may end with the feeling of satiety.

Factors involved in the modulation of appetite:

- taste (intensity and hedonics)
- volume and weight of food
- energy density
- osmolarity
- the presence of different proportions of macronutrients.

Biological responses include:

- oral stimulation
- gastric distension
- rate of gastric emptying
- release of hormones
- triggering of digestive enzyme secretions
- plasma concentrations of absorbed nutrients.

Satiation is the inhibition of hunger and eating, arising from the eating of sufficient food. Among the many elements that initiate appetite are food and its palatability. Palatability, a complicated sensation to define, is a mix of taste and smell. It is the hedonistic evaluation of the food under particular circumstances and cannot easily be measured. It is best perhaps measured with a visual analogue scale in which there is a line reading from 0 to 10. 0–4 is less and 6–10 more than expected. It is possible to rank a phenomenon by saying by how much it comes below or above expectations. Palatability is a rating of the pleasure experienced when a particular food is eaten. Salt and sweet foods are usually appreciated more than are bitter and sour.

Satiety is the inhibition of the sensation of hunger and as a consequence the limiting of food ingestion. The amount of food that is eaten should meet the needs of the individual, supplying the metabolic, reproductive and growth processes, and will vary with the individual in different phases and energy expenditures of life. There are also

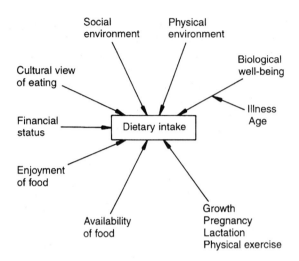

Fig. 23.2 Determinants of dietary intake are social, physical and biological.

strong social and cultural influences on food intake (Figure 23.2). Eating behaviour may be determined by an interaction between the availability and choice of food, satiation signals and the biological responses to food ingestion.

It is possible to fast, to eat sufficient or to eat in excess of requirement or that which is felt to be appropriate or desirable. If there is insufficient money or food available it may be imperative for a mother to reduce her energy intake to feed her children. If there is an excess of food available then this may lead to obesity and accumulation of body fat. These extremes of behaviour override the controls of appetite or dietary intake.

AGE AND APPETITE

Food preferences and hence the wish to consume particular foods begin at a very young age and are influenced by the mother, in choices made both before and after delivery. Later social interactions are important, as the preference repertoire increases.

In the process of growing from childhood to adult life, there is steady reduction in sweet taste preference, less sugar consumption and reduced energy intake.

Ageing is a process of decline and in physiological ageing as opposed to ageing complicated by illness, there is a decline in the ability to respond to changes in the internal and external environment to obtain optimal homoeostatic functioning. The rate of recovery to homoeostasis is also delayed in ageing. There is declining energy intake, smaller, sometimes less varied meals and fewer snacks. Ageing is associated with an added acceptance of bitter tastes. Gastric emptying, a contributor to the feeling of satiety is slower in the elderly. The elderly feel thirsty less readily. Yet levels of sensory acuity do not lessen with age. Dementia has a varied effect on weight and appetite. The demented elderly person often loses weight but may have a voracious appetite.

However, there is no causal relationship between age-related changes in sensory function and the selection of a more bulky, energy-diminished diet.

SATIETY AND NUTRITION SELECTION

There are two approaches to studies on eating behaviour.

- A behavioural approach measures qualitative aspects of eating. These include food choice, preference and the sensory aspects of food and hunger, fullness and hedonic sensations that accompany eating. The behavioural profile is the relationship between the pattern of intake of meals and snacks, and the sensory attributes of the foods.
- A quantitative approach measures dietary nutrient and energy intake. Quantitative aspects include the amount and energy value of food, nutrient value, composition of food, impact and energy balance. A quantitative profile is the total food consumed over a 24 h period, total energy intake, the proportions of macronutrients and micronutrients ingested, and the overall fuel balance.

BEHAVIOURAL AND QUALITATIVE ASPECTS OF FOOD INTAKE

Relationship between mood and appetite

The relationship is complex, but eating in a convivial environment has a stimulatory effect on appetite. This effect may be central, i.e. in the brain. The *satiety cascade* may be summarised as follows:

1. **Sensory** (taste and chewing): this includes palatability of the food and the pleasure in eating.
2. **Cognitive** (gastric phase, distension and hormones): gastric emptying time is important and can control the feeling of satiety.
3. **Post-ingestive** (oxidative metabolism): the rate of metabolism influences the feeling of satiety; protein is metabolised more rapidly than carbohydrate, which is in turn is metabolised more rapidly than fat. It is assumed that fat is not metabolised immediately, in contrast to protein and carbohydrate.
4. **Post-absorptive** (central effects): the central effects of food may be mediated by a series of hormones and biologically active substances, e.g. cholecystokinin (CCK), glucagon-like peptide-1,5-hydroxytryptamine (5-HT), opioid peptides, caffeine and leptin.

Sensory control of eating

Eating is generally organised into meals that are taken at particular time intervals. At least three distinct phases of the meal can be distinguished: meal initiation, associated largely with hunger; meal maintenance, which involves the act of eating; and meal termination, associated with satiety.

Meal initiation

The transition from the non-eating to the eating state includes the mechanisms involved in wanting to eat and anticipatory to eating. An animal ensures adequate nutrition by consuming a widely varied range of foods. Experiments in newly weaned infants and in adults show that when more than one food is available there is a natural tendency to switch between foods rather than to consume only the favourite meal. A nutritious but monotonous diet, given to military personnel or even starving refugees, may eventually be refused. The aversion may persist for several months. It is possible that the decline in acceptability of a particular food, when consumed in excess, is due to some innate automatic mechanism directing food variety selection, a sensory-specific satiety.

Food craving is one of the strongest sensations involved in eating. Among a normal population more than two-thirds of men and almost all women report intense desires for specific food items. Food cravings during pregnancy can be so profound that there are reports of pregnant women stealing food. Over 70% of bulimic women attribute binge episodes to previous carbohydrate cravings. Craving for sweet foods, especially chocolate, is frequent in premenstrual obese women. There are several theories about craving. One is that cravings indicate the need for a substance necessary to correct homoeostatic imbalance, e.g. salt. Another theory is that cravings may reflect the desire for specific sensory, not pharmacological or physiological, stimulation.

Food-associated sensations such as the smell and sight of food promote the desire for food and eating. Environmental stimuli associated with food or eating are strong controllers of meal initiation. Sensations arising from the sight or smell of food make one want to eat and induce craving, as do the place or location, time of day and social environment. Another factor is what may be called energy depletion and the loss of vital short-term energy sources, e.g. glucose.

There are endogenous determinants of energy intake, such as gender: a male, growing to a greater height and weight, will eat more than a female at the same stage of life. As people grow older food intake declines, in part because of reduced physical activity.

Surveys of attitudes towards dietary fat show that fat intake is related more to the pleasantness of the taste than to any views on health. Favourite foods are often fatty foods, desired because of their smell, flavours and palatable textures. Low-fat diets are seen as being monotonous and bland. It has been shown that body weight is related to a liking for fatty foods. As body weight increases so does the

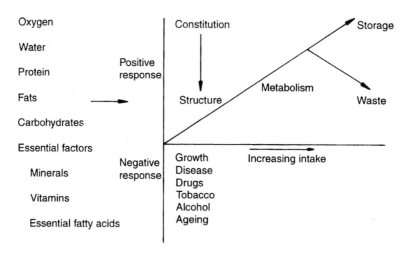

Fig. 23.3 Primary food sources. Increasing dietary intake meets the needs of metabolism. Excess dietary intake is stored or excreted. Metabolism and conversion of nutrients into structure are dependent on constitution. Possible negative effects on growth are shown.

liking for fatty foods. High-fat, energy-dense foods are associated with a greater reduction in hunger than low-energy-containing foods, at the same weight or volume intake. The weight of food eaten tends to remain constant; the variable is the energy content of the intake.

It is questionable whether food taste and palatability influence food intake. The chemical senses are crucial for the recognition and selection of food. Food may be selected or rejected on the basis of inborn preferences or aversions. Innate preferences for a sweet or salty taste may help in the identification of food that contains sugars, calcium, sodium and other minerals, i.e. essential nutrients. The aversion to bitter taste may help to reduce the risk of food poisoning. It has been suggested that there are alterations in taste for a number of nutrients, e.g. salt intake, in various conditions such as hypertension and cancer. Similar changes may be noted in eating disorders, and in gastrointestinal, liver and kidney disease. Corticosteroids may increase the appetite and food intake. Altered chemosensory responses have yet to be implicated as a contributory factor to changes in food intake.

Heavy sedation decreases food intake. Alcohol may decrease food intake because of gastritis or disordered social structure.

Endogenous and exogenous determinants of food selection

Society, religion and culture influence the choice of food. Delicacies for people in one part of the world may be regarded elsewhere with abhorrence. Finance may determine the availability of nutrients. Confusion over choice of food may occur after a period of deprivation. When the financial status improves and a wider range of food becomes available, factors in food choice other than nutrition, e.g. ignorance and inappropriate models, become important (Figure 23.3).

Meal maintenance
During eating the process progresses through a series of stages. The cephalic phase response includes secretory and motor reflexes related to digestion, e.g. insulin or gastric acid secretions and motility changes that are activated by the stimulation of receptors in the brain or oropharynx. Cephalic responses produced by brain receptors are often stimulated before eating, by the sight and smell of food. Such responses develop as a result of learning. In contrast, cephalic responses produced by oropharyngeal receptors arise from contact with the food within the mouth. There is a good

correlation between the palatability and the magnitude of the cephalic response produced.

Once eating has started, two types of sensory event are evoked, one excitatory and the other inhibitory. These are the main determinants of how much an individual eats at a meal, assuming that there is an excess of food available. The palatability of food is a major determinant of the duration of the meal and consequently the amount eaten. Palatability includes:

- the sensory properties of the food
- the physiological state of the person who is eating the food
- stimuli arising from previous associations with that particular food.

Other factors include particular dietary likes and dislikes, e.g. sweet or savoury food. The more pleasant the sensory properties of the food, the more is eaten.

Meal termination

A meal is usually completed with a feeling of satiation, when the excitatory stimuli which initiate the eating of the meal have been overcome. This occurs as a result of a suppression of the pleasant feeling for the food and is called *alliaesthesia*. The entire upper gastrointestinal tract produces sensory stimuli that signal that the eating process should stop. The stomach produces a whole range of sensations, including stomach distension, which are relayed by gastric stretch receptors to the brain. These signals are sent by the brain to suppress eating.

Food intake controls

Controls of food intake include:

- hunger, cravings and hedonic sensation
- energy and macronutrient intake
- peripheral physiology and metabolic events, concentration of neurotransmitters and metabolic interactions in the brain.

The cephalic phase responses are a result of events in many parts of the gastrointestinal tract. The effect of ingested food in the mouth results in positive feedback for eating, whereas from the stomach and small intestine there is negative feedback. The brain is informed about the amount of food ingested and its nutrient input through specialised chemoreceptors and mechanoreceptors that control physiological activity. This is followed by a post-absorptive phase after the nutrients have been digested and enter the circulation. These nutrients may be metabolised peripherally or even pass into the brain. It used to be thought that there were opposing hunger and satiety centres in the hypothalamus. Now it is thought that several neurotransmitters and neuromodulators, pathways and receptors are involved in the central neurological process. Foods of varying nutritional composition are thought to act differently with the regulating processes and have different effects on satiation and satiety.

BIOLOGICAL AND QUANTITATIVE BASIS OF HUNGER AND SATIETY

Food needs

The requirement to eat and food intake may be continuous, as in the ever-eating sparrow or field mouse, or intermittent. The eagle and lion appear quiescent between intense bursts of energy, during which the prey is caught and eaten before the resumption of sloth.

The basic vegetative activities of the cardiorespiratory, renal, endocrine, liver, nervous and brainstem systems are the 'housekeeping' functions of the body. To satisfy these needs, energy must be continuously available. The energy needs of intermittent activities range from trivial movements to activity at maximal capacity where brain and voluntary muscular systems are utilised to their limit. To satisfy these needs, additional energy must be provided.

In a freely eating society with readily available food, the intake of protein is tightly controlled between 11 and 14% of daily food intake. Fat and carbohydrate intake are less readily controlled. However, carbohydrate intake suppresses subsequent intake by an amount roughly equivalent to its energy content. The time-course of this suppressive action may vary according to the rate at which carbohydrates are metabolised. There is a relationship between energy intake and glucose, which is mediated through arterial – venous glucose concentration differences. The rate of hepatic glucose utilisation and the activation of glucoreceptive neurones in the brain are important controls. Cholecystokinin (CCK) is a hormone that affects the feeling of satiation and early-phase satiety. Protein or fat stimulates the release of CCK, activating CCK-A receptors in the pyloric region of the stomach. From there, signals to the vagal nerve afferents are passed to the nutrient nucleus of the tractus solitarius and to the medial zones of the hypothalamus. This is the mechanism by which dietary fat may trigger neurochemical responses and satiety. Dietary fat may also control satiety through enzyme systems responsible for fat digestion, e.g. pancreatic procolipase, with the release of an activation peptide, enterostatin. This may further decrease food intake. Oxidative metabolism of glucose and free fatty acids in the liver provides for the control of appetite. Alternatively, oxidation of fat may be an important signal initiating food intake.

Satiety can also be controlled through learned reflexes, although no centre controlling satiety has been identified in the brain. In humans the needs for metabolic fuels are substantial and continuous, yet eating is episodic. It is unlikely that there is a central receptor monitoring caloric flux and therefore controlling food intake. There may be important, non-central controls, e.g. the liver monitors gastric emptying and the distribution of insulin and energy sources.

The passage of energy-rich food from the stomach to the intestine is regulated. Concentrated solutions empty slowly, whereas dilute solutions empty rapidly, producing the same net delivery of calories to the intestine. Satiety may result from a feeling of gastric distension and from the rate of gastric emptying. After a meal, metabolism is stimulated by nutrients entering the circulation from the gastrointestinal tract, with excess energy being stored as glycogen or triglyceride. Intestinal absorption provokes insulin secretion and shifts hepatic metabolism from mobilisation to storage, thus providing a second signal of satiety. When both satiety signals have disappeared, liver and adipose tissue energy stores are mobilised and hunger recurs. Hunger may not reflect a biological need for food, as thirst does for water.

There may be individual differences in response to different nutrient intakes that determine the rate of metabolism and possibly satiation.

ROLE OF THE GUT IN CONTROLLING FOOD INTAKE

The mucosa of the gastrointestinal tract from the mouth to the terminal ileum is sensitive to chemical and mechanical stimuli of ingested food. A consequence is the release of gut hormones, and a negative feedback mechanism will signal the completion of feeding and make for post-prandial satiation.

Increased contractions in the stomach cause the sensation of hunger. There is a close association between epigastric fullness, observable abdominal protuberance, stomach distension and the cessation of eating. Receptors in the wall of the stomach are activated by distension. Distending the stomach with balloons or food stops eating. Removing recently ingested food restarts the ability to eat and leads to overeating. Romans, after a large feast, would induce vomiting by stimulating the oropharynx with a feather. After vomiting, the gorging of food would continue. Gastric emptying is slowed by neural and hormonal duodenal mechanisms. It has been suggested that gut peptides are important in the physiology of post-prandial satiety. Such gut hormones include CCK-8, bombesin, glucagon and somatostatin. Insulin and hypoglycaemia can provoke hunger contractions. However, neither hypoglycaemia nor decreased glucose utilisation occurs between meals. When the gastric motility response to insulin-induced hypoglycaemia is abolished by dividing the vagus below the diaphragm, the urge to eat still occurs. Patients who have had a total gastrectomy continue to experience hunger.

KEY POINTS

1. The amount of food eaten should meet the needs of the individual. Nutritional intake is important in supplying metabolic processes, which will vary with the individual, in different phases and energy expenditures of life. There is also a strong social and cultural influence on food intake.
2. Eating behaviour may be determined by an interaction between the choice of food, and the

satiation signals of the biological responses to food ingestion. Choice of food or taste, intensity and pleasure given (hedonistic response), volume or weight of food, energy density, osmolarity and the proportions of macronutrients are important factors in eating behaviour.

3. There are two approaches to eating behaviour studies: a behavioural approach measures eating patterns and food intake; a quantitative approach measures dietary nutrient and energy intake.

4. The behavioural approach to food intake looks at eating as being organised into meals that are taken at variable time intervals. A meal consists of a series of phases, each controlled by different mechanisms and associated with various emotional states. At least three distinct phases of the meal can be distinguished: meal initiation, meal maintenance and meal termination. Hunger is associated largely with meal initiation and satiety with meal termination.

5. The controls on food intake include: hunger, cravings and hedonic sensation; energy and macronutrient intake; peripheral physiology and metabolic events, and neurotransmitter and metabolic interactions in the brain.

6. The quantitative approach examines the requirement to eat as continuous or intermittent. The basic vegetative activities that ensure the housekeeping of the body require a continuous provision of energy.

7. No specific centre controlling satiety has been identified in the brain.

8. The passage of energy-rich food from the stomach to the intestine is regulated. Concentrated solutions empty slowly, whereas dilute solutions empty rapidly, producing the same net delivery of calories to the intestine. Satiety may result from a feeling of gastric distension and high rate of gastric emptying. Following the absorption of food, satiation may follow the storage of the absorbed nutrients.

THINKING POINTS

1. The elements that make for appetite and satiety are cultural, behavioural and chemical.

2. The response to particular foods and their ability to affect satiety are very varied.

NEED TO UNDERSTAND

1. The effect of age, mood and type of food on the four phases of satiation and the biological basis of these stages.

2. The different stages of a meal and the effect on hunger and satiation are important.

FURTHER READING

Birch, L.L. (1999) Development of food preferences. *Annual Review of Nutrition*, **19**, 41–63.

Blundell, J.E. and Tremblay, A. (1995) Appetite and energy (fuel) balance. *Nutrition Research Reviews*, **8**, 225–42.

Drewnowski, A. (2000) Sensory control of energy density at different life stages. *Proceedings of the Nutrition Society*, **59**, 239–44.

Hetherington, M.H. (1998) Taste and appetite in the elderly. *Proceedings of the Nutrition Society*, **57**, 625–31.

Levine, A.S. and Billington, C. (1997) Why do we eat? A neural systems approach. *Annual Review of Nutrition*, **17**, 597–620.

Rolls, B.J. and Shide, D.J. (1992) The influence of dietary fat on food intake and body weight. *Nutrition Reviews*, **50**, 283–90.

Rogers, P.J. (1995) Food, mood and appetite. *Nutrition Research Reviews*, **8**, 243–69.

Stubbs, R.J. (1998) Appetite, feeding behaviour and energy balance in human subjects. *Proceedings of the Nutrition Society*, **57**, 341–56.

Symposium on Social and Environmental Influences on Diet Choice (1999) *Proceedings of the Nutrition Society*, **58**, 755–63.

Yeomans, M.R. (1998) Taste, palatability and the control of appetite. *Proceedings of the Nutrition Society*, **57**, 609–15.

24

The gastrointestinal tract and food availability

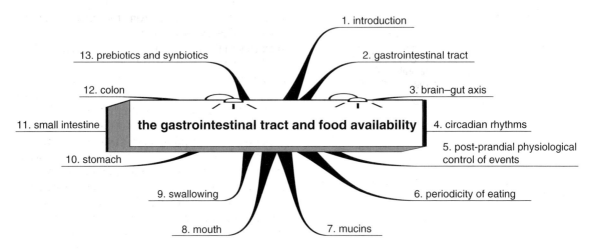

Fig. 24.1 Chapter outline.

INTRODUCTION

The uptake of food is dependent on the total intake and bioavailability, i.e. absorption. No food is of value to the individual until it has been absorbed.

An important function of the intestine is to regulate the intake of minerals that are essential but poisonous in excess. Some essential nutrients are very labile, and consequently there is the potential for nutritional deficiency.

The availability of foods for absorption from the lumen of the intestine (Figure 24.2) is dependent on a number of contributing factors, mucosal absorption, pathological factors altering intestinal absorption and alterations in luminal availability, e.g. interactions between accompanying nutrients within a meal. Other factors that may affect absorption include deficiency of necessary intestinal secretions, enteric bacteria, medicinal drugs and surgical procedures. Partial gastrectomy or gastroenterostomy will decrease gastric emptying time, accelerate absorption and endocrine response, and cause hypoglycaemia, i.e. dumping.

The uptake by the mucosa of various nutrients may depend on the individual's nutritional needs, whereby intestinal absorption may be either partially or totally controlled.

GASTROINTESTINAL TRACT

The gastrointestinal tract is a long length of tubing punctuated by reservoirs (mouth, stomach,

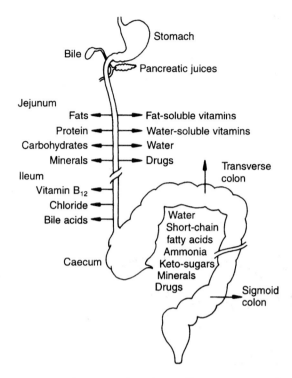

Fig. 24.2 Absorption along the small intestine, stomach, jejunum, ileum and colon.

caecum and rectum) and thickened regions of circular muscle or sphincters (oropharyngeal, lower oesophageal, pyloric, ileocaecal and rectal). Each of these reservoirs and sphincters slows the movement of food and chyle along the gastrointestinal tract, allowing digestion and absorption to take place. The sphincters have a high resting tone and relax under neuronal stimulus. The brainstem controls the basic reflex control of gastrointestinal function, receiving, integrating and sending information to higher brain centres or returning information to the gut.

The tract is lined by mucosa with specialised function in the various sections, i.e. protective, secreting and absorbing.

The control of gastrointestinal secretion is dependent on nervous, endocrine, immune and local factors. These integrate the effects of stimuli arising in the gut lumen and allow co-ordination of gastrointestinal secretion with the presence of food in the gut.

BRAIN–GUT AXIS

Function along the gastrointestinal tract is controlled by complex nervous pathways, with important contributions from the sympathetic and parasympathetic nervous systems. The innervation is intrinsic and extrinsic. The intrinsic nerves are arrayed in plexuses, the most important being the myenteric plexus, which is placed between the gastrointestinal longitudinal and circular muscle coats. The complexity of the myenteric plexuses is to some extent automonous and they act as a rudimentary brain, remote from the central nervous system. The extrinsic nerves connect the enteric plexuses to the central nervous system. All of these enable this long system to behave in a co-ordinated manner. The enteric nervous system controls and co-ordinates gastrointestinal function, motility, secretion, mucosal transport and blood flow, all of which are important for normal digestive processes. The vagal parasympathetic nervous system carries information from the gut to the brainstem, innervating the whole gut except for the terminal (distal) colon. Vagal nerves are believed to be involved in satiety and nausea. Gastrointestinal function works by a series of vagally controlled reflexes, including gastrogastric, enterogastric, hepatopancreatic and gastrocolic reflexes.

The eneteric nerves form three pharmacologically distinct groups: cholinergic parasympathetic, adrenergic sympathetic and non-adrenergic or cholinergic.

CIRCADIAN RHYTHMS

The body is tuned to a day–night rhythm. At the beginning of the day, serum cortisol and blood pressure rise and many people pass stool. Regular meals are eaten during the day, and at the end of the day people go to bed and to sleep, a state that takes up one-third of their life. The circadian rhythm is the cycle of life, which may be 24 h, seasonal or annual. The human steroid 24 h cycle and mood variations with season are examples. The clock for cell proliferation, migration, differentiation and structure in the various organs and tissues of the gastrointestinal tract and pancreas has a genetic basis but is mediated by hormones, e.g. cyclin. These rhythms are not present at birth and are established at weaning, when regular meals replace breast feeding on demand. The rhythms of the oesophagus and rectum are very rapid. The synchrony is different along the intestine, so the DNA synthesis is 6–8 h different along the intestine, as if to co-ordinate with the movement of food. The vulnerability of tissues to carcinogens, therapies and hormones is dependent on the time of day, and reflects tissue rhythms in cell proliferation, apoptosis and metabolism. The enzymes in the brush border of the epithelium also vary over time, influenced by cellular concentrations of specific messenger RNAs (mRNAs). One important circadian control system is the phosphorylation and suppression of action of key control enzymes. The whole system owes its rhythm as much to local peripheral control as to the brain, with its contact with the light/dark cycle.

POST-PRANDIAL PHYSIOLOGICAL CONTROL OF EVENTS ALONG THE GASTROINTESTINAL TRACT

There are three phases of the physiological control of gastric secretion, which also have consequences for other events along the gastrointestinal tract.

- **Cephalic phase**: as a result of the sight, smell and taste of food relayed through the brain the secretory process begins. The mouth waters and gastric and other juices begin to flow.
- **Gastric phase**: this begins once food reaches the stomach and gastric secretion is stimulated by neural reflex actions and liberation of hormones including gastrin. The stretch receptors of the stomach are influencing gastric emptying, along with hormonal control, in part controlled by the pH of the stomach.
- **The intestinal phase** of gastric secretion is inhibitory, but stimulates events further along the intestine.

Digestion and gastrointestinal hormone release

Endocrine cells are distributed along the length of the gastrointestinal tract.

The gut is the body's largest endocrine organ both in size and in the range of peptides produced. Three major groups of peptides are produced:

- acting locally within the gut, affecting gastric, pancreatic and biliary secretion, gut motility and gut mucosal proliferation
- neuroendocrine regulators, e.g. satiety
- extraintestinal action, e.g. influencing postprandial metabolism.

> The endocrine cells of the gut are distinct; they have similar staining properties to the adrenaline-producing chromaffin cells of the adrenal glands and therefore are called enterochromaffin cells. They have granules that are classified (G-, D-, I-, etc.) according to their shape, size, staining properties and number of granules. Endocrine cells are classified as open cells, in which part of the cell surface is in direct contact with the gut lumen, and closed cells, which are completely surrounded by other cells.

Some of the gut hormones are common to other tissues, such as the peripheral and central nervous system, e.g. CCK. These neuroendocrines and neuromodulators influence neurotransmission. They may also act as paracrine agents with effects limited to neighbouring cells. These are often spoken of as regulatory peptides, rather than gastrointestinal hormones, and can be considered in two groups: the gastrin group and the secretin group.

Gastrin group (gastrin and CCK): gastrin increases acid secretion in the fundus of the stomach, and is released by luminal dietary peptides and amino acids in the antrum and duodenum. Gastrin is released after a meal, probably as a result of direct contact of food with the open gastrin cells of the antrum. The extent of the response is dependent on the type of food, particularly how much protein is present. Dietary fat and carbohydrate have little effect on gastrin release. CCK is released by the digestion products of fat and by protein, and stimulates gallbladder contractions and pancreatic enzyme secretion. The best nutrient releasers of CCK are fatty acids of more than nine carbon atoms length. Glucose and amino acids may also be important in CCK release.

Secretin group [secretin, glucagon, glucagon-like peptides (GLPs), gastric inhibitory polypeptides

Sites of action of other gut regulatory peptides

- Pancreatic polypeptide (PP), peptide YY and neuropeptide Y: glucagon and PP exclusively in the pancreas; VIP, the enkephalins and neuropeptide Y are also found in neural tissue
- Gastrin (G-cells): predominantly in the antrum and duodenal mucosa
- CCK and secretin cells (I-cells and S-cells, respectively): in the duodenum and jejunum
- Somatostatin cells (D-cells): in all parts of the gut
- GIP-secreting K-cells: predominantly in the duodenum and jejunum, but also in the antrum and ileum
- M-cells, which secrete motilin: in the antrum, but also in the upper duodenum
- Glucagon-like peptide-secreting cells (L-cells) and neurotensin (N-cells): in the ileum

Pancreatic glucagon

Pancreatic glucagon formed in the pancreas consists of 29 amino acids. In the small intestine the three sequences initiate glucagon-like peptides.

Enteroglucagon, which is homologous to pancreatic glucagon, has an extra 32 amino acids.

Glicentin, which contains the enteroglucagon sequence, has a further 32 amino acid extension at the N-terminal.

- **Motilin**: released during fasting, and is related to specific intestinal contraction patterns, called the migrating motor complex. Motilin is excreted during the fasting period, but may also be involved in increasing gastric emptying.
- **GLPs** or pancreatic glucagon: present in the intestine. The original gene product gives three sequences and the enzymatic processes produce three different molecular forms.

(GIPs) and vasoactive intestinal polypeptide (VIP)]: secretin is released by acid and results in the flow of water and bicarbonate from the pancreas. Somatostatin is released postprandially and has an inhibitory effect on the secretion of growth hormone, insulin and glucagon. Neurotensin is released by fats and is important in the control of motility. GIP is released by sugars and some amino acids, and stimulates insulin secretion in the pancreas.

- **Secretin**: released by acid contact with the duodenal mucosa and causes bicarbonate secretion by the pancreas. Secretin also releases insulin, but glucose within the duodenum does not have any effect on secretin levels.
- **Somatostatin**: present in the cell walls of neurones of the central and peripheral nervous system, and in endocrine cells of the pancreas and gut. Its effect is largely inhibitory and it has an extremely short half-life. The somatostatin-containing endocrine cells are closely associated with the target cells, with effects on gastric acid secretion, pancreatic endocrine and exocrine secretion, and possibly gut motility. Somatostatin may inhibit amino acid and glucose absorption.
- **Neurotensin**: delays gastric emptying time.
- **GIP**: has an inhibitory effect on acid secretion and also increases insulin secretion under hyperglycaemic conditions.

PERIODICITY OF EATING

The frequency at which individuals eat has long been a topic of discussion, the grazer contrasting with the one-meal-a-day eater. In the one situation the body never recovers from one metabolic load and event before another arrives and in the other the body starts afresh after many hours. The usual advice in the Western world is three square meals a day, but this varies from two to nine. The range is partly cultural and religious and partly of necessity, e.g. a very physically active person needs to eat frequently, whereas a hunter is dependent on the availability of food. The timing of main meals varies from early to very late evening. The social importance of a meal varies and therefore times when everyone can gather together are important.

In contrast to circadian rhythms, ultradian rhythms reflect lifestyle and internal influences, and include opportunities to eat, work patterns and night shifts.

The hormonal and metabolic responses to small amounts of food eaten slowly are less than those to large amounts eaten quickly, although the type of meal and the physical nature of the food may be important.

MUCINS

The whole length of the gastrointestinal tract, from mouth to anus, is protected and lubricated by mucins produced by secretory glands. Mucins are high molecular weight glycoproteins with carbohydrate sugars attached by O-glycosidic linkages to serine or threonine. Secretory mucins form long polymers by end-to-end disulfide bonding, producing molecules that are very viscous in solution. The mucins are a product of distinct genes with considerable diversity in their structure of protein backbone and carbohydrate side-chains. There are nine mucin genes, *MUC1, 2, 3, 4, 5AC, 5B, 6, 7*, and *8* which, with the exception of *MUC7* and *MUC8*, are expressed at variable times in the development of the foetus. Mucins, except for *MUC7*, may be classified into membrane associated (e.g. *MUC1*) and secreted (gel-forming *MUC2* and *MUC5*). *MUC5* may protect the stomach against hydrochloric acid and peptic digestion. *MUC2* is found in the intestine and colon.

MOUTH

The mouth phase of food degradation has two components, mechanical food grinding by the teeth and enzyme digestion. The breakdown of the food into small particles is accompanied by the secretion of saliva, which lubricates the food and allows the entrance of salivary amylase to the bolus, to commence the digestion of starches.

SWALLOWING

Swallowing is a complicated process requiring the co-ordinated contraction of striated voluntary muscles in the pharynx and oesophagus. A brainstem swallowing centre is involved. Once swallowing begins with the entry of food into the hypopharynx, the continuous process unfolds until the food is moved by contractions down the oesophagus and through the relaxed lower oesophageal sphincter into the stomach. The stages of the process are as follows:

1. Closure of the nasopharynx and raising of the soft palate.
2. Upper oesophageal sphincter opening.
3. Laryngeal closure to prevent inhalation of food.
4. Tongue pushing food back and down the throat.
5. Pharyngeal clearing.

The process of converting the oropharynx from a respiratory to a swallowing pathway, by opening the inlet to the oesophagus and sealing the inlet to the larynx, lasts for less than 1 s.

Closure of the sphincter prevents the reflux of food back up the oesophagus. Vomiting and return of gas, of which there is a great deal swallowed during eating, are enabled by relaxation of the sphincter.

STOMACH

Gastric mucosa

The stomach is a reservoir that stores food. The rate of gastric emptying will influence the rate of release of food from the stomach to the small intestine for digestion and absorption. The gastric mucosa is maintained by a multitude of physical, chemical and physiological factors which join to form the gastric mucosal barrier and prevent hydrogen ions entering the tissues at quantities that produce injury. The integrity of the gastric mucosa exposed to the acid contents of the stomach is significantly dependent on the 100–400-μm-thick glycoprotein mucous barrier. The mucoprotein intrinsic factor is essential for vitamin B_{12} absorption. Acid secretions may pass in narrow channels through the mucous to the stomach lumen. The vagus nerve is involved in the resistance to injury and assisting repair.

Food ingestion results in an increase in heart rate, blood flow and metabolic rate. The physical nature of the meal, liquid or solid, affects the physiological response to food ingestion. Nutrient absorption may be slowed, with a consequent modulation in nutrient uptake, resulting in a reduction in plasma concentrations followed by a modified endocrine response and a possible reduction in the renal excretion of nutrient.

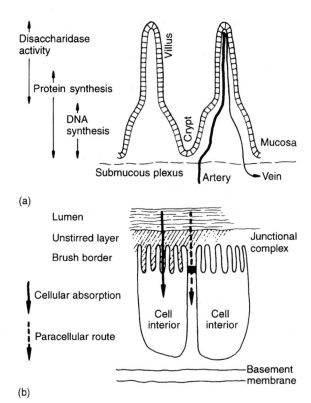

Fig. 24.3 The intestinal mucosa and enterocytes. (a) The villus and crypt of the small intestinal mucosa showing crypt, villus, blood supply, submucous plexus and enzymatic activity along the villus from DNA to disaccharidase activity. (b) Enterocyte and absorption showing the unstirred layer, brush border and basement membrane. There are two forms of absorption: cellular and paracellular through the functional complex.

SMALL INTESTINE

The small intestine is divided into the jejunum and ileum, a separation that partly reflects the absorptive capacity of the region.

Enterocytes

The small intestine has been described as an 'active interface' between the external environment and the blood and lymph, which distributes the absorbed materials for the metabolic needs of the body. The epithelial cells of the small intestine have

Enterocytes

The life of an enterocyte is approximately 48 h. Various constituents of food may alter enterocytes by:

- changes in the number of functional enterocytes
- changes in the carrier, enzymatic or metabolic process of the enterocytes
- changes in the rate of maturation or function in the enterocytes as they move from the crypts to the extrusion zone at the villus tip.

Transfer across the enterocyte from the lumen involves:

- movement from the bulk phase across the 'unstirred layer' to the enterocyte surface
- movement across the brush border membrane and across the cytoplasm
- removal to the bloodstream through the basolateral membrane.

three major functions: digestion, absorption and secretion. The enterocytes, that is the surface cells, are constantly being lost into the lumen from the tips of the villi and replaced (Figure 24.3).

Luminal factors, particularly nutrients and secretion, are necessary to maintain normal small intestinal enterocyte numbers. During starvation there is a progressive decrease in small intestinal enterocyte population, mucosal mass, enterocyte column number and villus height, particularly in the jejunum. The absorptive capacity of the small bowel is in part dependent on the number of enterocytes present. The maximum rate of absorption (J_{max} per unit length) is affected by the number of enterocytes.

The development of the intestinal mucosa and enzyme systems has been better studied in animals than in humans. The description given here is derived from such animal work in the expectation that the principles described will not be remote from what happens in humans.

Enterocytes produced in intestinal crypts express a genetically determined programme as they progress along the crypt. This can be affected by diet. Increasing intake or changing the protein content of the diet may alter enterocyte cell surface structure, as well as affecting crypt proliferation. Enterocytes change their structure and ability to digest and absorb nutrients during maturation. The lumenal chyme contains polyamines (putrescine, spermidine and spermine) that stimulate growth when absorbed by enterocytes.

Slowing enterocyte migration rates to less than 6 μm/h increases maximal microvillus length. Enzymatic activity increases rapidly as the enterocytes migrate over the lower parts of villi, activity declining as the tip is approached. Amino acid transport occurs only in the upper regions of villi, in keeping with dietary constituents affecting the expression of single or multiple genes at different stages of enterocyte development.

Weaning
As the child changes from a milk diet to a weaning and then an adult diet with a reduced lactose content, the enzymatic activity of the brush border membrane changes. Lactase activity, which is maximum at birth and during suckling, decreases to low adult levels with weaning; and sucrase activity, which is low at birth, begins to increase. These changes are driven by gene expression and regulated by dietary and hormonal activity.

Adult
To some extent the hydrolase activity of the intestinal brush border reflects the constituents of the diet.

Enteric absorption

The lipid layer of a cell membrane acts as a container that enables the cell to separate its internal environment from the surrounding fluids. This requires that the cell surfaces transport molecules into and out of the cells. The cells of the enteric border are particularly important in controlling the intake of molecules from the intestinal lumen and moving these molecules, either intact or modified, into the bloodstream or lymphatic system. Water-soluble nutrients of low molecular weight may pass through the intestinal epithelium by two major routes, paracellular and transcellular. Paracellular transport is mostly if not entirely through the highly permeable, tight junctions joining the brush border membranes of adjacent absorptive cells. This mechanism is by simple diffusion through pores or aqueous canals, the rate of transport being a function of concentration gradient. Paracellular trans-

port is mediated by solvent drag; solutes dissolved in the bulk flow of solvent are carried through the transepithelial channels. This system transports at a rate proportional to the concentration of the solution and to the rate of solvent flow, but becomes less effective as the radius of the solute molecules approaches that of the channel.

The transcellular route involves entry across the brush border membrane of the absorptive cells. In the case of amino acids entry is by translocation through the cytosol of the cell interior, by diffusion, and exit through basolateral membranes, by facilitated diffusion. There are two main methods of transport across the cell membrane (Figure 24.4):

- simple diffusion through minute aqueous canals in a predominantly lipid and protein cell membrane, although amino acids may diffuse through the lipid of a membrane. If the molecule is uncharged then the direction of flow is concentration dependent; if it is charged then an additional influence is the electrochemical gradient. Facilitated diffusion is enhanced diffusion, not requiring metabolic energy, and is dependent on a concentration gradient; the system can be fully loaded, i.e. it is saturable and affected by competitive inhibition. Simple and facilitated diffusion are *passive transport systems*.
- Mediated transport specific for each structurally related substance, e.g. amino acids across the membrane. Such a transport system involves a *specific carrier*.

Active transport transfers a substrate across a membrane against an electrochemical gradient driven by metabolic energy. Primary transport systems are directly dependent on metabolic energy, whereas secondary active transport is coupled to the re-entry of sodium across the brush border membrane. The extrusion of Na^+ across the membrane is energy dependent. When the transport of a substrate is linked to a metabolic energy supply, by a chain that involves transport of two ions, this is called *tertiary active transport*.

Facilitated and simple diffusion moves in one direction down a concentration differential, whereas active transport occurs in both directions.

Counter-transport occurs when a substance being transported in one direction accelerates the transport of another in the opposite direction.

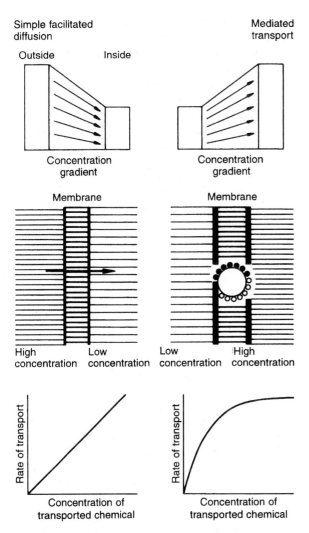

Fig. 24.4 Simple facilitated diffusion and mediated transport. Simple facilitated diffusion passes down a concentration gradient and is concentration dependent. Mediated transport passes up a concentration gradient and is dependent on carrier systems, which can become saturated.

Many active transport systems including amino acids, monosaccharides and many other substances passing across the brush border membrane are coupled to the passive re-entry of Na^+ into the absorptive cell down an electrochemical gradient. Active transport requires transport proteins, which belong to two categories. *Channel proteins* form hydrophilic pores, which allow a suitable solute, usually an ion, to pass along the channel.

V_{max} and J_{max}

Using Michaelis–Menten saturation kinetics it is possible to measure 'apparent' K_m and V_{max}:

$$v = \frac{V\,[S]}{K_m\,[S]}$$

where v is the velocity of transport, the maximal velocity of transport is V_{max}, [S] is the substrate concentration and K_m is the substrate concentration at which the velocity of transport is half-maximal. K_m is an inverse measure of apparent affinity for transport, so a high value means a low affinity for transport and vice versa. This relationship does not mean that an enzyme system is involved, only that a receptor system is involved that can be saturated.

Sometimes in the intestine the term Lax is used instead of V_{max}. Apparent K_m is an indicator of the affinity of the binding mechanism between the nutrient and its receptor carrier mechanism. The Lax is the transport equivalent of the maximum velocity of the enzymes. This allows comparison of the different transport mechanisms.

'Apparent K_m' = 'real K_{max}' + $J_{max}\,d/D$, where d is the thickness of the unstirred layer and D is the diffusion coefficient of the solution being transferred.

The active transport process also requires *carrier proteins*, which bind the substance being transported and undergo conformational change in order to cross the membrane. The activity of the carrier protein is geared to an energy production process, e.g. adenosine triphosphate (ATP) hydrolysis or an ion gradient. Carrier proteins have substrate-specific binding sites and follow Michaelis–Menten kinetics.

The unstirred layer, i.e. the structured water layers close to the mucosal surface, and the glycocalyx or fuzzy coat of the microvilli influence the saturation kinetics and passive permeability coefficients. The unstirred layer is a rate-limiting step for the diffusion of solutes from the luminal bulk to the surface of enterocytes through which solutes must diffuse to reach the surface. This retards the rate of diffusion towards and away from the surface. In the intestine the unstirred layer has an important role in dictating the absorption rate. There is no definite thickness of this boundary, but it varies from 100–300 μm to 400–650 μm depending on conditions and measurement. The effect of the unstirred layer is to reduce the concentration of a solute at the membrane surface relative to the luminal concentration, thus reducing the absorption rate. The rate of movement across this unstirred layer and reaching the intestinal mucosa influence the rate of absorption.

The carrier-mediated systems consist of:

- **uniport**: simple transport from one side of the membrane to the other
- **coupled transporters**: transport of one solute is dependent on the transport of a second solute. *Symport* is transport of both solutes in same direction; *antiport* is transport in opposite directions. An example of an antiport is the membrane Na^+/K^+ pump system; sodium out of and potassium into the cell.

Effect of nutrient interactions on bioavailability

Nutrients may interact both chemically and physically to increase or decrease bioavailability (Figure 24.5).

The underlying mechanism between these seemingly unrelated enhancements and inhibitions of absorption is water solubility. Insoluble calcium salts, e.g. calcium phytate, and fatty acids are not absorbed. If a trace mineral, e.g. zinc or magnesium, is bound to phytic acid then calcium can displace the trace element, which can then be absorbed, particularly if the latter is in the form of a soluble, readily absorbable amino acid salt.

Cooking may modify nutrient absorption; raw starch is poorly digested by amylase but during cooking starch granules are disrupted and become readily digested. Retrograde starch (see chapter 13), present in bread, potatoes and puddings, when stored in the cold after cooking is not readily hydrolysed by pancreatic amylase in the small intestine. This retrogradation is partially reversed by heating. Protein may have a reduced absorption efficiency after cooking through the formation of Maillard reaction products.

After absorption some substances are metabolised on first contact with tissues, e.g. liver or enteric mucosal cells. This is called the *first-pass metabolism*. Such metabolism of substances during absorption is important; an example is the immuno-

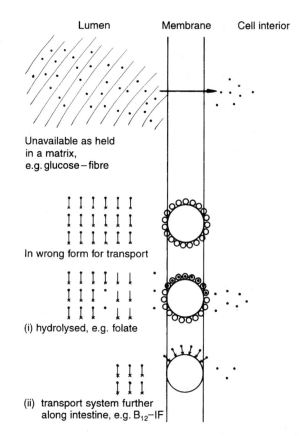

Fig. 24.5   Interaction between nutrients and absorption across the intestinal cell membrane.

suppressant drug cyclosporin, the efficacy of which is marred by poor and unpredictable bioavailability. This drug, and possibly erythromycin, lignocaine and oestrogen, may be metabolised by the enzyme system P450IIIA, which is found in the liver and also in enterocytes.

Competition for nutrients

Small-intestinal bacterial colonisation may develop in a surgically formed stagnant loop or in jejunal diverticulosis. There is nutrient competition between host and bacteria for vitamins, iron, proteins, fats and carbohydrates.

The most dangerous inhibitor of absorption is *Cholera vibrio*, the enterotoxin of which stimulates a cyclic adenosine monophosphate (cAMP)-

mediated secretory process with profound water loss.

Drugs may cause malabsorption and diarrhoea, e.g. neomycin precipitates bile acids, so that insufficient bile acids are available to reach a critical micelle concentration and steatorrhoea (fat malabsorption) results.

Specific amylase blockers in beans slow the hydrolysis of amylose and retard the absorption of starch breakdown products.

Factors affecting bioavailability

The complexing of vitamin B_{12} with intrinsic factor allows the vitamin to be absorbed from the ileum. In contrast, niacin is held in cereals in a bound form that is not absorbed unless released by dilute alkali or roasting, a factor in the development of pellagra (vitamin B_6 deficiency). Biotin is bound to avidin, a protein in raw eggs that renders biotin unavailable for absorption. The binding of calcium to oxalate and phytate reduces calcium absorption, because the human intestinal tract mucosa contains no phytase. Yeast cells contain phytase, which hydrolyses phytic acid during the leavening of dough. Calcium absorption is reduced in populations that habitually eat unleavened bread. Dietary fibre, a cation-exchange binder, may reduce mineral absorption.

Intestinal zinc absorption is reduced by cadmium, copper, calcium, ferrous iron, phytate and proteins that have undergone Maillard reactions. Zinc absorption is, however, increased by methionine, histidine, cysteine, citrate and picolinic acid.

Nutrient interactions may affect nutrient absorption. Alcohol may reduce thiamin absorption, particularly if there is coincidental folate deficiency. Intestinal calcium absorption is increased by lactose, unsaturated fatty acids, lysine, arginine and glucose polymers. Iron in the form of haem is readily taken up by the mucosal cells. Haem itself is poorly soluble in water, but when haemoglobin is digested the resultant peptides render the haem more soluble. Non-haem iron is absorbed by a separate transport system in an ionic form. Absorption is increased by a coincidental presence of meat, fish and vitamin C, and is inhibited by phytate and tannin. Selenium is better absorbed as the selenomethionine form than as sodium selenite.

COLON

The colonic epithelium presents a barrier protecting the body from a mass of molecules of varying molecular weight generated by the colonic bacteria. Some are useful to the body, e.g. bile acids, water and short-chain fatty acids, whereas others are toxic or potentially toxic and are not absorbed.

The crypt is the basic structure of the colonic mucosa and is involved in secretion and absorption. Extracellular signals, e.g. acetylcholine and vitamin D, are involved in the mobilisation of intracellular calcium, secretion of chloride, mucus secretion and increased cell turnover. Bicarbonate and chloride secretion in the colon are closely linked.

The right side of the colon is a fermenter of unabsorbed molecules that either originated from the diet, have been secreted in bile or by the intestine, or are sloughed off cells. The colon is a conserving organ, containing a large bacterial mass. The bacteria modify the enterohepatic circulation of chemicals secreted in bile, e.g. bile acids, hormones and drugs. The caecal bacterial breakdown of proteins is followed by the absorption of amino acid derivatives. Hydrogen, methane and other gases are also produced from fibre. Absorption from the colon is somewhat specific. Colonic bacteria are able to synthesise vitamin K_2 (multiprenylmenaquinones) and vitamin B_{12}, which are not absorbed. The faeces from subjects with pernicious anaemia contain vitamin B_{12} that would have been more than sufficient for their needs but is unavailable for absorption. The relatively modest large-bowel absorption of polar molecules, e.g. hormones, toxic bacterial products and drugs, is due to small colonic pores. Changes in colonic pore permeability can be induced by drugs and disease, e.g. colitis. Fatty acids and dihydroxy bile acids increase permeability and, pore size allowing, for example, oxalic acid to be absorbed.

Butyrate, a short-chain fatty acid derived from the bacterial degradation of dietary fibre, is an important fuel for colonic cells, induces cell arrest and apoptosis and reduces gut mucosal inflammation. Butyrate modulates the transcription expression of multiple enzymes. This includes effects on nuclear proteins, such as the inhibition of histone through deacetylase, phosphorylation and methylation processes. Butyrate may also act on the membrane signalling system by interactions with G proteins.

The unabsorbed material, along with water, bacteria and the residue of fibre, is lost from the body as faeces. Dietary fibre is the major dictate of faecal weight, but there are other influences, including mood and the menstrual cycle.

PREBIOTICS AND SYNBIOTICS

Functional foods are foods containing components that will affect functions in the body to give positive cellular and physiological effects. One area where this idea has been of interest is in the colon.

Prebiotics are non-digestible food ingredients that benefit the host by selectively stimulating the growth of one or more of a limited number of health-promoting bacteria in the colon.

An example of a prebiotic is chicory fructan (inulins and enzymatic hydrolysate oligofructans), a β-(2-1)-fructo-oligosaccharide, which has the potential to improve calcium availability and lipid metabolism.

A probiotic is a bacterium, e.g. *Lactobacillus* or *Bifidobacterium*.

A synbiotic is a product that is both a probiotic and a prebiotic combined in a single product. This could be a mixture of a probiotic, i.e. a bacteria normally present in the colon, a bifidobacterium and a chicory fructan.

KEY POINTS

1. In the gastric mucosa and small intestine the epithelial cells of the small intestine have three major functions: digestion, absorption and secretion. This process is under the control of hormones, the intestinal nervous network, and the stomach and intestinal contents.
2. The small intestinal enterocytes are constantly being lost into the lumen from the tips of the villi and are replaced every 48 h.
3. Absorption from the lumen involves movement from the bulk phase across the 'unstirred layer' to the enterocyte surface, movement across the brush border membrane, movement across the

cytoplasm, and removal to the bloodstream through the basolateral membrane.
4. Water-soluble nutrients of low molecular weight pass through the intestinal epithelium by two major routes, paracellular and transcellular. Paracellular transport is through highly permeable tight junctions joining the brush border membranes; the rate of transport depends on concentration gradient and solvent drag. The transcellular route is across the brush border membrane of the absorptive cells, followed by crossing the cytosol of the cell interior by diffusion and exit through basolateral membranes by facilitated diffusion.
5. There are two main methods of transport across the cell membrane: (i) simple and facilitated diffusion, which are passive transport systems; and (ii) mediated transport, which is specific for each structurally related substance, e.g. amino acid, across the membrane.
6. The availability of foods for absorption from the intestinal lumen depends on a number of contributing factors, mucosal absorption, pathological factors altering intestinal absorption and alterations in luminal availability, e.g. interactions between accompanying nutrients within a meal. Deficiency of necessary intestinal secretions and enteric bacteria, medicinal drugs and surgical procedures may also affect absorption.
7. The colon is a conserving organ containing a large bacterial mass.
8. Movement along and absorption from the gastrointestinal tract are dictated in part by local hormones.

THINKING POINT

The anatomical triad of 'in the lumen, in the wall and outside the wall' of the gut is helpful in understanding what is happening along the gastrointestinal tract.

NEED TO UNDERSTAND

The process of digestion and absorption is one in which an attractively laid out meal is eaten, reduced in mass by chewing and grinding in the stomach and reduced in molecular weight by digestion. The resultant bolus is released from the stomach to be digested and then absorbed. This process is controlled by the hormonal and nervous system of the gastrointestinal tract. The colon makes final adjustments to the absorption of nutrients. Finally, the residue of the meal is voided as faeces made of unabsorbed food and biliary and intestinal secretions, water and bacteria.

FURTHER READING

Aziz, Q. and Thompson, D.G. (1998) Brain–gut axis in health and disease. *Gastroenterology*, **114**, 559–78.

Borgnia, M., Nielsen, S., Engel, A. and Agre, P. (1999) Cellular and molecular biology of the aquaporin channels. *Annual Review of Biochemistry*, **68**, 425–58.

Dawson, D. (ed.) (1995) Intestinal mucins. *Annual Review of Physiology*, **57**, 547–658.

Dockray, G.J. (ed.) (1996) Regulation of gastrointestinal secretion: symposium. *Proceedings of the Nutrition Society*, **55**, 247–317.

Gilbney, M.J., Wolever, T.M.S. and Frayn, K.N. (1997) Periodicity of eating and human health. *British Journal of Nutrition*, **77**, (Suppl. 1), S1–128.

Habas, M.E. and Macdonald, I.A. (1998) Metabolic and cardiovascular responses to liquid and solid test meals. *British Journal of nutrition*, **79**, 241–7.

Hasler, C.M. (1998) Prebiotics and synbiotics: concepts and nutritional properties. *British Journal of Nutrition*, **80**, S195–233.

Hodin, R. (2000) Maintaining gut homeostasis: the butyrate–NF-κB connection. *Gastroenterology*, **118**, 798–801.

Holzer, P. (1998) Neural emergency system in the stomach. *Gastroenterology*, **114**, 823–39.

Johnson, L.R., Alpers, D.H., Christensen, J. *et al.* (1994) *Physiology of the Gastrointestinal Tract*. Raven Press, New York.

Kahrilas, P.J., Lin, S., Chen, J. and Logemann, J. (1996) Oropharyngeal accommodation to swallow volume. *Gastroenterology*, **111**, 297–306.

Kim, Y.S. and Gum, J.R. (1995) Diversity of mucin genes, structure, function and expression, *Gastroenterology*. **109**, 999–1013.

McLaughlin, J., Luca, G., Jones, M.N. *et al.* (1999) Fatty acid chain length determines cholecystokin secretion and effect on human gastric motility. *Gastroenterlogy*, **116**, 46–53.

Reuss, L. (ed.) (1998) Gastrointestinal physiology. *Annual Review of Physiology*, **60**, 105–78.

Roediger, W.E.W. and Babidge, W. (1997) Human colonocyte detoxification. *Gut*, **41**, 731–4.

Scheving, L.A. (2000) Biological clocks and the digestive system. *Gastroenterology*, **119**, 536–49.

Seal, C.J. and Puigserver, A. (1996) Regulation of gastrointestinal secretion. *Proceedings of the Nutrition Society*, **55**, 247–317.

Traber, P.G. and Silberg, D.G. (1996) Intestine-specific gene transcription. *Annual Review of Physiology*, **58**, 275–98.

Vlitos, A.L.P. and Davies, G.J. (1996) Bowel function, food intake and the menstrual cycle. *Nutrition Research Review*, **9**, 111–34.

25

Carbohydrate digestion and absorption

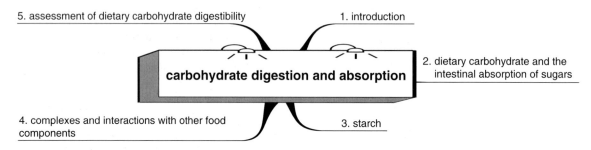

Fig. 25.1 Chapter outline.

INTRODUCTION

Dietary carbohydrate accounts for approximately half of the energy intake in the average Western diet. Some 60% of the carbohydrate is in the form of starch and glycogen; sucrose and lactose may contribute 30% and 10%, respectively. There may also be glucose and fructose in certain foods. Raffinose and stacchyose are present in small amounts in beans and are not absorbed in the upper intestine but are fermented in the colon. The polysaccharides are digested by salivary and pancreatic amylase in the lumen of the intestine. Starch digestion is intraluminal. There is further hydrolysis of the glucosyl oligosaccharides by the digestive, absorptive brush border enterocytes.

The osmolarity of a sugar solution influences gastric emptying and intestinal transit time. The higher the osmolarity the slower the gastric emptying time. Other determinants of gastric emptying include duodenal pH, fat and caloric intake, viscosity, the solid content of the meal and whether the carbohydrate is eaten as a monosaccharide or a disaccharide. Unabsorbed sugar results in an accumulation of fluid within the intestine and hence a shortened transit time.

DIETARY CARBOHYDRATE AND THE INTESTINAL ABSORPTION OF SUGARS

Oligosaccharides (glucose, galactose and fructose) are in general absorbed and metabolised after hydrolysis into the basic monosaccharides at the cell epithelial surface. Small amounts of larger molecular weight sugars may pass through the epithelial barrier. The enzymatic breakdown, with the exception of the hydrolysis of lactose, is extremely efficient. Sugar digestion and absorption is considerably influenced by the chemistry of the ingested sugar. Fructose as a constituent of sucrose is very readily absorbed, whereas fructose alone as the monosaccharide is not. Glucose may

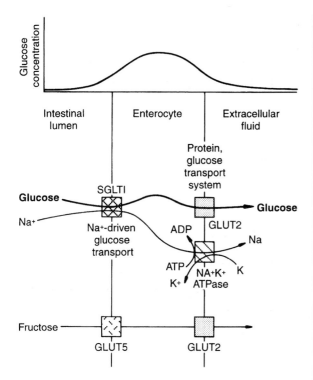

Fig. 25.2 Glucose absorption across the enterocyte. Glucose passes from the intestinal lumen into the interior of the enterocyte by a Na^+-driven glucose transport system (SGLTI). Glucose passes across the enterocyte and into the interior of the body across the basement membrane along a concentration gradient of facilitated diffusion and a protein glucose carrier system (GLUT2). Sodium passes into the interior of the body through a Na^+ gradient generated by Na^+/K^+-ATPase in the basal membrane of the enterocyte. Fructose is transported across the cell down a concentration gradient across the brush border (GLUT5 brush border fructose transporter). GLUT2 transports fructose across the basement membrane. Galactose is transported by the same transport system as glucose.

enhance fructose absorption by influencing the intestinal transport system or by stimulating water absorption.

Monosaccharide absorption

Monosaccharides pass across the epithelial lining of the small intestine by three processes: simple diffusion, facilitated diffusion and active transport.

Monosaccharides move along a concentration gradient by simple diffusion to the surface of the enterocyte, passing through the unstirred layer

Na$^+$ active hexose cotransporter SGLT1 system

This cotransporter has two binding sites, one for the hexose and the other for the Na^+ ion. The Na^+ ion bound to the cotransporter increases the affinity of the hexose site for glucose and galactose. On the inside of the enterocyte the Na^+ and the hexose diffuse into the cell. The cotransporter then undertakes another transfer cycle. When the glucose cotransporter transfers Na^+ ions across the brush border an electrical potential difference is created across the membrane, the enterocyte and the intestinal wall. This is electrogenic, i.e. potential producing, or rheogenic, i.e. current producing. The production of electrical activity allows the measurement of absorption across the brush border and intestinal wall. These transfer potentials follow Michaelis–Menten kinetics and can be characterised by apparent K_m. Electrical measurements are a measure of hexose kinetics. There may be more than one carrier in a membrane. The basolateral membrane is a barrier to free movement of hexoses in and out of the enterocyte. Glucose is transported from the cell to the blood by the unrelated GLUT2 transporter.

(Figure 25.2). The rate of diffusion and therefore rate of arrival of the nutrient at the brush border may affect absorption kinetics and confine the products of hydrolysis to the cell surface.

The epithelial lining of the small intestine is crossed by pores, of small radius (< 6 Å) and large radius (~ 50–60 Å). The pore system is localised in different parts of the epithelium, the larger pores being found in the crypts and the smaller at the tips. The absorbing passive transport of the villus contains the small pores, where monosaccharides pass through by solvent drag. Increased absorption is associated with an increase in the number of small pores. The water-soluble monosaccharides cross the lipid brush border membrane slowly and inefficiently. The Na^+ active transfer of hexoses has a specific membrane carrier system.

Hexoses move out of the cell by diffusion and a facilitated transfer process, which is Na^+ independent.

The transport systems for the absorption of sugars are found throughout biology, being similar in fish and humans. These are found in both the intestine and kidneys. Three major systems are known (Figure 25.2):

- brush border Na^+/glucose cotransporter (SGLT1)
- brush border fructose transporter (GLUT5)
- basolateral facilitated sugar transporter (GLUT2).

These are controlled by two gene families that govern a transporter system found in yeasts, plants and mammals. This transporter family includes 12 transmembrane transporters for a variety of sugars and organic acids. The activity and expression of SGLT1 are maintained by the presence of lumenal nutrients and decline in their absence.

The activity of SGLT1 is the basis of oral rehydration therapy for cholera. In the diarrhoea of cholera, a series of enterotoxins is released by the *Vibrio cholerae* organism, which initiate a loss of water from the intestinal cell, causing a secretory diarrhoea. An enterotoxin B subunit adheres to specific receptors on the cell surface and an A subunit enters the cell and permanently activates adenylate cyclase, resulting in chloride, sodium and then water loss in large amounts. This continues until the cell is sloughed off in the usual turnover of cells. This very serious and life-threatening condition can be treated by oral rehydration therapy, using a mixture of water with salt and carbohydrate added in equal amounts. The carbohydrate as sugar, or even starch, increases salt absorption and hence water absorption across the intestinal brush border.

In humans fructose transport is neither active nor dependent on sodium and is concentration dependent. The tranporter system is GLUT5.

Disaccharide absorption

The brush border disaccharidases hydrolyse maltose, sucrose and lactose to their constituent monosaccharides glucose, galactose and fructose. The rate of absorption of these monosaccharide products is the same as if they were monosaccharide solutions. However, there is a kinetic advantage to hexoses being liberated from disaccharides, leading to an enhanced absorption rate over that for free hexoses from the lumen. The transport mechanism for glucose, produced by sucrose hydrolysis,

Disaccharidases

The disaccharidases are all large protein heterodimers or single subunits, anchored with transmembrane domains, with most of the protein protruding into the intestinal lumen. These oligosaccharidases are synthesised as larger, glycosylated, precursor enzyme proteins. They pass to the apical membranes and are cleaved into active enzymes by the pancreatic enzymes. Large oligosaccharidases are removed from the enterocyte apical surface by pancreatic enzymes or by membrane shedding.

is Na^+ independent. The amount of substrate increases the activity of the disaccharidase in the brush border and even its specific activity. A high dietary intake of sucrose or fructose, but not glucose, increases sucrase and maltase but not lactase activity. Lactase activity does not appear to be regulated by lactose. The monosaccharides released by disaccharide hydrolysis act as inhibitors of the disaccharidases. The greater the amount of monosaccharide formed, the greater will be the inhibition of the carbohydrase and reduction of activity, i.e. a local negative feedback system.

The brush border enzymes, except for sucrase and isomaltase which hydrolyse both sucrose and maltose, are specific for specific glycoside linkages. Brush border enzymes are specific for α-1–4, α-1–6 and β-1–4 linkages.

Lactose

Lactose is split by the brush border enzyme lactase. Lactase is found in the small intestine in decreasing amounts along the intestine and in increasing amounts from the crypt to the apex of the villus. This is not an inducible enzyme. Surface hydrolysis appears to be rate limiting in rate of absorption of lactose. Both of the constituent sugars in lactose, galactose and glucose, are absorbed by active transport.

Lactase biosynthesis differs from other brush border hydrolases by initially being formed as a large precursor, which is cleaved intracellularly. Lactase is processed intracellularly and rapidly to a mature 160 kDa enzyme. Complex glycosylation of the large precursor occurs before proteolytic cleavage. The lactase is anchored to the brush border membrane by a hydrophobic segment of its protein structure. The regulation of lactase activity varies with species and race in humans.

Foetal intestinal lactase develops late in gestation and only achieves maximal activity at birth. Premature infants at 29–38 weeks have reduced lactase activities, whereas other intestinal carbohydrases achieve adult concentrations by the time of birth. Lactase levels remain constant during the suckling period in mammals, but decline after weaning, between the ages of 2 years and puberty. The jejunal brush border enzymatic activity decreases with age, whereas ileal activity increases.

Primary adult lactase deficiency is extremely common and is in the order of 87% in China, 75% in Greece, 100% in Japan, 100% in Thailand, 100% in Black Africans, 90% in South American Indians and 73% in Black Americans. This is in contrast to the Caucasian races, with 3% in Denmark, 5% in England, 16% in Finland, 20% in northern France, 40% in southern France, 50% in northern Italy, 70% in southern Italy and 3% in Sweden. The contrast between White and Aboriginal Australian primary lactase deficiency is evident: 5% in the European stock and 70% in the Aboriginal stock. The persistence of lactose absorption is an autosomal dominant characteristic. Lactase deficiency is inherited as a single autosomal recessive gene which in the homozygous state suppresses the synthesis of intestinal lactase. The presence of lactase along both the villus and the intestine is paralleled by the expression of lactase gene messenger RNA transcripts. Transcription of lactase gene is activated during enterocyte differentiation. A nuclear protein, NF-LPH1, recognises and binds to a short nucleotide sequence upstream of the transcriptional start site. There is an interaction with Cdx2, a homeodomain protein involved in regulating intestinal development and differentiation.

Similarly, congenital sucrase–isomaltase deficiency is inherited as an autosomal recessive defect. Heterozygotes have an enzyme capability intermediate between total inactivity and individuals with full activity. They may also have sucrase intolerance. The native people of the Arctic (Inuits or Eskimos) have the highest frequency of congenital sucrase–isomaltase deficiency, at 10% of the population.

Sucrose
Sucrose is absorbed by the brush border of the small intestine and is hydrolysed to glucose and fructose by sucrase. This is an inducible enzyme, dependent on the intake of sucrose. Fructose is absorbed by a facilitated diffusion mechanism and cannot be absorbed against a concentration gradient. It is absorbed at an appreciably slower rate than glucose.

Trehalase is the β-galactosidase enzyme that hydrolyses the disaccharide (two glucose molecules) in mushrooms. This was of little interest until trehalose was added to dried foods to increase quality during dehydration. Trehalose is important in the drying process of creatures that have to survive desiccation by replacing the water around proteins and membranes. In this way considerable dehydration is survived. Trehalase deficiency is found in 8% of native Greenlanders.

Sugar alcohols

Maltitol, isomaltol and lactitol, which are disaccharide sugar alcohols, are only partially hydrolysed in the small intestine. The absorption of the monosaccharide sugar alcohols xylitol, sorbitol and mannitol is by a passive diffusion process and they are absorbed less efficiently than glucose.

Vitamin C is absorbed by two transporters, SVCT1, and SVCT2, the former being the predominant transporter in the intestine. Large doses of ascorbic acid are associated with decreased transporter expression and consequent ascorbic acid absorption of significance for high ascorbic acid ingestion.

Oligosaccharides

The oligosaccharides raffinose and stacchyose are not hydrolysed and are absorbed in the large intestine after fermentation.

STARCH

The plant of origin and the chemistry of the starch digested determine the digestion of starches. Starch consists of two polysaccharides: (i) the linear 1–4-linked α-D-glucose (amylose); and (ii) the highly branched amylopectin with α-1–4 and α-1–6

Table 25.1 Classification of starch in foods by the ease of hydrolysis by amylase

Physical form of starch in food	Examples of food	Susceptibility to hydrolysis by amylase	Available to microflora in large intestine
Raw			
Granules: A structure	Most uncooked cereals	Readily hydrolysed	+
Granules: B and C	Potato and banana	Partially resistant to hydrolysis	++
Cooked			
Physically inaccessible	Granules within intact cell walls: whole or broken grains, many legumes	Resistant to hydrolysis	+++
Dispersed amorphous	Freshly cooked foods	Readily hydrolysed	+
Retrograded amylopectin	Cooled cooked potato	Partially resistant to hydrolysis	++
Retrograded amylose	White bread and many processed cereals	Resistant to hydrolysis	+++++
Gelatinised starch dried at high temperature	Some cooked cereal foods	Readily hydrolysed	+++++

Source: Englyst and Kingman (1990).

glycosidic links. Both are found in the plant as insoluble semicrystalline granules. Starch may be classified nutritionally by the ability of enzymes to hydrolyse the material (Table 25.1). The physical form of starch influences the resistance to hydrolysis by amylase and subsequently the potential substrate for colonic microflora. Starches resistant to amylase pass to the colon and become a substrate for large intestinal bacteria.

Ungelatinised starch

There is very variable pancreatic digestibility of ungelatinised starch granules. Cereal starches respond to pancreatic α-amylase more readily than legume and tuber starches. The digestibility of a raw starch is inversely related to the amylose content, although this difference is removed by cooking.

Gelatinised starch

Starch granules in water heated to 60–70°C swell, resulting in a weakening of intermolecular links. This allows amylose and amylopectin to form colloidal dispersions. When the starch cools there is reassociation to regions of varying polymer density. Cooking enhances the susceptibility of starch-

es to amylase hydrolysis. Amylose in corn (amylomaize) is poorly digestible after cooking, whereas waxy cereal starches are very digestible. Vegetables contain 30–40% of amylose starch. Starches from legume seeds (lentils and beans) are digested more slowly than starch from bread. This may be related to the entrapment of starch in the legume cell structure, preventing a complete swelling during cooking. The degree of milling is important in the digestibility of a cereal starch. Finely milled wheat flour is digested more quickly than the coarsely milled equivalent. While the presence of a fibrous cellular structure surrounding the starch is not sufficient to restrict carbohydrate digestion, the fibre may restrict access by the hydrolytic enzyme to the starch. Food processing with high temperatures and shear stress affects starch digestion, so that commercially canned beans hydrolyse more quickly than home-cooked preparations. Extrusion cooking and explosion puffing are food manufacturing processes that alter the digestibility of starch in corn, rice or potato. Some starchy foods may produce a viscous microenvironment in the intestinal lumen. This affects the access of amylase to starch and the diffusion of hydrolytic products towards the intestinal mucosa.

Salivary and pancreatic α-amylases act on the endo-α-1–4 links within starch, but do not digest the exo-glucose-glucose linkages (Figure 25.3). Salivary amylase is 94% identical to pancreatic

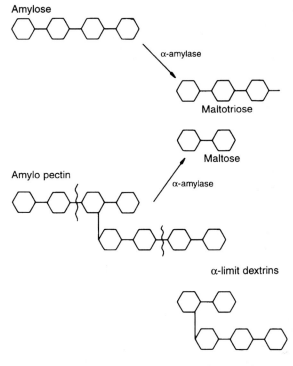

Amylose

Maltotriose

Maltose

Amylo pectin

α-amylase

α-amylase

α-limit dextrins

Fig. 25.3 Digestion of starch. Amylose and amylopectin are digested by α-amylase. Amylose yields maltotriose and maltose, amylopectin maltotriose, maltose and α-limit dextrins, the limitation being the α-(1–6) branch points.

amylase, is found in glycosylated and non-glycosylated forms, and cleaves α-1–4 glycosidic bonds. The free salivary amylase is inactivated at the low pH of the stomach. However, starch and its endproducts prevent this inactivation, partly by the bulk of the food preventing the gastric acid from permeating throughout the food complex in the stomach. There is a stabilisation of the pH above pH 4 in the stomach, which allows some salivary amylase to pass through the stomach without inactivation. Pancreatic α-amylase does not hydrolyse the α-1–6 branching unit or the α-1–1 links adjacent to these branching points. Consequently, large oligosaccharides (α-limit dextrins) with five or more glucose units, containing one or more α-1–6 branching links, are produced by amylase action (Figure 25.3). The products are maltose, maltotriose and α-limit dextrose, which have 5–10 glucose units, but not glucose. The amylase is unable to split at links near α-1–6 branch points. Consequently, α-1–4-linked disaccharides, maltose and trisaccharides (maltotriose) are final linear breakdown products. These small endproducts are cleaved by brush border enzymes. There are active carbohydrases in the columnar epithelial cells of the duodenum with reducing activity in the ileal villus. The glucoamylase removes single glucoses from the non-reducing end of α-linear α-1–4 glucosyl oligosaccharide. α-Limit dextrins are split by the combined action of glucoamylase and sucrase–isomaltase. The released glucose is absorbed by the intestinal mucosal cells by a carrier-mediated process.

Resistant starch

Starch may retrograde to a form that is highly resistant to hydrolysis by α-amylase. In this way, hydrogen bonds are re-formed and gelatinised starch partially recrystallises. Resistant starch passes to the colon as it is variably hydrolysed in the duodenum. The colon contains a large bacterial mass, which produces a wide range of enzymes to which most carbohydrates are susceptible. Under the conditions of the colon the major digestion products are carbon dioxide, hydrogen and methane, short-chain fatty acids, acetate, propionate, butyrate, organic acids such as lactic acid, pyruvic acid and possibly other breakdown products.

COMPLEXES AND INTERACTIONS WITH OTHER FOOD COMPONENTS

Inclusion complexes may be formed between the helices of amylose and polar lipids. These may occur during processing or naturally, as in cereal starches. Such amylose–lipid complexes may be formed during extrusion cooking, resulting in a relative resistance to amylase *in vitro*. In wheat flour there may be a complex physical or chemical interaction between starch and gluten that affects digestibility. The gluten matrix surrounding the gelatinised starch granules may limit access to amylase and reduce starch availability. Spaghetti has a high gluten content and is less readily digested than other wheat products with less gluten, such as bread. The digestibility of starch is decreased by Maillard reactions.

Food processing, toasting and excess heating storage all alter starch format and ideally enhance its digestibility by enteric enzymes. Other factors affecting starch digestibility include amylase inhibitors, lectins, phytic acid and tannins.

ASSESSMENT OF DIETARY CARBOHYDRATE DIGESTIBILITY

Tolerance tests

In these procedures, approximately 50 g of carbohydrate is ingested, then serial blood sugar estimations are taken and a blood–glucose curve is produced (Figure 25.4). Changes in blood glucose may be estimated for carbohydrates from different food sources. In this way a glycaemic index is calculated from the area under the blood–glucose curve after ingestion of 50 g of test carbohydrate, compared with the area under the blood–glucose curve following 50 g of standard carbohydrate (glucose or white bread). Glucose is the most potent sugar in its ability to increase blood glucose, and sucrose, lactose, galactose and fructose have an effect in descending order. Preformed maltose is absorbed from the intestine even more quickly than glucose, yet when maltose is formed as an intermediate in the intraluminal hydrolysis of starch, this difference in absorption of maltose is not discernible. There is, however, a large range of results.

The glycaemic response to plant foods depends on the source of the plant food, its physical form and the mode in which it is cooked. There are modifying effects on the absorption of starch by non-starch polysaccharides, fat and protein, through quite different mechanisms. Fats and proteins reduce the glycaemic response to carbohydrate by increasing insulin secretion in response to hyperglycaemia, and also by effects on gastric emptying. The hyperglycaemic effect of sweets and chocolates is reduced by the coincidental presence of fat and protein. Similarly, the glycaemic response to bread with butter is modified compared with bread on its own. These differences are due in part to changes in gastric emptying time and also to alterations in insulin response.

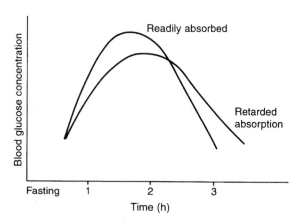

Fig. 25.4 Glucose tolerance test: readily absorbable and retarded absorption preparation of glucose. The readily absorbable glucose is absorbed in its free form, while the retarded absorption glucose is transported as a complex carbohydrate or in its natural form in food.

Dietary fibres, when they act on absorption, provide a mechanical barrier to the digestive juices acting on the starch granules, or interfere with the absorption of glucose through physicochemical mechanisms. This may involve interaction between the solid and soluble fibre and the glucoreceptor or the transporters on the surface of the enterocytes.

KEY POINTS

1. In many diets, the carbohydrate is 60% in the form of starch and glycogen, 30% as sucrose and 10% as lactose. Raffinose and stacchyose are present in small amounts in beans and are not absorbed in the upper intestine but are fermented in the colon.
2. The osmolarity of a sugar solution influences gastric emptying time and intestinal transit time. Other determinants of gastric emptying include duodenal pH, fat and caloric intake, viscosity, the solid content of the meal and whether the carbohydrate is a monosaccharide or a disaccharide.
3. Oligosaccharides in general are efficiently absorbed and metabolised after hydrolysis into the basic monosaccharides. The hydrolysis of lactose is relatively slow.

4. Fructose is not absorbed readily as the monosaccharide, but as a constituent of sucrose is very easily absorbed.

5. Monosaccharides cross the intestinal epithelium by one of three processes: simple diffusion, facilitated diffusion and active transport. The Na^+ active transfer of hexoses has a specific membrane carrier system, a cotransporter with two binding sites: one for the hexose and the other for the Na^+ ion.

6. Three major transfer systems are known: (i) a brush border Na^+/glucose cotransporter (SGLT1); (ii) a brush border fructose transporter (GLUT5); and (iii) a basolateral facilitated sugar transporter (GLUT2).

7. The brush border disaccharidases hydrolyse maltose, sucrose and lactose to the monosaccharides glucose, galactose and fructose. There is a kinetic advantage in hexoses being liberated from disaccharides, namely enhanced absorption rates from the lumen over those for free hexoses.

8. The brush border enzymes function on specific glycoside linkages. The disaccharidases are all large protein heterodimers or single subunits, anchored with transmembrane domains, with most of the protein protruding into the intestinal lumen.

9. Lactase is an unusual enteric enzyme that is present at birth and persists through life in Caucasian races, but not in most other races.

10. Starch consists of the linear α-1–4-linked α-D-glucose (amylose) and the highly branched amylopectin with α-1–4 and α-1–6 glycosidic links. Salivary and pancreatic α-amylases act on the endo-α-1–4 links within starch, but do not digest the exo-α-glucose–glucose linkages.

11. Starch may be classified nutritionally on the basis of its enzymatic hydrolysis: (i) rapidly digestible starch; (ii) slowly digestible starch; and (iii) resistant starch (which is not hydrolysed by pancreatic enzymes). Starch that is not digested in the intestine passes to the colon for fermentation by colonic bacteria.

12. Tolerance tests of carbohydrate loads allow changes in blood glucose to be estimated for carbohydrates of different food sources. When these are compared against a standard carbohydrate (glucose or white bread) a glycaemic index can be calculated.

THINKING POINT

For simplicity, the digestive and absorptive system is described in categories, but in reality many processes are going on at the same time.

NEED TO UNDERSTAND

1. A range of enzymes which hydrolyse complex to simple saccharides are secreted into the lumen of the intestine. The hydrolysis products are absorbed by very specific transport systems.

2. In the colon the hydrolysate system is provided by the colonic bacteria.

FURTHER READING

British Nutrition Foundation's Task Force Report (1990) *Complex Carbohydrates in Foods*. Chapman and Hall, London.

Crane, R.K. (1968) Digestive–absorptive circuits of the small bowel mucosa. *Annual Review of Medicine*, **19**, 57–68.

Cummings, J.H., Beatty, E.R., Kingman, S.M. *et al.* (1996) Digestion and physiological properties of resistant starch in the human large bowel. *British Journal of Nutrition*, **75**, 733–47.

Englyst, H.N. and Kingman, S.M. (1990) Dietary fiber and resistant starch. A nutritional classification of plant polysaccharides. In *Dietary Fiber* (eds D. Kritchevsky, C. Bonfield and J.W. Anderson). Plenum Publishing, New York.

Fang, R., Saantiago, N.A., Olds, L.C. and Sibley, E. (2000) The homoeodomain protein Cdx2 regulates lactase gene promoter activity during enterocyte differentiation. *Gastroenterology*, **118**, 115–27.

Feibusch, J.M. and Holt, P.R. (1982) Impaired absorptive capacity for carbohydrate in the ageing human. *Digestive Diseases Science*, **21**, 1095–100.

Fihn, B.-M., Sjoqvist, A. and Jodal, M. (2000) Permeability of the rat small intestinal epithelium along the villus–crypt axis: effect of the glucose transport. *Gastroenterology*, **119**, 1029–36.

Jenkins, D.J., Wolever, T.M.S., Taylor, R.H. *et al.* (1981) Glycemic index of foods: a physiological basis for carbohydrate exchange. *American Journal of Clinical Nutrition*, **34**, 362–6.

Johnson, L.R., Alpers, D.H., Christensen, J. *et al*. (1994) *Physiology of the Gastrointestinal Tract*. Raven Press, New York.

Levin, R.J. (1989) Dietary starches and sugars in man: a comparison. In *Human Nutrition Reviews; ILSI Europe* (ed. J. Dobbing). Springer, London.

MacDonald, L., Thumser, A.E. and Sharp, P. (2002) Decreased expression in the vitamin C transporter SVCT1 by ascorbic acid in a human intestinal epithelial cell line. *British Journal of Nutrition*, **87**, 97–100

Parsons, D.S. (1976) Closing summary, Appendix 2, Unstirred layer. In *Intestinal Ion Transport* (ed. J.WL. Robinson). MTP Press, Lancaster, pp. 407–30.

Symposium Nutrition Society (1996) Glucose transporters in the control of metabolism. *Proceedings of the Nutrition Society*. **55**, 167–78.

26

Protein absorption

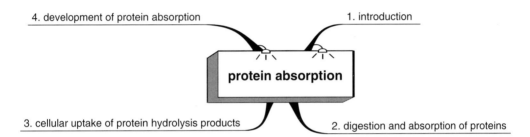

4. development of protein absorption

1. introduction

protein absorption

3. cellular uptake of protein hydrolysis products

2. digestion and absorption of proteins

Fig. 26.1 Chapter outline.

INTRODUCTION

The dietary protein intake is approximately 70–100 g/day, with approximately 50–60% of animal origin, except by vegetarians. In addition, 20–30 g of endogenous proteins, 30 g of desquamated cells and 1–2 g plasma proteins (1–2 g as albumin), enzymes and mucoproteins are secreted into the intestine. Protein of endogenous origin is in general digested and absorbed more slowly than that of exogenous origin. The faecal excretion of protein-derived nitrogen is about 10 g/day or less, demonstrating an effective absorption of protein, which in the small intestine is in the order of 95%. This efficiency is dependent on the type of protein, e.g. the absorption of cooked haricot bean protein is poor. Faecal protein is largely bacterial in origin, whereas faecal nitrogen is of endogenous origin.

Protein absorption involves the breakdown of protein to tripeptides, dipeptides and amino acids. The site of maximal peptide or amino acid absorption may differ along the intestine and is species dependent. The electrical gradient across the brush border is steeper in the jejunum than in the ileum. While most ingested protein is absorbed in the jejunum, some protein is absorbed in the ileum and some, albeit a small amount, passes on to the colon. Following a protein-containing meal there appear to be more intraluminal amino acids in the ileum than in the jejunum, suggesting that peptidases enter the ileal lumen. Absorption of amino acids from the ileum in humans may be more important than peptide absorption. The colonic mucosa appears to be an effective absorber of amino acids. Nitrogen absorption from the colon consists of the fermentation products of bacterial metabolism. It is possible that 3–24 g of protein passes into the colon each day and of this, perhaps 40–60% is endogenous.

DIGESTION AND ABSORPTION OF PROTEINS

There are six main phases in the digestion and absorption of proteins:

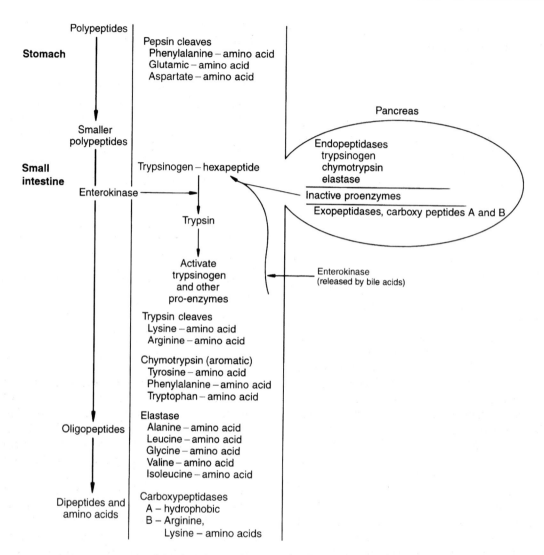

Fig. 26.2 Proteins are sequentially reduced in molecular size during passage through the stomach and the upper gastrointestinal tract. Pepsin initiates the enzymatic process. The pancreas excretes inactive proenzymes which are activated by enterokinase, a mucosal enzyme. This activates trypsinogen which, in turn, activates chymotrypsin, elastase and carboxypeptidases A and B. Enzyme activity with a specified amino acid–amino acid peptide linkage.

1. Whole protein absorption.
2. Intraluminal digestion of protein and its breakdown products, polypeptides, resulting from the sequential actions of the proteolytic enzymes of the stomach and pancreas.
3. Cellular uptake of protein hydrolysis products: (i) amino acids; (ii) peptides.
4. Brush border digestion of small peptides.
5. Intracellular metabolism.
6. Transfer of dipeptides and amino acids from the intestinal brush border to the bloodstream.

Whole protein absorption

It is possible that 2% of a dietary protein intake is absorbed as whole protein. The absorption of whole proteins involves pinocytosis and is thought to be unimportant in adults, but may be important in neonates. Pinocytosis is the binding of a substance to a membrane, and the membrane–substance complex is then brought into the cell interior as a whole vesicle that fuses with lysosomes. The pinocytotic vesicles formed from the brush border membrane fuse with lysosomes to form phagolysosomes, in which there is some protein hydrolysis. Proteins that have escaped hydrolysis enter the intercellular spaces by exocytosis and reach the bloodstream by the lymphatics.

Intraluminal digestion

Protein digestion begins in the stomach with the enzyme pepsin, which belongs to a class of enzymes aspartic proteinases, an enzyme group present in many forms of life (Figure 26.2). Another aspartic proteinase, chymosin (renin), is found in neonates. The precursor pepsinogen exists as multiple isoenzymes and its proteolytic activity requires a pH less than 4. Pepsin is activated by the acid conditions of the stomach and inactivated in alkaline conditions, e.g. in the duodenum or the stomach in which acid production is suppressed. The pepsin produced activates the precursor pepsinogen by cleavage of an N-terminal peptide (44 amino acids) from the pepsinogen. The result is a mixture of very large polypeptides with molecular weight of many thousands (Figure 26.2). There is no gastric protein absorption.

The physical form of the protein solid or liquid phase may alter the rate of gastric emptying. The rate of intraluminal digestion is a rate-limiting factor in protein absorption. Individual proteins are absorbed at very different rates. Casein disappears from the rat intestine three times more quickly than gliadin, which is slowly hydrolysed by trypsin. Gastric emptying time dictates the rate of release of protein into the small intestine and hence the rate of digestion and absorption. The size of the meal, chemical composition, presence of other nutrients and osmolality all affect the ease of digestion.

The next phase in protein digestion is the activation of proteolytic enzymes, secreted in an inactive form by the pancreas, and initiated by enterokinase (Figure 26.2). Enterokinase converts the precursor trypsinogen to trypsin by the cleavage of a small terminal peptide and the result-

Pancreatic enzymes

The proteolytic enzymes of the pancreas may be classified according to the bonds hydrolysed.

Endopeptidases split peptide bonds within the chain. Trypsin yields peptides with the basic amino acids (arginine, lysine) at the C-terminal end, while chymotrypsin A,B,C and elastin produce peptides with neutral amino acids at the C-terminal end.

Exopeptidases hydrolyse C-terminal bonds at the end of protein and peptide chains. The enzymes act in concert, producing oligopeptides and a proportion of free amino acids. The rate of release of individual amino acids varies widely. The release of arginine and lysine and many neutral amino acids is rapid; that of glycine, proline and the acidic amino acids, glutamate and aspartate is slow or very slow.

Carboxypeptidases release amino acids and oligopeptides 2–6 amino acids long, yielding 40% amino acids and 60% peptides.

ant trypsin activates more trypsin. The optimal pH is 7.5. Protein digestion involves hydrolysis of the peptide (CO–NH) bonds that link amino acids.

Brush border enzymatic activity is stimulated by trypsin and removed from the apical membrane assisted by the action of bile acids. In the duodenum intraluminal hydrolysis is far from complete. Some proteins are much less readily digested than others. Some are resistant to hydrolysis and their subsequent absorption is incomplete. In the proximal jejunum in humans the rate of release of amino acids from milk powder proteins varies depending on lysine being released 140 times more quickly than glycine and 14 times more quickly than glutamic acid. More distally the variations are smaller. There are very small differences between the appearance of free amino acids in the lumen and the amino acid composition of the protein.

Overheating of proteins during storage and preparation, Maillard reactions and other complex chemical changes result in digestive products of small peptides that are not only resistant to hydrolysis but also poorly absorbed. This may occur with dried milk that has been roller-dried. Gelatin is also resistant to later stages of hydrolysis. Many proteins that have been used in physiological studies are unusual in their digestive behaviour.

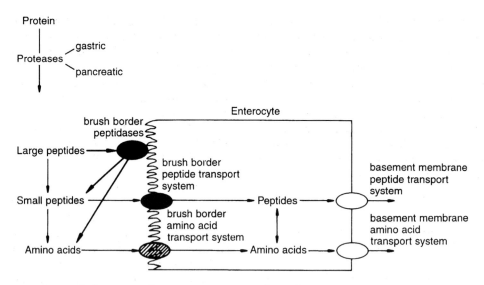

Fig. 26.3 Digestion and absorption of protein. Proteins are cleaved by proteases. Large peptides are split by brush border peptidases to produce small peptides and amino acids. Small peptides are absorbed by brush border peptide transport systems. Amino acids are absorbed by specific brush border amino acid transport systems. Peptides and amino acids are transported into the body by basement membrane peptide transport systems and amino acid transport systems.

Casein digestion liberates phosphopeptidases, which are initially absorbed but resist further cellular digestion. Raw egg white and soy and other varieties of beans contain a trypsin inhibitor. Cooking may well increase the digestibility of proteins, and also inactivate trypsin inhibitors.

Proteins of animal origin are more readily digested than vegetable proteins and yield a larger proportion of small peptides and amino acids. Egg protein is digested and absorbed with an efficiency of 85–90%; casein, like other phosphoproteins, is relatively resistant to hydrolysis. Proteins with a high proline content, e.g. gluten or casein, are relatively resistant to pancreatic enzyme action. While the nutritive value of a protein is dependent on its amino acid composition and digestibility, peptide bonds resistant to hydrolysis may be as important in ultimately determining the nutritive quality of a protein.

There is an enhanced peptide and amino acid absorption after starvation. There are changes in the thickness of the unstirred layer and possibly increases in the number of carrier proteins during starvation. There are diurnal and even seasonal changes in the intestinal ability to absorb nutrients. All of these changes may complicate experimental results.

CELLULAR UPTAKE OF PROTEIN HYDROLYSIS PRODUCTS

Proteins are absorbed from the intestinal lumen largely in the form of small peptides and the hydrolysis products, amino acids, resulting from intraluminal digestion. Small quantities of whole proteins are also absorbed and enter the circulation in trace amounts. The absorption of peptides and that of amino acids are complementary processes. Further hydrolysis of peptides occurs through the action of peptidases at the absorptive surface, the products being tripeptides, dipeptides and amino acids (Figure 26.3).

Ingesting a mixture of free amino acids is less efficient in maintaining nitrogen balance than an equivalent supply of amino acids in the form of peptides. This may in part be due to the amino acids being absorbed and delivered to, and thus utilised by tissues at individual and differing rates. This staggered delivery and utilisation pattern is not optimal for protein synthesis, where an abundant supply of amino acids is required.

In general, the rate of mucosal absorption of a partial hydrolysate of protein will be twice as fast as a mixture of equivalent amino acid content. It is possible that the absorption of peptides undergoes less intense competition than that of amino acids. The kinetics of brush border hydrolysis, rather than the kinetics of peptide or amino acid transport, govern the rate of absorption of the longer chain peptides.

The relative rates of absorption of amino acids from a peptide and from an equivalent mixture of amino acids are strongly influenced by concentration. The relative rates of absorption of peptides and amino acids are dependent on:

- the kinetics of mediated transport of peptides and amino acids
- the substantial uptake of amino acids released at the brush border; two independent transport systems become involved which accelerate total absorption, as the two systems are not readily saturated.

Glucose usually stimulates the intestinal transport of amino acids, possibly through an increase in water movement associated with glucose transport.

Amino acids have been reported to appear in the portal blood in proportions approximately equivalent to the amounts ingested. However, intraluminal digestion of protein releases amino acids in the free form at rates that differ very widely from and are not proportional to their content in the ingested protein. There is also the possibility of substantial dilution or even complete swamping of exogenous by endogenous protein. In addition, free amino acid absorption, a minor mode of absorption of protein hydrolysis products, progresses at a slower rate than that of peptides.

Amino acids

Free amino acids are transported into the absorptive cells by a number of well-defined mechanisms, which are mainly active and Na^+ linked. Several absorption mechanisms are specific for amino acids with common structural features. Amino acids, whether taken up as free amino acids or released from peptides in the absorptive cells after hydrolysis, pass from the cell to the blood by transport mechanisms using facultative diffusion. The amino acid transport system in the apical membrane is not the same as that of the basolateral membrane. The two transport systems are in contact with fluids and conditions of quite different composition. Some amino acids are extensively metabolised within the absorptive cell and all are utilised to some extent for protein synthesis.

> Basic amino acids lysine and arginine have a positive charge in the physiological pH range, so they concentrate in the cell as a result of differences in electrical potential between the electronegative interior and the exterior of the cell.

Charge is not important in dictating the rate of mediated transport. Multiple active transport systems are involved in the absorption of amino acids. There may well be five systems involved in the transport of neutral amino acids, imino acids and basic acids in the brush border. The system is complicated and incompletely understood.

The traditional 'main transport system' for neutral amino acids may possibly incorporate more than one system. The main transport system for most neutral amino acids requires a substrate with an uncharged side-chain and a primary amino acid in the α-position. Proline and hydroxyproline are exceptions to this rule. The system has a strong preference for L-amino acids, but does not transport basic or acidic amino acids, or β-alanine.

The larger and bulkier the side-chain of the amino acid, the stronger the lipophilic properties and the greater the apparent affinity for main system transport. Glycine and other amino acids with short aliphatic side-chains may use the imino system and some may use the basic system.

> The imino system carries proline, hydroxyproline and N-methylated forms of glycine and, to some extent glycine, β-alanine, γ-aminobutyric acid (GABA) and taurine. In humans a defect in this system leads to iminoglycinuria, with impaired absorption of glycine, proline and hydroxyproline. There is an active intestinal transport system for the basic lysine, arginine and ornithine, and for cystine. The investigation of the systems transporting acidic amino acids was hindered by the extensive transamination of glutamate and aspartate in the mucosa. They are transported by the same Na^+-coupled system.
>
> D-Isomers appear to use the same transport systems as their comparable L-form, but with reduced affinity characteristics and hence more slowly.

In general, the brush border transport of amino acids and that of peptides appear to be independent processes with little or no interaction between them.

All animal cell membranes contain a large number of transport systems for amino acids which differ in chemical and net charge. If one system is defective, there is another to retrieve the situation. There is a small role for non-mediated transport in the absorption of amino acids.

While much non-mediated transport takes place through water-filled channels, amino acids have a degree of lipid solubility that may allow some permeability through the lipids of the cell membrane. This is not likely to be of importance. Diffusion through water-filled channels is likely to be greater with lower molecular weight amino acids. In diffusion through lipid membranes the degree of lipid solubility of the amino acid is significant, especially a large molecular volume, a bulky side-chain and relatively lipophilic properties, e.g. phenylalanine > methionine > alanine > glycine. The transport of basic and acidic amino acids will be complicated by the effects of charge. Small lipid-insoluble molecules of sphere radius less than 0.4 nm and a range of larger hydrophilic molecules, e.g. hydrophilic cyanocobalamin (molecular weight 1357 Da), cross the epithelium more slowly by non-mediated transport.

> The paracellular pathways are believed to behave as water-filled channels with an equivalent pore radius of 0.4–0.8 nm. The pore size is said to be larger in the jejunum than in the ileum or colon (0.3 nm). Therefore, the permeability of the intestine to water and water-soluble substances is higher proximally than distally. On both the mucosal and serosal sides, there is a small number of electronegative pores with a larger size (6.5 nm) occupying 1% of the mucosal surface. There are also negatively charged, cationic-selective pores (0.7 nm) and electroneutral pores (0.4 nm in diameter) filled with water.

The absorption of some amino acids is through highly specific mechanisms, indicating a mediated absorption. The rate of absorption of amino acids from mixtures of free amino acids is related to their concentration, the kinetics of absorption transport of each amino acid, and mutual inhibitory and stimulatory effects. Methionine, leucine and isoleucine are absorbed quickly; glycine, threonine, glutamate and aspartate are absorbed relatively slowly, regardless of the mixture. The rates are determined by the relative affinity of transport, K_t.

Some of the amino acids with a strong transport affinity can inhibit the transport of amino acids with a lower affinity. It is not necessarily the essential amino acids or peptides containing essential amino acids that are absorbed the most quickly.

Transport defects of amino acids, e.g. Hartnup's disease (dipolar amino acid) and cystinuria (cationic amino acids and cystine), are overcome when the amino acids are incorporated into peptides. Amino acids do not competitively interfere with absorption of peptides of similar amino acid composition. The features that make peptides resistant to hydrolysis may be associated with poor transport, e.g. D-amino acid residues.

Dipeptides and tripeptides

The transport of peptides and amino acids is quite separate and independent. Peptide absorption is a process of peptide transport across the brush border, followed by hydrolysis at the brush border membrane and within the cell, and uptake of amino acids from the cell into the bloodstream.

Transmembrane transport of peptides involves active transport and is possibly limited to dipeptides and tripeptides. Chain length, rather than molecular volume, is the limiting factor. Lipophilic properties are not important in determining the rate of transport of peptides. Biologically active peptides of very long chain length may be absorbed, possibly by non-mediated transport or by mechanisms related to the uptake of whole proteins. Peptide transport is stereospecific, favouring peptides containing only L-amino acids or glycine. Peptides with D-amino acids are poorly transported and hydrolysed. Methylation, acetylation and other substitutions of the N-terminal group reduce the effectiveness of transport. Substitution of the C-terminal group may also reduce affinity for transport, whereas free amino acid absorption increases with increasing side-chain bulk. This relationship with size and ease of transport does not apply to dipeptides of those neutral amino acids.

Classification of the amino acid transport systems (Table 26.1)

System B: the major transport system for the transport of dipolar amino acids with the amino group in the α-position. Imino acids, β-dipolar, basic and acidic amino acids are not transported by this system. There is a transmembrane Na^+ gradient and an electrical potential. This system is found very early in foetal intestinal development.

System $B^{°,+}$: transports dipolar amino acids, basic amino acids and cystine. The system is dependent on a transmembrane Na^+ gradient and the transport system is electrogenic.

System $b^{°,+}$: a high-affinity, Na^+-independent system for dipolar and basic amino acids. This system is found throughout the small intestine but not the colon.

System y^+: transports basic amino acids by a Na^+-independent system.

Imino system: exclusively for imino acids, e.g. proline, hydoxyproline and pipecolic acid. It is found throughout the small intestine and is Na^+ and Cl^- dependent.

β-System: has a high affinity for taurine and other β-amino acids. There is no affinity for α-amino acids. The requirement is for Na^+ and Cl^- and it is very sensitive to the presence of calcium.

System X^-_{AG}: exclusively for the acidic amino acids aspartate and glutamate. The system is dependent on Na^+.

Table 26.1 Brush border enterocyte membrane absorption systems for amino acids

Substrate						Gradient	
Acidic amino acids	Dipolar α-amino acids	Basic amino acids	Cystine amino acids	Imino amino acids	β-Amino acids	Na^+	Other
	β					Yes	–
	$β^{°,+}$	$β^{°,+}$	$β^{°,+}$			Yes	–
	$B^{°,+}$	$b^{°,+}$	$b^{°,+}$			No	–
				Imino		Yes	Cl^-
					β	Yes	Cl^-
X^-_{AG}						Yes	K^+

Peptides are cotransported with protons, unlike in most other transport systems where Na^+ is the cotransporter. If the dipeptide carries a negative charge then two protons are cotransported; for a neutral dipeptide one proton and for an positively charged peptide there is no proton movement. This retains the electronegative environment of the cell cytoplasm (Figure 26.4). The peptides are then hydrolysed to amino acids at a site beyond the peptide transport mechanisms, probably in the cytosol of the absorptive cell.

The effect of the unstirred layer on peptide absorption is the same as for amino acids, i.e. to retard and hence to reduce the rate of absorption. The concentration of peptides at the absorptive surface will be greater than in the lumen.

Tertiary transport

The concentration of Na within the absorptive cells is kept low by the action of Na/K-ATPase, which pumps Na out of the cells across the basolateral membrane. The re-entry of Na down an electrochemical gradient through the Na/H system in the brush border membrane causes the extrusion of protons into the lumen. Protons re-enter the cells across the brush border membrane down an electrochemical gradient by a mechanism coupling their entry to the inward transport of peptides.

The dipeptides and tripeptides share a common transport system or systems, and compete for brush

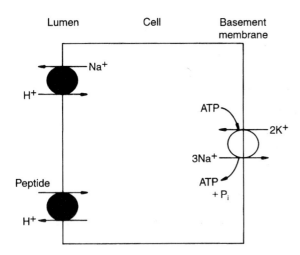

Lumen   Cell   Basement
                             membrane

Fig. 26.4   Peptide absorption across the enterocyte brush
border luminal surface using a Na⁺/H⁺ exchanger: peptide transporter. Basement membrane transport system
Na⁺/K⁺-ATPase.

border transport among themselves but not with
amino acids, as they use different mechanisms. The
dipeptide and tripeptide brush border system is relatively indifferent to the net charge on the side-
chains, transporting neutral, basic and acidic
peptides. Despite the enormous number of peptides and tripeptides resulting from the hydrolysis
of proteins, the peptide transporter PepT1 is able
to transport all peptides regardless of molecular
weight, charge or chemistry. Intestinal peptide
transfer varies in response to various factors, of
which dietary protein is the most important. The
promoter of the *PeP1* gene (localised on chromosome 13q24-q33) responds to particular amino acids
(phenylalanine, arginine and lysine) and dipeptides
(Gly-Sar, Gly-Phe, Lys-Phe and Asp-Lys).

Brush border digestion of small peptides

It may well be that only dipeptides and tripeptides
are transported into the absorptive cells. The
majority of the peptidases of the intestinal mucosa
are aminopeptidases, hydrolysing peptides sequentially from the N-terminal end of the molecule.
There are both brush border membrane and
cytosol peptidases. There is a very active dipepti-

dase with a very broad specificity. The cytosol of the
absorptive cells contains 90% of the total dipeptidase and less than 50% of the tripeptidase activity
of the mucosa. It is also possible that there
arc some proteases associated with the enteric
mucosa.

Peptides in which glycine is the N-terminal residue,
undergo little brush border hydrolysis and are
absorbed intact. The rate of hydrolysis is enhanced
when the substrate consists of amino acid residues
containing amino acids with large lipophilic side-
chains at the amino-terminus. Tripeptides and
tetrapeptides are absorbed at faster rates than
dipeptides. Peptidase activity against dipeptides
containing proline is nil. Less than 10% of the total
dipeptidase activity is to be found in the brush
border, 60% of tripeptidases and 100% of higher
peptidases. Individual dipeptidases and
oligopeptidases are integral membrane
glycoproteins with the carbohydrate-rich portion of
the molecule projecting from the luminal surface of
the brush border membrane.

Some of the large number of peptidases are
found only in the enteric mucosa, e.g. enterokinase,
and others are found in other cell membranes.
These peptidases are generally metalloenzymes
and are found in the intracellular apical membrane.
There are four families of peptidases:

- **endopeptidases**: the most important of these,
  neutral endopeptidase, cleaves dipeptides at
  non-amino-terminal hydrophobic amino acid
  residues
- **aminopeptidases** have a variety of specificities
  for neutral, acidic, proline, tryptophan amino-
  terminal residues yielding amino acids
- **carboxypeptidases** hydrolyse peptides at the C-
  terminal end
- **dipeptidases** hydrolyse over a wide range of
  amino acid residues.

Some peptidases in the brush border are glycosylated endopeptidases anchored at the amino-
terminal end. Some amino acids, e.g. histidine,
methionine, leucine, alanine and hydrophobic
amino acids, inhibit aminopeptidase activity. High
protein intake increases and starvation decreases
aminopeptidase activity.

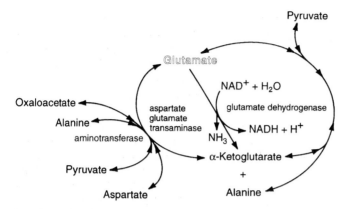

Fig. 26.5 Intracellular metabolism in enterocytes. Relationship between glutamate, α-ketoglutarate, oxaloacetate, pyruvate, alanine, aspartate and ammonia production.

Intracellular metabolism

After absorption free amino acids, whether absorbed as a free amino acid or peptide, enter a number of metabolic pathways, for degradation or conversion into other amino acids or proteins (Figure 26.5).

It is probable that at least 10% of amino acids taken up from the intestinal lumen in free or peptide form are synthesised into protein and another 10–20% (especially those rich in glutamate) undergo metabolic change. The synthetic activity of the small intestinal mucosa is intense, with rapid cell renewal, enzyme production, secretion of mucus and synthesis of apolipoproteins essential to the formation of chylomicrons.

Glutamine, glutamate and aspartate are important amino acids in intestinal metabolism. There is extensive transamination of glutamic acid (+ pyruvic acid → alanine + α-ketoglutarate) and aspartic acid (+ α-ketoglutarate → glutamic acid + oxaloacetic acid). This metabolism may be a detoxification mechanism, protecting from high concentrations of glutamic acid, which is then slowly metabolised by the liver. In some species glutamine and arginine are extensively metabolised in the small intestine which, together with the colon, is an important source of ammonia.

The unpleasant reaction to the savoury monosodium glutamate, the 'Chinese restaurant syndrome', is an idiosyncratic response that may be a result of a low level of intestinal alanine aminotransferase and hence an increased absorption of glutamate. When glutamic acid is given with glu-

cose the reduced increment in plasma glutamic acid that occurs may be a result of increased metabolic activity in the liver and intestine.

Transfer of dipeptides and amino acids from brush border to bloodstream

There is active transport of amino acids through the basolateral membrane by transport systems that are Na independent and probably mediated by facili-

---

Transport systems of amino acid transport

Na$^+$-dependent systems

System A transports all α-amino acids including imino acids. This allows transport of all amino acids from the bloodstream into the cells. System ASC is also Na$^+$ dependent and favours the transport of three- and four-carbon amino acids from the blood into the cell.

Na$^+$-independent systems

System asc is similar to ASC but is Na$^+$ independent. System L is the most important of these basolateral transport systems and favours dipolar amino acids, glutamine and cysteine, but not imino acids. System Y$^+$ transports basic amino acids, lysine, arginine, ornithine and histidine.

Peptides and pharmacological agents, e.g. β-lactam antibiotics, captopril, bestatin and renin inhibitors, are absorbed through a common pathway.

tated diffusion. A massive load of amino acids is imposed on this exit mechanism by the influx of ingested peptides that are hydrolysed in the mucosa in addition to the dietary amino acids. Amino acid concentrations in absorptive cells do not increase very much post-prandially as there is little impediment to flow from the cell to the blood.

Peptides, some of which are biologically active, may pass from the intestinal lumen to the blood; 10–30% of the absorbed partial hydrolysis products of protein have been estimated to cross into blood and red cells, the extent varying with the type of protein eaten. Of the 80% of protein digestion products that leave the lumen as peptides, approximately 50% may be transported across the brush border in peptide form. The proportion will vary with the protein, e.g. animal- or vegetable-derived proteins.

Amino acid transport from cell to bloodstream

There are five amino acid transport systems across the basolateral membrane. Two are Na^+ dependent and the other three Na^+ independent. The Na^+-independent systems transport amino acids from the cell into the blood; the Na^+-dependent systems supply the cells with amino acids between meals.

DEVELOPMENT OF PROTEIN ABSORPTION

In newborn animals whole proteins may be absorbed, which is of major immunological importance. Proteolytic enzymes develop rapidly in the newborn. The ability to transport amino acids develops at different rates in foetal and neonatal life. In the rabbit, the development of the active transport system for valine, methionine and lysine precedes that of proline and glycine. The absorption of peptides in the developing animal is very active. The foetus swallows large amounts of amniotic fluid (100–300 ml/kg/day in late pregnancy), which contains amino acids and glucose in similar concentrations to maternal blood.

KEY POINTS

1. Protein absorption involves the breakdown of protein to tripeptides, dipeptides and amino acids. The site of maximal peptide or amino acid absorption may differ along the intestine.
2. Most ingested protein is absorbed in the jejunum, some is absorbed in the ileum and a small amount in the colon.
3. There are six phases in the digestion and absorption of proteins: (i) whole protein absorption; (ii) intraluminal digestion of protein and its breakdown products polypeptides, resulting from the sequential actions of the proteolytic enzymes of the stomach and pancreas; (iii) cellular uptake of amino acids and peptides; (iv) brush border digestion of small peptides; (v) intracellular metabolism; and (vi) transfer of amino acids and dipeptides from the intestinal cell to the bloodstream.
4. Protein digestion begins in the stomach with the enzyme pepsin in the presence of hydrochloric acid. The next phase is the activation of proteolytic enzymes, a process initiated by enterokinase, which converts the precursor trypsinogen to trypsin by the cleavage of a small terminal peptide. Some proteins are resistant to hydrolysis, with the result that their subsequent absorption is incomplete. Whole protein absorption may be significant in newborn animals. This is of immunological importance. Proteolytic enzymes develop rapidly in the newborn.
5. Proteins are absorbed from the intestinal lumen largely in the form of small peptides and amino acids. Small quantities of whole proteins are also absorbed and enter the circulation in trace amounts. Intraluminal digestion of protein produces a mixture of small peptides and amino acids in which peptides predominate. The absorption of peptides and that of amino acids are complementary processes.
6. Free amino acids are transported into the absorptive cells by a number of well-defined mechanisms, which are mainly active and Na^+ linked. Several absorption mechanisms have defined specificity for certain groups of amino acids with structural features in common.

7. Active transport is a major mechanism of trans-membrane transport of peptides. Active transport is limited to dipeptides and tripeptides. Peptide transport by the PepT1 transporter is stereospecific, favouring peptides containing only L-amino acids or glycine. D-Isomers appear to utilise the same transport systems as their comparable L-form, but with reduced affinity characteristics. The transporter is unusual in having protons as the cotransporter.

8. The majority of the peptidases of the intestinal mucosa are aminopeptidases, hydrolysing peptides sequentially from the amino-terminal end of the molecule.

9. The synthetic activity of the small intestinal mucosa is intense, requiring absorbed amino acids for rapid cell renewal, enzyme production, secretion of mucus and synthesis of apolipoproteins essential for chylomicrons.

10. There is active transport of amino acids through the basolateral membrane by transport systems, which are Na^+ independent and probably mediated by facilitated diffusion.

THINKING POINT

There are differences in protein digestion between animal and vegetable proteins. What are the possible consequences for vegetarian and carnivorous diets?

NEED TO UNDERSTAND

1. The digestion of protein starts in the stomach and takes place mainly in the jejunum.

2. The breakdown products of protein digestion are primarily absorbed as peptides using a common transporter, PepT1, and the amino acids generated are absorbed by very specific pathways.

3. The peptides are further hydrolysed to amino acids in the brush border cells.

4. The small intestine is a very important protein synthetic organ.

FURTHER READING

Johnson, L.R., Alpers, D.H., Christensen, J. *et al.* (1994) *Physiology of the Gastrointestinal Tract.* Raven Press, New York.

Leibach, F.H. and Ganapathy, V. (1996) Peptide transporters in the intestine and the kidney. *Annual Review of Nutrition*, **16**, 99–119.

McNiven, M.A. and Marlowe, K.J. (1999) Contributions of molecular motor enzymes to vesicular-based protein transport in gastrointestinal epithelial cells. *Gastroenterology*, **116**, 438–81.

Matthews, D.M. (1991) *Protein Absorption, Development and Present State of the Subject.* Wiley-Liss, New York.

Shiraga T., Miyamoto, K.-I., Tanaka, H. *et al.* (1999) Cellular and molecular mechanisms of dietary regulation on rat intestinal H^+/peptide transporter PepT1. *Gastroenterology*, **116**, 354–62.

Symposium Nutrition Society (1995) Nitrogen transactions in the gut. *Proceedings of the Nutrition Society*, **54**, 519–23.

27

Lipid absorption

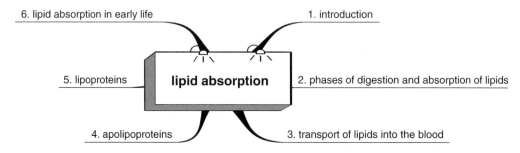

Fig. 27.1 Chapter outline.

INTRODUCTION

The absorption of lipids is different to that of carbohydrates and protein because of their poor solubility in water. The whole process, from mouth to body cell, requires fat-solvent systems. Fat digestion takes place in the small intestine and involves pancreatic esterase and lipase enzymes, which degrade the lipid into an absorbable form.

PHASES OF DIGESTION AND ABSORPTION OF LIPIDS

Gastric phase

The churning of stomach contents creates a coarse oil and water emulsion stabilised by phospholipids. Proteolytic digestion in the stomach releases lipids from food lipoprotein complexes (Figure 27.2). The digestion of dietary triglycerides

starts in the stomach with gastric or lingual lipase. This initial lipolysis accounts for 10–30% of the total hydrolysis of the ingested triglyceride. Fat in concentrations greater than 2–3% reduces proximal gastric tone by a lipid-specific mechanism, reduces antral contractions and increases pyloric tone. The effect is to slow gastric emptying.

Jejunal phase

On leaving the stomach the fat emulsion is modified by mixing with bile and pancreatic juice. The bile contains bile acids as glycine and taurine conjugates of the trihydroxylated cholic acid and the dihydroxylated chenodeoxycholic acid and phospholipids. Biliary secretion is proportional to the amount of fat in the diet.

The pancreas secretes enzymes which release fatty acids from triacylglycerols, phospholipids and cholesterol esters. Pancreatic lipase catalyses the hydrolysis of fatty acids from positions 1 and 3 of triacylglycerols, with little hydrolysis of the fatty

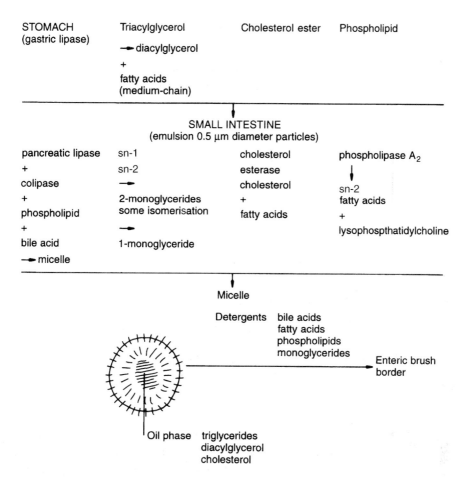

Fig. 27.2 Lipid digestion takes place in the stomach and small intestine. Gastric lipase initiates the digestion of tri-acylglycerol. Fats pass from the stomach into the small intestine as small emulsions. Micelles are created when pancreatic lipase, cholesterol esterase and phospholipase A₂ digest lipids to more polar substrates. Stable micelles are formed, which pass through the unstirred layer to the enteric brush border, where individual lipids are absorbed by specific pathways.

acid in position 2. There is some modest isomerisation to the 1-monoacylglycerols. The lipase hydrolyses triacylglycerol molecules at the surface of the large emulsion particles. If there are long-chain fatty acids (C20:5 and C22:6) in the 1 and 3 positions of the triacylglycerols then hydrolysis is less readily achieved by pancreatic enzymes than if there are shorter chain fatty acids in those positions. The pancreatic enzymes are modified to allow enzyme:lipid emulsion interaction to take place.

Bile acid molecules accumulate on the surface of the lipid droplet, displacing other surface-acting constituents. The bile acids give a negative charge to the oil droplets. This attracts colipase, a protein of 10 kDa molecular weight which binds the pancreatic lipase to the surface of the lipid droplets, creating a ternary complex containing calcium, bile salts, colipase and pancreatic lipase. Procolipase is secreted in a proform in both the stomach and pancreas, and is cleaved by trypsin or pepsin to colipase and enterostatin, which acts as a regulator of fat intake.

As digestion proceeds the large emulsified particles are converted into mixed micelles (Figures 27.3 and 27.4). The micelles are stable, small particles, which may be insoluble or soluble. They contain monoacylglycerols, lysophospholipids and

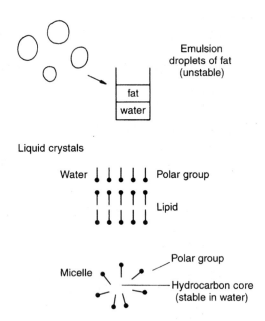

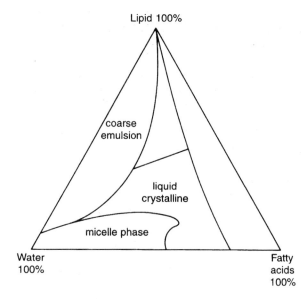

Fig. 27.3 Lipid interactions with water: emulsions, liquid crystals and micelles. When the concentration of amphiphiles (detergents) reaches a certain level a stable, small structure called a micelle is formed. This concentration is called a critical micelle concentration. The hydrocarbon groups protrude into the core of the micelle. The polar groups interact with water to give solubility. Micelles are very stable. Amphiphiles are lipids which are sited at water–lipid interphases and facilitate the solubility of one phase into the other.

Fig. 27.4 Micelle formation. If an insoluble lipid and a fatty acid are mixed in varying concentrations, a phase diagram can be drawn in which various mixtures are identified; with lipid (100%) at the apex and water (100%) and fatty acid (100%) at each base. Varying concentrations of each of these would be present at any mixture point shown in the interior of the diagram. When there is insufficient detergent and excess of lipid, a coarse emulsion is formed. If the amount of fatty acid increases, a liquid crystalline formation results. If the ratios of detergent, water and lipid are correct, a micelle is created. In the intestine, fatty acid monoacyl glycerols, phospholipids and bile acids are involved in micelle formation.

fatty acids. Fatty acids are in the form of soluble amphiphiles, since the pH in the proximal part of the small intestine is around 5.8–6.5. These soluble amphiphiles incorporate insoluble non-polar molecules such as cholesterol and vitamins into the micelles and consequently are important in absorption.

Phospholipase A_2 hydrolyses the fatty acid in position 2 of phospholipids, particularly phosphatidylcholine. The enzyme is an inactive proenzyme in pancreatic juice and is activated by the tryptic hydrolysis of a heptapeptide from the N-terminus. Lysophospholipids accumulate in intestinal contents. Cholesteryl esters are hydrolysed by a pancreatic cholesteryl ester hydrolase.

Lipid absorption in humans occurs largely in the jejunum. The lipids pass through the brush border membrane of the enterocytes as monoacylglycerol

and free-chain fatty acids (Figure 27.5). The rate-limiting step in the uptake of lipids is the unstirred water at the surface of the microvillus. Chain length can affect fatty acid absorption, e.g. partially hydrogenated fish oil contains a significant amount of *trans* fatty acids, but with hydrogenation there is an increase in very long-chain fatty acids, which are not well absorbed. Bile acids pass down to the ileum for absorption or into the caecum to be deconjugated and 7-α-dehydroxylated before reabsorption from the colon or excretion in the faeces.

Absorption into the enterocyte

Fat slows the movement of luminal contents (the 'ileal brake'). The process of absorption into the enterocyte involves an inward diffusion gradient of

Classification of lipids in terms of interaction with water

Non-swelling amphiphile lipids have little solubility in water in the bulk phase. They form a thin layer of lipid when added to water. Insoluble swelling amphiphiles in water form laminated lipid water structures called liquid crystals. The non-polar groups of the lipid molecules face each other, with water sandwiched between.

Non-polar:
- cholesteryl ester

- hydrocarbons
- carotene.

Insoluble non-swelling amphiphiles:
- triacylglycerols
- diacylglycerols
- fat-soluble vitamins.

Insoluble swelling amphiphiles:
- monoacylglycerols
- ionised fatty acids
- phospholipids.

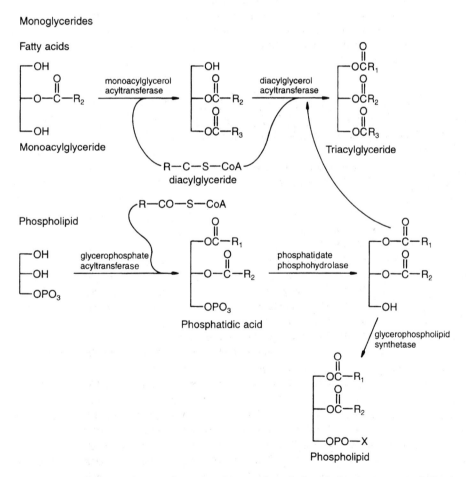

Fig. 27.5 Intracellular metabolism of monoglycerides, fatty acids and phospholipids. Post-prandially, the monoglyceride fatty acid pathway is the most important in the synthesis of triacylglycerol. During fasting the phospholipid pathway (α-glycerophosphate) becomes a major pathway for the formation of triacylglycerol. 2-Monoglyceride inhibits the α-glycerophosphate pathway.

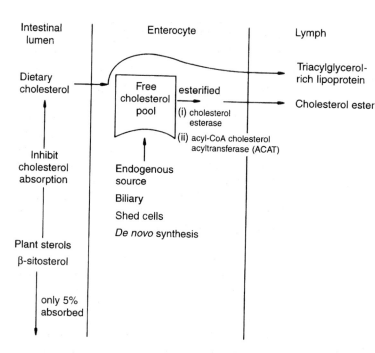

Fig. 27.6 Absorption of cholesterol and plant sterols. Dietary cholesterol and cholesterol of endogenous sources, biliary shed cells and cholesterol from *de novo* synthesis enter the enterocyte. Dietary cholesterol passes into lymph as triacylglycerol-rich lipoprotein. Free cholesterol is esterified by cholesterol esterase or acyl-CoA cholesterol acyltransferase, the cholesterol ester being transported into the lymph. Plant sterols, e.g. β-sitosterol, are minimally absorbed and inhibit cholesterol absorption in the small intestine.

lipid products. Fatty acids enter the cell and bind to a fatty acid binding protein. The protein binds long-chain and unsaturated fatty acids in preference to saturated acids. The next phase is an energy-dependent re-esterification of the absorbed fatty acids into triacylglycerols and phospholipids. The free fatty acids are converted into acyl-coenzyme A (CoA) thioesters. Long-chain fatty acids are the preferred substrate for esterification to 2-monoacylglycerols, the major forms of absorbed lipids through the monoacylglycerol pathway.

The major absorbed products of phospholipid digestion are monoacyl phosphatidylcholines. Fatty acids are re-esterified at position 1 to form phosphatidylcholine by an acyl transferase in the tips of the intestinal brush border. This phospholipid stabilises the triacylglycerol particles or chylomicrons.

Absorption of cholesterol is slower and less complete than that of other lipids (some 55% is absorbed). There is also a loss of absorbed sterol through desquamation of cells. Most of the absorbed cholesterol is esterified by cholesteryl esterase or acyl-CoA:cholesterol acyl transferase (Figure 27.6). Plant sterols, e.g. sitosterol, are not absorbed, their absorption being prevented at the intestinal mucosal level by sterolin-1 and sterolin-

2 proteins. Any plant sterol that is absorbed is rapidly excreted into bile by a sterolin-1 and 2 mechanism in the liver.

TRANSPORT OF LIPIDS INTO THE BLOOD

Many factors determine the post-prandial concentration of lipids, including age, gender, and the amount of fat, sucrose and fructose in the meal. Other factors include rate of intestinal digestion and absorption, rate of synthesis of chylomicrons and flow into the lymphatics. Dietary triglycerides enter the bloodstream relatively slowly and reach a peak over 3–5 h. The shape of the absorption curve is affected by the amount of carbohydrate present in the meal. The raised triglyceride concentration can persist from breakfast until 3 a.m., as a consequent of the cumulative effect of the regular meals through the day. The dietary fatty acids affect the rate of decline of the increased triglyceride concentration, with long-chain n-3 fatty acids being the most effective in reducing the raised concentration.

Table 27.1 Lipoprotein molecules

Lipoprotein	Source
Chylomicrons	Intestine
Very low-density lipoproteins (VLDL)	Liver
Intermediate-density lipoprotein (IDL)	VLDL catabolism
Low-density lipoproteins (LDL)	IDL catabolism
High-density lipoproteins (HDL)	Liver, intestine

Lipids are transported in blood as apolipoproteins, which stabilise the lipid particles with a coat of amphiphilic compounds of phospholipids and proteins. These vary in physical form, but their function is to transport lipids from one tissue to another. Lipoproteins contain a core of neutral lipids, cholesterol esters and triglycerides, and a surface coat of more polar lipids, unesterified cholesterol and phospholipids and apoproteins. The surface coat, which in many ways resembles the cell–plasma membrane, is an interface between the plasma and the non-polar lipid core. Lipoproteins differ in the ratio of lipid to protein, as well as having different proportions of lipids, triacylglycerols, free and esterified cholesterol and phospholipids. The biological function varies with the size of the lipoprotein molecule; these are shown in Table 27.1, from lowest to highest densities. None of these groups is a single entity and each contains a wide variety of particle sizes and chemical composition.

Fat dropules are found post-prandially in the smooth endoplasmic reticulum, where the enzymes of the monoacylglycerol pathways are found. Here, there is synthesis of phospholipids and apolipoproteins which coat the lipid dropules. Long-chain fatty acids are transported in chylomicrons. Fatty acids with a chain length of less than 12 carbon atoms are absorbed in the free form, pass into the portal vein and are metabolised directly by β-oxidation in the liver. This is because of their more ready hydrolysis from triacylglycerols and their solubility in water.

APOLIPOPROTEINS

The protein moieties of lipoproteins solubilise lipid particles and ensure continued structural integrity. They are important in determining the lipoprotein type and how it is metabolised. They are cofactors in the activation of enzymes involved in the modification of lipoproteins. They interact with specific cell-surface receptors which remove lipoproteins from the plasma. The lipoproteins are classified either by their density or by their electrophoretic mobility. ApoBs are the largest apolipoproteins. The complete amino sequences of all of these are known.

ApoAs (types A-I, A-II and A-IV) are synthesised by both liver and intestine, and are present in both chylomicrons and HDL.

ApoB exists as two variants of different molecular mass (approximately 100 and 48 kDa) designated as $apoB_H$ (heavy) and $apoB_L$ (light) or apoB-100 and apoB-48, respectively. Human VLDL contains the heavy variant, whereas rat VLDL contains both. ApoB-48 is of intestinal origin and forms part of the chylomicron. ApoB-100 is synthesised in the liver and forms part of the surface coat of the triacylglycerol-rich VLDL, IDL and cholesterol rich-LDL. ApoB has a β-sheet protein structure in addition to regions of random coil and α-helices. ApoB is a glycoprotein linked to glucosamine through asparagine residues.

ApoC is synthesised in the liver and contributes part of the chylomicrons, VLDL, IDL and HDL. There are three types, C-I, C-II and C-III, of low molecular weight 5800–8750 Da.

The apoproteins E, E-2, E-3 and E-4 are synthesised in the liver and peripheral tissues, have a molecular weight of 35 kDa and differ only in the

The isoforms of apoE are genetically transmitted, an isoform from each parent. Six genotypes exist: E-3/E-3 is found most frequently (two-thirds of the US population); E-3/E-4, 22%; E-3/E-2, 12%; and E-4/E-4, E-4/E-2 and E-2/E-2, less than 2%. These apoproteins are involved in chylomicrons, VLDL, IDL and HDL. The $apoE_4$ isoform has an increased serum cholesterol and LDL concentration and risk of cardiovascular disease, late-onset Alzheimer's disease and gallstone formation.

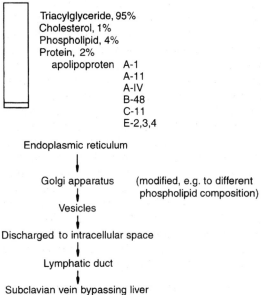

(a) CHYLOMICRON (80–500 nm diameter;
                 predominant post-prandially)

Triacylglyceride, 95%
Cholesterol, 1%
Phospholipid, 4%
Protein, 2%
    apolipoproten A-1
                   A-11
                   A-IV
                   B-48
                   C-11
                   E-2,3,4

Endoplasmic reticulum
          ↓
Golgi apparatus   (modified, e.g. to different
          ↓   phospholipid composition)
     Vesicles
          ↓
Discharged to intracellular space
          ↓
   Lymphatic duct
          ↓
Subclavian vein bypassing liver

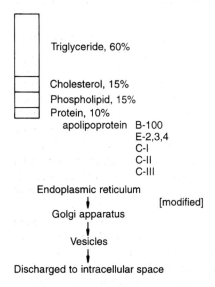

(b) VERY LOW-DENSITY LIPOPROTEIN (30–80 nm diameter;
                                 produced during fasting)

Triglyceride, 60%

Cholesterol, 15%
Phospholipid, 15%
Protein, 10%
    apolipoprotein B-100
                    E-2,3,4
                    C-I
                    C-II
                    C-III

Endoplasmic reticulum
          ↓   [modified]
Golgi apparatus
          ↓
     Vesicles
          ↓
Discharged to intracellular space

Fig. 27.7 (a) Intestinal lipoprotein assembly. Chylomicrons are produced post-prandially: 95% triacylglycerol, 1% cholesterol, 4% phospholipid and 2% apolipoprotein. Apolipoproteins are assembled as pre-chylomicrons in the endoplasmic reticulum, and pass to the Golgi apparatus to be modified. The phospholipid composition is altered before discharge into the intracellular spaces by vesicles. (b) Very low-density lipoproteins (VLDL) are produced in the liver, predominantly during fasting. VLDL are formed as 60% triglycerol, 15% cholesterol, 15% phospholipid and 10% protein. The assembly of VLDL passes through different pathways to chylomicrons. VLDL pass through the endoplasmic reticulum and Golgi apparatus and are excreted via vesicles.

amino acid-occupying position 112 and 158. ApoE is found in all plasma lipoprotein fractions except for LDL. Cholesterol metabolism is different in subjects with different isoforms. $ApoE_4$ is associated with increased intestinal cholesterol absorption and faster chylomicron remnant clearance from the circulation. This suppresses the expression of LDL receptors and 3-hydroxy-3-methylglutaryl-coenzyme A (HMG-CoA) reductase activity and increased serum LDL cholesterol concentration. Individuals with $apoE_2$ have the opposite responses.

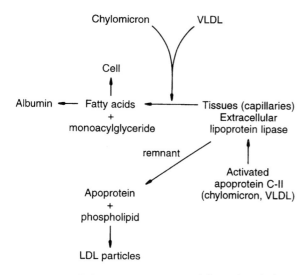

Fig. 27.8 Chylomicrons carry triacylglycerol and cholesterol ester from the intestine to other tissues in the body. Very low-density lipoproteins (VLDL) similarly carry lipids from the liver and the intestine. In tissue capillaries, extracellular lipoprotein lipase is activated by apoprotein C-II and hydrolyses triacylglycerol to produce fatty acids and monoacyl glycerides, which are absorbed into the cell. Some fatty acids may bind to albumin to be transported to other tissues. The chylomicron and VLDL remnants, apoproteins and phospholipids become LDL particles.

LIPOPROTEINS

Chylomicrons

Chylomicrons (Figure 27.7a) are the largest and least dense of the lipoproteins (diameter 80–500 nm). Their function is to transport lipids of exogenous or dietary origin (Figure 27.8). Chylomicrons can be measured in the plasma after a fatty meal, their size depending on the rate of lipid absorption and the type of dietary fatty acids that predominate. Larger chylomicrons are produced after the consumption of large amounts of fat at the peak of absorption or when apolipoprotein synthesis is rate limiting. They contain triacylglycerols with small amounts of phospholipids and sufficient protein to cover the surface. The core lipid contains some cholesteryl esters and fat-soluble substances, fat-soluble vitamins, etc.

Several apoproteins are present in the chylomicron surface layer: apoB-48, apoA$_1$, apoA$_4$, the apoC group and apoE. The apoB-48 and apoA series apolipoproteins are synthesised in the endoplasmic reticulum of the intestinal epithelial cells, whereas apoCs and apoE are acquired from other lipoproteins once the chylomicrons have entered the blood. The apoE and apoCs are important in the catabolism of the chylomicron.

The chylomicrons pass initially into the lymph and hence to the thoracic duct and into the bloodstream. In the circulation, lipoprotein lipase, an enzyme on the capillary endothelium cell surface, hydrolyses the triglyceride fatty acids. Large amounts of free fatty acids, apoA and apoC are released. The chylomicron remnant returns to the liver and is removed from circulation. The released fatty acids are held in solution in the plasma bound to albumin. They are subsequently metabolised in two main ways:

- transported to adipose tissue for incorporation into triglycerides; when required, these can be released through the action of adipose tissue lipase
- used by the liver as a fuel source or stored as triglyceride.

The triacylglycerols release the fatty acids; apoC$_2$ plays a key role in activating lipoprotein lipase. The peptide facilitates an interaction of the enzyme with the lipoprotein interphase catalysing hydrolysis of long-chain rather than short-chain fatty acids. This is a rapid hydrolysis, taking only 2–3 min; the apolipoprotein and the remaining apoC are transferred to HDL with the phospholipids. The remnant chylomicron particle, although reverting to the same basic structure, contains fewer triacylglycerols and is rich in cholesterol esters. These are not able to compete for lipoprotein lipase and circulate in the plasma to be taken up by liver cells by a receptor-mediated endocytosis. The receptors in the liver bind to the apoE component of the remnant. There is then a complete hydrolysis of the lipid and protein component.

The regulation of lipoprotein lipase is crucial to the control of lipoprotein metabolism in different tissues in the body. The enzyme is synthesised in the parenchymal cells of the tissues and secreted into the capillary endothelium, bound to the cell surface by sulfated glycosaminoglycan, the activities of which are regulated by diet and hormones, particularly insulin. The secretion of insulin results in increased adipose tissue lipoprotein lipase activity. The equivalent muscle enzyme is suppressed. In fasting, the adipose tissue lipoprotein lipase activity is suppressed and the hormone-sensitive lipase activated, allowing the mobilisation of free fatty acids. Muscle lipoprotein lipase activity is raised and fatty acids from circulating lipoproteins can be used as fuel.

During lactation, lipoprotein lipase is regulated by prolactin, which promotes the utilisation of chylomicron triacylglycerol fatty acids for milk synthesis.

Very low-density lipoproteins

These consist predominantly of triacylglycerols and transport triacylglycerols of endogenous origin derived from the liver and intestine (Figure 27.7b). They are spherical particles (30–80 nm), smaller than chylomicrons. There is a core of predominantly triacylglycerols and some cholesteryl esters, with cholesterol, phospholipids and proteins on the surface. The composition and the classification depend on the method of isolation, the species, nutrition and physiological state of the animal. The major apoprotein is apoB-100; the amount of apoB per VLDL is dependent on the particle mass and is similar to the composition of LDL. Other lipoproteins include apoC-I, C-II and C-III and apoE.

> As the apoB-100 passes towards the smooth endoplasmic reticulum, there is admixing with the triglyceride and cholesteryl esters at the junction of the smooth and rough endoplasmic reticulum. This creates nascent VLDL particles; these pass from the smooth endoplasmic reticulum to the Golgi apparatus. Secretory vesicles bud off and migrate to the surface with VLDL for release into the plasma.

Glucose is converted into the lipid precursor glycerol-3(sn) phosphate through the glycolytic pathway and long-chain fatty acids through the malonyl-CoA pathway. Some fatty acids arise from circulating free fatty acids bound to albumin. The triglycerides and small amounts of cholesteryl ester are synthesised by membrane-bound enzymes in the smooth endoplasmic reticulum.

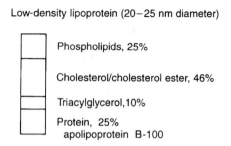

Low-density lipoprotein (20–25 nm diameter)

Phospholipids, 25%

Cholesterol/cholesterol ester, 46%

Triacylglycerol, 10%

Protein, 25%
apolipoprotein B-100

Fig. 27.9 Low-density lipoproteins (LDL) transport cholesterol to the tissues. The coat, which is hydrophobic, consists of cholesterol and phospholipids, and the hydrophobic core consists of cholesterol esters and triglycerides. Surface apoprotein B is important in LDL receptor recognition. The LDL are produced from very low-density lipoproteins (VLDL). Lipoprotein lipase removes triglyceride from the core of the VLDL to form intermediate-density lipoprotein (IDL), which may be further metabolised by lipoprotein lipase and hepatic lipase to LDL. Triglycerides are removed from LDL to produce VLDL and cholesterol esters pass from VLDL to LDL. The LDL lipoproteins belong to several classes: the smaller particles have a higher protein/lipid ratio; the larger particles have more triglyceride.

The major site of synthesis of VLDL is in the liver, although some is produced in the enterocyte. VLDLs receive their full complement of apoproteins by synthesis in the liver or from enterocyte rough endoplasmic reticulum.

The VLDL circulating in the bloodstream is converted into mature VLDL through incorporation of cholesterol esters, apoC-II and apoC-III, and possibly apoE. These are transferred from HDL.

At the same time there is release of phospholipids, most apoCs and some apoEs, which move onto HDL. Remnant VLDL is now rich in cholesterol esters which include some transferred from HDL. The remnant VLDL may be removed by the liver through receptors on liver cells, including those for chylomicron remnants and LDL. The latter recognises apoB-100 or apoE. Some VLDL remnant triglycerides are hydrolysed by hepatic triglyceride lipase, producing a cholesterol-rich LDL. This involves the release of fatty acids, apoE and apoC.

Low-density lipoproteins

The function of LDLs is to transport cholesterol to tissues. They have a diameter of approximately

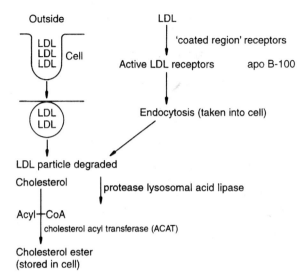

Fig. 27.10 LDL catabolism. LDL is taken up by receptors in the liver and extrahepatic tissues. The LDL particles bind to coated regions which contain active LDL receptors. This is followed by the LDL particles being taken up into the cell by endocytosis. The LDL particle is degraded by protease and lysosomal acid lipase. Cellular cholesterol inhibits HMG-CoA reductase and stimulates cholesterol acyltransferase. The cholesterol ester produced is stored in the cell. The cholesterol ester inhibits the production of LDL receptors and limits the uptake of LDL.

20–25 nm and a lipid core that is essentially cholesterol. The surface of the particle comprises unesterified cholesterol, phospholipids and apoB-100. The cholesterol is available for incorporation into membrane structure or conversion into various metabolites, e.g. steroid hormones. Each lipoprotein particle contains the same mass of apoB-100, but differs in the amount of bound lipid (Figure 27.9).

LDL is derived from VLDL by a series of steps that remove triacylglycerol, through the VLDL remnant which originates from the VLDL particle. This results in particles with progressively smaller proportions of triacylglycerol and increasing amounts of cholesterol and phospholipids. Such reactions take place initially in adipose tissue capillaries and subsequently in the liver. The apoB-100 remains with the LDL particle, and apoC and apoE are progressively lost. The synthesis of LDL is dependent on the amount of VLDL produced by

the liver and the proportion of VLDL removed by the liver. This latter reaction is dependent on the number of LDL receptors that remove VLDL remnants. These same receptors dictate the concentration of LDLs and their removal from the circulation.

ApoB-100 is important in that it interacts with specific cell-surface receptors before the LDL particle is taken up and metabolised by the cells. Macrophage receptors recognise modified LDL and are responsible for the degradation of LDL particles that are not recognised by normal cell-surface LDL receptors. ApoE plays a role in receptor binding, while the C group apolipoproteins are involved in reactions by which the particles are sequentially degraded by lipases.

LDLs are principally removed by specific extrahepatic LDL receptors. LDLs are less efficiently removed by hepatic receptors, which take the receptor–ligand complex into the cell lysosomes (Figure 27.10). The distribution of LDL to various tissues depends on the rate of transcapillary transport as well as the number of LDL receptors on the cell surface. Adipose tissue and muscles have few LDL receptors and take up LDL only slowly. The adrenal gland is important in the synthesis of steroid hormones and takes up LDL avidly. The LDL receptor has a recognition site for both apoE and apoB.

About 80% of the LDL receptors are concentrated in the clathrin-coated pits which, nevertheless, represent only 2% of the cell surface. Negatively charged residues bind electrostatically with the positively charged region of apoE. This lipoprotein binds at several receptor sites, apoB having a single site. Once bound to the receptor, the LDL receptor complex is taken into the cell and the LDL degraded by lysosomal enzymes. The receptor is recycled within minutes and reutilised many times before eventual catabolism. The number of LDL receptors is regulated by regulatory proteins and genes, according to the amount of cholesterol in the cell.

In the cell, cholesterol esters are hydrolysed by cholesteryl ester hydrolase. The incorporation of cholesterol into the endoplasmic reticulum membrane inhibits HMG-CoA reductase, the rate-limiting enzyme in cholesterol biosynthesis. The cholesterol may be stored within the cell as the cholesterol ester, incorporated into membranes or

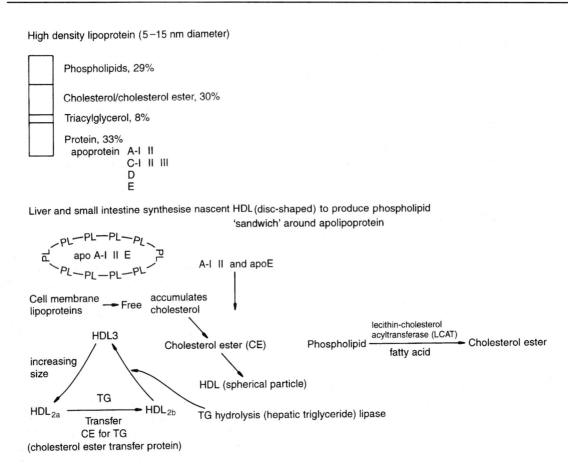

Fig. 27.11 Formation of high-density lipoprotein (HDL). HDL are spheres consisting of phospholipids (29%), cholesterol and cholesterol ester (CE; 30%), triacylglycerol (8%) and protein (33%). They are formed in the liver and small intestine from nascent HDL and accumulate cholesterol, which is converted to cholesterol esters by lecithin–cholesterol acyltransferase (LCAT), the fatty acid being obtained from phospholipid. The smallest spherical form of HDL is HDL_3. As cholesterol accumulates, HDL_{2a} is formed. HDL_{2a} is converted into HDL_{2b} by the addition of triglyceride (TG) from triglyceride-rich lipoproteins, catalysed by cholesterol ester transfer protein. HDL_{2b} is converted to HDL_3 by triglyceride hydrolysis through hepatic triglyceride lipase.

exported to the plasma. In liver cells there is conversion to bile acids for excretion in bile.

High-density lipoproteins

The function of HDL (Figure 27.11) is to remove unesterified cholesterol from peripheral tissues and transport it to the liver to be degraded and excreted, possibly in the form of bile acids.

HDL particle size is 5–15 nm. HDLs are usually grouped into two classes, HDL_2 and HDL_3. The smallest spherical form of HDL is HDL_3. HDL_2 appears to have a stronger inverse relationship with

cardiovascular disease than HDL_3. The major apolipoproteins of HDL are $apoA_1$ and $apoA_2$. The former is a monomer of molecular weight 28 kDa; the latter is a dimer of this monomer, linked by a disulfide bond. The surface coat also contains some apoC, apoE and apoD, the latter being found only in HDL. Additional surface components, phospholipids and cholesterol are acquired by transfer from chylomicrons and VLDL during their catabolism by lipoprotein lipase. The first step is the synthesis of nascent HDL in both liver and intestine. Nascent HDL accepts unesterified cholesterol from cells or other lipoproteins. ApoA synthesised in the intestine and some apoC are transferred

Low-density lipoprotein receptors

These consist of a number of domains. The domain that binds LDL consists of 292 amino acids and comprises a number of 40 amino acid repeat sequences. It is orientated to the luminal side of the cell membrane and is able to bind both apoB and apoE simultaneously. The second domain is approximately 400 amino acids and is similar in sequence structure to epidermal growth factor. The third, which is 58 amino acids, is where the carbohydrate residues are linked. The fourth domain (22 amino acids in size) crosses the plasma membrane, i.e. it is a transmembrane domain. The fifth (50 amino acids) projects into the cytoplasm and may have a role in the clustering of the receptors into coated pits. These migrate in the plane of the membrane until they reach a pit coated with the protein clathrin.

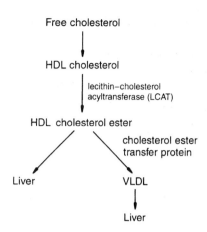

Fig. 27.12 High-density lipoprotein (HDL) carries cholesterol to the liver by reverse cholesterol transport. Free cholesterol attaches to the HDL sphere. The cholesterol is esterified by lecithin–cholesterol acyltransferase (LCAT). Some cholesterol ester is transferred to the VDL and LDL to be carried to the liver by cholesterol ester transfer protein. HDL also carries cholesterol to the liver.

during the breakdown of chylomicrons. Further apoC is transferred from VLDL breakdown products.

As cholesterol accumulates in the plasma, subfractions of HDL containing $apoA_1$ and apoD become associated specifically with the enzyme lecithin–cholesterol acyltransferase (LCAT). This enzyme catalyses the transfer of fatty acids from phosphatidylcholine to cholesterol to form a cholesterol ester. The phospholipid substrate is transferred from chylomicron remnants or IDL during the degradation of chylomicrons or VLDL. LCAT, by consuming cholesterol, enables its transfer from non-hepatic cells from plasma and other lipoproteins to a site of esterification. Molecules of cholesterol ester are transferred to lipoproteins containing apoB-100 or apoE, and are taken up by the liver. This transfers fatty acid from phosphatidylcholine to cholesterol on the surface of the disc-shaped HDL to form cholesterol esters, which accumulate in the core of the HDL particle.

Lysophosphatidylcholine is transferred to plasma albumin, from which it is rapidly removed from blood and reacylated with fatty acids. During this distribution of lipid the particle changes from dis-. coid to spherical in shape.

As HDL_3 increases in size, HDL_2 develops, initially as HDL_{2a} which, in turn, is converted into HDL_{2b}, wherein cholesterol ester is exchanged for triglycerides. These triglycerides are obtained from VLDL lipoproteins which, in turn, are replenished with cholesterol ester from the HDL. This exchange is facilitated by cholesterol ester transfer protein. HDL_{2b} is converted back to HDL_3 through the loss of triglycerides by hepatic triglyceride lipase. This whole process is called reverse cholesterol transport (Figure 27. 12). A single protein, ABCA1, regulates HDL production and cholesterol absorption. ABCA1 protein is one of a superfamily of membrane transporters that binds and hydrolyses adenosine triphosphate (ATP) to drive substances across membranes. The efflux of cholesterol from a cell is aided by the binding of apoA-1 ABCA1. This is the first stage in the transport of cholesterol on HDL to the liver, conversion to bile acids and excretion. The cholesterol-induced increase in ABCA1 expression is affected by two nuclear receptor family members, which are intracellular transcription factors activated by steroid hormones and metabolites.

Other lipoproteins

Serum albumin binds many types of molecule, including free fatty acids. As such, it is the main transporter of free fatty acids released by lipases from adipose tissue into the blood. There are three classes of binding sites, which bind two, five and 20 molecules of fatty acids, respectively. Other fatty acid-binding proteins such as z protein transport fatty acids and acyl-CoA within cells, rather than in the blood. Phospholipids may be transported in cells by binding to phospholipid exchange proteins, which introduce lipids into plasma membranes and organelle membranes remote from their sites of synthesis.

LIPID ABSORPTION IN EARLY LIFE

The newborn animal adapts rapidly to a diet of breast milk with a relatively high fat content. The pancreatic secretion of lipase is rather low and the immature liver secretes insufficient bile salts for lipid digestion. This is particularly marked in the premature infant. However, the infant is able to digest fat as a result of the activity of a lipase secreted by the tongue, This is active in the stomach at a pH of 4.5–5.5, and does not require bile salts. Secretion of oral lipase is stimulated by sucking and the presence of fat in the mouth. The products are mainly 2-monoacylglycerols, the free fatty acids being predominantly medium-chain fatty acids. Milk fat in most mammals is relatively rich in medium-chain fatty acids. There may also be a lipase in human milk that facilitates the digestion of milk lipids.

On weaning, the site of fat digestion changes from the stomach to the duodenum.

KEY POINTS

1. Fat digestion takes place in the small intestine. Pancreatic esterase and lipase enzymes are involved in the degradation of the lipid before it is absorbed.
2. The fat emulsion, on entering the stomach, is modified by mixing with bile and pancreatic juice. The pancreas secretes enzymes which release fatty acids from triacylglycerols (lipase), phospholipids (phospholipase A_2) and cholesterol esters (cholesterol esterase).
3. Lipid absorption in humans occurs largely in the jejunum by passing through the brush border membrane of the enterocytes as mono-acylglycerol and free-chain fatty acids. Fatty acids enter the cell and bind to a fatty acid binding protein (or z protein), followed by an energy-dependent re-esterification of the absorbed fatty acids into triacylglycerols and phospholipids.
4. The major absorbed products of phospholipid digestion are monoacylphosphatidylcholines, which are re-esterified to form phosphatidylcholine.
5. Cholesterol absorption is slower and less complete than that of other lipids.
6. Lipids are transported in the blood within apolipoprotein complexes, classified by their densities as chylomicrons, very low-density lipoproteins (VLDL), low-density lipoproteins (LDL) and high-density lipoproteins (HDL).
7. Fatty acids with a chain length of less than 12 carbon atoms are absorbed in the free form and pass to the liver, where they are metabolised by β-oxidation.
8. The protein moieties of lipoproteins solubilise lipid particles, are cofactors in the activation of enzymes involved in the modification of lipoproteins and interact with specific cell-surface receptors which remove lipoproteins from the plasma.
9. Chylomicrons are the largest and least dense lipoproteins; they transport lipids of exogenous or dietary origin to adipose tissue for incorporation into triglycerides. These can be released through the action of adipose tissue lipase; alternatively, fatty acids may be used by the liver as a fuel source or stored as triglyceride.
10. VLDL consists predominantly of triacylglycerols and transports triacylglycerols of endogenous origin derived from the liver and intestine. The major site of synthesis of VLDL is the liver or enterocytes.
11. LDL transports cholesterol to tissues; it is derived from VLDL, initially in adipose tissue capillaries and subsequently in the liver. LDLs are removed by specific extrahepatic LDL receptors and less efficiently by hepatic receptors. The LDL receptor complex is taken into the cell and the LDL degraded by lysosomal enzymes.

12. In the cell, cholesterol esters are hydrolysed by cholesterol ester hydrolase. Cellular cholesterol inhibits β-hydroxy-β-methyl glutaryl-coenzyme A reductase (HMG-CoA reductase), the rate-limiting enzyme in cholesterol biosynthesis.

13. HDL removes unesterified cholesterol from peripheral tissues for transport to the liver. HDL is synthesised in both liver and intestine and accepts unesterified cholesterol from cells or other lipoproteins. Lecithin–cholesterol acyltransferase (LCAT) catalyses the transfer of fatty acids from phosphatidylcholine to cholesterol to form a cholesterol ester.

14. The newborn adapts rapidly to a diet of breast milk with a relatively high fat content. The pancreatic secretion of lipase is rather low and the immature liver secretes insufficient bile salts for lipid digestion; this is particularly marked in premature infants.

THINKING POINTS

1. The absorption and handling of fat in the body necessitates complex systems to make the fats water soluble.
2. The complicated system is achieved by detergents in the intestine and proteins in the blood.

NEED TO UNDERSTAND

1. Triglycerides are the most significant contributor to fat in the diet.
2. In the intestine fat is reduced to a slightly more water-soluble form and further solubilised by bile acid and phospholipids.
3. Following absorption the fats are solubilised for transport to and from the liver by incorporation into lipoproteins and by binding to albumin.

4. This complex system is of great significance in health and disease.
5. Other lipids are dealt with in a similar manner.

FURTHER READING

Bruce, C., Chouinard, R.A. and Tall, A.R. (1998) Plasma lipid transfer proteins, high density lipoproteins and reverse cholesterol transport. *Annual Review of Nutrition*, **18**, 297–330.

Frayn, K.N. (1998) Dietary factors and postprandial lipaemia. *British Journal of Nutrition*, **80**, 409–10.

Griffin, B.A. (1997) Low-density lipoprotein subclasses: mechanisms of formation and modulations. *Proceedings of the Nutrition Society*, **56**, 693–707.

Johnson, L.R., Alpers, D.H., Christensen, J. *et al.* (1994) *Physiology of the Gastrointestinal Tract*. Raven Press, New York.

Lairon, D. and Frayn, K.N. (1996) Lipid absorption and metabolism. *Proceedings of the Nutrition Society*, **55**, 1–154.

Livesey, G. (2000) The absorption of stearic acid from triacylglycerols: an enquiry and analysis. *Nutrition Research Reviews*, **13**, 185–214.

McLaughlin, J.T., Troncon, L.E., Barlow, J. *et al.* (1998) Evidence for a lipid specific effect in nutrient induced human proximal gastric relaxation. *Gut*, **43**, 248–51.

Symposium (1996) Lipid absorption and metabolism: physiological and molecular aspects. *Proceedings of the Nutrition Society*, **55**, 1–155.

Van Erpecum, K.J. and Carey, M.C. (1996) Apolipoprotein E4, another risk factor for cholesterol gallstone formation. *Gastroenterology*, **111**, 1764–6.

Wade, D.P. and Owen, J.S. (2001) Regulation of the cholesterol efflux gene *ABCA1*. *Lancet*, **357**, 161–3.

Williams, C.M. (1997) Post prandial lipid metabolism: effects of dietary fatty acids. *Proceedings of the Nutrition Society*, **56**, 679–92.

28

Foetal and placental nutrition

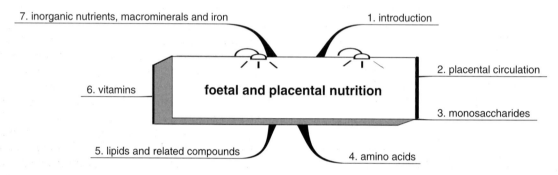

7. inorganic nutrients, macrominerals and iron

1. introduction

6. vitamins

foetal and placental nutrition

2. placental circulation

3. monosaccharides

5. lipids and related compounds

4. amino acids

Fig. 28.1 Chapter outline.

INTRODUCTION

The foetus is a separate unit from the mother; they are attached by the placenta, an important organ which serves both as a protector of, and source of nourishment for the developing foetus. During the first days following conception and implantation of the fertilised human ovum, nutrition is from local sources. Thereafter, the nutrition of the foetus is dependent on nutrition from the mother through the placenta. For the first 4–5 months, placental growth is greater than that of the foetus, but thereafter foetal growth exceeds that of the placenta. By full term at 40 weeks, the weight of foetus, placenta and liquor amnii is 5 kg, 3.5 kg of which is the baby and 0.5 kg the placenta.

The placenta is a defined, transporting organ by the fourth week of pregnancy, which not only transports nutrients, but also is a source of oxygen to the foetus. The placenta is the means whereby carbon dioxide and substances excreted by the bowel and kidneys of the foetus are eliminated into the maternal circulation.

It is increasingly appreciated that the health of the baby is a determinate of the well-being of the mother. The diet of the pregnant mother may be the most important contribution to the health of a population.

PLACENTAL CIRCULATION

There are three features to the circulation of the placenta:

- the relationship between the maternal and foetal circulation within the placenta
- the uterine circulation, which supplies maternal blood to the placenta
- the umbilical circulation, which supplies blood to the foetus.

At the onset of pregnancy, the maternal blood vessels under the developing embryo become dilated. Small projections from the blastocyst, the chorionic villi, grow into these blood vessels. The foetal mesoderm invades the chorionic villi with the development of a blood-filled intervillous space and a core of capillaries and connective tissue. The chorionic villi dip into the maternal blood, separated by three thin layers: the foetal vascular epithelium, the connective tissue of the villus and the trophoblast. The trophoblast is tissue that attaches the ovum to the uterine wall. The maternal blood supply enters the intervillous space under pressure, spreads to the chorion plate and passes laterally and downwards past the capillary bed of the foetal villi to the basal plate. The blood then drains into the uterine veins.

In a multiple pregnancy there may be different rates of growth, so one twin or triplet may be malnourished in comparison with the others.

MONOSACCHARIDES

Glucose is the principal substrate of the foetus and placenta. The placental transfer system is stereospecific, GLUT1 and GLUT3 can be saturated, and is a mediated process, i.e. not a sodium-dependent concentrating glucose transporter. These transporters respond in activity to maternal glucose concentrations. Thus, the placenta cannot concentrate glucose against a concentration gradient, and maternal plasma glucose concentration determines the transfer of glucose to the placenta and foetus. This placental transfer capacity increases as the foetus matures. Glucose transfer in the foetus is regulated by membrane localised glucose transporters, GLUT1. In the brain the foetus uses GLUT3 for neuronal glucose uptake and glial cells use GLUT1. Cardiac and skeletal cells use GLUT1, as do adiopocytes, which change to GLUT4 later in gestation.

Foetal hypoglycaemia may occur as the foetus develops. It is secondary to increased insulin concentrations and more foetal tissue being insulin sensitive, and hence increased demands by the foetus. This is due to insulin-induced GLUT1 and possibly GLUT4 expression.

Monocarboxylates and dicarboxylates

The metabolism of glucose within the placenta produces lactate at a high rate, which is delivered into the foetal and maternal circulation. The lactate carrier of the brush border membrane is sodium independent. The system is specific for monocarboxylates, e.g. lactate, pyruvate and β-hydroxybutyrate. There is a separate high-affinity transport system for dicarboxylic acids that requires a transmembrane electrical sodium gradient.

Insulin regulates glucose metabolism and transport, as well as foetal growth, by increasing glucose, lipid and amino acid in tissues. Insulin-like growth factors (IGFs) and IGF-binding proteins are important in foetal and post-partum life. They respond to foetal glucose supply, concentration and insulin production, responding to intracellular glucose concentration for gene transcription control. IGF-1 limits protein breakdown. There is a positive relationship between foetal plasma IGF-1 concentration, foetal growth, size at birth and growth of individual organs. IGF-1 has important effects on brain development and the myelination process, and increases the number of oligodendrocytes.

AMINO ACIDS

Amino acid transport across the placental membrane involves mediated transport through both the microvilli and basal membrane.

Monoamino, monocarboxy amino acids

The microvillous membrane of the placenta uses transport systems common to many cell types. This is quite different from intestinal brush border systems, which use specialised amino acid systems. Placental systems include:

- system A: a sodium-dependent transporter for alanine, serine, methyl amino isobutyric acid and proline
- system N: a sodium-dependent system for histidine and glutamine

- various sodium-independent systems, including leucine, tryptophan, tyrosine and phenylalanine.

There is a second sodium-independent system for alanine, serine and branched-chain and aromatic amino acids. Cellular regulation of amino acid transport involves regulation of transport systems with either of the maternal or foetal surface membranes.

Anionic amino acids

These are not concentrated in the foetal circulation and are not transferred between maternal and foetal circulations. Anionic amino acids are taken up from either or both circulations. Millimolar concentrations of aspartate and glutamate are present within the placenta, whereas concentrations in the maternal and foetal blood are in micromolar concentrations. There does not appear to be transport between mother and foetus.

Basic amino acids

The cationic amino acids, lysine and arginine, are concentrated in the foetal circulation and within the placenta. This concentration effect appears to be due to two sodium-independent transport systems in the basal membrane of the placenta.

β-Amino acids

The amino acid with the highest concentration in the placenta is the β-amino acid taurine, of which the foetus requires an exogenous supply. The active transport of taurine by the placenta results in foetal concentrations that are greater than maternal concentrations.

In conditions of foetal growth retardation, e.g. starvation in the mother, and consequent foetal hypoglycaemia, foetal protein breakdown increases, releasing amino acids which are then oxidised. Under these adverse conditions there is a shift from placental to foetal metabolism, with impoverishment of the placenta.

LIPIDS AND RELATED COMPOUNDS

Lipid uptake and metabolism are relatively mod-

est. Specific transporters transfer fatty acids. The foetus is very dependent on the maternal delivery of some essential long-chain polyunsaturated fatty acids important for brain development.

Lipoprotein lipase on the maternal surface of the placental membrane hydrolyses triacylglycerol carried by maternal very low-density lipoprotein (VLDL). The free fatty acids are taken up by the trophoblasts and may be used by the trophoblast or transferred to the foetus. The rate of fatty acid synthesis in the placenta is very high. Low-density lipoprotein (LDL)-cholesterol is taken up by receptor-mediated endocytosis and released in lysosomes. The liver, skeletal muscle and adipose tissue fatty acid synthase is active in the foetus, stimulated by glucose-enhanced production of malonyl-coenzyme A (CoA).

The cells of the growing foetus incorporate lipids into developing membranes. The foetus is dependent on the placental transfer of substrates from the mother, which can then be metabolised into lipids through:

- biosynthesis from glucose in foetal tissue
- incorporation of fatty acids transferred from maternal to foetal circulation
- incorporation of fatty acids from circulating maternal lipoproteins after release by a placental lipoprotein lipase
- biosynthesis of lipids in the placenta itself, which are then transferred to the foetal circulation.

In the foetus, glucose is a substrate for conversion into fatty acids and the glycerol moiety of glycerides. The placenta of most mammals is permeable to non-esterified fatty acids. There is a concentration of arachidonic acid in the placental circulation greater than that on the maternal side, a form of biomagnification. The ratio of n-3 to n-6 fatty acids may have implications for individual tissue development, for study in embryology.

The development of human fat cells begins in the last third of the gestation period. At birth, a baby weighing 3.5 kg contains between 500 and 600 g of adipose tissue. An important source of foetal fat reserves is circulating maternal lipids; consequently, the adipose tissue composition of the foetus and newborn infant reflects the fatty acid composition of the maternal diet. Concentrations of all lipoprotein classes increase in the maternal circulation during pregnancy, mediated by the sex hormones. Brown adipose tissue is present before white adipose fat in the foetus.

Many of the essential fatty acids required during the perinatal period are for brain growth. Of these, 50% are long-chain polyunsaturated fatty acids (PUFAs), e.g. arachidonic acid (C20:4, n-6), adrenic acid (C22:4, n-6), docosapentaenoic acid (C22:5, n-6) and docosahexaenoic acid (C22:6, n-3) (DHA). The maximum rate of brain development in humans is in late gestation and in the early postnatal period. Long-chain derivatives of linoleic acid increase in the brain from mid-gestation to term. Little linoleic acid accumulates until after delivery, when the concentration increases three-fold. It is possible that linoleic acid is metabolised in the brain and neural tissue to long-chain PUFAs throughout the perinatal period. The foetus obtains these fatty acids by placental transfer.

> The chemistry of the brain phospholipids is similar in most species. The concentration of essential fatty acids is low, at C18:2, n-6, 0.1–1.5%; and C18:3, n-3, 0.1–1%, while arachidonic acid C20:4, n-6 and docosahexaenoic C20:6, n-3 acids predominate, 18–27% and 13–29 %, respectively. This contrasts with the liver, where there is a great variety. The precursor essential fatty acids are present in greater concentrations in the brains of carnivores and omnivores than in vegetarians, with C22:6 predominating.

Phospholipids make up one-quarter of the solid matter of the brain and are important for brain functioning. There appears to be no blood–brain barrier to fatty acid transfer in the foetus and infant. Variations in composition of dietary PUFAs may lead to different concentrations of long-term PUFAs in brain tissue. There appears to be powerful genetic control on the incorporation of these fatty acids into the cerebral cortex, which overrides the effects of the wide variations in saturated and unsaturated fatty acid content of milk feeds for infants. It is thus predictable that human breast milk with higher DHA and dietary n-3 fatty acids concentrations will be reflected in higher concentrations of long-chain PUFAs in brain cortical tissue. This may be beneficial to infant neurodevelopment. Excessive intake of linoleic acid should be avoided as there may be inhibition of α-linolenic metabolism.

It is possible that deficiencies in maternal fatty acids that should have been provided to the foetus *in utero* will have consequences for brain and neurological development that may never be retrieved in later development. Maternal nutrition, especially in the early months of development, is crucial. In premature infants appropriate brain lipid development may not have been achieved. The diet after birth may be poorer in terms of long-chain fatty acids than that provided across the placenta.

At birth, the sole source of nutrition for the newborn baby is milk; some 50% of the available energy of milk is derived from fat. The baby's enzymes for fatty acid synthesis are suppressed and fat becomes the main source of energy and structure. Human fat contains a high proportion of long-chain PUFAs and this may be a response to the needs of the still-developing brain and nervous tissue. There are, however, wide differences in milk fat composition, depending on the mother's diet.

VITAMINS

Water-soluble vitamins

Dehydroascorbate is taken up more rapidly than ascorbate, by a sodium-independent transport system by the syncytiotrophoblast membrane. After absorption the dehydroascorbic acid is metabolised to ascorbic acid and released into the foetal circulation.

Folic acid is probably transported by a specialist protein system. A low-capacity riboflavin transport system, which is saturable, results in a concentration in the placenta and partial metabolism to flavin adenine dinucleotide (FAD) and flavin mononucleotide (FMN). Thiamin transport has many of the features of riboflavin transport. Concentrations of vitamin B_{12}, biotin, vitamin B_6, pantothenic acid and nicotinic acid are higher in umbilical cord blood at delivery than in maternal blood. Water-soluble vitamins are actively transported across the placenta.

Lipid-soluble vitamins

Vitamin A is normally transported in the blood as a complex of retinol and retinol-binding protein. It is probable that maternal retinol-binding protein crosses the placenta. Foetal retinol-binding protein production occurs late in gestation. A considerable fraction of retinol is esterified and stored by the human placenta, and subsequently hydrolysed and released into the foetal circulation unesterified. Concentrations of both 25(OH)-vitamin D_3 and 1,25(OH)$_2$-vitamin D_3 are similar between maternal and cord blood. This suggests a diffusion of vitamin D across the placenta. Concentrations of lipid-soluble vitamins E and K are higher in maternal plasma than in umbilical cord plasma.

INORGANIC NUTRIENTS, MACROMINERALS AND IRON

Increasingly large quantities of calcium are required to support the development of the growing foetal skeleton. Concentrations of total and ionic calcium in cord blood exceed those in maternal blood, which indicates that there is an active placental transfer system. The transport system is similar to that in the intestine and kidney, with partial saturation at physiological concentrations of maternal blood.

Little is currently known about the transfer of magnesium across the placenta.

Foetal serum concentrations of phosphate are higher than maternal concentrations. The substantial requirements of phosphate needed by the foetus in the last 3 months of pregnancy are transported against the concentration gradient.

Sodium transport across the brush border membrane of the placenta occurs by three mechanisms:

• Na^+/H^+ exchange
• cotransport with inorganic anions and organic solutes
• Na^+ conductants.

The Na^+/H^+ exchange produces an electroneutral coupling of sodium influx from the maternal circulation into the placental membrane cells, with H^+ reflux in the opposite direction.

The Na^+/H^+ exchange at the placental brush border may participate in functions that are essential to the normal growth and development of the placenta. The removal of H^+ from the cell by the exchanger is a significant factor in maintaining the intracellular concentration of H^+ and the regulation of intracellular pH.

The movement of hydrogen across the placenta is important for the maintenance of acid–base balance in the foetus and the placenta. Four potential mechanisms have been identified:

• the Na^+/H^+ exchange at the placental brush border membrane, which transports H^+ along the Na^+ gradient across the brush border membrane
• a proton pump
• the coupled transport of H^+ and organic iron, e.g. lactate
• a protein-mediated H^+ transfer.

The foetus obtains its supply of iron from the maternal circulation in a receptor-mediated endocytosis of ferric transferrin.

There are two distinct mechanisms in the transfer of Cl^- across the placental brush border:

• an anion exchanger that accepts Cl^- as a substrate, the exchange ion is HCO_3^-
• a functional coupling between this transport system and the Na^+/H^+.

Sulfate, selenium, chromium, molybdenum and trace elements appear to be transported by active transport.

Swallowing: spontaneous intrauterine swallowing is important in regulating amniotic fluid volume. The underlying controls are unknown. The foetus swallows 100–300 ml/kg/day.

KEY POINTS

1. The foetus is separated from the mother by the placenta, an important organ that serves as both a protector and nourishment source for the developing foetus. For the first 4–5 months, placental growth is greater than that of the foetus; thereafter, foetal growth exceeds that of the placenta.
2. The placenta is a defined, transporting organ by the fourth week of pregnancy. It not only transports nutrients and is the source of oxygen, but also is the means of excretion via the bowel and kidneys, and route of elimination of carbon dioxide.

3. Glucose is an important foetal and placental fuel. The transfer system is stereospecific, can be saturated and is a mediated process.
4. Amino acid transport across the placental membrane involves mediated transport mechanisms through both the microvilli and the basal membrane.
5. There is metabolism of glucose within the placenta, producing lactate at a high rate.
6. Lipoprotein lipase on the maternal surface of the placental membrane hydrolyses triacylglycerol carried by maternal VLDL. The free fatty acids are taken up and may be used by the trophoblast or transferred to the foetus. The foetus is dependent on the placental transfer of substrates from the mother; these can then be used for lipid synthesis.
7. Many of the essential fatty acids required during the perinatal period are for brain growth. Of these, 50% are long-chain polyunsaturated fatty acids (PUFAs). The maximum rate of brain development in humans is in late gestation and in the early postnatal period.
8. Phospholipids comprise 25% of the brain's solid matter and are important for brain function. There appears to be no blood–brain barrier to fatty acid transfer in the infant or foetus. Variations in the composition of dietary PUFAs may lead to different concentrations of long-term PUFAs in brain tissue.
9. Water- and lipid-soluble vitamins and inorganic nutrients are transported across the placenta by specific transport systems.

THINKING POINT

Maternal nutrition and health is critical to the future health of the baby.

NEED TO UNDERSTAND

1. The relationship between the foetus and the mother is mediated through the placenta.
2. Glucose is the main energy source, supplemented by essential nutrients derived from the maternal diet, transferred by exchanges across the placenta.
3. There are great benefits of a full term *in utero*.

FURTHER READING

Battaglia, E.C. and Meschia, G. (1988) Fetal nutrition. *Annual Review of Nutrition*, **8**, 43–61.

Farquharson, J., Cockburn F., Patrick, W.A., *et al.* (1992) Infant cerebral cortex phospholipid fatty-acid composition and diet. *British Medical Journal*, **340**, 810–13.

Hay, W.W. Jr (1999) Nutrition–gene interactions during intrauterine life and lactation. *Nutrition Reviews*, **57**, S20–30.

Ross, M.G. and Nijland, M.J. (1998) Development of ingestive behaviour. *Am. J. Physiology*, **274**, 879–93.

Zaret, K.S. (1996) Molecular genetics of early liver development. *Annual Review of Physiology*, **58**, 231–52.

29

Thermodynamics and metabolism

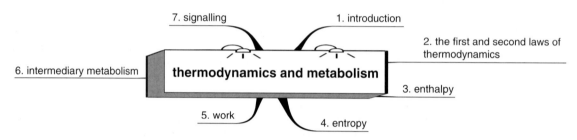

Fig. 29.1 Chapter outline.

INTRODUCTION

An important role of ingested nutrients, separate from their roles in growth and other functions, is to provide energy to the body. This provision of energy has many similarities to other energy-using systems, such as were originally studied in machines. Consequently, energy provision and utilisation in the body have been described in the concepts used in thermodynamics. This section gives a simple, non-mathematical introduction to thermodynamics, the laws of which are obeyed by all biochemical processes. Through such systems are determined: (i) whether or not a reaction will proceed spontaneously; (ii) how the reaction is designed; and (iii) how complex structures are folded.

Organisms can use carbohydrates, fats and proteins to produce energy by oxidation. Metabolic oxidation during respiration consumes oxygen and produces energy. Energy is stored work or the capacity to do work. Thermodynamics describes the difference in energy between the reactants and products, but not the mechanism whereby the reaction takes place. The latter part of this chapter incorporates the concepts of thermodynamics into the processes of intermediary metabolism.

The internal energy (E) of a molecule may be translational, rotational or vibrational. There are also electronic energies, which involve electron–electron interactions, electron–nucleus interactions and nucleus–nucleus interactions.

THE FIRST AND SECOND LAWS OF THERMODYNAMICS

The first law of thermodynamics states that the total amount of energy is constant. The energy, however, may transform from one form to another. While the overall energy remains constant, energy may flow from the system to the surroundings, or from the surroundings to the system. Chemical energy may be translated into thermal, electrical or mechanical energy. Heat and work are equivalent and are mechanisms whereby the system may gain

Definitions in energy and units of energy

$\Delta E = q - w.$

ΔE is the change in the energy of the system, q is the heat flow, and w is the work done.

Definitions
joule: $1 J = 1 kg\, m^2\, s^{-1}$
$1 kg\, m^2 = 1 N\, m$ (Newton metre)
$= 1 W\, s$ (Watt second)
$= 1 CE$ (Coulomb volt)

Thermochemical calorie
$1 cal = 1 kcal = 4.184 kJ$

1 kilocalorie (kcal) is the amount of heat required to raise the temperature of 1 kg of water from 14.5 to 15.5°C

1 kilojoule (kJ) is the amount of energy needed to move 1 Newton of force over a distance of 1 km.

or lose energy to its surroundings. The change in energy is equivalent to the difference between the heat absorbed by the system and the work performed by it.

The second law of thermodynamics has been expressed in a number of ways, but the gist is of an inevitable progression throughout the universe from a more ordered to a disordered state. This is the phenomenon of entropy, and is an index of the number of different ways in which a system can be arranged without changing its energy state. An irreversible process is accompanied by an increase in entropy. A reversible process is a finely balanced change, always in equilibrium with the surroundings. There is no loss of energy in a chaotic manner, nor an increase in entropy. A system requires a certain amount of energy to be at any particular state, i.e. perpetual motion is impossible.

ENTHALPY

The enthalpy of a compound is its internal energy. The enthalpy of a reaction is measured as the heat absorbed by the system at constant pressure. Chemical and biochemical reactions take place usu-

ally at constant pressure rather than at constant volumes. In most biochemical reactions there is little change in either pressure or volume. If a reaction absorbs heat, the surroundings will cool and the change in the enthalpy of the system is positive. If, however, heat is created by the system then the enthalpy (ΔH) of the reaction is negative, energy being lost from the system to the surroundings.

The change in the chemical internal energy is equal to the heat produced or consumed plus the work done on or by the reaction. The change in enthalpy in the reaction is:

Heat absorbed – Work done.

This is independent of the reaction mechanism, concentration of the substrate or product. The number of moles transferred in the reaction is significant.

ENTROPY

The first law of thermodynamics cannot predict whether a reaction will take place. Some spontaneous reactions may absorb heat. Natural systems allow only a proportion of their total potential energy to be available for work.

Entropy (S) is the randomness or disorder in a system. As S increases the disorder increases. Entropy measures the extent to which the total energy of the system is unavailable for the performance of useful work.

Structural changes that make molecules more rigid reduce rotational and vibrational energy and reduce entropy, e.g. double-bond or ring formations. This becomes important in the formation of comparatively rigid macromolecules from flexible polypeptide and polynucleotide structures. When a molecule is converted to a dimer the entropy is reduced, and this is a function of the molecular weight.

The physical state is a very important factor in the entropy of a compound. A gas has much more translational and rotational freedom than a liquid, which in turn has more freedom than a solid. In a reversible reaction there is a slow progression through intermediate states wherein the system is always in equilibrium. Entropy is increased on evaporation and melting; this can be measured from the heat of vaporisation and from the heat of fusion. There is a greater increase in translational and rotational freedom in progressing from a liquid to a gas than in going from a solid to a liquid.

The entropy of solutions is affected by mixing two solvents, by placing solutes into solution, and by hydrogen bonding and other associations within the solvent or between solute and solvent. Each compound resulting from mixing will make a positive contribution to the entropy. An ideal solution is one in which there is no interaction between the molecules. Any intermolecular interaction causes a decrease in the entropy of mixing as the translational and rotational freedom of the individual molecules will be reduced. Solvation is the interaction between solute and solvent molecules, and this is an important factor in the negative entropy of a compound in solution.

When a solute is added to a solvent, entropy decreases. This is due to the restricted movement of the solute and the restrictive movement of the solvent in the vicinity of the solute. The consequence is that small molecules become more highly hydrated than larger ones with the same charge. Anions are more readily hydrated than cations. The entropy of hydration becomes a larger negative number with increasing charge or decreasing radius.

Molecules and ions that have bipoles or hydrogen bond donor or acceptor groups interact strongly with water. Consequently, this restricts the mobility of the water. An apolar molecule in water causes a decrease in entropy. The water is held on the surface of the molecule, forming a rigid structure of hydrogen bonds. Such an orientation of water is a feature of the apolar areas of proteins and other biological macromolecules.

These entropy changes are caused by binding or absorption of molecules on the surface of a macromolecule. This is important in the function of enzymes, substrates and inhibitors. When a substrate is bound onto an enzyme, water molecules are displaced and this results in a positive entropy change. Another entropy effect between enzyme and substrate is called the chelation effect: if a molecule binds at several points to a protein the binding is stronger than through one point of attachment. This is important in enzyme kinetics. Any system tends to move towards the lowest enthalpy and the highest entropy. Entropy increases spontaneously.

Gibbs showed that for reactions occurring in equilibrium and at a constant temperature, the change in entropy is numerically equal to the change in enthalpy divided by the absolute temperature. Gibbs described the phenomenon of free energy. There is free or available energy and total energy in a system:

Δ Free energy =
Δ Enthalpy – (Absolute temperature ×
Δ Entropy)

where Δ = change. Free energy consists of enthalpy and entropy, and determines whether or not a reaction can occur. This requires, however, that a chemical pathway is also possible and that the free energy change is negative and hence favourable.

The standard free energy of formation of a compound is the free energy difference between a compound and the state of the elements of which the compound is composed. If the system produces energy then it is negative or exergonic and will proceed without an external energy source, e.g. heat. If the system requires free energy to proceed (i.e. positive) then the reaction can only take place with the addition of external energy; it is an endergonic reaction.

A reaction is only spontaneously possible if there is negative free energy. The molecules must, however, be in a reactive state. This reactivity is created by enzymatic activity in biological systems. Enzymes accelerate a reaction that is possible on energetic grounds. Proteins are highly ordered and have a defined constrained conformation. Amino acids are in a state of increased entropy and are more reactive than native proteins.

Free energies

Free energies are expressed in units of kilocalories per mole or kilojoules per mole. By subtracting the sum of the free energies of formation of the reaction from the total free energy of formation of the products, it is possible to calculate the free energy change of any reaction for which the free energies of formation of all reactants and products are known. Tables are available of the free energies of formation of many compounds.

The standard free energy for a reaction can be calculated by adding or subtracting the standard free energies of two other reactions that will combine to give the desired reaction. When the concentrations of reactants and products are at their equilibrium values, there is no change in free energy for the reactants to go in either direction. In biological systems, concentrations of compounds are maintained at values below their equilibrium values. This is achieved by removal of the endproducts, either physically or by conversion to other compounds, so considerable free energy is generated by their reactions.

The free energy change of a system gives a measure of the maximum amount of useful work that can be obtained from a reaction. The larger the amount of work obtainable from a reaction, the further the reaction is from equilibrium. An important concept is the maximum amount of useful work that can be obtained from a reaction.

WORK

The amount of work that is actually obtained depends on the pathway that the process takes. Work that can be derived from biological systems is of three types.

- **Mechanical work**: this is work that involves movement, e.g. muscle contractions or movement of chromosomes towards the opposite pole of a mitotic spindle.
- **Osmotic and electrical work** (changes in concentration): this involves the movement of chemical compounds or ions against a concentration gradient. These processes include active absorption and movement of chemicals from the blood into the cell.
- **Synthetic work** (changes in chemical bonds): this is involved in the formation of the chemical bonds for complex organic molecules. Such large molecules are more complex and have a higher energy content than the molecules from which they are derived.

Some reactions are only possible by using the high negative free energy of one reaction (exergonic reaction) to drive another reaction that has a low negative free energy (endergonic reaction).

An enzyme may catalyse two reactions sequentially.

An example is the phosphorylation of glucose by hexokinase/glucokinase, in which adenosine triphosphate (ATP) gives a phosphate to the glucose to yield adenosine diphosphate (ADP) and glucose-6-phosphate. The reaction of glucose to phosphoric acid to form glucose-6-phosphate has an unfavourable equilibrium constant. The hydrolysis of ATP has a quite favourable equilibrium. When these reactions are coupled, the overall reaction is favourable:

Glucose + ATP = Glucose-6-phosphate + ADP

This is the main source of free energy in energy-producing and energy-consuming systems. ATP can be hydrolysed by two quite different reactions. The α,β-linkage can be hydrolysed to form adenosine monophosphate (AMP) and pyrophosphate ion, or the β,γ-linkage can be hydrolysed to form ADP and phosphate ion. AMP can subsequently be hydrolysed in an irreversible reaction. This occurs in nucleic acid synthesis. ADP is involved in irreversible reactions. Less free energy is required to rephosphorylate the ADP product than that required for AMP. Considerable free energy is released on the hydrolysis of ATP or ADP, but not from AMP. The α,β and the β,γ phosphate links are high-energy linkages. Any compound can be phosphorylated by compounds that have a greater phosphate group transfer potential. Therefore, ADP can be phosphorylated to ATP from glycerate-1,3-disphosphate (producing –11.8 kcal/mol) but not from glucose 6-phosphate (–2.2 kcal/mol). ATP has a standard free energy of hydrolysis of –7.5 kcal/mol. The ATP–ADP system is an acceptor and a donor of phosphate groups. ADP accepts phosphate from high-energy compounds, e.g. phosphoenolpyruvate (–14.8 kcal/mol), glycerate-1,3-disphosphate (–11.8 kcal/mol) and phosphocreatine (–10.3 kcal/mol), and the lower energy compounds that ATP donates to phosphates, e.g. glucose-1-phosphate (–5.0 kcal/mol); glucose-6-phosphate (–3.3 kcal/mol) and glycerol phosphate (–2.2 kcal/mol). Regeneration of ATP is a requirement for all cells as part of the energy system of the cell.

This means that there are many reactions happening at the same time, which are acting synergistically within a biological system. Reactions can occur simultaneously or rapidly in sequence without build-up of intermediate substrate.

The shortcoming of thermodynamic theory is that this applies to a closed system. In biology there is an 'open system', in so far that there is removal and loss of compounds from a series of biologically and anatomically different areas.

In cells or organisms it is relevant that there is a high degree of collaboration between reactions. This results in diverse and highly specific reactions taking place rapidly and with the generation of heat. The reactions require energy and use starting materials which are, in general, provided by nutrition.

INTERMEDIARY METABOLISM

This supplies the energy needed for:

- synthesis of molecules
- transfer of molecules across membranes
- movement of molecules in tissues.

Homoeostasis or the development of a steady state requires a constant and reliable supply of nutrients for the cell. The Japanese industrial system of 'just-in-time' is an artificial system equivalent to the cellular manufacturing system. That is, little is stored and just sufficient components are provided alongside the working station. The rate of flow of compounds along metabolic sequences is regulated to meet functional needs. The system, however, has to be economic in order not to spend excessive time or energy in wasteful processes. A series of reactions provides intermediates for initiating other reactions that branch from the overall reaction. The overall reaction passes along a pathway with a defined endproduct. The conversion of glucose with six carbons to the 3-carbon pyruvate provides energy in the form of ATP in ten discrete, enzymatically catalysed steps (Figure 29.2). In the first six reactions of this metabolic pathway ATP is consumed, and in the last four steps ATP is regenerated.

Anabolic pathways, synthesis of proteins and polysaccharides always require energy (endergonic) and involve a decrease in entropy. *Catabolic pathways* are energy liberating (exergonic), and increase entropy. Acetyl-coenzyme A (CoA) is a chemical unit where many of the intermediate products of proteins, polysaccharides and lipids

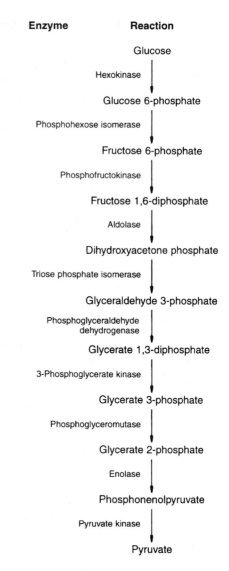

Fig. 29.2 Metabolic pathway: the conversion of glucose to pyruvate.

converge or emerge in new pathways. At the same time, acetyl-CoA is a source of raw material for the synthesis of amino acids, sugars or fats. In general, catabolic pathways follow a converging pattern that results in common intermediates. Anabolic pathways start from common intermediates and end with quite different endproducts, i.e. a diverging pattern.

Just as reactions are organised into reaction sequences, enzymes that function in the different steps of this reaction are clustered together in the cell. Three groupings can be found.

- In the simplest, grouping all enzymes for a particular pathway are different, independent, soluble proteins in the same cellular compartment. The reaction intermediates pass from one enzyme to another by diffusion through the cytoplasm or by transfer after contact with the sequential enzymes.
- All enzymes involved in a sequence of reactions form a complex. The intermediates are held in this complex until synthesis is complete.
- Functionally related enzymes are bound to a membrane. This applies to enzymes in the electron transport processes associated with oxidative phosphorylation.

An important aspect of biochemistry is that the direction of reactions in living cells is dictated in response to metabolic needs, rather than to thermodynamic factors. The direction of such changes must be independent of changes in concentrations of metabolic intermediates. The direction of the conversions, as well as their rates, are regulated by metabolic signals, e.g. the concentration of special local metabolites, available ATP or controlling hormones. Any reaction may be made thermodynamically possible by being coupled to a sufficient number of ATP to ADP conversions.

Various systems regulate metabolism. The amount of enzyme in a cell or compartment is regulated by protein synthesis and degradation. Enzymes are produced in greatest amounts when they are needed. Some are produced at moderate levels all the time and are constitutively expressed. Such enzymes include the enzymes involved in coenzyme synthesis.

Enzyme activity may be regulated by non-covalent interactions with small molecular regulatory factors, or by reversible covalent reactions, e.g. phosphorylation or adenylation of an amino acid side-chain. Enzymes that are directly regulated occupy key positions in metabolic pathways. Often the first enzyme in a pathway is used to regulate the subsequent pathway. In a branched chain pathway, endproduct inhibition results in inhibition of the first enzyme after the point of branching in this reaction system.

The ATP–ADP and occasionally ATP–AMP systems couple energy into biosynthetic sequences; this system is involved in controls that reflect the energy status of the cell. The energy status of the cell is called the energy charge and is the effective mole fraction of ATP in the ATP/ADP/AMP pool.

$$\text{Energy charge} = \frac{\text{ATP} + 0.5\,\text{ADP}}{\text{ATP} + \text{ADP} + \text{AMP}}$$

The 0.5 in the numerator allows for ADP being half as effective as ATP in carrying chemical energy. The values for energy charge vary from 0 to 1. Some reactions in anabolic and catabolic pathways respond to variations in the value of the energy charge. The enzymes in catabolic pathways respond in an opposite manner from enzymes in anabolic pathways.

SIGNALLING

Cells and organs have to be aware of the environment in which they are functioning. They need to be informed of what is happening and what are the requirements of similar cells, related cells, cells that function in a network of activity and dependent cells. The same applies to organs, in order to create a co-ordinated whole. The nervous system and hormones are significant in such an intelligence system. This intelligence system carries information from detectors (receptors) through intermediary molecules within the cell to the effector system, whether this be a gene or an enzyme. Receptors on the cell surface or membrane receive stimuli or evidence of change, whether this be quantitative or qualitative, more or less of the same or a different stimulus. Nutrients may bind to receptors. Such binders to receptors are ligands. Following such binding a signal passes through the membrane, using a receptor. Such receptors may be arranged across the membrane. The relationship of the receptor with intracellular mediators or the localisation or function of these mediators may then alter. Enzymes may be stimulated, e.g. the kinases which transfer phosphate to proteins and hence activate or inhibit their activity. Alternatively, the receptor may act as an ion channel or pump, allowing the transfer of ions, e.g. calcium, which alters cell activity. Other signalling proteins may be

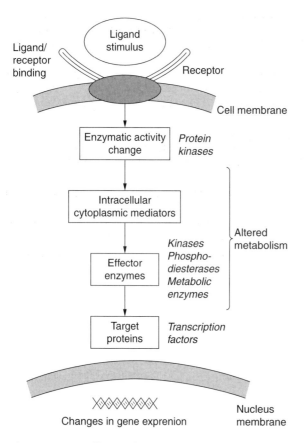

Fig. 29.3 Signalling pathway transmitting information from the cell surface to gene expression.

alerted. Another system uses the special lipid system phosphatidylinositol-3,4,5-triphosphate which initiates another cascade of information. Often considerable information is provided at the same time and the result is a compromise that meets the needs of the cell, organ and body (Figure 29.3).

The intracellular stimulation may then progress to the nucleus to affect gene activity and transcription and hence the gene expression programme of the cell.

KEY POINTS

1. An important role of ingested nutrients is to provide energy to the body. Energy provision and utilisation in the body has been described in the concepts used in thermodynamics, which describe the difference in energy between the reactants and products, but not the mechanism whereby the reaction takes place.

2. The total amount of energy is constant and this is described in the first law of thermodynamics. While the overall energy remains constant, energy may flow from the system to the surroundings, or from the surroundings to the system.

3. The enthalpy of a compound is its internal energy.

4. The second law of thermodynamics describes a transition from an ordered to a disordered state (change in entropy).

5. Only a proportion of total potential energy is available for work. There is free or available energy and total energy in a system: Free energy = Enthalpy – absolute temperature × Entropy. Entropy measures the extent to which the total energy of the system is unavailable for the performance of useful work.

6. A reaction is only spontaneously possible if there is negative free energy. The molecules must, however, be in a reactive state. This reactivity is created by enzymatic activity in biological systems. Enzymes accelerate a reaction that is possible on energetic grounds.

7. When a substrate is bound to an enzyme, water molecules are displaced and this results in a positive entropy change. Another entropy effect between enzyme and substrate is called the chelation effect; this is important in enzyme kinetics.

8. Three types of work can be derived from biological systems: (i) mechanical work, which involves movements; (ii) osmotic and electrical work, changes in concentration, or movement of chemical compounds or ions against a concentration gradient; and (iii) synthetic work with changes in chemical bonds.

9. Some biological reactions are only possible by using high negative free energy of one reaction (exergonic reaction) to drive another reaction that has a low negative free energy (endergonic reaction).

10. The direction of reactions in living cells is dictated in response to metabolic needs, rather than to thermodynamic factors. The direction of such changes must be independent of

changes in concentrations of metabolic inter-mediates. The amount of enzyme in a cell or compartment is regulated by protein synthesis and degradation.

11. Enzyme activity is regulated by non-covalent interactions with small molecular regulatory factors, or by reversible covalent reactions, e.g. phosphorylation or adenylation of an amino acid side-chain. Enzymes that are directly reg-ulated occupy key positions in metabolic pathways.

THINKING POINTS

1. This is a critical area in nutrition, the point where the energy created by metabolism is con-verted into work.

2. The efficiency of this system is important and may be affected by a number of factors, e.g. age, gender, exercise and nutrients.

NEED TO UNDERSTAND

The mechanism whereby energy is moved about within the cell, organ and the whole body, all described by the laws of thermodynamics.

FURTHER READING

Atkins, P.W. (1998) *Physical Chemistry*, 6th edn. Oxford University Press, Oxford.

Harold, F.M. (1986) *The Vital Force. A Study of Bioen-ergetics*. Freeman & Co., New York.

Nicholls, D.G. and Ferguson, S.J. (2002) *Bioenergetics*. Academic Press, New York.

30

Mitochondria

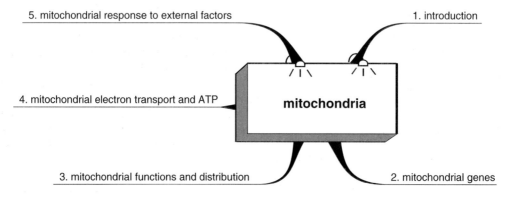

Fig. 30.1 Chapter outline.

INTRODUCTION

Mitochondria are elongated cylinders, 0.5–1.0 μm in diameter (Figure 30.2). They are important in metabolism, carry out most cellular oxidation reactions and produce most of the animal cell's adenosine triphosphate (ATP). The energy available in the form of reduced nicotinamide-adenine dinucleotide (NADH, NADH$_2$) and flavin adenine dinucleotide (FAD) is harnessed by electron transport chains to the synthesis of ATP. Energy is provided by the oxidation of nutrients.

Mitochondria consist of internal membranes, a smooth outer and a folded inner membrane. The infoldings of the inner membrane are called cristae and increase the surface area of the inner membrane. The space within a crista connects to the intermembrane space through five or six tubu-lar channels at the edges. The inner membrane sep-arates the mitochondria into two distinct spaces:

- the internal or matrix space
- the intermembrane space.

The outer membrane has few enzymatic activities, but is permeable and involved in transmembrane transport of molecules with a molecular weight of up to 5 kDa. The inner membrane is impermeable to ions and polar molecules and limits the move-ment of energy-rich compounds between the mitochondrial matrix and the intermembrane space. The inner membrane is rich in enzymes.

The number of mitochondria in a tissue reflects the tissue's requirement for ATP: the more mito-chondria, the more ATP is produced. The mito-chondrial enzymes and enzyme complexes are organised in defined positions in the different com-partments of the organelle.

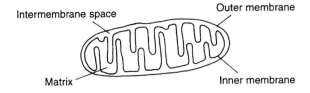

Matrix: mix of enzymes including: citric acid cycle
                                             DNA genes
                                             ribosomes
                                             tRNA

Inner membrane: folded into cristae to increase
                    surface area. Functions include
                    (i) Oxidative reaction of the
                        respiratory chain
                    (ii) ATP synthase
                    (iii) Transport protein for metabolites
                    (iv) Impermeable to small ions

Outer membrane: (i) Permeable to substances of molecular
                      weight <5000 Da
                  (ii) Lipid synthesis

Intermembrane space: enzymes using ATP

Fig. 30.2 Mitochondria consist of an outer membrane, an inner membrane and a matrix. Two-thirds of the mitochondrial proteins are in the matrix, 20% in the inner membrane and 6% in the outer membrane. The matrix contains enzymes involved in the citric acid cycle and DNA genes, ribosomes and tRNA. The inner membrane is folded into cristae and is involved in oxidative reactions in the respiratory chain; it contains ATP syntase and transport proteins for the transfer of metabolites . The outer membrane is permeable for substances with a molecular weight < 5 kDa and contains enzymes involved in lipid synthesis. The intermembrane space contains enzymes using ATP.

MITOCHONDRIAL GENES

The mitochondrion is unusual in that it contains its own DNA (mtDNA). Mitochondrial genes are derived entirely from the mother through the ovum's contribution to the gamete. This means that the inheritance of the genes is non-Mendelian. The organelle DNA will evolve independently at its own rate. Organelle DNA is replicated by a DNA polymerase that differs from the nuclear DNA polymerase. Most organelle genomes take the form of a single molecule of DNA (mtDNA). Since there

are several mitochondria in a cell there is a number of organelle genomes. Mitochondrial genomes in the human are of the order of 16 kilobases (kb). There may be 750 organelles in a cell, but the amount of DNA relative to the nuclear cell DNA is < 0.1%. The mitochondria do not synthesise much protein; the enzymes encoded for include cytochrome *b*, cytochrome oxidase, NADH dehydrogenase and some units of ATPase.

The mitochondria contain 10% of the body's protein pool and all but a few proteins are imported from the cell cytosol. Most proteins are encoded by nuclear genes in free cytosolic ribosomes, enter the mitochondria by vectorial processing by binding to a chaperoning protein and are transported through a molecular pontoon bridge, Tom and Tim. These proteins undergo covalent modification, interact with coenzymes and are thereby activated. As both mitochondrial and nuclear gene products are required for effective mitochondrial activity, the expression of gene products must be co-ordinated. A failure to provide a necessary nutrient or mineral may distort this co-ordination.

MITOCHONDRIAL FUNCTIONS AND DISTRIBUTION

Functions

The principal function of the mitochondria is to produce energy, through the electron transport chain and oxidative phosphorylation. These processes include the synthesis of ATP, terminal oxidation of pyruvate from carbohydrate and amino acid catabolism, β-oxidation of fatty acids and oxidation of acetate [acetyl-coenzyme A (CoA)] from ethanol and fatty acid, protein and carbohydrate oxidation. Mitochondria are also involved in the oxidation of branched-chain amino acids, maintenance of nitrogen homoeostasis and urea formation, oxidation of sulfite, activation of vitamin D_3 and synthesis of many important compounds, e.g. bile acids.

New mitochondria are formed by growth and division. Energy from oxidative reactions in the mitochondria is devoted entirely to ATP synthesis. The control of this system includes rate limitation of the adenine nucleotide transporter system [delivery of adenosine monophosphate (ADP) and removal of ATP from the matrix], supply of NADH from dehydrogenases and transfer of electrons through cytochrome oxidase (O_2).

Distribution

Mitochondria are distributed in distinct patterns, which are characteristic for different cell types and provide ATP as required. In transport epithelia, e.g. renal proximal tubule cells and gastric parietal cells, mitochondria are located next to the membrane pump transport systems; in muscle and sperm cells, next to the contractile elements; at gap junctions in cardiac myocytes and synaptic terminals in neurones; and between hepatocytes in the periportal region of the liver sinusoid and centrilobular region. Cells with different positions relative to blood supply are exposed to different nutrient provision. The nutrient supplies are a major factor in determining the enzyme content and metabolic characteristics of the cells. In smooth muscle, glycolytic activity is separate, so that the overall supply of nutrients to the mitochondria is independent of the supply of nutrients for glycolysis.

MITOCHONDRIAL ELECTRON TRANSPORT AND ATP

The outer membrane of the mitochondria has little enzymatic activity and is involved in the transmembrane transport of substances with a molecular weight of up to 5000 Da. The inner membrane contains the pathway for the electron transport and oxidative phosphorylation in five multisubunit complexes. The inner membrane, although somewhat impermeable, allows protons or cofactors to move freely between the mitochondrial matrix and the intermembrane space. The membrane contains proteins for oxygen consumption and the formation of ATP (Figure 30.3). The phospholipids of the inner membrane have a high content of unsaturated fatty acid; cholesterol is found in the outer but not in the inner membrane.

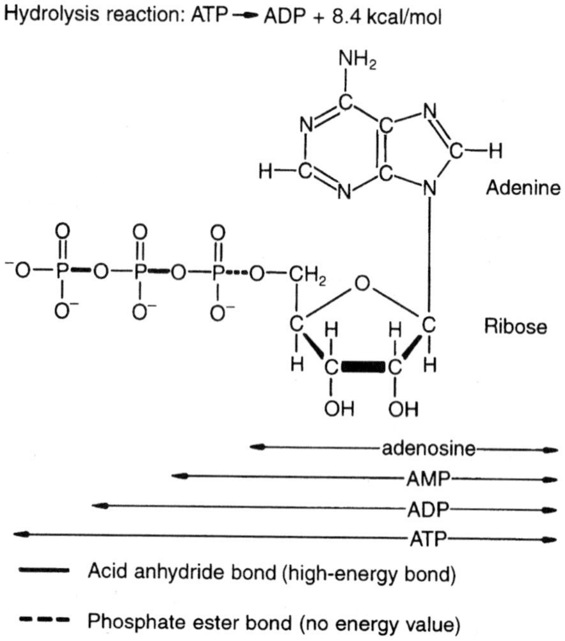

Hydrolysis reaction: ATP → ADP + 8.4 kcal/mol

Fig. 30.3 ATP (adenosine 5′-triphosphate). Adenosine monophosphate has no energy store, but adenosine 5′-diphosphate, and particularly ATP, contain high-energy acid anhydride bonds. The conversion of ATP to ADP releases at least 8.4 kcal/mol.

The respiratory chain
NADH and $NADH_2$ are generated by glycolysis, β-oxidation and the tricarboxylic acid cycle. NADH and $NADH_2$ undergo oxidation–reduction reactions, which provide a mechanism whereby electrons move from reduced coenzymes (NADH and $FADH_2$) to oxygen (Figure 30.4). Electrons are not passed directly from coenzymes to oxygen but progress through reversible oxidisable electron acceptors. Prosthetic groups that possess electrons or H^+ pass from one reversible oxidisable electron acceptor to another along the inner mitochondrial membrane. These reactions are coupled with the synthesis of ATP. At each step the electrons fall to a lower energy level until they are transferred to oxygen, which has the highest affinity of all of the carriers of electrons. Electrons bound to oxygen are in their lowest energy state. The free energy converted into an electrochemical gradient is harnessed for ATP synthesis.

The electron carriers include flavins, quinone, iron–sulfur complexes and copper atoms.

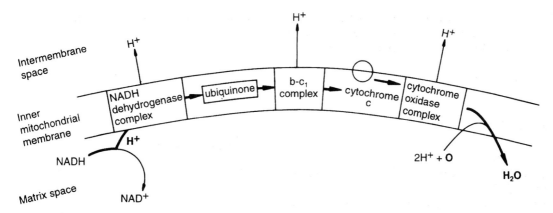

Fig. 30.4 Respiratory chain across the inner mitochondrial membrane. NADH transfers an H^+ into the respiratory chain. The respiratory chain carries electrons from reduced coenzymes NADH and $FADH_2$ to oxygen. These reactions create a high energy difference between the two sides of the membrane, which enables ATP synthase and other energy-requiring reactions to take place.

Flavins: the dehydrogenases that catalyse the loss of an electron from succinate or NADH dehydrogenase require FAD. There are many other flavoprotein dehydrogenases within the mitochondrial matrix. These transfer electrons to other membrane-bound flavoproteins. Some dehydrogenases (NADH dehydrogenase, succinate dehydrogenase and flavoprotein ubiquinone oxidoreductase) contain iron atoms bound to the sulfur atoms at the cysteine of the protein. These are non-haem iron proteins.

Ubiquinone: this is a benzoquinone with a long side-chain. The hydrocarbon tail makes the molecule strongly hydrophobic. Ubiquinone is reduced by the loss of two electrons to form dihydroquinone. Ubiquinone accepts electrons from the enzymatic activity of dehydrogenases and these electrons move on to the cytochrome system. Most of the major electron carriers, with the exception of cytochrome c and ubiquinone, are found as large complexes. These contain polypeptide subunits, some of which have no electron-carrying groups. These enzymes also acquire some of the free energy released during the reaction.

The electron carriers include the cytochromes a, b and c, complexes of iron and porphyrin. Cytochrome c is found in the inner membrane of the mitochondria. The b- and a-type cytochromes are attached to large complexes on the membrane. The iron is attached to four pyrrole nitrogens in the porphyrin ring. The b cytochromes contain Fe-

protoporphyrin IX in the same form as haemoglobin and myoglobin. The a cytochromes include a modified prosthetic group, haem A. The c, cytochromes contain haem C, wherein the vinyl groups of protoporphyrin IX are bound covalently to the protein by thioether links to cysteine residues. Cytochrome c is a globular protein with a molecular weight of 12.5 kDa and consists of a planar haem group in the centre of the molecule, surrounded by hydrophobic amino acids, including a strongly basic cluster of eight lysine residues. This positively charged area may be important in the activity of the cytochrome. The iron of the haem is bound to the sulfur atom of the methionine residue and the other to a histidyl nitrogen. The methionine is replaced by a second histidine residue, leaving space for oxygen, water and carbon monoxide to bind to the iron. The iron atoms of the cytochromes are oxidised and reduced, cycling between the ferrous (Fe^{2+}) and ferric (Fe^{3+}). During anaerobic conditions the cytochromes become reduced. In the presence of oxygen they become oxidised.

The movement of electrons from NADH to the cytochrome bc_1 complex appears to progress by the diffusion of ubiquinone from one complex to another within the phospholipid bilayer of the mitochondrial inner layer. From here, there is movement of electrons to the cytochrome oxidase by the diffusion of reduced cytochrome c along the surface of the bilayer. Cytochrome c is a water-

Mitochondrial electron transport

Complex I: the NADH dehydrogenase complex
This is the largest complex in the mitochondrial inner membrane (26 different polypeptides). The total molecular weight is 10^6 Da. The complex consists of flavoprotein subunits with the iron–sulfur clustered at the centre, surrounded by a shell of hydrophobic proteins. Electrons move from one iron–sulfur centre to another and eventually to ubiquinone. This complex is placed very specifically between the two surfaces of the membrane of the mitochondria. The binding site for NADH faces the mitochondrial matrix space. This allows the oxidation of NADH, which is produced in the matrix by the enzymes of the tricarboxylic acid cycle. This forms an enzymatic shuttle system. The ubiquinone then passes to the second complex, complex III, the cytochrome bc_1 complex in the central hydrophobic area of the membrane.

Complex II: the succinate dehydrogenase complex
Succinate dehydrogenase is embedded in the mitochondrial inner membrane, and consists of two iron–sulfur proteins, of molecular weights 70 and 27 kDa. Oxidation takes place on the larger of the subunits, on the matrix side of the membrane. It possesses a 4-Fe centre and a molecule of FAD bound to a histidine residue of the protein.

Complex III
This consists of two different b-cytochromes and has a molecular weight of 450 kDa. The subunits of complex III consist of stretches of hydrophobic amino acids, which are transmembrane α-helices extending from one side of the inner membrane to the other. The oxidation of ubiquinone by the cytochrome bc_1 complex is related to the uptake of proteins from the matrix side of the mitochondrial inner membrane, and to the release of protons on the cytoplasmic side. This is called the *Q cycle*.

Complex IV: cytochrome oxidase
This contains atoms of copper in addition to the haems of cytochromes a and a_3. The copper in cytochrome oxidase may be important in preventing the production of superoxide in this reaction. Cytochrome oxidase consists of six to 13 subunits with a molecular weight range of 5 to 50 kDa. Copper atoms are found in two of the large subunits. The three largest subunits are synthesised in mitochondria, the smaller ones in the cytoplasm.

soluble protein attached to the membrane surface by electrostatic weak interactions. NADH dehydrogenase can only oxidise NADH within the mitochondrial matrix. Protons are bound and released on either side of the inner membrane of the mitochondria when electrons progress down the respiratory chain. This is known as *chemiosmosis*.

Two electrons are used for every atom of oxygen that is reduced from O^{2-} to H_2O. The flow of two electrons through the complex of I, III, IV supports phosphorylation of ADP to ATP. This does not happen in the succinate dehydrogenase complex II.

There is a close relationship between respiration and phosphorylation. Respiratory control is the regulation of the rate of electron transport by ADP. Phosphorylation coupled to electron transfer in the respiratory chain is quite different to the mechanism of energy coupling in soluble enzymes.

The *chemiosmotic coupling* system was first described by Peter Mitchell. Chemical reactions drive or are driven by the movement of molecules or ions between osmotically distinct spaces separated by membranes. Protons are pumped out of

the mitochondria during respiration. The flow of electrons from reducing substrates to oxygen causes protons to move out of the matrix space to create a small pH gradient and an electrical potential difference across the mitochondrial inner membrane (Figure 30.5). The electrochemical potential gradient for protons across the mitochondrial inner membrane is the mechanism by which electron transfer is coupled to phosphorylation; ten to twelve protons are pumped out of the mitochondria for each pair of electrons that moves down the respiratory chain from NADH to oxygen, while six to eight protons are pumped for a pair of electrons from succinate. This creates an electrochemical potential gradient for protons across the membrane. Enzymatic reactions in such an organised situation as the membrane have what is called vectorial or a directional character. Protons move back into the matrix by ATP synthase activity and the formation of ATP. When mitochondria are oxidising and form ATP at a constant rate, protons move inwards at a rate that balances the rate at which protons are pumped out by the

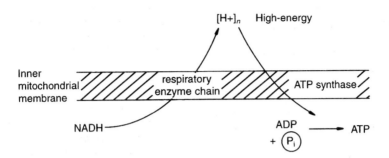

Fig. 30.5 Reversible coupling. NADH releases hydrogen through the respiratory enzyme chain and enables a high energy state to be created, whereby ATP synthase can generate ATP.

electron transport reaction. Three molecules of ATP are formed for each pair of electrons that pass along the whole system to oxygen. The oxidation of succinate involves the extrusion of eight protons per pair of electrons.

Proton ATP synthase
This enzyme uses electrochemical energy derived from the proton gradients, produced by respiration, to the ATP chemical form for storage. This is the point where the energy created by metabolism can be stored in ATP, which acts as a storage system akin to a battery for electricity. The transfer of energy to be stored is by means of protein motors which act in much the same way as when the energy of movement provided by wind, petrol combustion or steam is used to generate electricity to be stored in a battery. A multiprotein complex, F_1, is embedded on the mitochondrial inner membrane and includes five different polypeptide units with a total molecular weight of 370 kDa. A second complex, F_0, has five hydrophobic polypeptides, is an integral component of the inner membrane and holds F_1 to the membrane. This $F_1 F_0$-ATPase complex is located on the side of the mitochondrial inner membrane that faces the matrix. Such an orientation is very important for the function of this complex. ATP synthase is charged by these two rotatory motors, F_1 and F_0, which are coupled through a drive shaft, using rotational motion in 120° rotary sweeps to convert energy from metabolism to ATP in three stages from electrochemical (through protons supplied by metabolic processes) to motion to chemical stored energy. The F_0 motor is bound to the energy-generating mitochondrial structures and channels protons through its rotor

and non-rotating stator to drive rotation. F_1 catalyses the production of ATP from ADP and P, provided F_0 drives the F_1 rotor sufficiently strongly. Other enzymes use the rotary co-operative interaction system, including the motor protein kinesin.

ATP synthesis

ATP synthesised in mitochondria is transported from the mitochondria in exchange for ADP by an electrogenic process. The enzyme ATP/ADP exchange protein is the most abundant protein in the mitochondrial inner membrane. In contrast, the mitochondrial inner membrane does not transport NAD^+ or NADH. NADH is produced in the mitochondrial matrix by the tricarboxylic acid cycle or the oxidation of fatty acids. Electrons are transferred on the cytoplasmic NADH to the respiratory chain by a chain reaction that involves the conversion of dihydroxyacetone phosphate to glycerol-3-phosphate in the cytoplasm and the reoxidation of the glycerol-3-phosphate to dihydroxyacetone phosphate by the mitochondrial glycerol-3-phosphate dehydrogenase. Another shuttle involves oxaloacetate and malate, malate being carried across the inner membrane by a specific transport system. The reverse reactions are important in gluconeogenesis. Oxaloacetate within the mitochondria can undergo transamination with the amino acid glutamate to form aspartate and α-ketoglutarate. The endproducts can be transported from the mitochondria. Overall, the complete oxidation of glucose yields 36–38 molecules of ATP. Two molecules of ATP are formed in glycolysis and two more in the tricarboxylic acid cycle. Two molecules of NADH are produced in the cytoplasm by glycolysis. Eight molecules of NADH are generated in the mitochondrial matrix by the pyruvate dehydrogenase complex and the tricarboxylic acid cycle.

Succinate reduces two molecules of FADH to $FADH_2$. Reoxidation of the eight mitochondrial NADHs and two $FADH_2$ generates 28 molecules of ATP and two of $FADH_2$. The glycerol-3-phosphate shuttle provides two electrons ($FADH_2$), allowing the formation of four molecules of ATP. The malate shuttle leads to the formation of six molecules of ATP. This gives a total of 36 or 38 molecules of ATP. However, the system is not 100% efficient, perhaps owing to non-specific leakage of protons and other ions through the membrane. NADH from the cytoplasm may also be involved in other reductive biosynthetic reactions, e.g. formation of fatty acids.

MITOCHONDRIAL RESPONSE TO EXTERNAL FACTORS

Mitochondria respond to metabolic and environmental conditions in ageing, training and pathological processes.

Giant mitochondria at least 10 μm in diameter develop during nutrient deficiency, when there are also degenerative changes in cristae structure and decreased oxidation of many oxidisable substances.

Riboflavin is an essential component of the prosthetic group of mitochondrial flavoproteins in the citric acid cycle, the respiratory chain and β-oxidation of fatty acids. In riboflavin deficiency, the mitochondria increase in size and volume. The structure of the cristae alters, increasing in number and size. Similar changes take place with protein-poor diets.

Variations in the protein content of the diet affect mitochondrial volume and number. The amount of hepatic urea cycle enzymes is directly proportional to the daily consumption of protein. Starvation also results in a net increase in the urea cycle enzymes.

Both the expression of the enzymes involved and the rate of degradation are important. Variations

in carbohydrate diet can affect enzymes that relate to triglyceride synthesis.

The biochemical and morphological characteristics of skeletal muscle mitochondria change in response to submaximal endurance exercise training, increasing in number and size in those muscles involved in training. This means that this change is local and not the result of circulating hormones or metabolites. Pyruvate oxidation, citric acid cycle enzymes, electron transport, cytochrome content and fatty acid oxidation all increase during activity. Substrate utilisation moves from carbohydrate to fat, thereby sparing glucose and allowing greater use of energy-utilising processes with less glucose depletion and improved efficiency of energy expenditure. Efficiency of coupling of the mitochondrial proton motive force from biological oxidation with ADP phosphorylation is variable and under physiological control. Metabolism is inherently less efficient as ATP concentration increases relative to the concentration of ADP and activated phosphorus (P_i). ATP production increases before an increase in demand for ATP, thereby anticipating increased energy need, e.g. by secretion, phagocytosis or cell division. This may mean the release of the inhibition of ATP synthase by an endogenous inhibitor and stimulation of the activity of critical NAD^+-linked dehydrogenases. Exercise or inactivity affects energy efficiency. High ATP concentration means greater and immediately available utilisable energy, but at a reduced energy efficiency. More oxidisable substrate is needed to do the same productive work. Mitochondrial function is also affected by thyroid hormones and probably by the carbohydrate relative to the protein content of the diet.

Thermogenesis in brown fat

Brown fat cells use electron transport that is uncoupled from phosphorylation for the generation of heat rather than for the formation of ATP. The heat produced by brown fat mitochondria is important for maintaining body temperature in the newborn. Brown fat produces heat at approximately 450 W/kg, which contrasts with 1 W/kg from other resting mammalian tissues. The inner membrane of brown fat mitochondria has a protein *thermogenin*; this is a channel for anions (OH^-, Cl^-). Thermogenin acts as an uncoupler, in that free energy is released in the electron transfer reaction in an electrochemical potential gradient and then dissipated as heat. This requires ATP, ADP and guanosine diphosphate (GDP), which bind to the protein and inhibit anion transport. This appears to be affected by fatty acid concentrations.

Mitochondrial genoype and longevity

Accumulations of mtDNA mutations in cells may contribute to ageing and degenerative diseases. The rate of mutation in these mitochondrial DNA is said to be five to ten times faster that of nuclear DNA. An advantageous mitochondrial genotype may be significant in longevity. Mutations in the mitochondria of subjects over the age of 65 years make the mitochondria less efficient at generating ATP. It has been suggested that exercise that increases the mitochondrial mass may reduce the impact of ageing.

KEY POINTS

1. Mitochondria are elongated cylinders, important in metabolism and cellular oxidation reactions and the production of ATP. The energy provided by nutrient oxygenation in the form of NADH, $NADH_2$ and FAD is harnessed by electron transport chains to the synthesis of ATP.
2. Mitochondria contain internal membranes, a smooth outer and a folded inner membrane. The inner membrane separates the mitochondria into two distinct spaces, the internal or matrix space and the intermembrane space. The outer membrane has few enzymatic activities, but is permeable to molecules with a molecular weight of up to 5 kDa. The inner membrane is impermeable to ions and polar molecules, limits the movement of energy-rich compounds and is rich in enzymes.
3. The mitochondrion is unusual in that it contains its own DNA and the genes are derived entirely from the mother.
4. The number of mitochondria in a tissue reflects that tissue's requirement for ATP.
5. Mitochondrial functions include the synthesis of ATP, terminal oxidation of pyruvate from carbohydrate and amino acid catabolism, β-oxidation of fatty acids and oxidation of acetate, fatty acids, protein and carbohydrate. Mitochondria are also involved in the oxidation of branched-chain amino acids, maintenance of nitrogen homoeostasis and urea formation, oxidation of sulfite, activation of vitamin D_3 and synthesis of many important compounds, e.g. bile acids.
6. The processes of glycolysis, β-oxidation and the tricarboxylic acid cycle generate NADH and $NADH_2$. These undergo oxidation–reduction reactions, which provide a mechanism whereby electrons move from reduced coenzymes (NADH and $FADH_2$) to oxygen.
7. NADH dehydrogenase can only oxidise NADH within the mitochondrial matrix. Protons are bound and released on either side of the inner membrane of the mitochondria when electrons progress down the respiratory chain. This is known as chemiosmosis.
8. Mitochondria respond to metabolic and environmental conditions in ageing, training and pathological processes.

THINKING POINTS

1. Critical to metabolism is the storage of energy.
2. ATP is such a store and hence provides the energy for metabolic needs. This is a system analogous to the battery, which revolutionised the use of motors.

NEED TO UNDERSTAND

The mechanism by which mitochondria, the mother's gift to the child, convert electrochemical energy derived from nutrients into stored chemical energy that is available for use.

FURTHER READING

Boyer, P.D. (1997) The ATP synthase – a splendid molecular machine. *Annual Review of Biochemistry*, **66**, 717–50.

Brierley, E.J., Johnson, M.A., James, O.F.W. and Turnbull, D.M. (1996) Effects of physical activity and age on mitochondrial function. *Quarterly Journal Medicine*, **89**, 251–8.

Chinnery, P.F. and Turnbull, D.M. (1997) Mitochondrial medicine. *Quarterly Journal of Medicine*, **90**, 657–67.

Denton, R.M. and McCormack, J.G. (1995) Fuel selection at the level of mitochondria in mammalian tissues. *Proceedings of the Nutrition Society*, **54**, 11–22.

Dulloo, A.G. and Samec, S. (2001) Uncoupling proteins: their role in adaptive thermogenesis and substrate metabolism reconsidered. *British Journal of Nutrition*, **86**, 123–39.

Harold, F.M. (1986) *The Vital Force; A Study of Bio-energetics*. W.H. Freeman & Co., New York.

Leonard, J.V. and Schhapira, A.H.V. (2000) Mitochondrial respiratory chain disorders I. Mitochondrial DNA defects. *Lancet*, **356**, 583–7.

Schatz, G. (1997) Just follow the acid chain. *Nature*, **388**, 121–2.

Schnitzer, M.J. (2001) Molecular motors. Doing a rotary two-step. *Nature*, **410**, 878–80

Shoffner, J.M. (1996) Maternal inheritance and evaluation of oxidative phosphorylation diseases. *Lancet*, **348**, 1283–8

Shadel, G.S. and Clayton, D.A. (1997) Mitochondrial DNA maintenance in vertebrates. *Annual Review of Biochemistry*, **66**, 409–36.

Tanaka, M., Gong, J.-S., Zhang, J. *et al.* (1998) Mitochondrial genotype associated with longevity. *Lancet*, **351**, 185–6.

31

Cytochrome P450

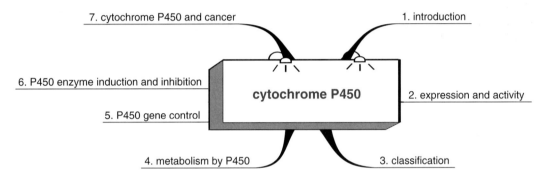

7. cytochrome P450 and cancer

1. introduction

6. P450 enzyme induction and inhibition

cytochrome P450

2. expression and activity

5. P450 gene control

4. metabolism by P450

3. classification

Fig. 31.1 Chapter outline.

INTRODUCTION

Cytochrome P450 is the collective term for a family of haemoproteins found predominantly in the hepatic endoplasmic reticulum and which possess mixed function oxidase activity. Cytochrome P450-dependent mono-oxygenases are a supergene family of enzymes that catalyse the oxidation of lipophilic chemicals through the insertion of one atom of molecular oxygen into the substrate. The enzyme systems include epoxide hydrolase, uridine diphosphate (UDP)-glucuronyltransferases, sulfotransferases and glutathione-S-transferases. They are largely responsible for the metabolism of a wide range of endogenous and exogenous compounds before excretion from the body in urine or bile, or further metabolism.

EXPRESSION AND ACTIVITY

While abundant in the liver, P450 complex enzymes are also expressed at lower concentrations in almost all tissues in the body, with the exception of striated muscle and erythrocytes. Within a given species, different tissues may vary in their overall pattern of expression and activity of different cytochrome P450 enzymes. All have characteristic ferrous carbon monoxide complexes and molecular weights of approximately 50 kDa. Their spectroscopic appearances show complex peaks near 450 nm. The P450 molecule is formed from an apoprotein and a haem prosthetic group (iron protoporphyrin IX), linked by a cysteine residue. To date, ten families of P450 enzymes (some with subfamilies) have been found in mammals and there are probably 20 or more different mammalian P450 proteins, all with distinct gene origins.

The activities of individual P450 enzymes are altered by administration of, or exposure to, a wide variety of chemicals, including carcinogens.

The P450 enzymes show catalytic specificity determined by structural features in the substrate binding site. The specificity rests in the apoprotein region, which is unique in each P450 type. Different P450 types vary in their rate of catalysis of a single reaction involving a particular substrate. Several can metabolise a single substrate, but selectively catalyse reactions at different side-chains of the molecule. Furthermore, enantiomeric pairs of a single substrate may be transformed at different rates by each P450. When presented with a prochiral substrate a P450 enzyme complex can selectively use one group, e.g. one hydrogen, as opposed to another. Catalytic specificity has important consequences. Oxidation of a single compound may render the product more electrophilic and hence capable of reacting with macromolecules. Other oxidation reactions may result in products that are less biologically active and facilitate their elimination from the body.

P450 oxidation is often sufficient for the elimination of a chemical, but sometimes the generation of a more hydrophilic metabolite is required for elimination in bile or urine e.g. glucuronide or sulfate. The cytochrome P450 family contains microsomal enzymes that convert environmental organic compounds (xenobiotics) to either stable metabolites or intermediate compounds that undergo additional metabolism by other enzyme systems. Some compounds are converted to highly reactive intermediates that covalently bind to cellular macromolecules.

CLASSIFICATION

Individual P450 enzymes are classified on the basis of amino acid sequence similarities, those displaying less than 40% sequence homology being assigned to different families. In this way, 14 P450 families can be isolated, some of which contain more than one subfamily. There are 29 subfamilies, CYP II has eight subfamilies.

Of the 14 families, four are involved in steroidogenesis, two metabolise cholesterol in bile acid synthesis and one family is concerned with fatty acid and prostaglandin metabolism. The remaining three families (CYP I, CYP II, CYP III) are responsible for the metabolism of a wide variety of foreign compounds and xenobiotics, including drugs and environmental carcinogens.

METABOLISM BY P450

The cytochromes P450 IA are responsible for the metabolism of compounds including phenacetin (O-de-ethylation), caffeine (3-demethylation) and carcinogenic arylamines (N-oxidation).

Cytochromes P450 IA1 (CYP IA1) and IA2 (CYP IA2) are members of the CYP IA gene family. This is an inducible enzyme system and induction is by many of its substrates, as well as xenobiotics found in cruciferous vegetables, e.g. flavones and indoles. Aryl-hydrocarbon hydroxylase activity, an enzymatic reaction characteristic of CYP IA enzymes, is one such inducible reaction. Such an enzyme system also exists in the small intestine. The proton pump enzyme inhibitor omeprazole has been shown to induce CYP I genes in tissues such as the human duodenum.

Polymorphism in human P450 activity exists, most notably in the metabolism of debrisoquine (by CYP IIB6), which may vary in activity by several thousand-fold between individuals. Variant RNAs from defective IID genes are responsible for the poor metabolism of debrisoquine seen in some subjects. The clinical importance of this is unclear, but rapid metabolisers of debrisoquine may be at increased risk of smoking-induced lung cancer.

There are at least three cytochrome P450 IIIA proteins and these appear to be important in the metabolism of drugs such as nifedipine, cyclosporin A and many others. Omeprazole has been shown to be an inducer of human cytochrome P450 IA and affects the clearance of diazepam and phenytoin.

Cigarette smoking can also induce members of this family. Substrates for cytochrome P450 enzymes often bind to and are metabolised by the same proteins that they induce in the course of prolonged exposure to cigarette smoke. Another mechanism is down-regulation of cytochrome P450 II proteins, i.e. a reduction in synthesis or activity that can occur with agents that induce members of the CYP IA family.

P450 GENE CONTROL

There is significant genetic polymorphism in the genes controlling the synthesis of the P450 enzyme system. The diversity of P450 enzymes appears to be controlled at the level of single genes, coding for single proteins and not by gene rearrangements.

P450 ENZYME INDUCTION AND INHIBITION

These P450 enzyme systems may be induced and inhibited in many ways. There is competition between chemicals for processing by these enzymes. The imidazoles inhibit P450 activity through a ligand interaction with the P450 haem iron, thereby impeding the rate of P450 reduction reactions. Cimetidine, used to reduce gastric hydrochloric acid production, is an imidazole derivative that inhibits P450 activity, and this effect resides in the hydrophobic nature of its side-chain. In contrast, exposure to lipophilic substances may lead to an adaptive response by the P450 system which, in turn, enhances the elimination of these substances. During induction of P450 IA1, for example, there is an interaction of the hydrocarbon with a hydrophobic cytosolic receptor (the 'Ah', i.e. aromatic hydrocarbon receptor). The substrate–ligand complex translocates to the nucleus and there is increased specific P450 enzyme complex synthesis. Other inducers include glucocorticoids, e.g. dexamethasone and macrolide antibiotics also induce P450 IIIA1 activity. Phenobarbitone induces P450 IIB1, IIC6 and IIA1, while ethanol is a potent inducer of P450 IIE1 activity.

CYTOCHROME P450 AND CANCER

The majority of known procarcinogens are converted by P450-dependent reactions into electrophiles that bind covalently to DNA.

The cytochrome P450 IA family appears to be particularly important in the biotransformation of procarcinogens and carcinogens. They activate or inactivate a broad range of procarcinogens, including polyaromatic hydrocarbons, e.g. benzopyrene, arylamines and aflatoxin B_l. Enhanced activity of these enzyme systems may be important in the risk of cancer formation through bioactivation of procarcinogens; however, they may reduce this risk by the detoxification of carcinogenic parent molecules. Such bioactivation reactions include epoxidation and hydroxylation of the procarcinogen benzo[a]pyrene and related polyaromatic hydrocarbons. In contrast, protective pathways include 4-hydroxylation of the carcinogen aflatoxin to an inactive metabolite. The degree of induction of cytochrome P450 IA depends on many factors, including dietary components and endogenous hormones. The extent of environmental exposure to particular chemicals is important, as is the variable extent of induction in individual subjects.

KEY POINTS

1. Cytochrome P450 is the collective term for a family of haemoproteins found predominantly in the hepatic endoplasmic reticulum, which possess mixed function oxidase activity. This supergene family of enzymes catalyses the oxidation of lipophilic chemicals through the insertion of one atom of molecular oxygen into the substrate. The enzyme systems include epoxide hydrolase, UDP-glucuronyltransferases, sulfotransferases and glutathione-S-transferases.
2. P450 oxidation may be sufficient for the elimination of a chemical, but sometimes the generation of a more hydrophilic metabolite, e.g. glucuronide or sulfate, is required.

3. In the genes controlling the synthesis of the P450 enzyme system, there is significant genetic polymorphism. These P450 enzyme systems may be induced and inhibited in many ways.
4. The cytochrome P450 1A family is important in the biotransformation of procarcinogens and carcinogens.

THINKING POINT

Many potentially toxic chemicals present in the diet, e.g. from plant secondary metabolites and agricultural chemicals, are detoxified by the P450 system, an important protective system. The stimulation of these enzymes by plant secondary metabolites and agricultural chemicals is an unexplored area.

NEED TO UNDERSTAND

1. This large superfamily encodes more than 55 enzymes which act as oxidases in mixed function oxidase reactions.
2. The metabolism of many exogenous substances, drugs and plant secondary metabolites is undertaken in this system.

FURTHER READING

Guengerich, F.P. (1988) Roles of cytochrome P450-enzyme in chemical carcinogenesis in cancer chemotherapy. *Cancer Research*, **48**, 2946–54.

Jokanovic, M. (2001) Biotransformation of organophosphate compounds. *Toxicology*, **166**, 139–60.

Lin, J.H. and Lu, A.Y.H. (2001) Interindividual variability in inhibition and induction of cytochrome P450 enzymes. *Annual Review of Pharmacology and Toxicology*, **41**, 535–68.

McDonnell, W.M., Scheiman, J.M. and Traber, P.G. (1992) Induction of cytochrome P450 IA genes (CYP IA) by omeprazole in the human alimentary tract. *Gastroenterology*, **103**, 1509–16.

Miles, J.S. and Wolf, C.R. (1991) Developments and perspectives on the role of cytochrome P450 in chemical carcinogenesis. *Carcinogenesis*, **12**, 2195–9.

Murray, G.I., Melvin, W.T., Greenlee, W.F. and Burke, M.D. (2001) Regulation, function and tissue-specific expression of cytochrome P450 CYP1B1. *Annual Review of Pharmacology and Toxicology*, **41**, 297–316.

Park, B.K. (2000) Cytochrome P450 enzymes in the heart. *Lancet*, **355**, 945–6.

Vaz, A.D. (2001) Multiple oxidants in cytochrome P450 catalyzed reactions: implications for drug metabolism. *Current Drug Metabolism*, **2**, 1–16.

32

Free radicals

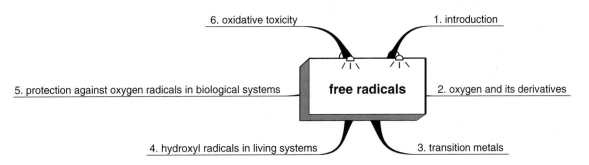

Fig. 32.1 Chapter outline.

INTRODUCTION

Metabolism is a balance of oxidation and reduction. Oxidative processes have to be contained through defence mechanisms that are developed through an antioxidant system that nullifies excess free radicals produced by oxidative processes. The antioxidant system includes mineral-dependent enzymes and small molecules, usually vitamins, which act as scavengers of reactive oxygen species. The enzymes include the selenium-dependent free-radical scavenger glutathione peroxidase. The low molecular weight molecules include the water-soluble ascorbic acid, glutathione and uric acid, and the lipid-soluble carotenoids and vitamin E.

Radicals are groups of atoms that behave as a unit. A free radical is any chemical type capable of independent existence that contains one or more unpaired electrons. An unpaired electron is one that occupies an atomic or a molecular orbital by itself. Radicals can easily be formed by homolytic fission when a covalent bond is split, when one electron from each shared pair remains with each atom.

In a compound where A and B are two covalently bonded atoms, $_x{}^x$ represents the electron pair. Homolytic fission can be written as:

$$A_x{}^xB \rightarrow A^x + B_x$$

A^x is an A-radical, often written as A·, and B_x is a B-radical (B·). Homolytic fission of one covalent bond in a water molecule produces a hydrogen radical (H·) and a hydroxyl radical (OH·). In heterolytic fission, however, one atom receives both electrons when a covalent bond breaks, i.e.

$$A_x{}^xB \rightarrow A_x{}^{x-} + B^+$$

This extra electron gives A a negative charge and B is left with a positive charge. Heterolytic fission of water gives a hydrogen ion (H^+) and a hydroxyl ion (OH^-).

OXYGEN AND ITS DERIVATIVES

Oxygen is a good oxidising agent, being a radical with two unpaired electrons, each located in a different π^* antibonding orbital. These two electrons have the same spin quantum number or parallel spins. This is the stable or *ground state* of oxygen.

- **Oxidation** is the loss of electrons by an atom or molecule, e.g. the conversion of a sodium atom to the ion Na^+.
- **Reduction** is the gain of electrons by an atom or molecule, e.g. the conversion of a chlorine atom to the ion Cl^-.
- An **oxidising agent** absorbs electrons from the molecule that it oxidises, whereas a reducing agent is an electron donor.

When oxygen accepts electrons these electrons must be of antiparallel spin so as to fit in the vacant spaces in the π^* orbitals. Electrons in an atomic or a molecular orbital would not meet this criterion as they have opposing spins. This restricts electron transfer, which tends to make oxygen accept electrons one at a time, resulting in oxygen reacting slowly with many non-radicals. More reactive forms of oxygen, known as *singlet oxygen*, can be generated in pairs. There are thus no unpaired electrons; therefore, this is not a radical. In both pairs of singlet oxygen the spin restriction is removed and the oxidising ability is increased. If a single electron is added to the ground-state oxygen molecule it enters one of the π^* antibonding orbitals, producing a superoxide radical, O_2^-. With only one unpaired electron, superoxide is actually less of a radical than oxygen itself. Adding one more electron creates O_2^{2-}, the peroxide ion. As the extra electrons O_2^- and O_2^{2-} enter antibonding orbitals the strength of the oxygen bond decreases. Adding two extra electrons to the O_2^{2-} would remove the bond as they pass into the δ^*2p orbitals, so giving $2O^{2-}$ species.

Ozone

Ozone (O_3) is produced by the photodissociation of molecular oxygen into oxygen atoms:

$$O_2 \xrightarrow{\text{solar energy}} 2O$$

$$O_2 + O \longrightarrow O_3$$

Photodissociation of fluorinated hydrocarbons, e.g. CF_2Cl_2 and $CFCl_3$, produces chlorine atoms in the atmosphere which cause the breakdown of ozone. Nitric oxide (NO) and nitrogen dioxide (NO_2) can also affect ozone. These also involve free radicals.

Oxidation and reduction

$$O_2 \xrightarrow[\text{reduction}]{\text{one-electron}} O_2$$

$$O_2 \xrightarrow[\substack{\text{reduction} \\ \text{(plus } 2H^+)}]{\text{two-electron}} H_2O_2 \text{ (protonated form of } O_2^{2-})$$

$$O_2 \xrightarrow[\substack{\text{reduction} \\ \text{(plus } 4H^+)}]{\text{four-electron}} 2H_2O \text{ (protonated form of } O^{2-})$$

O–O is relatively weak and hydrogen peroxide readily decomposes with homolytic fission:
$$H_2O_2 \longrightarrow 2OH^+$$

TRANSITION METALS

All of the metals in the first row of the d-block in the Periodic Table contain unpaired electrons and are radicals, with the exception of zinc. Copper is not exactly a transition element as the 3d orbitals are full, but form the Cu^{2+} ion by loss of two electrons: one from the 4s and one from the 3d orbital, leaving an unpaired electron. The transition elements have a variable valency, which allows changes in oxidation state involving one electron. Examples are iron, iron(II) ferrous ion and iron(III) ferric ion; copper(I) cuprous ion and copper(II) cupric ion. Iron(III) is stable, whereas iron(II) salts are weak reducing agents. Manganese can exist as Mn(III), Mn(IV) and Mn(VII). Zinc has only one valency, Zn^{2+}, and does not promote radical reaction.

Reactions of a free radical with a non-radical species may produce a different free radical which is more or less reactive than the original radical.

Radicals of OH^+ may be due to hydrogen removal, addition and electron transfer. Radicals produced by reactions with OH^+ usually have reduced reactivity. An example of hydrogen removal is

$$CH_3OH^{\bullet} \longrightarrow {}^{\bullet}CH_2OH + H_2O$$
$${}^{\bullet}CH_2OH + O_2 \longrightarrow {}^{\bullet}O_2CH_2OH$$

This may lead to two radicals joining to form a non-radical product joined by a covalent bond. $OH\cdot$ may react with aromatic ring structures and with the purine and pyrimidine bases in DNA and RNA. A thymidine radical may undergo a series of reactions.

HYDROXYL RADICALS IN LIVING SYSTEMS

Ionising radiation

The major constituent of living cells is water. Exposure of such water to ionising radiation results in hydroxyl radical production and possibly damage to cellular DNA and to membranes.

Detection of hydroxyl radicals

Electron spin resonance (ESR) detects the presence of unpaired electrons. An unpaired electron has a spin of either $+1/2$ or $-1/2$ and behaves like a small magnet. When exposed to an external magnetic field an unpaired electron can align itself in a direction either parallel or antiparallel to that field and thus can have two possible energy levels. Electromagnetic radiation of the correct energy is absorbed and moves the electron from the lower energy level to the upper one. An absorption spectrum is obtained.

ESR spectrometers show not the absorption but the rate of change of absorption. ESR is very sensitive and can detect radicals at concentrations as low as 10^{-10} mol/l, provided that there is some stability. For very unstable radicals several other techniques are available. Flow systems are used whereby the radicals are continuously generated in the spectrometer so as to maintain a steady-state concentration. An alternative procedure is spin-trapping. A highly reactive radical is allowed to react with a compound to produce a long-lived radical, e.g. nitroso compounds ($R\cdot NO$) in reaction with radicals may produce nitroxide radicals that have a prolonged lifetime.

Spin-trapping methods are often used to detect the presence of superoxide and hydroxyl radicals in biological systems, e.g. the formation of organic radicals during lipid peroxidation. Trapping molecules include *tert*-nitrosobutane, α-phenyl-*tert*-butylnitrone, 5,5-dimethylpyrroline-*N*-oxide, *tert*-butylnitrosobenzene and α-(4-pyridyl-1-oxide)-*N*-*tert*-butylnitrone. The ideal trap reacts rapidly and specifically with the radical under study to produce a stable product with a highly characteristic ESR. However, reactions with such radicals may inhibit the process and dynamics.

Aromatic hydroxylation

Aromatic compounds react rapidly with hydroxyl radicals to produce hydroxycyclohexadienyl radicals. Such a radical may undergo dimerisation to give a product that may decompose to give biphenyl or result in a mixture of phenol and benzene. This is called a disproportionation reaction. Disproportionation is a reaction in which one molecule is reduced and an identical molecule oxidised. One radical molecule is reduced to benzene and another oxidised to phenol. The attack of $OH\cdot$ on phenol produces a mixture of hydroxylated products.

Production of singlet oxygen

Two singlet states of oxygen exist when the spin restrictions are removed, resulting in increased reactivity. The singlet state of oxygen is energetic. The singlet oxygen produced on illumination with light of the correct wavelength can react with other molecules or may attack the photosensitiser molecule. These are known as photodynamic effects. Photosensitisation reactions involving singlet oxygen may be important in biological systems, e.g. chloroplasts of higher plants and the retina of the eye.

Singlet oxygen can interact with other molecules, to combine chemically or transfer its excitation energy, by returning to the ground state while the other molecule enters an excited state. This is known as quenching. The most important of these reactions of singlet oxygen involves compounds that contain carbon–carbon double covalent bonds. Such bonds are present in carotenes, chlorophyll and the fatty acid side-chains in membrane lipids. Such double bonds separated by a single bond (conjugated double bonds) often react to give endoperoxides. If one double bond is present, a reaction can occur in which the singlet oxygen adds on and the double bond shifts to a different position. Damage to proteins by singlet oxygen is often due to oxidation of methionine, tryptophan, histidine or cysteine residues.

Reactions of the superoxide radical

Superoxide dismutase specifically catalyses removal of the superoxide O_2^-. The concept of the free radical suggests that O_2^- formation is a major factor in oxygen toxicity. Superoxide dismutase enzyme activity is an essential defence. Superoxide chemistry depends on whether the reaction is in aqueous solution or in organic solvents.

Superoxide in aqueous solution acts as a base, i.e. acceptor of protons (H^+ ions). When O_2^- accepts a proton, it forms the hydroperoxyl radical ($HO_2\cdot$). $HO_2\cdot$ can dissociate to release H^+ ions again. There is a supply of protons, i.e. it is an acid. When O_2^- and H^+ ions are mixed, an equilibrium is established:

$$HO_2 \longleftrightarrow H^+ + O_2^-$$

Superoxide in aqueous solution is also a very weak oxidising agent, i.e. an electron acceptor, and oxidises ascorbic acid. In contrast, there is no significant oxidation of reduced nicotinamide adenine dinucleotide (NADH) or reduced NAD phosphate (NADPH). It will, however, interact with NADH, bound to the active site of the enzyme lactate dehydrogenase, but not other dehydrogenases.

When superoxide is dissolved in organic solvents the ability to act as a base and as a reducing agent is increased and may reduce dissolved sulfur dioxide in organic solvents (which it does not do when in aqueous solution). O_2^- has a longer life, is able

to act as a nucleophile and is attracted to centres of positive charges in a molecule. Superoxide can displace chloride ion from chlorinated hydrocarbons such as chloroform.

The disappearance of O_2^- in aqueous solution is a dismutation reaction:

$$O_2^- + O_2^- + 2H^+ \rightarrow H_2O_2 + O_2$$

This dismutation reaction is most rapid at acidic pH values needed to protonate O_2^- and will become slower as the pH rises and becomes more alkaline.

As well as acting as a weak base, O_2^- in aqueous solution is a reducing agent, i.e. a donor of electrons, and may reduce cytochrome c. Iron is reduced from the Fe^{3+} to the Fe^{2+} state.

Any biological system generating O_2^- may produce hydrogen peroxide by the dismutation reaction. However, the O_2^- may be intercepted by some other molecule, e.g. cytochrome c. Hydrogen peroxide, through O_2^-, may be formed in mitochondria and microsomes. Enzymes that produce hydrogen peroxide without the free O_2^- radical include glycollate oxidase, D-amino acid oxidase and urate oxidase.

PROTECTION AGAINST OXYGEN RADICALS IN BIOLOGICAL SYSTEMS

This is referred to as the superoxide theory of oxygen toxicity.

Protection by enzymes

It is important for cells to control the amount of hydrogen peroxide in the cell. This may be achieved enzymatically:

catalase: $2H_2O_2 \rightarrow 2H_2O + O_2$
peroxidases: $SH_2 + H_2O_2 \rightarrow S + 2H_2O$

where SH_2 is the substrate being oxidised. Catalase is present in all major organs, particularly the liver and red cells, and in modest amounts in the brain, heart and skeletal muscle.

Catalases

Catalases consist of four protein subunits containing a haem [Fe(III) protoporphyrin] group bound to the active site.

The catalase reaction is:

$$Fe(III) + H_2O_2 \rightarrow Compound\ I$$
$$Compound\ I + H_2O_2 \rightarrow Catalase\text{--}Fe(III) + 2H_2O + O_2$$

Glutathione peroxidase is found in animal tissues but not in higher plants or bacteria. The substrate is the thiol compound glutathione (GSH). Most GSH exists as the free compound but approximately one-third of the total cellular GSH may be present as mixed disulfides, with the remainder present as other compounds that contain –SH groups, e.g. cysteine, coenzyme A and the –SH of the cysteine residues of proteins. Glutathione peroxidase enzymatically assists the oxidation of GSH to GSSG at the expense of hydrogen peroxide:

$$H_2O_2 + 2GSH \rightarrow GSSG + H_2O$$

This enzyme is found particularly in the liver, less in the heart, lung and brain, and hardly at all in muscle.

Glutathione oxidase consists of four protein subunits containing selenium at the active site. Selenium belongs to group VI of the Periodic Table and has properties intermediate between a metal and a non-metal. Selenium may well be at the active site as selenocysteine, wherein the sulfur atom is replaced by a selenium atom.

The GSH reduces the selenium and the reduced form of the enzyme reacts with hydrogen peroxide. The reduction of GSSG to GSH is by glutathione reductase:

$$GSSG + NADPH + H^+ \rightarrow 2GSH + NADP^+$$

The NADPH is derived from the oxidative pentose phosphate pathway. The pentose phosphate pathway is controlled by the supply of $NADP^+$ to glucose-6-phosphate dehydrogenase.

Superoxide dismutase

The superoxide radical is believed to be a major factor in oxygen toxicity and the superoxide dismutase enzymes are an essential defence mecha-

Glutathione reductase reduces the NADPH: $NADP^+$ ratio. The enzyme contains two protein subunits with flavin adenine dinucleotide (FAD) at the active site. NADPH reduces the FAD and the electron moves to a disulfide bridge (–S–S–) between the two cysteine residues on the protein. The two –SH groups interact with GSSG, which results in the reduction to 2GSH.

In mammalian red blood cells, the pentose phosphate pathway is important in providing NADPH for glutathione reduction. However, red cell glucose-6-phosphate dehydrogenase deficiency results in haemolysis, which commonly occurs in populations in tropical and Mediterranean areas. Curiously, this enzymatic deficiency is protective against infestation with the malarial parasite.

nism. In general, oxidative metabolism results in water and carbon dioxide. A few enzymes, e.g. glycollate oxidase, produce hydrogen peroxide. Other enzymes reduce oxygen to O_2^-.

The copper–zinc enzymes

The copper–zinc-containing superoxide dismutases are specific for the superoxide radical. These enzymes are found in all animal cells and have a molecular weight of approximately 32 kDa. They contain two protein subunits, each bearing an active site containing one copper ion and one zinc ion. The reaction catalysed is:

$$O_2^- + O_2 \longrightarrow + 2H^+ \rightarrow H_2O_2 + O_2$$

The copper ions undergo alternate oxidation and reduction. The zinc does not appear to function in the catalytic cycle but stabilises the enzyme.

The amino acid structure of the copper–zinc superoxidase dismutase from yeast, human red cells, horse liver and bovine red cells appears to be similar and consists of eight antiparallel strands of β-pleated sheet structure forming a flattened cylinder and three external loops.

The copper ion is held at the active site by interactions with the nitrogens in the imidazole ring structure, of four histidine residues. Zinc is connected by a bridge to the copper by interaction with the imidazole of histidine. The surface of each protein is largely negatively charged, repelling O_2^-, although there is a positively charged channel leading into the active site.

Manganese enzymes
The manganese superoxide dismutase is a tetramer and contains 0.5 or 1 ion of manganese per subunit, which is essential for catalytic activity. The amino acid sequence of all manganese superoxidase dismutases is similar in animals, plants and bacteria.

Protection by small molecules

Ascorbic acid
Ascorbic acid is a cofactor for the enzymes proline hydroxylase and lysine hydroxylase, which are involved in the biosynthesis of collagen. These enzymes contain iron at their active sites. Ascorbic acid is necessary for the action of dopamine-β-hydroxylase, which is involved in the conversion of dopamine to noradrenaline. Ascorbic acid acts as a reducing agent, e.g. in the reduction of Fe(III) to Fe(II). The loss of one electron by ascorbic acid results in the semidehydroascorbate radical, which then oxidises to dehydroascorbate. Dehydroascorbate is unstable and spontaneously converts into oxalic and L-threonic acid. Ascorbic acid scavenges ringlet oxygen.

Glutathione
GSH is a substrate for glutathione peroxidase and for dehydroascorbate reductase. Glutathione is also a scavenger of hydroxyl radicals and ringlet oxygen. Glutathione is a cofactor for such enzymes as glyoxylase, malonylacetoacetate isomerase and prostaglandin endoperoxide isomerase, and may be involved in the synthesis of thyroid hormones.

Uric acid
Uric acid is present in plasma. It is a scavenger of ringlet oxygen and hydroxyl radicals and may, for example, inhibit lipid peroxidation.

OXIDATIVE TOXICITY

It has been suggested that in tissue deprived of oxygen there is a rapid conversion of xanthine dehydrogenase to oxidase activity. During ischaemia there is degradation of adenosine triphosphate (ATP) in the ischaemic cells and accumulation of hypoxanthine. However, when oxygen is restored there is reperfusion damage. The accumulated hypoxanthine is oxidised by xanthine oxidase and the excessive O_2^- causes further damage. Other molecules that oxidise in the presence of oxygen to yield O_2^- include glyceraldehyde, the reduced forms of riboflavin, adrenaline and thiol compounds, e.g. cysteine.

Lipid peroxidation

Lipid peroxidation is the oxidative deterioration of polyunsaturated lipids. Superoxidation of a polyunsaturated fatty acid involves the removal of a hydrogen ion from a methylene ($-CH_2-$) group. This leaves an unpaired electron on the carbon $-CH-$ and the production of a conjugated diene to give a peroxy radical, $R-OO^+$. The propagation stage of lipid peroxidation is the addition of a hydrogen atom from another lipid molecule so that a chain reaction develops to yield a lipid hydroperoxide, $R-OOH$. An alternative is the production of cyclic peroxides.

Vitamin E

Vitamin E concentrates in the interior of membranes and in tissues where lipid antioxidant activity is important. Vitamin E quenches and reacts with ringlet oxygen and reacts with the superoxide radical, although this reaction is slow. Vitamin E can react with lipid peroxy radicals to form vitamin E radicals, thereby interrupting the chain reaction of lipid peroxidation, i.e. it is a chain terminator. It is possible that the vitamin E radical is reduced back to vitamin E by vitamin C.

Glutathione peroxidase

This enzyme disposes of hydrogen peroxide. It has an important role in protection against lipid peroxidation in lipoproteins.

KEY POINTS

1. Metabolism is a balance of oxidation and reduction. Oxidative processes have to be contained through defence mechanisms, using an antioxidant system which nullifies excess free radicals engendered by oxidative processes. The antioxidant system includes mineral-dependent enzymes and small molecules (usually vitamins), which act as scavengers of reactive oxygen species.

2. A free radical is any species capable of independent existence that contains one or more unpaired electrons. An unpaired electron is one that occupies an atomic or molecular orbital by itself.

3. Oxidation is the loss of electrons by an atom or molecule, e.g. the conversion of a sodium atom to the ion Na^+. Reduction is the gain of electrons by an atom or molecule, e.g. the conversion of a chlorine atom to the ion Cl^-. An oxidising agent absorbs electrons from the molecule that it oxidises, whereas a reducing agent is an electron donor.

4. The major constituent of living cells is water. Exposure of such water to ionising radiation results in hydroxyl radical production and possibly damage to cellular DNA and membranes.

5. It is important for cells to control the amount of hydrogen peroxide in the cell. This may be achieved enzymatically, e.g. catalase, peroxidases, superoxide dismutase, and copper–zinc and manganese enzymes.

6. Protection against oxygen radicals is provided by small molecules, e.g. ascorbic acid, glutathione and uric acid. Lipid peroxidation is the oxidative deterioration of polyunsaturated lipids. Superoxidation of a polyunsaturated fatty acid involves the removal of a hydrogen ion from a methylene ($-CH_2-$) group. Protection is given by vitamin E and glutathione peroxidase.

7. It has been suggested that in tissue deprived of oxygen there is a rapid conversion of xanthine dehydrogenase to oxidase activity. During ischaemia there is degradation of ATP in the ischaemic cells and accumulation of hypoxanthine. However, when oxygen is restored there is reperfusion damage. The accumulated hypoxanthine is oxidised by xanthine oxidase and the excessive O_2^- causes further damage.

THINKING POINTS

1. Antioxidants have differing solubilities in lipid and water.
2. This implies that the different phases of the cell, water soluble and fat soluble, will be protected by lipid-soluble and water-soluble antioxidants.
3. This requires a mix of antioxidants in the diet.

NEED TO UNDERSTAND

The chemistry behind the antioxidant phenomenon.

FURTHER READING

Aruoma, O.I. and Halliwell, B. (eds) (1998) *Molecular Biology of Free Radicals in Human Diseases*. OICA International, Saint Lucia.

Eastwood, M.A. (1999) Interaction of dietary antioxidants *in vivo*: how fruit and vegetables prevent disease? *Quarterly Journal of Medicine*, **92**, 527–20.

Fridovich, I. (1995) Superoxide radical and superoxide dismutases. *Annual Review of Biochemistry*, **64**, 97–112.

Halliwell, B. (1996) Antioxidants in human health and disease. *Annual Review of Nutrition*, **16**, 33–51.

Halliwell, B. and Gutteridge, J.M.C. (1999) *Free Radicals in Biology and Medicine*. Oxford University Press, Oxford.

33

Carbohydrate metabolism

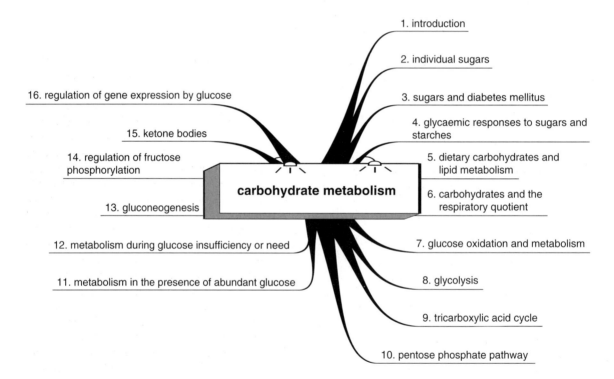

Fig. 33.1 Chapter outline.

INTRODUCTION

Despite their central importance for metabolic processes, carbohydrates are not in the strict sense essential nutrients. Nevertheless, glucose is an important constituent in the provision of energy to the body and in that respect is essential. If the carbohydrate content of the diet is reduced or low then more expensive and less immediately utilisable

energy sources such as fat and protein have to be used. This is expensive both nutritionally and metabolically.

Dietary carbohydrates, whether eaten as starches, glycogen or glucose, are metabolised as their constituent monosaccharides. The presence of the monosaccharides glucose, galactose and fructose in tissues is essential for normal nutritional development.

INDIVIDUAL SUGARS

Glucose

Dietary carbohydrates are 70–90% glucose. Starch that is absorbed in the jejunum is metabolised largely as glucose. The metabolic differences between different physical types of starch result from their digestion and absorption in different parts of the lumen of the gut.

Glucose in the blood is derived from food, from the breakdown of preformed glycogen in the liver or by glucose molecules formed in the liver from circulating intermediate metabolites. Dietary glucose is absorbed, enters the body through the portal vein and crosses the liver, where some of it is removed and converted by phosphorylation into glucose-6-phosphate and glycogen. A reliable blood glucose concentration is important for tissue metabolism. Controls on carbohydrate metabolism depend on whether there is an abundance or a shortage of carbohydrate. Glucose may be taken up by tissues, particularly skeletal muscles. Insulin facilitates the active transport of glucose into the muscle and fat cells, where glucose is converted into glucose-6-phosphate by hexokinase. At the same time glucose production by the liver is suppressed. Insulin increases the uptake of glucose into the fat or muscle cell through the redistribution of the glucose transporter GLUT4 on the cell membrane. The glucose membrane cell transport systems of the brain, the haematopoietic system, bone marrow and red cells, liver and endocrine pancreas do not require insulin.

Glucose is the prime fuel source for the red cell, the kidney medulla and the central nervous system. The liver and skeletal and cardiac muscle can use alternative fuels such as ketone bodies and fatty acids. Adipose tissue converts glucose to α-glycerol phosphate for triglyceride formation.

Post-prandially in humans there is massive glycogen synthesis. Following a high protein meal much of the glucose incorporated into glycogen originates from pyruvate and oxaloacetate. The amino acids absorbed by the intestinal mucosa pass into the blood and are taken up by a variety of tissues, including the liver. The carbon skeleton from the amino acids may be stored as glycogen. In con-

trast, during fasting glycogen may be converted to glucose-1-phosphate and then to pyruvate. The liver is central to this process, exporting glucose to the blood from the glycogen which is stored post-prandially. When the blood glucose concentration begins to fall, the liver supplies glucose to the blood following the breakdown of glycogen. When the blood glucose level is further reduced, the hexose phosphate pool is supplemented from glycogen and from pyruvate and oxaloacetate. Glucose-6-phosphate is hydrolysed and glucose supplied to the blood.

Galactose

Galactose is absorbed through the same active transport system in the small intestine as glucose. Galactose enters the portal venous blood but is almost entirely removed by the liver at first pass so that little enters the peripheral circulation. The blood concentration of galactose is rarely greater than 1.0 mmol/l. Alcohol inhibits galactose uptake and metabolism by the liver and galactosaemia can occur. Galactose in the cells is converted by the specific enzyme galactokinase to galactose-1-phosphate and then to glucose-1-phosphate, catalysed by an epimerase. This is in contrast to fructose, which can enter the glycolytic pathway directly without being converted into glucose. While there are enzymes throughout the body that metabolise galactose, most galactose metabolism takes place in the liver through the utilisation of dietary galactose. Any galactose that is required for structural purposes in body cells and connective tissue, e.g. galactosamine, a constituent of glycoprotein and mucopolysaccharides, is produced by the reversal of the normal galactose–glucose interconversions.

Galactose, when present in the blood, is taken up by specific tissues, particularly the lens of the eye. The galactose is converted by aldehyde reductase into galactitol. This may accumulate in tissues and is a factor in the development of cataracts. Cataracts are a complication of diabetes mellitus and may also occur in inborn errors of galactose metabolism caused by a deficiency of galactose-1-phosphate uridyltransferase and in galactokinase deficiency. Galactokinase deficiency is not associated with any clinical problems other than galactosaemia, galactosuria and cataracts.

Galactose-1-phosphate uridyltransferase deficiency usually has a fatal outcome in the first few days of life or results in mental retardation. Treatment depends on instant recognition and the exclusion of galactose in the form of lactose in human or animal milk. In these instances it is necessary to give soya milk supplemented by sucrose, glucose or fructose. This deficiency condition is very rare. The heterozygotes have a reduced galactose-1-phosphate uridyltransferase activity and make up 1% of the population.

Fructose

In humans, fructose enters the portal venous system unchanged and is taken up by the liver; little passes to the systemic circulation. Within the liver, fructose is phosphorylated to fructose 1-phosphate by a hepatic fructokinase. Fructokinase requires ATP and inorganic phosphate, which is regenerated when fructose-1-phosphate is split into glyceraldehyde and dihydroxyacetone phosphate. The splitting of fructose-1-phosphate is catalysed by hepatic aldolase (aldolase B). The hepatic aldolase differs from the muscle aldolase in having an equal affinity for fructose-1-phosphate and fructose-1,6-diphosphate. Fructose-1,6-diphosphate is an important intermediary in the glycolytic and gluconeogenic pathways of the liver and kidney. Dihydroxyacetone phosphate is an intermediate in metabolism in both the glycolytic and gluconeogenic pathways.

Glyceraldehyde is a substrate for a number of enzymes before glycolytic intermediary metabolism. Much of the glyceraldehyde from fructose is converted to glyceraldehyde-3-phosphate, which can then be converted to glycogen. Alternatively, glyceraldehyde can be converted to glycerol-3-phosphate to be esterified as fatty acids to triglycerides. The activity of these reactions is dictated by the nutritional and hormonal state of the individual.

Following the ingestion of fructose or sucrose in substantial amounts, there is an increase in the peripheral blood pyruvate and lactate as a result of intermediates entering the glycolytic rather than the gluconeogenic pathways of the liver. Fructose can increase the rate of alcohol metabolism by 10% when given intravenously with alcohol. This occurs through the inhibition of gluconeogenesis from pyruvate and lactate. Fructose, unlike glucose, does not require insulin to be transported into muscle and fat cells. Consequently, glucose and fructose have a different role in fat metabolism and insulin release.

In contrast to glucose, fructose can enter cells regardless of the insulin concentration and can be used as a substrate for hexokinase and conversion into fructose-6-phosphate and glycerol-3-phosphate. This is available for re-esterification of free fatty acids produced by intra-adipocyte lipolysis. Production of fructose-1-phosphate leads to an increase in adenosine triphosphate (ATP) turnover and intrahepatic depletion of inorganic phosphate.

This may occasionally lead to a rise in body urate production, which may occur in chronic alcohol abuse with a predisposition to the development of gout. However, it is possible that there is increased urate production in hereditary fructose intolerance in the heterozygous state. This has led to the occasional treatment of gout by a fructose-restricted diet.

Polyols

Sorbitol is a sweetener that is absorbed more slowly from the gut than any of the monosaccharides and is removed from the portal blood by the liver. Sorbitol is converted into fructose by sorbitol dehydrogenase and then into fructose-1-phosphate by fructokinase. Sorbitol can be formed from glucose in the body by the action of aldose reductase.

Xylitol is an intermediate in the glucuronic acid pathway and is involved in vitamin C synthesis in some animals. In the benign inborn error pentosuria, L-xylulose is excreted into urine. L-Xylulose reductase deficiency does not allow the conversion of L-xylulose into xylitol, xylitol being further metabolised to glucose-5-phosphate or glucose-6-phosphate. Xylitol is sweeter than sorbitol.

Carbohydrates and vitamins

Most of the enzymes involved in carbohydrate metabolism require vitamin B metabolites as essential coenzymes. This requirement increases the dietary requirement for these vitamins. The coenzymes from vitamin B are cofactors in the glycolytic pathway, pentose phosphate shunt and tricarboxylic acid (TCA) cycle. For example, thiamin pyrophosphate is the coenzyme for pyruvate dehydrogenase, transketolase and α-ketoglutarate dehydrogenase.

Non-enzymatic glycosylation

Sugars may react with free amino groups on proteins to produce a readily chemically reversible glycosylated product (a Schiff base), which may then undergo internal rearrangements to produce a more stable and possibly reversible Amadori-type glycosylation product. This can be converted irreversibly into an advanced glycosylation endproduct that may interact with other proteins.

Both aldose and ketose sugars can react with proteins to form Schiff bases when in the chair form. Glucose has only 0.002% in the chair form, whereas 0.7% of fructose is in the chair form. Fructose is thus more significant in the development of non-enzymatic glycosylated proteins.

SUGARS AND DIABETES MELLITUS

The products of some metabolic pathways of glucose and galactose may result in many of the diabetic complications. Muscle tissue, fat cells and connective tissue require insulin for the transmembrane passage of glucose. Neurones, epithelial and endothelial cells do not require insulin for glucose entry and depend on the concentration of glucose in the plasma. At high glucose concentration glucose and other aldoses are reduced to the corresponding sugar alcohols, glucose forming glucitol and galactose forming galactitol. Diabetics have an increased concentration of an abnormal haemoglobin, HbA_I, which results from the attachment of a molecule of glucose to the N-terminus of the β-ring, an Amadori rearrangement. Many proteins will condense with sugars even at normal concentrations of glucose. Collagen, crystallin in the lens, serum proteins, nerve myelin, all membrane proteins, transferrin and fibronectin, all form glucose adducts. All of these incorporations are increased in diabetics.

HbA_I

The HbA_I concentration is dependent on the mean blood glucose concentration. In the normal non-diabetic population on average 4–5% of the haemoglobin is of the A_I variant, but in diabetics this may increase to 8–15%, depending on the previous blood glucose concentrations. Measurement of HbA_I enables a history to be obtained of the recent glucose control during the weeks preceding the assay.

GLYCAEMIC RESPONSES TO SUGARS AND STARCHES

A carbohydrate meal, other than fructose, produces an increase in blood glucose. The blood glucose concentration is also a factor in the feeling of hunger. The capillary blood glucose concentration increases in response to starch and glucose.

Factors affecting measurements of the glycaemic response to meals:

These include:

- the method of measuring the blood sugar concentration
- whether arterial or venous blood is sampled
- whether the long-term or acute response is taken into account
- the chemical nature of the carbohydrate under study, and especially the constituent monosaccharides
- whether the carbohydrate is taken alone or with other dietary constituents
- the physical form and texture of the ingested carbohydrate
- the amount of carbohydrate eaten at one sitting
- whether the carbohydrate is eaten raw, cooked or processed
- the energy content and composition of the normal diet
- the rate of gastric emptying
- the health status of the individual being studied.

In the fasting state arterial and venous bloods contain equivalent amounts of glucose. Post-prandially, however, the arterial blood concentration of glucose rises rapidly and then falls to fasting levels. Venous blood concentrations rise more slowly and a peak is achieved within 2 h of ingestion. This arterial–venous (A/V) blood glucose difference is a measure of the uptake of glucose by the tissues under the influence of insulin secreted in response to the diet. It is a useful indicator of the peripheral utilisation of glucose.

In diabetes the rise in blood glucose concentration, particularly of venous blood, bears little relationship to the size of the glucose load. When large amounts of more than 50 g are taken there is a saturation of the system in the normal subject. In diabetics, the blood glucose concentration continues to rise with the glucose load until there is overflow and renal excretion.

Blood glucose measurements are usually taken for 2–3 h after a test meal. This permits the calculation of a glycaemic response or a graph of glucose concentration over time. The results indicate the difference in the rate at which glucose enters the body glucose pool and the rate at which it is removed.

Capillary blood obtained from the hand is equivalent to arterial blood throughout the post-absorptive phase. This gives a more appropriate indication of the true glycaemic response to food than that of mixed forearm venous blood. Insulin is secreted in response to a meal, and the more insulin sensitive the tissue the greater the A/V glucose difference. In healthy young subjects with good glucose tolerance the A/V glucose difference can be 3.0 mmol/l or more.

It is possible in diabetic subjects to obtain a measure of fluctuations in blood glucose over the preceding few months by measuring of HbA_{Ic} and glycosylated albumin.

There is often a hypoglycaemic period after the fall in blood glucose, when the blood glucose falls to below fasting concentrations. This is particularly pronounced if venous, rather than arterial, blood is measured, but does not appear to occur following ingestion of mixed meals. The site of sugar absorption may be in the duodenum, jejunum or ileum. Therefore, the effects of glucose may be seen as a hormone releaser or as a simple provision of metabolic fuel at each intestinal site.

DIETARY CARBOHYDRATES AND LIPID METABOLISM

The long-chain fatty acids in the body, stored as triglycerides, are derived from the diet. However, they can also be synthesised from metabolites from the glycolytic pathway of carbohydrates and 'reducing equivalents' from the pentose phosphate shunt. These routes become important when dietary carbohydrates are eaten in excess of daily requirements. Fatty acids are either metabolised to carbon dioxide and water or stored as triglycerides. Glycerol is phosphorylated to be brought back into the metabolic pool. Glycerol-3-phosphate, an intermediate in the glycolytic pathway, is used to re-esterify fatty acids. Glucose enters adipocytes from the blood when insulin is present in the extracellular fluid in excess of a critical concentration, which depends on the number and affinity of insulin receptors on the surface of the adipocytes. Below this insulin concentration, glucose does not enter the cells, glycolysis decreases and insufficient glycerol-3-phosphate is available for re-esterification of the free fatty acids produced by lipolysis.

Free fatty acids, therefore, are released into the bloodstream, where they can be used by heart and striated muscle as fuel or passed to the liver for con-

Glucose given hourly to men reduces serum triglycerol concentrations, with less marked reductions in phospholipid and cholesterol concentrations. Glucose given intravenously has the same effect. This is a direct effect, not an effect mediated by the absorption process. If insulin is added to the glucose infusion, the post-prandial lipaemia is further decreased. Fructose, in contrast, increases the post-prandial hypertriglyceridaemia. All of this may be due to increased removal of plasma triglycerides as a result of increased lipoprotein lipase activity, stimulated by insulin. However, this effect is not uniform. Variables include the age and gender of the individual; pre-menopausal women react to sucrose differently to men and post-menopausal women. It is possible that females clear plasma triglycerides more rapidly than males.

version into ketone bodies (acetoacetate and β-hydroxybutyrate) or back to triglycerides in the form of very low-density lipoprotein (VLDL).

Prolonged exposure to sucrose diets raises the fasting serum triglyceride concentration, owing to endogenous production of triglycerides. The triglyceride concentration after a 12–14 h fast is a good indicator of triglyceride status. A substantial dietary sucrose intake results in an increase in the concentration of triglycerides compared with starch. This effect of sucrose is independent of the previous triglyceride concentrations. Plasma triglyceride concentrations are reduced when the unsaturated fat content of the diet is increased.

There may be a synergistic effect of sucrose on plasma triglycerides that is not shown by starch and animal fat. There is also a very individual response to these dietary changes, which presumably has a genetic basis, e.g. individuals with type IV hyperlipoproteinaemia have a more pronounced increase in plasma triglycerides following sucrose ingestion than with starch, compared with non-type IV individuals.

Adipose tissue

Dietary carbohydrate can be converted to fat, an energy-consuming process that uses some 10–15% of the ingested glucose. Adipocytes convert glucose to fatty acids, a process that is less energy consuming during fasting and following a high-fat meal, although energy consumption is increased by a high-carbohydrate diet. The process is controlled by insulin.

Fructose may also be taken up by the adipocyte, but transport across the cell membrane is slow as the carrier system for fructose has a relatively high K_m.

Glucose is not converted to glycogen or fatty acid directly, but through a C_3 molecule formed in tissues other than the liver. This C_3 unit is then recycled to the liver. Over two-thirds of glucose absorbed escapes uptake by the liver and is transported to the peripheral tissues.

Diets rich in dietary fibre produce a reduced stimulus to insulin secretion compared with diets free of fibre. This, depending on the type of fibre, may decrease cholesterol and triglyceride concentrations.

CARBOHYDRATES AND THE RESPIRATORY QUOTIENT

The ratio of carbon dioxide in the breath to oxygen, the respiratory quotient (RQ), gives an indication of the type of substrate being metabolised and a hint as to which metabolic route is being followed. The RQ should be 1. After the ingestion of fructose or galactose it is greater than after glucose. In the release of energy after fructose digestion it is possible that more of the carbohydrate is broken down than with other sugars. The more rapid metabolism of fructose may be because it follows first-order reactions, with the utilisation being proportional to concentration. There is an increase in plasma uric acid, lactate and pyruvate concentrations after fructose ingestion.

> The mean percentage increase in metabolic rate following glucose ingestion over a 3 h period is 10%, with the response in women being less than that in men. The metabolic response to the ingestion of a simple sugar may vary with the previous diet of the individual. Thermogenesis is greater after a high-carbohydrate diet than after a high-fat diet. Much of the carbohydrate load is deposited in glycogen rather than in fat. The metabolic cost of dietary carbohydrate may vary between 7 and 23%, depending on whether the carbohydrate is stored as glycogen or fat.

The metabolism of dietary protein requires a greater energy expenditure than dietary carbohydrate or fat. Dietary fat and carbohydrate undergo less metabolism before being stored in adipose tissue. The resting metabolic rate measured for 3 h after the ingestion of various disaccharides and monosaccharides and mixtures shows a greater increase in metabolic rate than with sucrose. This increase is greater than with the constituent glucose:fructose (0.90, compared with glucose, 0.87, and the disaccharide lactose, 0.86).

GLUCOSE OXIDATION AND METABOLISM

Glucose is a major energy source, especially for the brain, nerve cells and red blood cells. This means

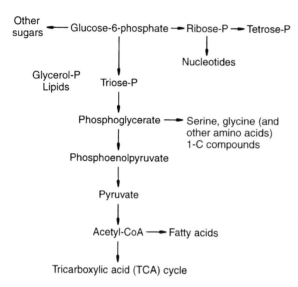

Fig. 33.2 Glycolysis. The oxidative cleavage of glucose to pyruvate, acetyl-CoA and other metabolites.

that control of blood glucose concentrations is very important. This is achieved through a balance of

- hormone control
- glucose production by the liver and kidneys
- peripheral uptake of glucose by muscle, and fat.

The liver produces glucose from stores as glycogen and by gluconeogenesis from lactate, pyruvate, glycerol and alanine.

In aerobic metabolism, organic carbon can be fully oxidised to carbon dioxide using oxygen as an electron acceptor. The ATP yield for each glucose molecule metabolised under oxidative conditions, for example, is almost 20 times greater than that under anaerobic conditions. The amount of energy that can be liberated from nutrients by anaerobic oxidation is limited. Every such anaerobic oxidation reaction involves an electron being removed and taken up by another organic compound. The energy difference between such coupled oxidations is very small.

Aerobic respiratory metabolism involves:

- oxygen being the ultimate electron acceptor
- complete oxidation of organic chemicals to carbon dioxide and water
- the free energy being conserved as ATP.

At the same time, there is a continuous reoxidation of reduced coenzyme molecules, e.g. reduced nicotinamide dinucleotide (NADH) and flavin adenine dinucleotide ($FADH_2$), which link into the respiratory chain to produce ATP. These coenzyme molecules in their oxidised form are involved in the oxidation of organic intermediates from pyruvate. Therefore, under aerobic conditions a glycolytic pathway is the initial phase of glucose catabolism, following which are:

- the TCA cycle
- the oxidative phosphorylation of adenosine diphosphate (ADP) to ATP.

This leads to the formation of 36–38 molecules of ATP for each molecule of glucose metabolised by this process.

GLYCOLYSIS

Glycolysis is the pathway in which glucose is metabolised before splitting into two interconvertible three-carbon molecules (Figure 33.2). These reactions take place in the cell cytoplasm. The first three steps involve reactions that lead to a doubly phosphorylated fructose derivative.

Glucose-1-phosphate, glucose-6-phosphate (G6P) and fructose-6-phosphate (F6P) readily interconvert and thereby form a single metabolic pool. Glucose-1-phosphate is the first product in the catabolism of storage polysaccharides, e.g. starch. G6P is the first hexose phosphate generated when free glucose is metabolised, and F6P is the first hexose phosphate formed when the carbohydrate is derived from non-carbohydrate precursors.

G6P and F6P readily interchange through the action of the enzyme glucose phosphate isomerase. The available amount is dependent on the phosphorolysis of storage polysaccharides, yielding glucose-1-phosphate, by the phosphorylation of glucose yielding G6P or by gluconeogenesis of F6P. The subsequent catabolic steps are:

- glycolysis with F6P as the starting point
- the pentose phosphate pathway, which uses G6P.

Alternatively, G6P and F6P can be converted into storage polysaccharides with G6P acting as the starting point. G6P can also be hydrolysed to yield

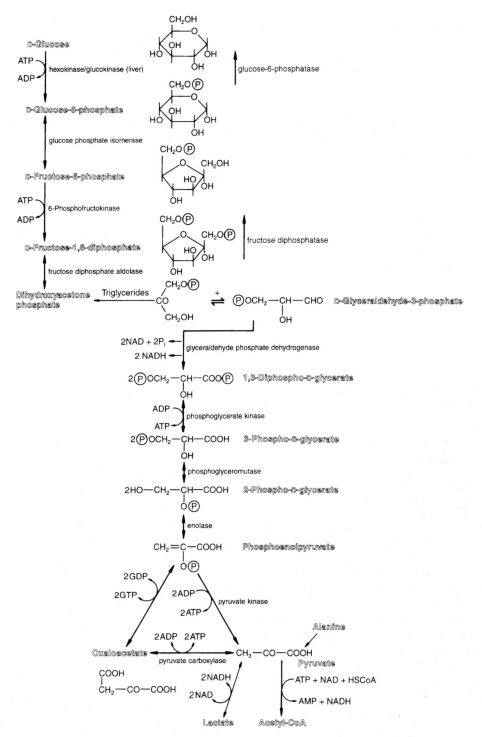

Fig. 33.3 Glycolytic (Embden–Meyerhof) pathway from glucose to pyruvate. Some of the enzymatic pathways are irreversible, e.g. glucose to glucose-6-phosphate, fructose-6-phosphate to fructose-1,6-diphosphate, fructose-1,6-diphosphate to dihydroxyacetone phosphate and glyceraldehyde-3-phosphate, phosphoenolpyruvate to pyruvate, and pyruvate to acetyl-CoA.

free glucose to be transported in the blood to peripheral tissues.

The steps in glycolysis are listed below (Figure 33.3).

1. Glucose is phosphorylated on the carbon 6 position by hexokinase or glucokinase. Both are Mg^{2+}-dependent enzymes. Hexokinase has a wide number of substrates: glucose, fructose, mannose and galactose. Hexokinase activity is affected by the concentration of the products G6P and ADP. Hexokinase exists in several isoenzyme forms with varying affinity for glucose. Glucokinase is a hepatic enzyme, specific for D-glucose, and is unaffected by the product concentration. The K_m is 5–10 mM, compared with 0.1 mM for hexokinase.

2. G6P is isomerised to F6P. The generation of fructose gives a primary hydroxyl group on carbon 1 for subsequent phosphorylation. The carbonyl on carbon 2 is important for subsequent β-cleavage to produce two three-carbon products. The enzyme is phosphoglucoisomerase.

3. The 1-carbon position is phosphorylated by phosphofructokinase (PFK), a Mg^{2+}-dependent enzyme, and ATP. This reaction is rate limiting. The product is fructose-1,6-diphosphate. ATP inhibits PFK, an effect counteracted by ADP and AMP. Citrate increases ATP inhibition, which is significant in this feeder system for the TCA cycle.

4. Fructose-1,6-diphosphate is reversibly split into two isomers, dihydroxyacetone phosphate (carbons 3, 2,1 of the fructose-1,6-diphosphate) and glyceraldehyde 3-phosphate (carbons 4, 5, 6 of the fructose-1,6-diphosphate). The enzyme involved is aldolase and the reaction is driven by the rapid removal of the glyceraldehyde-3-phosphate. There are isoenzymes of aldolase in muscle, liver and brain.

5. The two three-carbon isomers are interconvertible by the action of the enzyme triosephosphate isomerase. The removal of glyceraldehyde-3-phosphate affects the equilibrium of this enzymatic reaction. This series of reactions is energy consuming, in that two ATPs are used per glucose molecule.

6. Glyceraldehyde 3-phosphate is converted to 1,3-diphosphoglycerate with the creation of a high-energy phosphoanhydride bond on carbon-1. The enzyme is glyceraldehyde-3-phosphate dehydrogenase. The reaction passes through a high-energy thioester stage, which accounts for the inhibitory effect of alkylating agents and heavy metals on the reaction. The phosphate is organic phosphate.

7. The carbon-1 phosphate of the 1,3-diphosphoglycerate is used to phosphorylate ADP to ATP, a substrate phosphorylation reaction. As two three-carbon derivatives of glucose pass through this stage, the two ATPs used in stages 1 and 2 are regenerated.

8. The phosphate on carbon 3 of 2-phosphoglycerate is moved to carbon 3. The enzyme is phosphoglyceromutase, a Mg^{2+}-requiring enzyme.

9. The removal of water by enolase produces a high-energy phosphate bond at carbon 3 next to a double bond, in phosphoenolpyruvate.

10. The high-energy phosphate is used to convert ADP to ATP with the production of pyruvate. This is an irreversible reaction requiring the enzyme pyruvate kinase. The enzyme is K^+ and Mg^{2+} or Mn^{2+} dependent, and is inhibited by high ATP concentrations. The enzyme is activated by fructose-1,6-diphosphate and phosphoenolpyruvate.

The overall yield over the ten stages of the process is two ATP molecules per glucose oxidised. The final steps in the oxidation of glucose require the transfer of the pyruvate into the mitochondria. Pyruvate plays a major role as an intermediary metabolite and is central to the interconversion of glucose fatty acids and amino acids.

Pyruvate interconversion

The pathways that pyruvate may follow include conversion to:

- L-malate to oxaloacetate, then to the TCA cycle
- acetyl-coenzyme A (acetyl-CoA), which is the substrate for (i) fatty acid synthesis; (ii) oxyacids; (iii) cholesterol; and (iv) the TCA cycle.

Pyruvate is the most important source of acetyl-CoA in the TCA cycle. Other sources include fatty acids and amino acids (PDH, pyruvic dehydrogenase):

$$\text{Pyruvate} + \text{CoA} + \text{NAD} \xrightarrow[\text{PDH}]{} \text{Acetyl-CoA} + \text{NADH} + CO_2$$

Pyruvic acid is converted to acetyl-CoA in the mitochondria, where the TCA cycle takes place. The first step is the transport of pyruvate into the mitochondria. The reaction is irreversible, very complicated, and dependent on three different enzymes and five coenzymes. The first step is the removal of a carbon dioxide by a decarboxylase, which requires thiamin pyrophosphate. The next is a transfer to a lipoic acid cofactor and dehydrogenation using a dehydrogenase. The acetyl group is then transferred by a transacetylase to form acetyl-CoA. In this reaction NADH is generated. This enzyme complex is very cofactor dependent and sensitive to deficiencies of thiamin.

Pyruvate dehydrogenase (PDH) is inactivated by phosphorylation by PDH kinase and PDH phosphatase. In the presence of ATP the kinase phosphorylates the PDH enzyme. The process is inhibited by ADP and pyruvate, so that at times of nutrient shortage the enzymatic system is ready for the generation of acetyl-CoA. Inactivated PDH is activated by a phosphatase, which requires Mg^{2+} or Ca^{2+} as cofactors. These may be chelated by ATP or citrate, which are also controlling systems. The nutritional and endocrine status dictates the activity of PDH. The availability of PDH is very tissue dependent, being independent of nutrition in the brain and activated post-prandially in heart and kidneys. Liver and fat PDH are largely present in the inactive form, regardless of nutritional status. Elsewhere in the body PDH is converted to the inactive form during starvation. The only other nutritional sources available for gluconeogenesis are proteins and glycerol.

TRICARBOXYLIC ACID CYCLE

The TCA cycle is a mitochondrial system that starts with acetyl-CoA. This is derived either by oxidative decarboxylation of pyruvate which results from glycolysis, or oxidative cleavage of fatty acids, or from amino acids. Acetyl-CoA donates the acetyl group to oxaloacetate, which is a four-carbon acceptor. This produces citrate, which has six carbons. Citrate subsequently passes through two successive decarboxylation processes and a number of oxidative processes to yield oxaloacetate. While passing through the cycle two carbons are introduced from

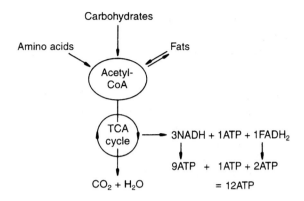

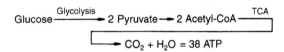

Fig. 33.4 Overall scheme of the tricarboxylic acid (TCA) cycle. Amino acids, carbohydrates and fats in the form of acetyl-CoA enter the TCA cycle. Each rotation of an acetyl-CoA through the cycle yields 12 ATP. One molecule of glucose, after passing through the oxidative process of glycolysis and the TCA cycle, yields 38 ATP.

acetyl-CoA and two are released as carbon dioxide.

The TCA acid cycle is the main common oxidative process for the three major nutritional elements, carbohydrates, fats and proteins (Figure 33.4). The cycle is regulated to provide for cell needs. This is important because the cycle's function is to:

- provide NADH and $FADH_2$ for the electron transport chain
- provide substrates for biosynthesis.

The cycle depends on the availability of acetyl-CoA, the ratio of $NADH/NAD^+$ and the ATP/ADP ratio.

The decarboxylation of pyruvate requires an intermediate, stabilised by prior condensation of carbonyl with thiamin pyrophosphate. The PDH complex has a molecular weight of 9×10^6 Da. This enzyme system is regulated and is sensitive to the ATP/ADP ratio and the concentration of acetyl-CoA. The enzyme complex is also subject to regulation by enzyme modification in which a protein kinase catalyses the phosphorylation of specific

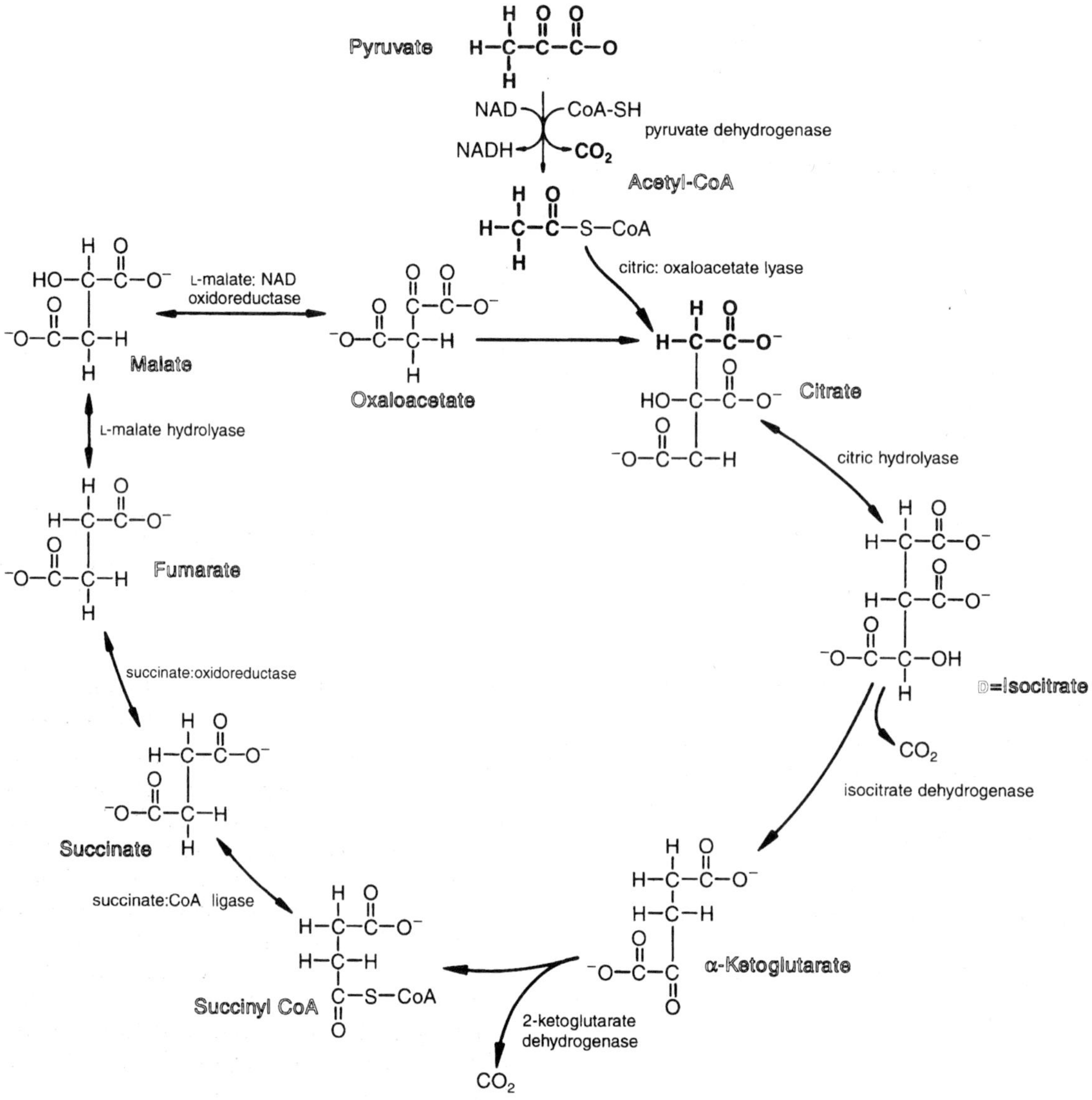

Fig. 33.5 Tricarboxylic acid (TCA) cycle showing the detailed pathways. Most of the enzymes of the TCA cycle are found in the matrix of the mitochondria. Succinate dehydrogenase is a membrane protein on the inner mitochondrial membrane. The enzyme has a covalently linked flavin β-histidyl FAD. Succinate dehydrogenase is reoxidised by the electron transport chain.

serine –OH groups on the pyruvate carboxylase section of the enzyme complex. A phosphorylase removes these phosphoryl groups. The phosphorylated enzyme is relatively inactive. The action of the kinase and the decrease in the activity of the pyruvate complex are controlled by the ATP/ADP and NADH/NAD$^+$ ratios and by a high acetyl-CoA concentration (Figure 33.5)

$$\text{acetyl-CoA} + \text{oxaloacetate} \xrightarrow[\text{citrate synthase}]{} \text{citrate} + \text{CoA}$$

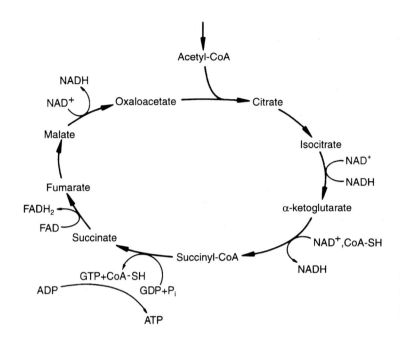

Fig. 33.6 Tricarboxylic acid (TCA) cycle and electron carriers NAD^+ and FAD, the subsequent oxidation of which results in the synthesis of ATP.

Citrate is isomerised to isocitrate by the action of aconitase. Isocitrate dehydrogenase is the enzyme for the conversion of isocitrate to α-ketoglutarate. NAD^+ is the electron acceptor in this oxidative step and Mg^{2+} and Mn^{2+} are required for the decarboxylation.

α-Ketoglutarate $+ NAD^+ + CoA \longrightarrow$ Succinyl-CoA $+ NADH + H^+ + CO_2$

Succinyl-CoA is an activated intermediate.

Succinyl-CoA $+$ GDP $\xrightarrow[\text{succinate thiokinase}]{}$ Succinate $+$ GTP

The reaction involves an intermediate in which a phosphate group is attached to a histidine residue of the enzyme. The next stage is:

Succinate $+$ FAD $\xrightarrow[\text{succinate dehydrogenase}]{}$ Fumarate $+$ $FADH_2$

This is a flavoprotein enzyme and is attached to the inner mitochondrial membrane:

Fumarate $+ H_2O \longrightarrow$ L-Malate

This is a stereospecific addition of water to the double bond. The cycle is completed by

L-Malate $+ NAD^+ \longrightarrow$ Oxaloacetate $+$ $NADH + H^+$

There is considerable stereochemistry in the reaction between enzymes and substrates in the TCA cycle, and therefore the enzymatic reactions are very stereospecific. The result of acetyl-CoA entering the TCA cycle is to yield one ATP molecule. However, there is storage of free energy as NADH and $FADH_2$ (Figure 33.6). Consequently, oxidation of one mole of acetyl-CoA leads to the overall production of 12 moles of ATP. In addition to this, pyruvate metabolism leads to 15 moles of ATP per mole of pyruvate, or 38 moles ATP per mole of glucose (Figure 33.4).

The metabolites in the TCA cycle are major starting materials for a number of biosynthetic pathways (Figure 33.7):

• Acetyl-CoA supplies the carbon atoms for fats and lipids, and for the synthesis of some amino acids.
• Oxaloacetate is the start of the synthesis of aspartate, asparagine, threonine, isoleucine and methionine.
• α-Ketoglutarate is the start of the synthesis of glutamate, glutamine, proline and arginine.
• Succinyl-CoA is part of the synthetic path in the synthesis of haem.

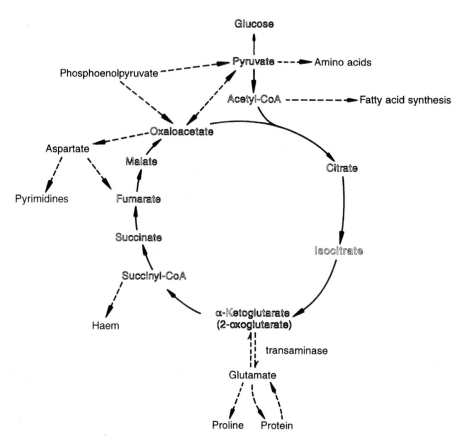

Fig. 33.7 Tricarboxylic acid (TCA) cycle in relationship to other nutrients. Pyruvate can be synthesised to amino acids, acetyl-CoA synthesised to fatty acids, α-ketoglutarate transaminated to glutamate, and oxaloacetate synthesised into aspartate and phosphoenol pyruvate.

This means that most of the starting materials required for the biosynthetic pathways of a cell can be derived from aerobic pathways fuelled by carbohydrates.

Most of these reactions are reversible, so the TCA cycle can be replenished at points other than acetyl-CoA. Acetyl-CoA is an important biosynthetic material, providing the carbon atoms of lipids, cholesterol and some amino acids within the cytosol of the cell. The acetyl-CoA results from fat degradation and pyruvate from carbohydrate degradation. In the mitochondria the acetyl-CoA required for synthesis in the cytosol is derived from citrate, which passes from the mitochondria to the cytosol. In the cytosol the citrate is cleaved to acetyl-CoA and oxaloacetate. Some of the oxaloacetate is converted to aspartate, a precursor for

asparagine synthesis. The excess is reduced to malate, which diffuses readily into the mitochondria and is convertible into pyruvate.

Citrate has a double role: to supply the carbon atoms of fatty acids and also to regulate fatty acid synthesis. The beginning of fatty acid synthesis is the carboxylation of acetyl-CoA to form malonyl-CoA. Citrate is an important regulator of this reaction. Citrate also indirectly inhibits PFK activity and hence the rate of glycolysis. PFK is inhibited by ATP and accentuated by citrate. Consequently, increases in citrate concentration in the cytosol result in increased production of storage fats and reduce the rate of carbohydrate breakdown. Reduction in citrate concentration has the reverse effect.

The reduction of the carbonyl group of pyruvate

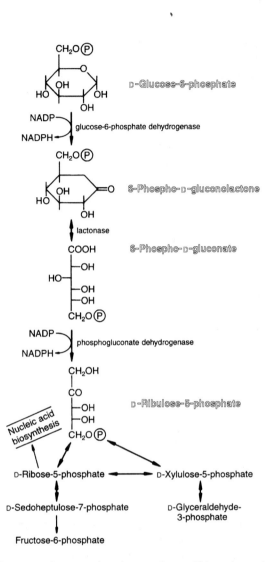

Fig. 33.8 Pentose phosphate pathway. This pathway is a series of interrelated reactions providing a series of end-products. It is also an alternative pathway for glucose oxidation with the formation of the reduced coenzyme NADPH. NADPH can be used to drive reductive anabolic pathways, e.g. synthesis of fatty acids and steroids. This pathway is a prime source of NADPH for biosynthetic reactions in most cells. The pathway also allows the interconversion of hexoses and pentoses. The end products fructose-6-phosphate and glyceraldehyde-3-phosphate then pass into the glycolytic pathway. Ribose-5-phosphate is available for nucleic acid biosynthesis.

to form lactate maintains supplies of NAD under anaerobic conditions. The enzyme is lactic dehydrogenase, existing in five isoenzyme forms, with various arrangements of A and B subunits, each with different K_m values. Lactic dehydrogenase isoenzymes with low K_m values are found in muscles where a high enzyme affinity for glycolysis is important for energy production. Cardiac muscle lactic dehydrogenase enzyme affinity is low. Lactate utilisation is important during severe anaerobic skeletal exercise. Lactate may return to the liver and is converted back to pyruvate and then to glucose in the gluconeogenic pathway.

PENTOSE PHOSPHATE PATHWAY

This is an alternative metabolic pathway to the glycolytic system (Figure 33.8). The initial reaction requires glucose-6-phosphate dehydrogenase as an enzyme and generates NADPH for other reductive reactions in fatty acid and cholesterol synthesis. The next product is D-ribulose-5-phosphate (enzyme, transaldolase), another NADPH-generating reaction. NADPH production is important in the reducing conditions for some biosynthetic reactions, especially lipids.

Several ribose phosphates can be produced from ribulose-5-phosphate, e.g. xylulose-5-phosphate (enzyme: phosphopentose epimerase) and ribose-5-phosphate (enzyme: phosphopentose isomerase). These pentose phosphates are the starting point for the formation of a whole array of three- to seven-sugar phosphates, from which are produced triose phosphate, e.g. erythrose-4-phosphate which is converted to fructose-6-phosphate, ribose-5-phosphate for nucleic acid synthesis or generation of NADPH. NADPH is important in a variety of biosynthetic systems, e.g. oxidation of malate to pyruvate.

METABOLISM IN THE PRESENCE OF ABUNDANT GLUCOSE

Here, the emphasis is on anabolic processes and storage (Figure 33.9). The liver converts some glucose to stored glycogen and some to fatty acids

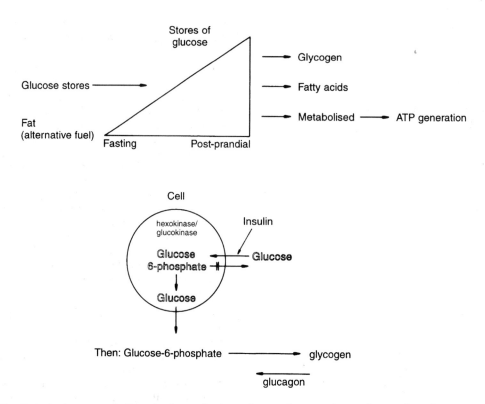

Fig. 33.9 Carbohydrate metabolism. In times of excess dietary glucose, glucose is stored as glycogen, synthesised into fatty acids or metabolised to produce ATP. When dietary glucose is deficient glucose stores are mobilised and fat is used as an alternative fuel. Glucose enters the cell by a transport system increased by insulin. In the cell, glucose is metabolised into glucose-6-phosphate which in turn can be synthesised into glycogen.

to be used as a fuel. Peripherally, glucose is metabolised to generate ATP. Excess is stored as glycogen and adipose tissue.

Glycogen synthesis

Glycogen is a convenient way to store sugar until it is required. Glycogen has low osmotic properties, it is stable and its metabolism can be controlled. Insulin stimulates the uptake of glucose by various tissues and the synthesis of glycogen in the liver, and reduces blood glucose concentrations. Glycogen is synthesised, using the enzyme glycogen synthase, by an addition reaction of uridine diophosphate (UDP)-glucose with an existing glucose polymer (Figure 33.9).

The resultant polymer structure is an α-(1–4) with α-(1–6) branch points (Figure 33.10). The branched chains of α-(1–6) are synthesised by the branching enzyme amylo-(1–4,1–6) *trans*-glycosylase. The enzyme adds a chain of six to seven carbons to the C6 group of a glucose in a glycogen chain.

Glycogen synthase is inactive when phosphorylated; it is activated by insulin and high concentrations of G6P. This latter control is important in the liver, but not in muscle where the enzyme hexokinase controls G6P concentrations.

METABOLISM DURING GLUCOSE INSUFFICIENCY OR NEED

Mobilisation of tissue glucose

In times of glucose shortage, glucose stores in the form of glycogen and free glucose are mobilised. Glucose synthesis from non-glucose sources (gluconeogenesis) is stimulated in the liver and kidney.

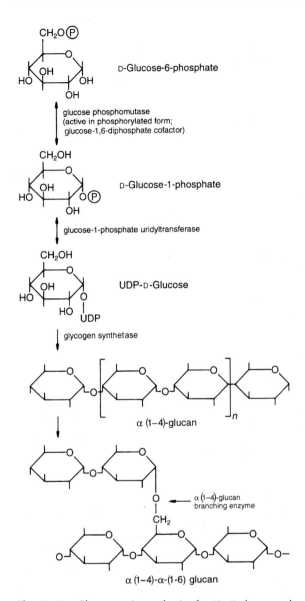

Fig. 33.10 Glycogenesis: synthesis of α-(1–4) glucan and α-(1–4)-α-(1–6) glucan.

Glycogen breakdown

Phosphorylase (Figure 33.11) releases glucose in the form of G1P:

$$\text{Glycogen} + P_1 \xrightarrow{\text{phosphorylase } a} \text{Glycogen} + G1P$$
$$\longrightarrow G6P$$

This enzyme is active when phosphorylated and inhibited by insulin.

Phosphorylase *a* and *b* cascade

Skeletal muscle phosphorylase consists of two or possibly four identical proteins. A serine at position 14 in each constituent protein of the enzyme is phosphorylated by phosphorylase kinase *b*, which requires ATP to yield the active phosphorylase *a* form. The inactive form phosphorylase *b* is produced by phosphorylase a phosphatase (Figure 33.12). The phosphorylase kinase is kept in an active and inactive form by protein kinase, which is increased by noradrenaline and glucagon. The enzyme activity is affected by covalent modification of the enzymes. An increase in AMP is associated with a decrease in ATP, and activation of glycogen phosphorylase due to an increase in AMP. An increase in the amount of glucose-1-phosphate leads to an increase in the rate at which ATP is regenerated.

As the glucose concentration falls, glucagon and adrenaline increase the conversion of phosphorylase *b* to phosphorylase *a*. This is independent of AMP control. This overriding system is a membrane-bound enzyme, adenylate cyclase, which converts ATP to cAMP. Activation of the cyclase requires guanosine triphosphate (GTP) and a GTP binding protein called the G protein. cAMP activates protein kinase A. The inactive form of this enzyme consists of two catalytic (C) and two regulatory subunits (R). cAMP binds to the two regulatory subunits (R), causing a dissociation of the (R) and the (C) subunits. The C dimers dissociate to give two active monomers that catalyse a transfer of a phosphoryl group from ATP to specific sites of many proteins, including phosphorylase kinase, which results in activation of the phosphorylase kinase which then converts phosphorylase *b* to phosphorylase *a* by phosphorylation of a specific serine residue.

The phosphorylase cascade begins with and amplifies an initiating, regulatory signal followed by production of many molecules of cyclic adenosine monophosphate (cAMP) so there is amplification at every enzymatic step. Thus, low concentrations of hormones have profound effects on metabolism.

Noradrenaline converts phosphorylase *b* to phosphorylase *a*, both in the liver and in muscle. In contrast, glucagon only affects the conversion of hepatic phosphorylase *b* to phosphorylase *a*, as glucagon is a gentle modulator of blood glucose concentrations.

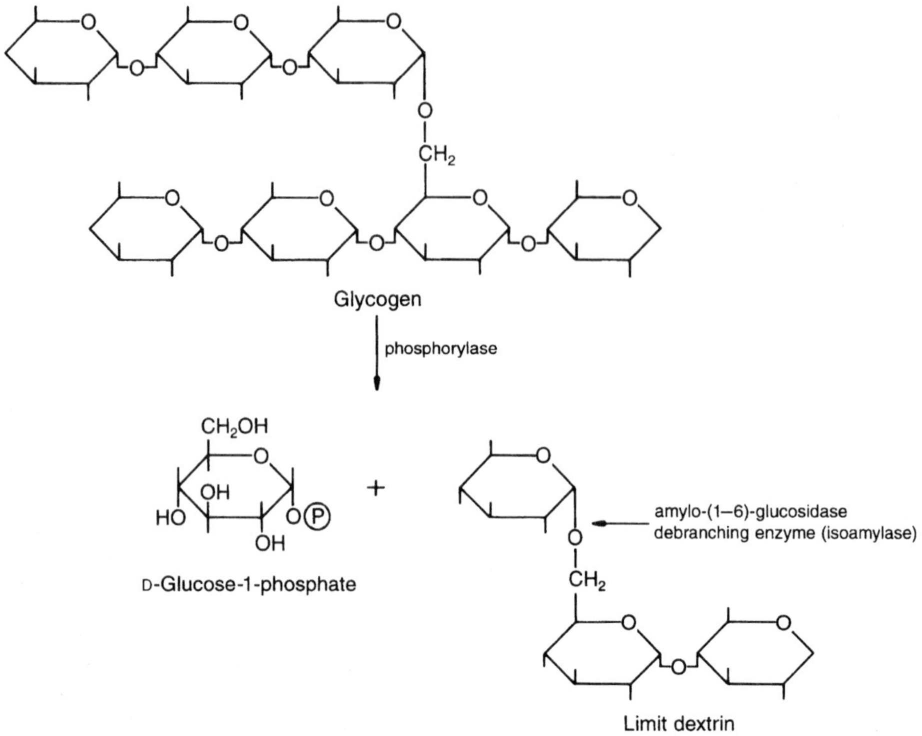

Fig. 33.11 Glycogenolysis: the enzyme phosphorylase removes glucose units from the non-reducing ends as glucose-1-phosphate as far as 2–3 glucose units from an α-(1–6) branch unit. The α-(1–6) linkage-releasing enzyme is amylo-(1–6)-glucosidase, debranching enzyme or isoamylase.

GLUCONEOGENESIS

Glucose synthesis

Glucose has a central role in the production and harnessing of energy and in the synthesis of other sugars. The ability to synthesise glucose is equally important, as the brain and red cells are restricted to glucose as an energy source. While an individual is fasting the brain uses 80% of the glucose metabolised. The liver only contains sufficient glucose to meet the requirements of the brain for 12 h; the ability to synthesise glucose is therefore important.

Several systems are available:

- production of sugars from non-sugar sources, e.g. lactate, pyruvate, fatty acids or amino acids
- synthesis of free glucose by the liver for transmission in the blood.

Gluconeogenesis is activated under different conditions and serves different functions in different species. Glycolysis and gluconeogenesis are directly opposed reaction sequences (see Figure 33.3). Most of the enzymes that function in glycolysis are also reversed in gluconeogenesis. This is an important property of carbohydrate metabolism, which can feed into all elements of carbohydrate, lipid and amino acid metabolism, except for the essential fatty acids and essential amino acids. Fatty acids are not capable of gluconeogenesis.

The intermediates in the gluconeogenic and glycolysis pathways are the same, are in near equilibrium concentrations, and can move in either direction, dependent on small changes in concentration. All of these processes are coupled to the ATP/ADP system, and regulate the direction of subsequent metabolic pathways. A problem that has to be overcome within this process is that some steps in metabolic pathways are irreversible.

In glycolysis (see Figure 33.3) these are:

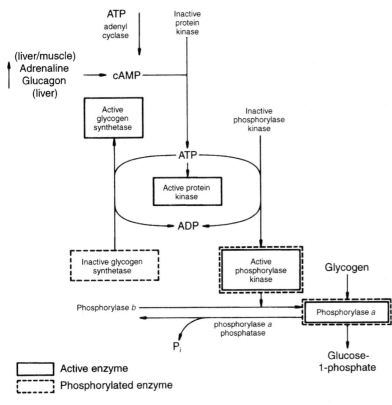

Fig. 33.12 Synthesis of glycogen by glycogen synthase acts in the opposite direction to phosphorylase *a*, which cleaves glycogen to yield glucose-1-phosphate. This reciprocating enzyme activity is controlled by phosphorylation by protein kinase and phosphorylase kinase. Active phosphorylase *a* is phosphorylated. Active glycogen synthase is dephosphorylated.

- the phosphorylation of glucose and F6P, which are ATP-dependent reactions. The irreversible nature of this reaction is due to the kinases involved. In the reverse reaction in gluconeogenesis this problem is bypassed by the enzymes being phosphatases, which remove the phosphate in an inorganic form. These are cytosolic enzymes, remote from the mitochondrial enzymes of the TCA cycle;
- pyruvate to phosphoenolpyruvate: the bypassing of the enzymatic barrier imposed by the pyruvate kinase barrier is a two-step reaction involving ATP and GTP hydrolysis. Pyruvate is converted to oxaloacetate using pyruvate carboxylase and ATP in the mitochondria. This enzyme requires Mg^{2+} and biotin. The CO_2 donor is a carboxylated derivative of the cofactor biotin. Oxaloacetate cannot gain access to the next enzymes, which are cytosolic, as it cannot pass across the mitochondrial membrane. Such passage is achieved by conversion to malate and conversion back to oxaloacetate in the cytosol.

The merit of these stages is that oxaloacetate and malate are therefore usable as substrates in gluconeogenesis. Oxaloacetate is a product of deamination of aspartate and both are constituents of the TCA cycle.

Oxaloacetate is converted to phosphoenolpyruvate from phosphoenolpyruvate carboxykinase and a GTP–guanosine diphosphate (GDP) conversion. The regeneration of GTP is at the expense of ATP; consequently, two molecules of ATP are used to reverse the conversion of pyruvate to phosphoenolpyruvate. The phosphorylated three-carbon acids phosphoenolpyruvate, glycerate-2-phosphate and glycerate-3-phosphate are interrelated. These may be converted to the fructose-1,6-disphosphate/triosephosphate pool following the conversion of glycerate-3-phosphate to glyceraldehyde-3-phosphate. This is a reversible, concentration-dependent reaction.

Fructose-1,6-disphosphate is hydrolysed to F6P by the enzyme fructose disphosphate phosphatase at the phosphoryl ester bond at C1. When F6P

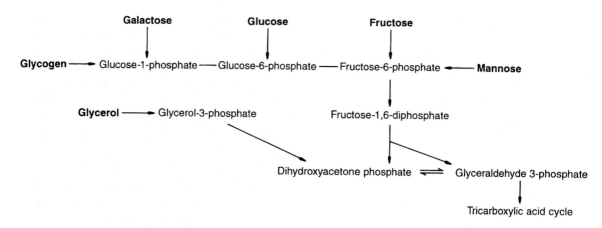

Fig. 33.13 Interrelationship of the carbohydrates glycogen, galactose, glucose, fructose, mannose and glycerol.

is produced by gluconeogenesis an equivalent amount of glucose-1-phosphate is usually removed from the hexose monophosphate pool by conversion to glycogen, which requires a nucleoside triphosphate. Such activation is achieved by UDP-glucose, an important and perhaps critical hexose derivative in mammalian metabolism.

Of the enzymes involved in gluconeogenesis, only pyruvate carboxylase functions in the mitochondria.

The energy difference between glycolysis and gluconeogenesis is four ATP molecules per hexose metabolised. This means that regulation of the glycolysis/gluconeogenesis systems is of prime importance to cellular metabolism. The direction of the flux is very sensitive to the needs of the animal.

REGULATION OF FRUCTOSE PHOSPHORYLATION

The conversion of F6P to fructose-1,6-bisphosphate is catalysed by PFK and is affected by the ATP/ADP ratio in the opposite direction to the responses of typical kinases (Figure 33.13). When ATP binds at the regulatory site the enzyme activity decreases. Citrate also increases the influence of ATP by increasing the ease of binding of ATP to the regulatory site. This means there is a direct effect of concentrations of metabolites within the TCA cycle on PFK activity. The kinase that catal-

yses the production of fructose-2,6-disphosphate in the liver is inactivated by phosphorylation. This inactivation is mediated through the same cAMP-dependent protein kinase that is responsible for the phosphorylation of phosphorylase kinase. The phosphorylated kinase is the enzyme hydrolysing the conversion of fructose-1,6-bisphosphate to F6P (Figure 33.13). As the blood glucose decreases, glucagon is secreted and increases the intracellular concentration of cAMP. This, in turn, activates the cAMP-dependent protein kinase that phosphorylates and inactivates the enzyme that generates fructose-1,6-bisphosphate. Glycolysis is inhibited and gluconeogenesis is stimulated, resulting in glucose being secreted into the blood.

During starvation or intake of high-protein or high-fat diets, the amount and activity of phosphoenolpyruvate carboxykinase increase and decrease when there is a restoration of carbohydrate to the diet.

Glucose is regenerated by gluconeogenesis (the Cori cycle), in the liver and kidney cortex, consuming six ATP molecules, so this is not an energy-creating system.

KETONE BODIES

Ketone bodies are small molecules with a molecular weight less than 104 Da; they are water soluble and weakly acidic. They include acetoacetate (AcAc), β-hydroxybutyrate (BHB) and acetone.

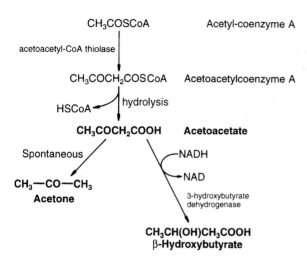

Fig. 33.14 Ketone bodies include acetoacetate, acetone and β-hydroxybutyrate. They are produced when large amounts of acetyl-CoA are synthesised, as in uncontrolled diabetes and starvation with consequent fat mobilisation.

AcAc and BHB are interconvertible, catalysed by α-hydroxybutyrate dehydrogenase within mitochondria and using the $NAD^+/NADH_2$ couple as a cofactor. The conversion of AcAc to acetone is a non-enzymatic reaction, which is followed by conversion to glucose (Figure 33.14).

Ketone bodies are synthesised almost entirely in the liver, but occasionally also in the muscle and kidneys. Fatty acids, released from adipose tissue, pass to the liver, enter the liver cells and are transported to the mitochondria as carnitine ester. There is oxidative cleavage of long-chain fatty acid acyl-CoA to acetyl-CoA by β-oxidation. Two acetyl-CoA molecules condense to form acetoacetyl-CoA. Deacylation and reduction then result in 3-hydroxybutyrate. These diffuse from the liver cell into the plasma. Because the liver cell does not have the enzyme 3-ketoacid CoA-transferase, the liver is unable to metabolise ketone bodies, which are either metabolised in peripheral tissues or excreted in urine. Ketone bodies, as well as free fatty acids and glucose, supply non-nitrogenous substrates to most tissues. Ketone bodies have an energy content of 4.2 kcal/g. The metabolism of ketone bodies is dependent on the concentration available.

Glucose is the principal endogenous substrate post-prandially, while free fatty acids are the principal endogenous substrates during fasting conditions. Ketone bodies are intermediate in timing and substitute for amino acids.

After the meal has been digested and absorbed, glucose disappears from the portal system, and there is a small lowering in the systemic plasma glucose level and an increase in insulin concentrations. At this point ketone body synthesis begins and plasma concentrations of AcAc and BHB become detectable. Overnight fasts result in ketone bodies being the predominant fuel for muscles, with only the brain using glucose. At this stage one-third of glucose requirements is derived from gluconeogenesis.

If fasting continues the plasma concentrations of ketone bodies gradually increase. After 3 weeks of fasting, plasma glucose concentrations fall slightly and the concentrations of free fatty acids increase. The concentration of ketone bodies is four times that at the outset, with BHB concentrations twice those of the AcAc. At this stage hepatic ketone body production is maximum, at 130 g/per day. The brain increases its oxidation of ketone bodies and the muscles use free fatty acids.

During a prolonged fast the kidney removes more BHB than AcAc from the plasma. There is a reduced loss of urinary ketone bodies and some reduced losses of ammonia/nitrogen, thereby conserving protein. This is called starvation adaptation, the main effects being on nitrogen metabolism.

In the early stages of fasting, ketone bodies replace carbohydrates during the onset and reduce carbohydrate requirement, even when the free fatty acids become the predominant metabolic fuel. Later, ketone bodies are used by the brain, while muscles use free fatty acids. In this way there is a conservation of glucose of 60 g/day and muscle sparing of 55 g/day. Prolonged starvation and diabetes result in very high concentrations of ketone bodies in blood, a condition known as ketosis. The high concentration of ketone bodies leads to serious related metabolic problems.

REGULATION OF GENE EXPRESSION BY GLUCOSE

Gene expression reflects the demands of the external environment. Such gene expression modulation enables the cell and organ to cope with a changing world. If there is plenty of one nutrient then there is no necessity for the genes encoded for the metabolism of related nutrients to be fully expressed. Hormones communicate with cells in organs about the concentration of nutrients in the blood, and changes in gene expression follow.

Glucose, a central source of energy for all tissues, is essential for the brain. The liver and kidneys are the prime sources of endogenous glucose, due to their being the only organs possessing G6P.

Glucose enters and leaves liver cells by a high-capacity glucose transporter, GLUT2. The expression of GLUT2 decreases with starvation and increases with a high carbohydrate intake. Insulin has the opposite effect. When there is a flux of glucose into the cell there is increased glucokinase activity, G6P is produced and a concentration gradient is maintained. Starvation or the feeding of a high-fat or high-protein, low-carbohydrate diet reduces messenger RNA for aldolase B and L-type pyruvate kinase. A high-carbohydrate feed and insulin will have the opposite effect.

Insulin is necessary for glucose stimulation of pyruvate kinase and fatty acid transcription, which also requires a high glucokinase expression. This allows a rapid transport of glucose into the cell, 6-phosphorylation and the movement of the glucose into the metabolic system. Glucokinase activity is increased by reduced fructose concentration, which is mediated through F6P and a glucokinase regulatory protein. Glucokinase activity is important in gene expression relating to monosaccharide metabolism. Both mannose and fructose can be metabolised to G6P. It is likely that G6P is the signal for insulin-dependent, glucose-regulated genes. The GLUT2 transport gene activity is controlled by glucose, mannose, fructose, dihydroxyacetone and sorbitol. Glucose increases GLUT2 transport gene activity.

The genes encoding the enzymes involved in gluconeogenesis, phosphoenolpyruvate carboxykinase, fructose-1, 6-bisphosphatase and glucose-6-phosphatase, are controlled at the transcriptional level by insulin, glucagon and glucocorticoids. A protein coactivator of nuclear receptors and other transcription factors, PGC-1, is a powerful stimulant of the key genes of the gluconeogenesis pathway as well as being important in cellular respiration and adaptive thermogenesis in brown

fat and skeletal muscle. PGC-1 is controlled by insulin and the other hormones controlling gluconeogenesis.

In the pancreas the insulin gene produced by the pancreatic β-cells is regulated by glucose.

Lactose and galactose regulate the expression of gene coding for the enzymes involved in their metabolism. The overriding by glucose over lactose and galactose gene expression is called catabolite repression. This follows an increase in cell cAMP and a catabolite gene activator protein (CAP). This is activated with its gene when glucose concentrations are low.

KEY POINTS

1. Glucose is an important energy source to the body. Blood glucose is derived from food, liver glycogen and intermediary metabolites.
2. Glucose may be taken up by tissues, particularly skeletal muscles. Insulin facilitates the active transport of glucose into the muscle and fat cells. Post-prandially, there is massive glycogen synthesis. During fasting glycogen may be hydrolysed to glucose-1-phosphate and then to pyruvate in the liver.
3. Galactose is absorbed through the same active transport system in the small intestine as glucose. A small amount enters the peripheral circulation as galactose, and is converted in the small intestine epithelium cells to galactose-1-phosphate and then to glucose-1-phosphate. Galactose is required for structure in body cells and connective tissue, e.g. galactosamine is produced from glucose.
4. Dietary fructose is taken up by the liver and enters directly into the glycolytic pathway. Within the liver fructose is phosphorylated to fructose-1-phosphate, which is split into glyceraldehyde and dihydroxyacetone phosphate; the latter is an intermediate in both the glycolytic and gluconeogenic pathways. Glyceraldehyde is converted to glyceraldehyde-3-phosphate, then to glycogen, a source of glucose. Glyceraldehyde can also be converted to glycerol-3-phosphate and esterified to fatty acids in triglycerides. These reactions are

dictated by nutrition and hormonal state. Fructose enters cells regardless of the insulin concentration.

5. Most of the enzymes involved in carbohydrate metabolism require vitamin B metabolites as essential cofactors in the glycolytic pathway, pentose phosphate shunt and tricarboxylic acid cycle.

6. Sugars may react with free amino groups on proteins to produce a chemically reversible glycosylated product (a Schiff base), and by internal rearrangement to produce a more stable Amadori-type glycosylation product, an advanced glycosylation endproduct.

7. A carbohydrate meal (e.g. starch or glucose, but not fructose) increases blood glucose. Several factors affect the measurement of the glycaemic response to meals.

8. Triglyceride long-chain fatty acids come from the diet or are synthesised from products of the glycolytic pathway and the pentose phosphate shunt. Blood-borne glucose requires insulin to enter adipocytes. Without insulin stimulation, glucose does not enter the cells and glycolysis decreases. Prolonged exposure to high-carbohydrate diets raises the fasting serum triglyceride concentration.

9. The ratio of carbon dioxide to oxygen in the breath (the respiratory quotient, RQ), indicates the substrate being metabolised and which metabolic route is being followed. The RQ after ingestion of fructose is greater than that after glucose.

10. ATP yield for each glucose molecule metabolised aerobically is 20-fold greater than anaerobically. The free energy is conserved as ATP and there is continuous reoxidation of reduced coenzymes, e.g. NADH and $FADH_2$, which link into the respiratory chain to produce ATP. The oxidised coenzymes are involved in the oxidation of pyruvate intermediates.

11. During aerobic conditions the glycolytic pathway is the initial phase of glucose catabolism leading to the tricarboxylic acid cycle and the oxidative phosphorylation of ADP to ATP, yielding 36–38 moles of ATP for each mole of glucose.

12. Glycolysis is the pathway in which glucose is metabolised before splitting into two inter-convertible, three-carbon molecules in the cell cytoplasm.

13. The catabolic steps are glycolysis with fructose-6-phosphate (F6P) as the starting point, or the pentose phosphate pathway, which uses glucose-6-phosphate (G6P). Alternatively, G6P and F6P can be converted into storage polysaccharides with G6P acting as the starting point. Fructose-1,6-diphosphate is reversibly split into dihydroxyacetone phosphate and glyceraldehyde-3-phosphate.

14. Glyceraldehyde-3-phosphate is converted into 1,3-diphosphoglycerate with a high-energy phosphoanhydride bond on carbon 1. Two ATP molecules are regenerated, with the coincidental production of pyruvate, which is transferred into the mitochondria. Pyruvic acid must be converted to acetyl-CoA in the mitochondria, where the tricarboxylic acid (TCA) cycle takes place.

15. Pyruvate plays a major role as an intermediary metabolite and is central to the interconversion of glucose, fatty acids and amino acids.

16. In the TCA cycle the most important supply of acetyl-CoA is from pyruvate, fatty acids and amino acids.

17. The TCA cycle is regulated to provide for cell needs. The function of the cycle is to provide NADH and $FADH_2$ for the electron transport chain and to provide substrates for biosynthesis.

18. Acetyl-CoA entering the TCA cycle yields one ATP molecule and storage of free energy as NADH and $FADH_2$. Oxidation of 1 mole of acetyl-CoA leads to the overall production of 12 moles of ATP. In addition, pyruvate metabolism provides 15 moles of ATP per mole of pyruvate or 30 moles per mole of glucose. The metabolites in the TCA cycle are major starting materials for a number of biosynthetic pathways.

19. The pentose phosphate pathway is a an alternative metabolic pathway. The initial reaction of glucose-6-phosphate dehydrogenation generates NADPH for fatty acid and cholesterol synthesis. The NADPH production throughout the pathway is important for some biosynthetic reactions, especially lipids.

20. In the presence of abundant glucose the emphasis is on anabolic processes and storage.

The liver converts some glucose to stored glycogen and some to fatty acids to be used as a fuel. Peripherally, glucose is metabolised to generate ATP and excess is stored as glycogen and adipose tissue.

21. Insulin stimulates the uptake of glucose by various tissues and the synthesis of glycogen in the liver.
22. Glycogen is an α-1–4 polysaccharide with α-1–6 branch points. Glycogen synthase is inactive when phosphorylated, and is activated by insulin and high concentrations of G6P.
23. Glucose stores in the form of glycogen are mobilised when needed. Glucose synthesis from non-glucose sources, lactate, pyruvate, fatty acids or amino acids (gluconeogenesis) is stimulated in the liver and kidney.
24. Phosphorylase releases glucose from glycogen in the form of G6P. The enzyme phosphorylase *a* is active when phosphorylated. The inactive form, phosphorylase *b*, is produced by phosphorylase *a* phosphatase. The phosphorylase kinase is kept in an active and inactive form by protein kinase, and the process is controlled hormonally.
25. Glucose has a central role in the production and harnessing of energy and in the synthesis of other sugars. While an individual is fasting the brain uses 80% of the glucose consumed. The liver only contains sufficient glucose (as glycogen stores) to meet the needs of the brain for 12 h.
26. Glycolysis and gluconeogenesis are directly opposed reaction sequences. Most of the enzymes that function in glycolysis are reversed in gluconeogenesis. Fatty acids are not capable of undergoing gluconeogenesis.
27. The intermediates in the gluconeogenic and glycolysis pathways are the same and are coupled to the ATP–ADP system. Some steps in metabolic pathways are irreversible, and hence alternative pathways are necessary.
28. The energy difference between glycolysis and gluconeogenesis is four ATP molecules per metabolised hexose. This means that regulation of the glycolysis and gluconeogenesis systems is of prime importance to cellular metabolism. There is a direct effect of concentrations of metabolites within the TCA cycle on phosphofructokinase activity.

29. During starvation or high-protein or high-fat diets, the amount and activity of phosphoenolpyruvate carboxykinase increase and they decrease when there is a restoration of carbohydrate to the diet.
30. Ketone bodies are acetoacetate (AcAc), β-hydroxybutyrate (BHB) and acetone. AcAc and BHB are interconvertible within mitochondria, using the $NAD^+/NADH_2$ couple as a cofactor.
31. Ketone bodies are synthesised almost entirely in the liver, resulting in 3-hydroxybutyrate. There is diffusion from the liver cell into the plasma. The brain, but not the liver, is able to metabolise ketone bodies.
32. During starvation ketone body synthesis begins and plasma concentrations of AcAc and BHB become detectable. During prolonged starvation and diabetes mellitus high concentrations of ketones appear in the blood; this condition is called ketosis.
33. The genetic control of transport of sugars and the subsequent metabolism is mediated through the transported sugar or by a metabolite and hormones, e.g. insulin.

THINKING POINTS

1. Begin to form a view on how the major nutrients, carbohydrates, fats and amino acids, interact and interconvert.
2. Glucose is a major and flexible source of energy.

NEED TO UNDERSTAND

1. Carbohydrates are major nutrients for energy.
2. Their absorption, control and storage by the liver and subsequent release for entry into cells around the body, and their rapid removal by metabolic processes, are important to understand.

FURTHER READING

Birnbaum, M.J. (2001) Diabetes. Dialogue between muscle and fat. *Nature*, **409**, 672–3.

Coleman, L. (1980) Metabolic interrelationships between carbohydrates, lipids and proteins. In *Metabolic Control and Disease* (eds. P.K. Bondy and L.E. Rosenberg). W.B. Saunders, Philadelphia, PA, pp. 161–274.

Hanson, R.W. and Reshef, L. (1997) Regulation of phosphoenolpyruvate carboxykinase (GTP) gene expression. *Annual Review of Biochemistry*, **66**, 581–612.

Harold, F.M. (1986) *The Vital Force; A Study in Bioenergetics*. W.H. Freeman & Co., New York.

Picard, F. and Auwer, X. (2002) PPARγ and glucose homeostasis. *Annual Review of Nutrition*, **22**, 167–97.

Rencurel, F. and Girard, J. (1998) Regulation of liver gene expression by glucose. *Proceedings of the Nutrition Society*, **57**, 265–75.

Rich, A.J. (1990) Ketone bodies as substrates. *Proceedings of the Nutrition Society*, **49**, 361–73.

Salati, L.M. and Amir-Ahmady, B. (2001) Dietary regulation of expression of glucose-6-phosphate dehydrogenase. *Annual Review of Nutrition*, **21**, 121–40.

Worth, H.G.J. and Curnow, D.H. (1980) *Metabolic Pathways in Medicine*. Edward Arnold, London.

34

Lipid metabolism

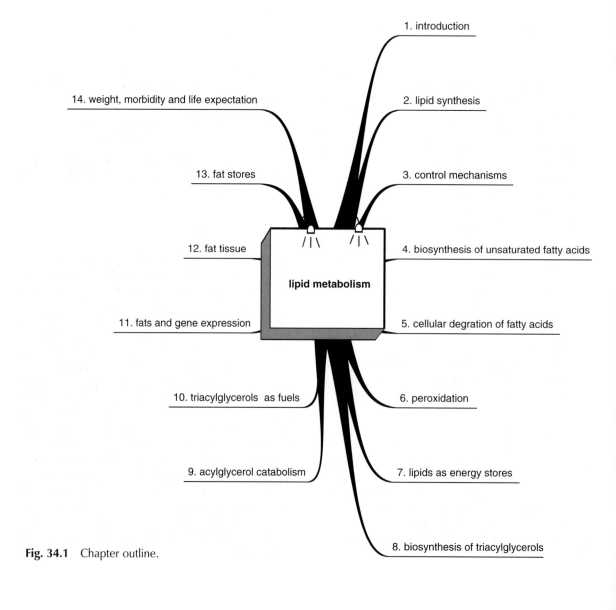

1. introduction
2. lipid synthesis
3. control mechanisms
4. biosynthesis of unsaturated fatty acids
5. cellular degration of fatty acids
6. peroxidation
7. lipids as energy stores
8. biosynthesis of triacylglycerols
9. acylglycerol catabolism
10. triacylglycerols as fuels
11. fats and gene expression
12. fat tissue
13. fat stores
14. weight, morbidity and life expectation

lipid metabolism

Fig. 34.1 Chapter outline.

INTRODUCTION

Most naturally occurring fatty acids are formed from even numbers of carbon atoms. The entire chain of synthesised fatty acids derives from acetic acid. The major biosynthetic route to long-chain fatty acids is different from fatty acid degradation through β-oxidation. Most fatty acids are synthesised in the liver and transported to the periphery for storage.

LIPID SYNTHESIS

Acetyl-coenzyme A carboxylase

The first step in fatty acid synthesis is the carboxylation of the two-carbon fragment acetate, acetyl-coenzyme A (CoA), to malonate, catalysed by acetyl-CoA carboxylase, a biotin-containing and important control enzyme in fatty acid synthesis (Figure 34.2). Most of the acyl-CoA is derived from the oxidation of pyruvate in mitochondria from lactate, glucose and amino acids. Pyruvate dehydrogenase is a mitochondrial enzyme, so acetyl-CoA is formed within the mitochondria, remote from fatty acid synthesis in the cytoplasm. The mitochondrial membrane is impermeable to acetyl-CoA. The transfer may be mediated by conversion of the acetyl-CoA within the mitochondria to citric acid as an intermediary:

Acetate + ATP + HS-CoA $\longrightarrow$
Acetyl-CoA + AMP + 2P$_i$

Acetyl-CoA + Oxaloacetate + ADP + P$_i$ $\longrightarrow$
Citrate + ATP + HS-CoA

(ATP: adenosine triphosphate; HS-CoA: coenzyme A; AMP: adenosine monophosphate; ADP: adenosine diphosphate; P$_i$: inorganic phosphate).

In the cytosol the reverse reaction takes place. Oxaloacetate is not readily transferred across membranes, so there is a further conversion to malate and then pyruvate by the catalytic activity of malate dehydrogenase. This is the pyruvate–malate shunt (Figure 34.3). This series of reactions generates reduced nicotinamide adenine dinucleotide phosphate (NADPH) for fatty acid synthesis.

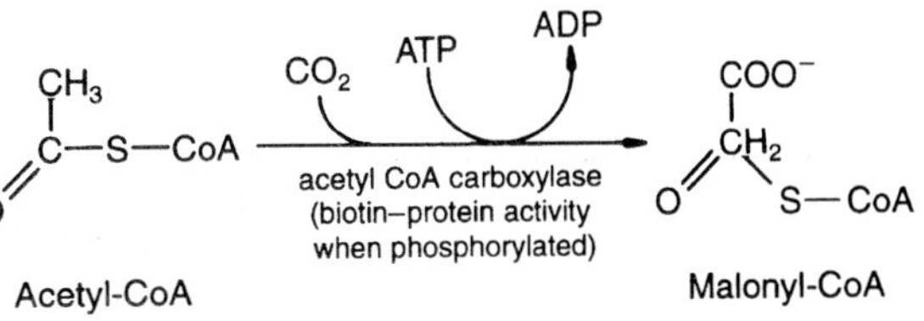

Fig. 34.2 The first step in the synthesis of fatty acids is the synthesis of malonyl-CoA from acetyl-CoA (enzyme acetyl-CoA carboyxlase, a biotin-requiring enzyme).

Citrate is also an activator of acetyl-CoA carboxylase, a rate-limiting enzyme in fatty acid synthesis:

Acetyl-CoA + CO$_2$ + ATP $\longrightarrow$
Malonyl-CoA + ADP + P$_i$

Citrate is converted to oxaloacetic acid by citrate lyase, and the oxaloacetate reduced by NADH to form malate:

malate + NADP $\longrightarrow$ pyruvate + CO$_2$ +
NADPH

In the conversion of acetyl-CoA to fatty acids, NADPH is required and is obtained from the citrate/malate/pyruvate pump.

Fatty acid synthase

Fatty acid synthesis from malonyl-CoA is a series of condensation additions and reductions from carbonyl to methylene groups, catalysed by the multienzyme system, fatty acid synthase. There is a transfer of intermediates within the system from one active site to another during chain elongation.

The malonyl-CoA generated by acetyl-CoA carboxylase is the source of the atoms of the fatty acyl chain, except for the first two atoms derived from acetyl-CoA. In some instances butyryl-CoA is the initiating molecule. Propionyl-CoA and branch primers allow the formation of odd chain length and branched-chain fatty acids, respectively.

Acetyl-CoA synthase enables acetate transport from the liver to be activated and oxidised in mitochondria of other tissues. Butyryl-CoA synthetase, a mitochondrial enzyme, is used in the heart for acids with chain length in the range 3–7 carbons. In the liver there is also a special propionyl-CoA synthetase.

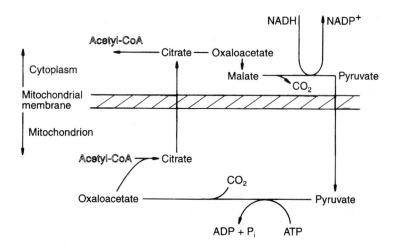

Fig. 34.3 Pyruvate–malate shunt. Acetyl-CoA does not cross the mitochondrial membrane. This shunt system allows the effective transport of acetyl-CoA from the mitochondria to the cytoplasm.

The medium-chain acyl-CoA synthase is found in heart mitochondria and is active for acids with a chain length of 4–12 carbons.

densation and reduction product is temporarily moved. A maximum of seven malonyl groups condenses with the fatty acid chain.

Fatty acid synthase

The fatty acid synthase family can be divided into type I, II and III enzymes.

- Type I synthases are multifunctional enzymes that catalyse individual reactions.
- Types II and III are complexes of molecular weight 450–550 kDa. The multifunctional forms of fatty acid synthase result from gene fusion. The genes for type II fatty acid synthase, found in lower bacteria and plants, fuse to give two genes that code for a yeast-type fatty acid synthase. The latter then fuse to give a single gene coding for the mammalian type I fatty acid synthase.

Stages by which the malonyl groups condense with the fatty acid chain

- Acetyl transferase: the acetyl CoA is transferred first to the 4'-phosphopantetheine arm and then to a second site, leaving the 4'-phosphopantetheine arm free.
- Malonyl transferase: each incoming malonyl group is transferred to the 4'-phosphopantetheine arm.
- 3-Ketoacyl synthase: the malonyl group on the 4'-phosphopantetheine arm is added to the acetyl group, followed by decarboxylation to give 3-ketobutyryl derivatives.
- D-Hydroxybutyrate is produced by reduction using NADPH.
- 3-Hydroxyacyl dehydratase removes a water molecule.
- This enoyl intermediate is reduced by NADPH, resulting in a fatty acid attached to the 4'-phosphopantetheine arm. This fatty acid is then transferred to the second active site 3-ketoacyl synthase, leaving the 4'-phosphopantetheine arm free for the next malonyl-CoA.
- Thioester hydrolase releases palmitic acid from the 4'-phosphopantetheine arm.

Fatty acid synthase (Figure 34.4) contains a functional 4'-phosphopantetheine group, a flexible chain of 14 atoms that joins to the synthase protein through a serine residue. Endproducts are transferred from one active site (4'-phosphopantetheine arm) to another (3-ketoacyl reductase). This has a terminal cysteine group on the acyl protein carrier protein (ACP), to which each successive con-

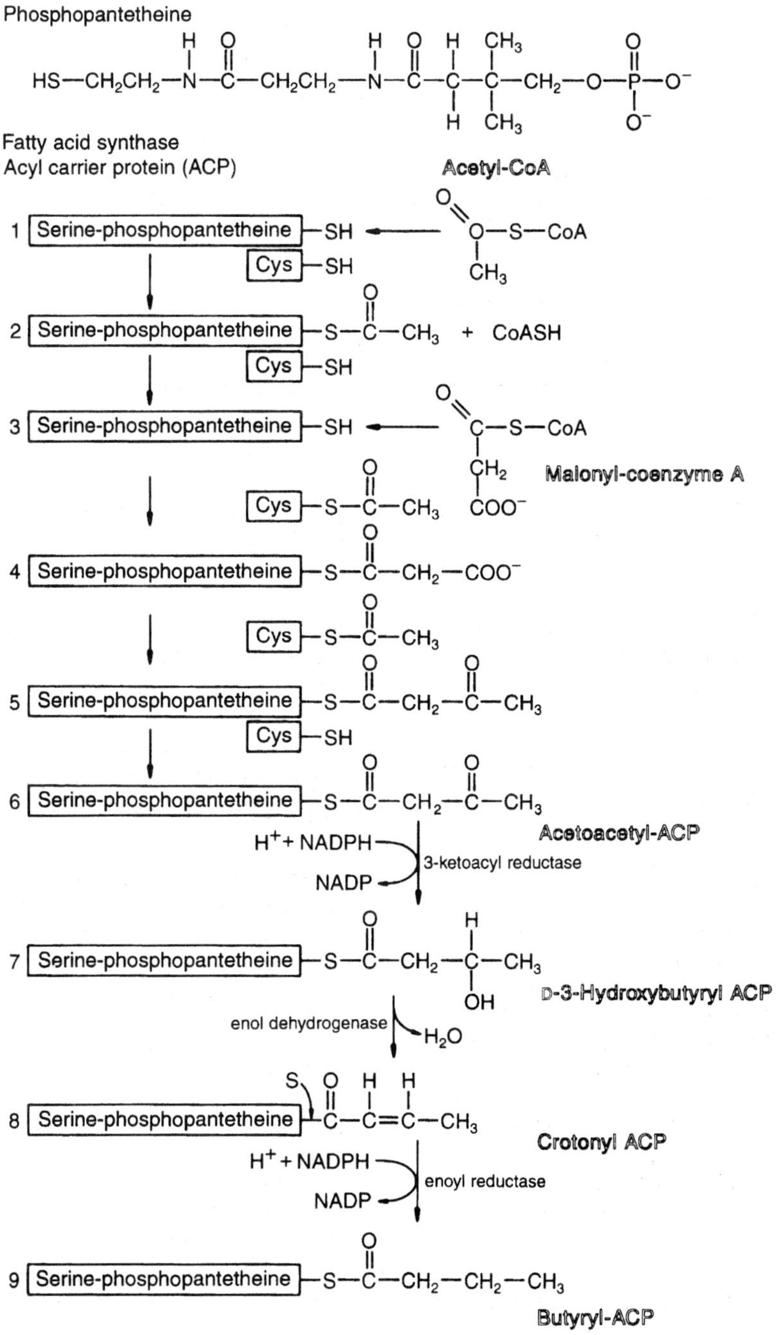

Fig. 34.4 Fatty acid synthase. Fatty acid synthesis begins with the binding of an acetyl group to fatty acid synthase, followed by incremental additions of malonyl-CoA. The active sites on the fatty acid synthase are phosphopantotheine and a cysteine grouping. There is an incremental addition of malonyl-CoA. The second active site (Cys-SH) binds the previous metabolite, ready for the addition of further malonyl-CoA. The 3-ketoacyl product is reduced to the corresponding saturated acyl group, ready for the next addition of malonyl-CoA.

The endproduct of animal fatty acid synthase enzyme activity is free palmitic acid. The cleavage of this acid from the enzyme complex is catalysed by a thioesterase, an integral part of the enzyme complex.

The rate of fatty acid synthesis is determined by the availability of malonyl-CoA, the concentration of palmitoyl-CoA and possibly citrate.

Fatty acids have to be converted into metabolically active thiol esters before further anabolic or catabolic metabolism. The active form is usually the thiol ester of the fatty acid with the complex nucleotide coenzyme (CoA) or the small protein ACP. This makes the acyl chains water soluble. The formation of acyl-CoA is by acyl-CoA synthetases, dependent on chain length specificity and tissue distribution.

Fatty acid elongation

Fatty acid elongation is catalysed by the type III synthases or elongases present in the endoplasmic

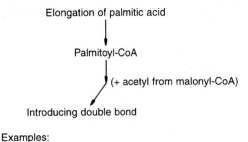

Reaction: occurs in endoplasmic reticulum and mitochondria

Double bonds: can only be added after C:16

Fig. 34.5 Elongation of some monounsaturated fatty acids is possible by elongating the palmitoyl carbon chain and introducing double bonds, e.g. oleic acid C18:1. This reaction takes place either in the endoplasmic reticulum or in mitochondria. Humans can introduce double bonds at C9, C6 and C3, but not towards the tail. Double bonds result from the catalytic activity of acyl-CoA desaturases in the endoplasmic reticulum, the enzymes being mixed-function oxidases.

reticulum (Figure 34.5). They catalyse the addition of malonyl-CoA to preformed acyl chains requiring NADPH as a reducing coenzyme. Two carbon units can be added as far as 24 carbon atoms. Saturated fatty acids less than C16 are preferred as the initial substrate. The important function of elongation is to transform dietary essential fatty acids to higher polyunsaturated fatty acids (PUFAs). The starting point is linoleoyl-CoA, which is first desaturated to a trienoic acid.

CONTROL MECHANISMS

The activity of the enzymes involved in fat synthesis decreases during starvation or a high dietary fat intake. The enzymes involved in fatty acid biosynthesis are most active while a low-fat, high-carbohydrate diet is being eaten. PUFAs are effective in reducing fatty acid synthesis. Sucrose ingestion, probably as a result of the fructose content, results in an increase in the liver lipogenesis enzymes.

Insulin is important in determining adipose tissue cell permeability. When fat is ingested, whether in the form of fatty acids or other lipids, blood insulin concentrations remain low. On an enriched fatty diet, the metabolic responses are those of a starved animal, with increased plasma concentrations of free fatty acids and low insulin, whereas there is increased glucose and insulin after a more balanced nutrient intake. Acetyl-CoA carboxylase, the rate-limiting step enzyme for fatty acid synthesis, is inhibited by fatty acyl-CoA and by free fatty acids. Following a high-carbohydrate meal, blood glucose and insulin concentrations rise.

Glucose enters the cell and may be converted to fatty acids and glycerol, and hence triglycerides. In contrast, on a high fat intake, a limiting factor is the limited glucose available for glycerol synthesis.

Fatty acid synthesis is controlled by acetyl-CoA carboxylase, which requires a hydroxy tricarboxylic acid, e.g. citrate or isocitrate, as substrate. Citrate, being a precursor of acetyl-CoA, is a positive feedforward activator. Acetyl-CoA carboxylase, the dephosphorylated enzyme form, is much more active than the phosphorylated form. The main role of citrate in this catalytic process is to keep the carboxylated form of the enzyme in its active form by shifting the equilibrium from the inactive to the active species of the enzyme. Long-chain acyl-CoA inhibits mammalian acetyl-CoA carboxylase.

Synthesis and degradation

Acetyl-coenzyme A carboxylase

Long-term regulation of key enzymes, in part, depends on changes in enzyme amounts, affected by nutritional and hormone state and genetic factors. There is a decrease in enzyme activity and amount during fasting owing to diminished synthesis or accelerated breakdown. Unesterified fatty acids are the metabolite responsible for controlling the synthetic rate of the enzyme.

Fatty acid synthase

The amount of liver fatty acid synthase is decreased by starvation, glucagon, increased feeding, insulin, β-oestradiol, hydrocortisone and growth hormone. The increase in fatty acid synthase between the starved and refed state is about 20-fold.

Dietary factors that affect fatty acid synthetase levels do not affect all tissues equally. Fatty acid synthase activity in the liver is highly influenced by diet, yet the enzyme's activity in the brain is unaffected. The fatty acid turnover rate of the brain changes over a much longer time-scale than that of the liver. Differences in fatty acid synthase activity result from changes in enzyme amounts rather than changes in enzyme activity. These alterations result from changes in the balance of enzyme synthesis and degradation as a result of the amount of cell fatty acid synthase messenger RNA (mRNA). NADPH production is adjusted to cope with the altering amounts of fatty acid synthesis. Fatty acid synthase activity increases in mammary gland tissue during mid to late pregnancy and early lactation. The synthase level in the brain is highest in the foetus and neonate and decreases with maturity. The supply of malonyl-CoA by acetyl-CoA carboxylase activity is a major factor in the regulation of overall fatty acid formation.

Fatty acid desaturases

Unsaturated fatty acids are present in all living cells. They are important:

- in regulating the physical properties of lipoproteins and membranes

- in regulation of metabolism in cells
- as precursors for physiologically active compounds, e.g. eicosanoids.

When diet causes an increased synthesis of fatty acid synthase there are similar increases in activity of the enzyme Δ^9 desaturase, but not of Δ^4, Δ^5 or desaturase (the Δ numbering being the chemical numbering of the unsaturated bond; see below). Insulin influences desaturase activity. However, dietary fructose, glycerol or saturated fatty acids can also increase enzyme activity, which means that the influence of insulin activity is modest or indirect.

BIOSYNTHESIS OF UNSATURATED FATTY ACIDS

The most important pathway is an oxidative mechanism by which a double bond is introduced directly into a saturated long-chain fatty acid, using a reduced compound, e.g. NADH, as cofactor. Most of the acids produced have a Δ^9 double bond, e.g. palmitic into palmitoleic acid. The double bond

n-9 series

Oleic acid 18 : 1 Δ^9

→ 18 : 2 $\Delta^{6,9}$

→ 20 : 4 $\Delta^{5,8,11}$

n-6 series (essential fatty acids)

Linoleic acid 18 : 2 $\Delta^{9,12}$

γ-linolenic acid 18 : 3 $\Delta^{6,9,12}$

Arachidonic acid 20 : 4 $\Delta^{5,8,11,14}$

n-3 series (essential fatty acids)

α-Linolenic acid 18 : 3 $\Delta^{9,12,15}$

18 : 4 $\Delta^{6,9,12,15}$

20 : 4 $\Delta^{8,11,14,17}$

Eicosapentaenoic acid 20 : 5 $\Delta^{5,8,11,14,17}$

n-system: count from CH_3 end

Δ-system: count from COOH end

Fig. 34.6 Fatty acid synthesis. Elongation of polyunsaturated fats in n-9 (Δ^9), n-6 (Δ^6) and n-3 (Δ^3) series, the n-6 and n-3 series being essential fatty acids. From a dietary point of view linoleic and α-linolenic acids are essential. If these are present in the diet, the other longer fatty acids can be synthesised from these precursors.

is introduced between carbon atoms 9 and 10, counting from the carboxyl end of the fatty acid chain (Figure 34.6).

Monounsaturated fatty acyl-CoA esters can be substrates for the cell membrane Δ^6-desaturase. Oleic acid is converted to a series of n-9 fatty acids. Oleic acid 18:1, n-9 becomes 18:2, n-9. The enzyme is more usually involved in the reaction 18:2, n-6 to 18:3, n-6 and 18:3, n-3 to 18:4, n-3. When an 18-carbon chain is extended by two carbon atoms, an extra double bond may be added between the carboxyl group and the first double bond. Linoleic acid is the precursor of a series of n-6 fatty acids. Δ^5-Desaturase can yield arachidonic acid 20:4, n6 and eicosapentaenoic acid 20:5, n-3. Further fatty acids for membranes and eicosanoid production yield Δ^4-desaturase, which adds a double bond to produce docosapentaenoic acid 22:5, n-6 and docosahexaenoic acid 22:6, n-3.

The Δ^6-desaturase enzyme introduces a double bond at position 6 in the three families, n-3, n-6, n-9. There is competition between the enzymes, which have affinities greatest for Δ-linolenic acid, 18:3, n-3, less for linoleic acid 18:2, n-6 and least for oleic acid 18:1, n-9. The Δ-linoleic family can be converted to a series of n-3 fatty acids.

Introduction of a double bond into a saturated fatty acid

Humans can introduce a double bond at the C9 position (Δ^9 desaturase) and C6 and C3, but not beyond C9. The double bonds are introduced with the catalytic action of mixed function oxidases and acyl-CoA desaturase on the endoplasmic reticulum. Oxygen is activated through NADH or NADPH and cytochrome b_5 or cytochrome P450. To synthesise fatty acids with fewer than seven carbons beyond the double bond, the reactant has to use a fatty acid of plant origin.

linoleate 18:2 (9,12) $\longrightarrow$ arachidonate 20:4 (5,8, 11,14)

But palmitate cannot be so transformed:

Palmitoleoyl 16:1 (9) $\longrightarrow$ 20:4 (4,7,10,13)

PUFAs of the same family can be recognised by subtracting the number of the last unsaturated bond from the number of carbons, and these will be equal in a fatty acid family.

Introduction of a double bond into a polyunsaturated fatty acid

In plants, double bonds are introduced at the 12,13 position to form linoleate, followed by further desaturation of the 15,16 position to form α-linolenic acid. The most abundant PUFA synthesised by plants, linoleic acid (cis,cis-9,12 C18:2) cannot be synthesised by animals, yet this acid is necessary to maintain animals in a healthy state. Consequently, linoleic acid is an essential fatty acid for animals.

The inability of animals to desaturate oleic acid towards the methyl end of the chain gives rise to distinct families of PUFAs that are not interconvertible. Polyunsaturation in animals requires three separate desaturases, designated as Δ^4, Δ^5 and Δ^6 because they introduce double bonds between carbon atoms 4–5, 5–6 and 6–7. These reactions involve cytochrome b_5 and NADH-cytochrome b_5 reductase, molecular oxygen and reduced nicotinamide nucleotide. Substrates for the first polydesaturation are oleic acid (n-9), linoleic acid (n-6) and α-linolenic acid (n-3).

Dietary *trans* acids can be incorporated into the lipids of most tissues of the body, including liver, adipose tissue, brain and milk. The incorporation of *trans* fatty acids into tissues is dependent on the amounts present in the diet, particularly for *trans*-octadecenoates. However, this is also affected by the other constituents in the diet, e.g. the presence of essential fatty acids that reduce the accumulation of *trans* fatty acids in tissues.

Trans fatty acids are incorporated into all major classes of complex lipids, particularly triacylglycerols in adipose tissue. These are esterified at glycerol carbon positions 1 and 3. In the heart, liver and brain *trans* fatty acids are incorporated into phospholipids. The *trans*-octadecenoic acids behave as saturated fatty acids and are esterified preferentially into position C1 of the phosphoglycerides. Oleic acid is distributed randomly among the carbons of the glycerol.

Trans fatty acids are catabolised as any other fatty acids, and are readily removed from tissues and oxidised. They are of no distinctive physiological or pathological significance except in the proportions of non-essential and essential fatty acids in the diet.

CELLULAR DEGRADATION OF FATTY ACIDS

Fatty acid breakdown is by oxidation at defined bonds in the acyl chain or oxidation at defined double bonds in unsaturated fatty acids. The main pathways are α, β and ω oxidation, depending on the position of the carbon of the acyl chain that is oxidised (Figure 34.7).

β-Oxidation

β-Oxidation is quantitatively the most important form of fatty acid oxidation (Figure 34.8). Long-chain fatty acids are degraded as two-carbon (acetyl-CoA) fragments by β-oxidation. The reaction takes place in mitochondria, peroxisomes and glyoxysomes. The latter two are particularly important in liver and kidney. Microbodies oxidise long-chain fatty acids to medium-chain fatty acids, which are then transported to mitochondria to complete the degradation.

Two carbon atoms as acetyl-CoA are removed from the fatty acid by the successive action of four enzymes: acyl-CoA dehydrogenase, enoyl-CoA hydrolase, 3-L-hydroxyacyl-CoA dehydrogenase, and thiolase.

1. The first step in the β-oxidation cycle is the introduction of a *trans* α, β-double bond to the hydrocarbon chain of the activated fatty acid by the flavoprotein enzyme acyl-CoA dehydrogenase.
2. Enoyl-CoA hydrolase then catalyses the addition of water across the *trans* double bond of the unsaturated acyl-CoA to form 3-L-hydroxy-acyl-CoA.
3. L-3-Hydroxyacyl-CoA dehydrogenase converts the L-hydroxy fatty acid into 3-ketoacyl CoA.

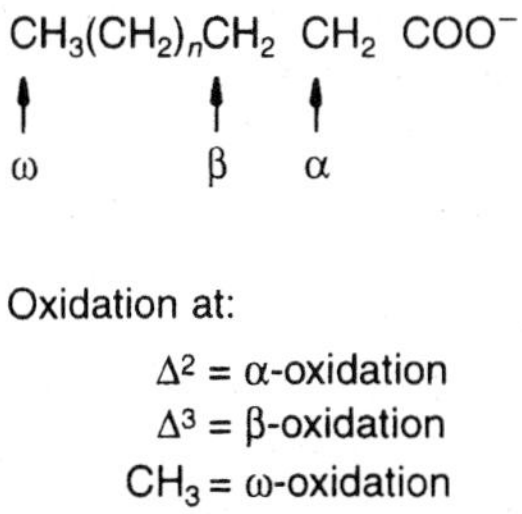

$$CH_3(CH_2)_nCH_2 \quad CH_2 \quad COO^-$$

$$\omega \qquad\qquad \beta \quad \alpha$$

Oxidation at:

$$\Delta^2 = \alpha\text{-oxidation}$$
$$\Delta^3 = \beta\text{-oxidation}$$
$$CH_3 = \omega\text{-oxidation}$$

Fig. 34.7 Degradation of fatty acids. Nomenclature of oxidation: α, β and ω.

4. Acyl-CoA:acetyl-CoA acyl transferase (or thiolase) catalyses a thiolytic cleavage of the keto acid, removing an acetyl-CoA to be replaced with an –SH group from CoA.

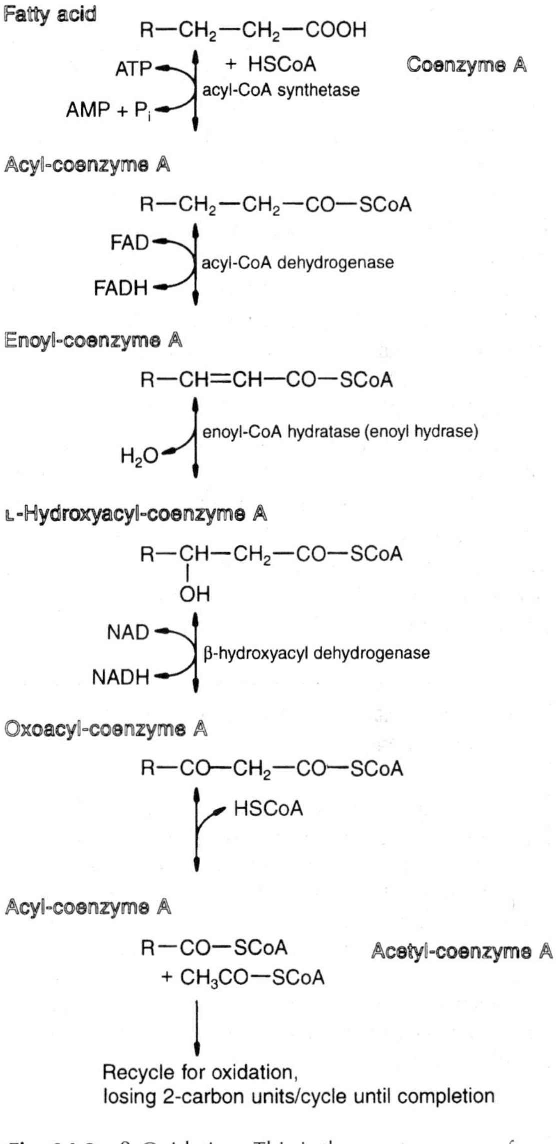

Fatty acid

$$R-CH_2-CH_2-COOH$$

ATP → + HSCoA   Coenzyme A
acyl-CoA synthetase
AMP + P_i →

Acyl-coenzyme A

$$R-CH_2-CH_2-CO-SCoA$$

FAD →
acyl-CoA dehydrogenase
FADH →

Enoyl-coenzyme A

$$R-CH=CH-CO-SCoA$$

enoyl-CoA hydratase (enoyl hydrase)
H_2O →

L-Hydroxyacyl-coenzyme A

$$R-CH-CH_2-CO-SCoA$$
$$\quad\ |$$
$$\quad OH$$

NAD →
β-hydroxyacyl dehydrogenase
NADH →

Oxoacyl-coenzyme A

$$R-CO-CH_2-CO-SCoA$$

HSCoA

Acyl-coenzyme A

$$R-CO-SCoA$$ Acetyl-coenzyme A
$$+ CH_3CO-SCoA$$

Recycle for oxidation,
losing 2-carbon units/cycle until completion

Fig. 34.8 β-Oxidation. This is the most common form of fatty acid oxidation as the acyl-CoA form. This is oxidised to unsaturated enoyl-CoA by a flavoprotein, followed by hydration to an alcohol group which is oxidised by NAD to a ketone. The ketoacyl-CoA is cleaved with another CoA, producing acetyl-CoA and a new acyl-CoA compound that is two carbons shorter than the original. This shorter acyl-CoA can then undergo the same reaction sequence.

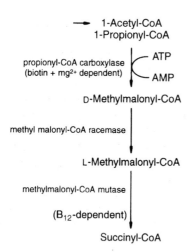

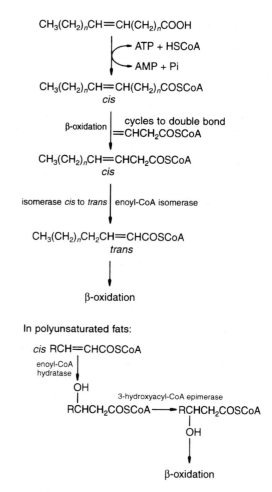

Fig. 34.9 Oxidation of fatty acids with an odd number of carbon atoms. The final products of β-oxidation are one molecule of acetyl-CoA and one molecule of propionyl-CoA. The propionyl-CoA is metabolised to D-methyl malonyl-CoA and L-methyl malonyl-CoA. The final reaction proceeds to succinyl-CoA. The enzyme (methyl malonyl-CoA mutase) has an absolute requirement for vitamin B$_{12}$.

The shortened acyl fatty acids repeatedly pass through this sequence of oxidation, hydration, oxidation and cleavage until the entire chain is reduced to two-carbon lengths and enters the tricarboxylic acid (TCA) cycle.

Acids of odd chain length yield propionic acid through oxidation in some tissues, e.g. in the liver, but not myocardial tissue (Figure 34.9). Branched-chain fatty acids with an even number of carbon atoms can also produce propionate.

Many natural fatty acids are unsaturated, with most double bonds being *cis*-orientated. When unsaturated fatty acids are β-oxidised, the unsaturated acids have *cis* double bonds and this may prove difficult for β-oxidation. An isomerase converts the *cis*-3 compound into the necessary *trans*-2 fatty acyl-CoA. β-Oxidation then continues, with removal of a further two carbons and then dehydrogenation to 2-*trans*,4-*cis* decadienoyl-CoA from linoleoyl-CoA (Figure 34.10).

The acetyl-CoA produced enters the TCA cycle. Acetoacetate and β-hydroxybutyrate may accumulate as ketone bodies. Acetoacetyl-CoA may convert to the free acid and CoA. Alternatively, acetoacetyl-CoA may convert into hydroxymethyl-glutaryl-CoA (HMG-CoA), which is cleaved to free

Fig. 34.10 Oxidation of unsaturated fatty acids. Unsaturated bonds cannot act as substrates for the acyl-CoA dehydrogenase enzyme. This is overcome by an isomerisation of the double bond from the *cis* to the *trans* conformation. A substrate for enoyl-CoA hydratase and the normal β-oxidation results. In polyunsaturated fats, 3-hydroxyacyl-CoA epimerase hydrates and inverts the configuration of the hydroxyl at carbon 3 from the D-isomer to the L-isomer.

acetoacetic acid. HMG is important in cholesterol synthesis. Ketone bodies are metabolic substrates for brain and liver metabolism (see Chapter 33). Acetyl-CoA can therefore be involved in the citric acid cycle or ketogenesis. The particular pathway that is followed depends on the rate of β-oxidation and on the redox state of the mitochondria controlling the oxidation of malate to oxaloacetate.

The overall rate of β-oxidation is dependent on:

- the availability of free fatty acids
- the rate of utilisation of β-oxidation products
- feedback mechanisms.

The concentration of plasma free fatty acids is controlled by the inhibitory effect of insulin, the stimulating effect of glucagon and the breakdown of triacylglycerols, and varies from tissue to tissue. In muscle, the rate of β-oxidation is dependent on the plasma free fatty acid concentration and energy requirements. A decrease in energy demand by muscles results in increased concentrations of NADH and acetyl-CoA. An increase in NADH/NAD$^+$ ratios inhibits mitochondrial TCA cycle activity.

Liver metabolism of lipids is much more complicated because of the conflicting influences of lipids, carbohydrates and ketone bodies. Malonyl-CoA inhibits carnitine palmitoyltransferase and reduces the movement of acyl groups into mitochondria for oxidation. Malonyl-CoA is produced by acetyl-CoA carboxylase, which is regulated by hormones. Fatty acid synthesis and degradation are both regulated by liver hormonal concentrations.

Under normal conditions peroxisomes contribute up to 50% of the overall fatty oxidation activity of the liver. Such oxidation is increased by

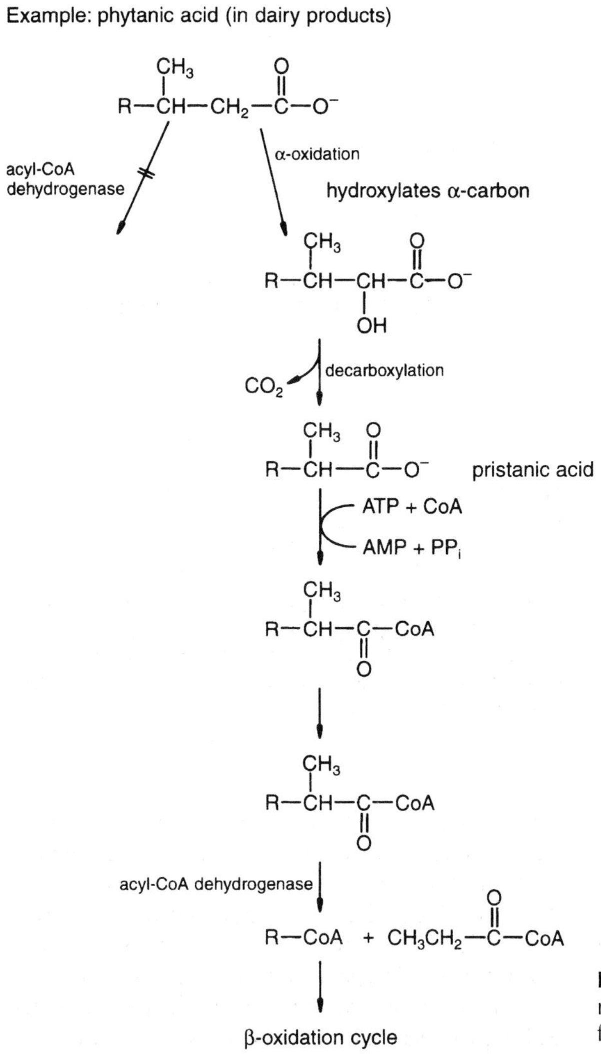

Fig. 34.11   α-Oxidation is important in fatty acids with methyl substitutions at carbon 3. These are not substrates for acyl-CoA dehydrogenase.

hypolipidaemic drugs, high-fat diets, starvation or diabetes, and is limited to medium-chain and acetyl-CoA moieties. Peroxisomal β-oxidation generates less adenosine triphosphate (ATP) than mitochondrial β-oxidation. Peroxisomes also oxidise pristanic acid, derived from phytol, the long-chain alcohol attached to chlorophyll.

α-Oxidation

α-Oxidation is so called because only one carbon, the carboxyl, is lost at each step and the α-carbon becomes oxidised to the new carboxyl group (Figure 34.11). This fatty acid oxidation occurs in the microsome; the fatty acids do not have to be oxidised, and non-esterified fatty acids are permitted as substrates. This system is not linked to high energy production.

α-Oxidation is important in α-hydroxy fatty acid formation and one-carbon chain shortening. This is important for molecules that cannot be directly metabolised by β-oxidation. For example, brain cerebrosides and other sphingolipids contain α-hydroxy fatty acids. A mixed function oxidase breaks down α-hydroxy fatty acids, requires NAD and oxygen and results in one-carbon loss and the liberation of carbon dioxide.

An α-oxidation system in liver and kidney is important for the breakdown of branched-chain fatty acids, e.g. phytanic acid derived from phytol in animals. Methyl fatty acids, where the methyl group is β to a carboxyl group, cannot be β-oxidised, are shortened by one carbon by α-oxidation, after which β-oxidation can continue, with the release of propionyl-CoA. In the brain it is probable that free fatty acids are the substrates for α-oxidation.

ω-Oxidation

ω-Oxidation of straight-chain fatty acids produces dicarboxylic products. This is an oxidative process at the opposite end from the fatty acid carboxyls producing ω or (α, β and ω) or (ω-1) hydroxy acids and then dicarboxylic acids. This is a slower process than β-oxidation. However, in substituted derivatives ω-oxidation is an important first step to the subsequent β-oxidation. An ω-hydroxy fatty acid requires cytochrome P450, oxygen and NADPH, and is an intermediate for the mixed-function oxidase enzyme.

PEROXIDATION

Lipids, when exposed to oxygen, form peroxides. If this occurs in membranes then membrane disintegration occurs. Lipid peroxidation occurs in three separate processes: initiation, propagation and termination.

Peroxidation products are important, e.g. short- or medium-chain aldehydes from unsaturated fatty acids give rise to rancidity and the spoilage of frozen foods. The pleasant tastes of fresh green leaves, oranges and cucumbers are also derived from aldehydes.

LIPIDS AS ENERGY STORES

Lipids are a long-term form of stored energy, particularly as triacylglycerols. Animals store the fat in adipose tissue, whereas fish use their flesh or liver as a lipid store.

Fatty acids are transported from organ to organ as either:

- non-esterified fatty acids bound to albumin
- triacylglycerols associated with lipoproteins, particularly chylomicrons and very low-density lipoproteins (VLDLs).

Triacylglycerol is hydrolysed by lipoprotein lipase, which is predominantly an adipose tissue enzyme. Free fatty acids are transported bound to albumin and cross the cell membrane into cells by active transport. Inside the cells, fatty acid acyl-CoAs are generated, by an ATP-dependent acyl-CoA synthetase. Free fatty acids and acyl-CoA fatty acids bind to distinct cytosolic fatty acid proteins. Such small molecular weight (14 kDa) proteins include the z-protein of liver. Acyl-CoA groups cannot cross the mitochondrial membrane. Transport occurs as an acyl carnitine derivative (Figure 34.12), which crosses the membrane to be reconstituted as acyl-CoA. The transport of fatty acids from the cytosol into the mitochondria requires acylcarnitine

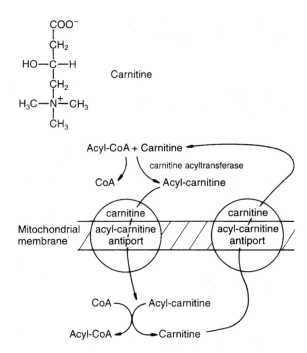

Fig. 34.12 Acyl-CoA is unable to cross the mitochondrial membrane. Transport of fatty acids into mitochondria occurs as acyl carnitine, through the acyl carnitine antiport and resynthesis to acyl-CoA.

translocase. Fatty acids of fewer than ten carbons can be taken up by mitochondria.

Within an adipose cell the hydrolysis of triglyceride yields diglyceride, monoglycerides, glycerol and free fatty acids. Triglycerides may be re-formed or metabolised and the free fatty acids may enter the bloodstream. This process is controlled by the concentration of glucose and cellular cyclic AMP (cAMP) and is therefore an important element in adipose tissue control. During starvation, cAMP concentrations increase and triglycerides are hydrolysed; the fatty acids then pass into the bloodstream, to be bound to albumin. This complex passes to other tissues for utilisation as a fuel. The permeability of glucose through cell membranes is inhibited; hence glucose metabolism is protected. Fatty acid metabolism creates raised concentrations of citrate and ATP which, in turn, inhibit glycolysis by inhibiting phosphofructokinase (PFK) activity.

BIOSYNTHESIS OF TRIACYLGLYCEROLS

The fatty acid composition of animal acylglycerols is dependent on the diet and particularly the vegetable oils eaten. Such metabolism varies between species and between organs within a species.

The glycerol phosphate pathway for the synthesis of triacylglycerol is the progressive esterification of glycerol-3-sn-phosphate and 1-acylglycerol-3-sn-phosphate with long-chain acyl-CoA fatty acids. Critical to this pathway is phosphatidic acid in both phospholipid and triacylglycerol biosynthesis. The diacylglycerol originating from phosphatidic acid forms the building block for triacylglycerols as well as phosphoglycerols. The transfer of acyl (fatty acids) groups from acyl-CoA to glycerol-3-phosphate requires two enzymes, specific for positions 1 and 2. The enzyme responsible for position 1 exhibits marked specificity for saturated acyl-CoA thiolesters, whereas the second enzyme shows

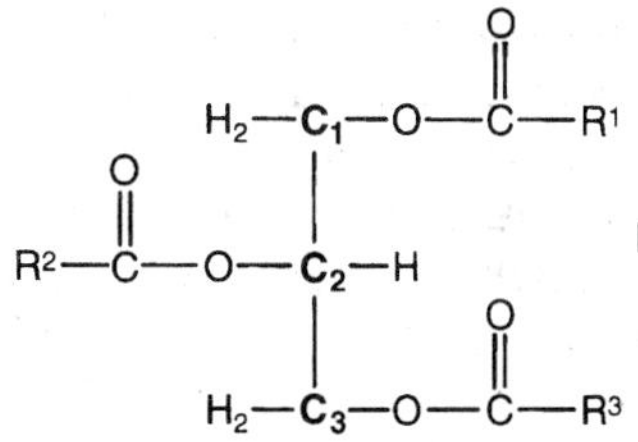

Predominant fatty acids, palmitic, stearic, oleic, linoleic
There is stereospecificity of distribution of fatty acids between C1, C2, C3,

milk fat
    short-chain fatty acid   ⟶ C3

animal fat
(not human milk)
    short-chain fatty acids
    unsaturated fatty acids   ⟶ C2
    polyunsaturated fatty acids
        mammals   ⟶ C3
        fish   ⟶ C2

seed oils
    acetate   ⟶ C3

Fig. 34.13 Lipids as an energy store: acyl glycerols. There is stereospecificity in the distribution of fatty acids between Cl, C2 and C3.

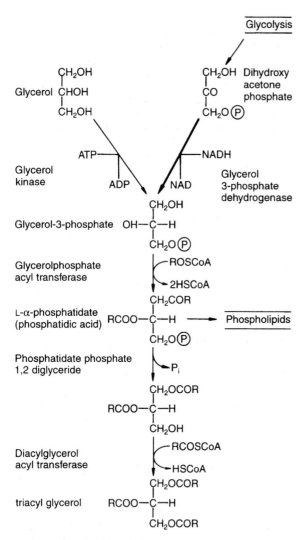

Fig. 34.14 Synthesis of triacylglycerol. Glycerol-3-phosphate is metabolised to L-α-phosphatidate (phosphatidic acid). L-α-Phosphatidate can be further metabolised to phospholipids or 1,2-diglycerides and triacylglycerol. Of major importance is the availability of diacylglycerol and fatty acyl-CoA. The supply of fatty acid is increased post-prandially and from biosynthesis of carbohydrate. Increased insulin post-prandially stimulates the synthesis of malonyl-CoA, increasing fatty acid synthesis. Phosphatidic acid phosphatase activity may be increased by glucocorticoids.

specificity towards mono- and dienoic fatty acyl-CoA thiolesters. This explains the saturated and unsaturated difference between positions 1 and 2 (Figure 34.13).

The conversion of phosphatidic acid to diacylglycerol is a rate-limited step catalysed by phosphatidate phosphohydrolase. The final step in synthesis is the transfer of fatty acid from acyl-CoA to diacylglycerol; the enzyme for which, diacylglycerol acyltransferase, can catalyse reactions over an extensive range of fatty acids (Figure 34.14).

An alternative precursor for 1-acylglycerol-3-sn-phosphate uses the dihydroxyacetone phosphate pathway; 1-acyl dihydroxyacetone phosphate acts as an intermediate. The conversion of glucose into triacylglycerol through the dihydroxyacetone phosphate (DHAP) pathway requires NADPH. The glycerol phosphate pathway consumes NADH. NADPH is associated with fatty acid biosynthesis. The activity of DHAP is enhanced under conditions of increased fatty acid synthesis and relatively reduced with starvation or a relatively high-fat diet.

Enteric triacylglycerols

Triacylglycerols are resynthesised from monoacylglycerols that have been absorbed after hydrolysis in the small intestinal lumen. The reactions are catalysed by enzymes in the enterocytes of the endoplasmic reticulum. The 2-monoacylglycerols are more readily esterified than the 1-monoacylglycerols. The rate of the initial esterification depends on which fatty acid is esterified in C2. Short-chain saturated or longer chain unsaturated fatty acids are favoured. Diacyltransferase has a specificity for 1,2-sn-diacylglycerols. Diacylglycerols with two unsaturated or mixed acid fatty acids are preferred as substrates to disaturated compounds.

ACYLGLYCEROL CATABOLISM

Lipases split fatty acids from the acylglycerol ester formed with the primary hydroxyl groups of glycerol.

Different tissues contain different lipases that vary in their substrate specificity. Lipoprotein lipase hydrolyses triacylglycerols complexed with proteins, and is involved in the catabolism of serum lipoproteins. Adipose tissue triacylglycerol lipase is activated by phosphorylation by hormones such as catecholamines (Figure 34.15). There is a mono-acylglycerol lipase in many cells. Fatty acids of chain length less than 12 carbon atoms, especially the very short chain lengths of milk fats, are cleaved more rapidly than the C14–18 chain length fatty acids. The very long-chain polyenoic acids (C20:5 and 22:6 of fish oils and marine mammals) are hydrolysed slowly.

For most free fatty acids the relative proportion in the plasma is different from the adipose tissue stores, containing more polyunsaturates than long-chain saturates and monounsaturated fatty

> The fatty acids at positions 1 and 3 are initially removed at equal rates. Once one fatty acid has been removed, hydrolysis of the resulting diacylglycerol is slower than for the original triacylglycerol. Similarly, monoacylglycerol hydrolysis is slow once the fatty acids are racemised to position 1. This means that there is an accumulation of monoacylglycerols and non-esterified fatty acids. Some lipases hydrolyse both the fatty acids in the primary position of acylglycerols and the fatty acids esterified in position 1 of phosphoglycerides.

acids. There is a 15-fold range of mobilisation, from the highest 18:5, n-3 to the lowest 24:1, n-9. Mobilisation is determined by chain length; short-chain and unsaturated are preferred to long-chain and saturated. The selectivity of release is not due to the position in the triacylglycerol, i.e. 1, 2 or 3. The adipose tissue type or chemistry does not appear to be a factor.

Animals are unable to convert lipid directly into carbohydrate because of the irreversible decarboxylation steps in the TCA cycle (isocitrate dehydrogenase) and α-ketoglutarate dehydrogenase. Each of the two fatty acid carbons entering the Krebs cycle as acetyl-CoA is lost as carbon dioxide.

TRIACYLGLYCEROLS AS FUELS

Triacylglycerols in animals are a source of fatty acids and form a metabolic fuel. This is a controlled system. Blood glucose concentrations are normally maintained at a constant level and if this should alter it is restored rapidly to that level. Glycogen is stored as an emergency fuel in liver and muscle. When these stores are replete, excess carbohydrate is converted to fats and stored in adipose tissue. Optimal supplies of protein are needed for growth, tissue repair and enzyme synthesis; excess protein amino acids are converted into fat. Carbohydrate and protein are interconvertible and can be converted into fat. Fat, however, is only stored or oxidised but not converted into protein or carbohydrate.

Humans require continued access to nutrient energy, regardless of times of eating. Following a meal, plasma glucose concentrations are initially

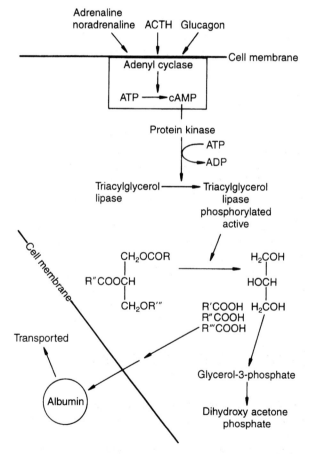

Fig. 34.15 Acylglycerol catabolism. The rate of hydrolysis of triacylglycerol is dictated by lipase activity (phosphorylated form). The activity of lipase is controlled by a protein kinase that is controlled by cAMP. This is under hormone control by adrenaline, noradrenaline, ACTH, glucagon and probably other hormones.

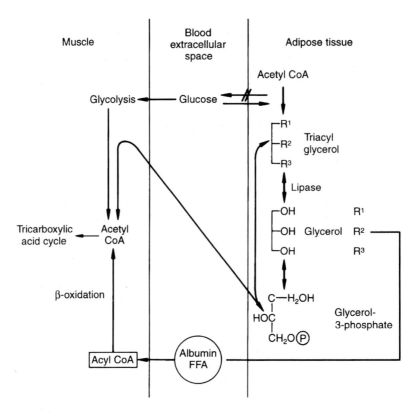

Fig. 34.16   Glucose and fatty acids in muscle and adipose tissue. Triacylglycerol is metabolised to glycerol and glycerol-3-phosphate, which can pass into the tricarboxylic acid cycle. Triacylglycerol fatty acids can pass from the cell and are transported bound to albumin to supply cells throughout the body. The fatty acid is converted to acyl-CoA, undergoes β-oxidation to acetyl-CoA and enters the tricarboxylic acid cycle. Glucose is oxidatively degraded to acetyl-CoA to glycerol-3-phosphate. Acetyl-CoA enters the tricarboxylic acid cycle. Glycerol is oxidised to glycerol-3-phosphate which enters the glycolysis pathway to acetyl-CoA. Acetyl-CoA, however, cannot reverse the process to glucose. There is hormonal control of glucose entry into the muscle and adipose tissue and of lipase-catalysed triacylglycerol hydrolysis.

derived from the meal, glycogen breakdown and to some extent from muscle protein. Additional energy comes from adipose tissue in the form of glycerol (converted into glucose in the liver) and fatty acid oxidation, particularly in muscles (Figure 34.16). Triacylglycerol synthesis increases when energy demands exceed immediate requirements. When there is a preponderance of fat in the diet, tissue fat synthesis from carbohydrate is depressed. Absorbed triacylglycerols are converted into lipoproteins and circulate in the blood. The fatty acids are released from the acylglycerols at the endothelial surfaces of cells, are catalysed by lipoprotein lipase and enter the cells. The fatty acids are then re-esterified into acylglycerols.

Acylglycerol synthesis is most important in the small intestine, where the resynthesis of triacylglycerols follows fat digestion.

The concentration of acyltransferases in cells is influenced by nutritional status. Glycerol-3-phosphate, which is important for acylglycerol synthesis, is regulated by similar factors to those responsible for glycolysis and gluconeogenesis. Starvation reduces the glycerol-3-phosphate cell concentrations, which are restored by refeeding. The intracellular concentration of acyl-CoA is increased during starvation (Figure 34.17).

The main metabolic alternative to acylglycerol synthesis is β-oxidation. The relative activities of glycerol phosphate acyltransferase and carnitine

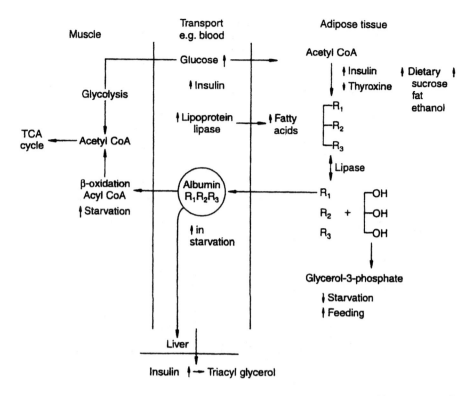

Fig. 34.17 Controls on carbohydrate and lipid metabolism by feeding, starvation and hormones. When there is an abundance of energy available, triacylglycerols are synthesised in adipose tissue, liver, heart and skeletal muscle. Fatty acids are mobilised from adipose tissue as a fuel during starvation.

palmitoyl transferase control the interaction of these two pathways. The underlying control mechanism is still poorly understood. The rate-limiting enzyme in mammalian acylglycerol biosynthesis is phosphatide phosphohydrolase, the activity of which increases with dietary sucrose and fat, ethanol and starvation, all of which result in high concentrations of plasma free fatty acids. This enzyme is also increased during liver regeneration following partial hepatectomy, in obese individu-

als, in diabetes and in association with drugs that result in reduced plasma lipid concentrations.

When there is an increased supply of saturated and monounsaturated fatty acids to the liver, phosphatide phosphohydrolase activity increases. When this enzyme activity is low, the phosphatidic acid becomes a substrate for the biosynthesis of acidic membrane phospholipids, e.g. phosphatidylinositol. This requires a supply of unsaturated fatty acids greater than could be used in acylglycerol metabolism.

The biosynthesis of phospholipids takes precedence over triacylglycerols when the synthesis of diacylglycerol is relatively reduced, membrane turnover and biosecretion being biologically more important than the accumulation of storage triacylglycerol. The relatively low K_m of choline phosphotransferase for diacylglycerols is an important factor in such metabolic control.

> The liver is important in relation to the synthesis of triacylglycerols or carbohydrates. Adipose tissue is involved in longer term storage and the mammary gland synthesises milk fat during lactation. In the intestine, dietary fatty acids are the main source of lipids. Elsewhere in the body the glycerol phosphate pathway is important.

> Phosphatidate phosphohydrolase is physiologically inactive until adsorbed onto the membrane on which the phosphatidate is being synthesised. This adsorption is regulated by both hormones and substrate. cAMP displaces the enzyme from the membranes. Increasing concentrations of non-esterified fatty acids and their CoA esters promote attachment. This has the effect of decreasing the intracellular concentrations of cAMP, which ensures more effective adherence at lower fatty acid concentrations. Metabolic control, in this instance, is dependent on enzyme activity, which in turn is dependent on location in the cells.
> Phosphorylcholine cytidyl transferase, which regulates the biosynthesis of phosphatidylcholine, is another enzyme whose activity is dependent on location in the cell.

The ratio of circulating insulin to glucagon influences the fate of fatty acids entering the liver. High ratios favour esterification of fatty acids into acylglycerols with a low rate of β-oxidation. Insulin increases the rate of glucose transport into fat cell membranes, and also increases the synthesis of the enzyme lipoprotein lipase, thereby catalysing fatty acid and glycerol release from triacylglycerol. Within the cell, insulin stimulates the synthesis of lipids by increasing the activity of lipogenic enzymes in general. Insulin also inhibits fat globule triacylglycerol breakdown and inhibits the hormone-sensitive triacylglycerol lipase activity by causing a decrease in the production of cAMP. Thyroid hormones stimulate triacylglycerol biosynthesis in the liver and suppress triacylglycerol synthesis in fat. This may be a general effect on metabolic turnover rather than a specific enzyme effect. The control of phosphatide phosphohydrolase is also controlled by glucocorticoids.

FATS AND GENE EXPRESSION

Fatty acids are important mediators of gene expression in the liver and adipose tissue. The mechanism of the influence of fatty acids is different in adipose tissue and the liver and includes:

- fish oil fatty acids, which suppress fatty acid synthesis, reduce esterifying enzyme activity and increase mitochondrial and peroxisomal oxidation of fatty acids in the liver
- a reduction in the plasma lipid concentration of fish oil fatty acids, which reduces the activity of fatty acid synthase, acetyl-CoA carboxylase, glucose-6-phosphate dehydrogenase and malic enzyme
- regulation of the key hepatic enzymes, diacylglycerol acyl transferase and phosphatide phosphorylase, and the control of apolipoprotein secretion
- n-6 and n-3 polyunsaturates diverting acyl-CoA towards oxidation. Eicosapentaenoic acid (20:5, n-3) reduces the plasma acyltriglycerol concentration by acting on mitochondria and increasing β-oxidation activity. Lipoprotein lipase activity may also be affected, as well as the transport of glucose into the adipocyte cell. Polyunsaturates result in a higher diet-induced thermogenesis than other fatty acids.

Genes regulated by dietary polyunsaturated fatty acids

Hepatic

- Fatty acids appear to act directly on hepatocyte gene transcription, but may also affect the insulin signalling pathway.
- Peroxisome proliferator-activated receptors (PPAR) are modulated by PUFA.
- Fatty acid synthase gene transcription is suppressed by PUFA.
- Glycolytic enzymes:
  L-pyruvate kinase PUFA reduces transcription.
- Lipogenic enzyme encoded genes:
  PUFA (chain length > C18 and = at C9 and C12) repress transcription.
- Fatty acid oxidation:
  acyl-CoA dehydrogenase mRNA increases with fish oils
  carnitine palmitoyltransferase I mRNA increases with long-chain fatty acids
  stearoyl-CoA desaturase is suppressed by PUFA.

Adipose tissue

- Fatty acid effects on gene expression are site dependent.
- n-3 PUFAs reduce fat storage by down-regulating prostaglandin synthesis.

- PUFA acts directly on adipocyte gene expression.
- Adipocyte lipid binding protein aP2 gene is induced by long-chain fatty acids, prostaglandins and leukotrienes, increasing expression of CCAAT/enhancer-binding protein, and thereafter is involved in the activation of adipogenic genes. This effect varies with different tissues. Peroxisome proliferator activated receptors (PPARs) have three distinct forms, α, δ and γ, each encoded by a different gene. The PPARs are associated with the nuclear receptor retinoid X (RXR) and are activated by different fatty acids.
- Fatty acid synthase gene is suppressed by arachidonic acid.
- Angiotensin gene is regulated by fatty acids.
- The human hormone-sensitive lipase gene is located on the long arm of chromosome 19(q13.1–13.2 region). Activity is increased with increased plasma free fatty acid concentrations, in pregnancy, and reduces with age.

FAT TISSUE

In response to day-to-day food intake, amino acid oxidation adjusts to amino acid intake, carbohydrate oxidation adjusts to carbohydrate intake, but fat balance is not regulated and nutrient excess goes into stores.

The function of fat tissue is to receive, store and release lipids. Adipose tissue is the tissue both quantitatively and qualitatively most directly affected by diet. Storage of triacylglycerol fatty acids reflects dietary intake. Fat-soluble xenobiotics and cholesterol accumulate in fatty tissue.

Membranes

The fatty acid composition of plasma and different cellular membranes is in part determined by the diet.

Brain and nervous tissue

The lipid content of the brain, retina and nervous tissue is high and rich in arachidonic acid (20:4, n-

6) and docosahexaenoic acid (22:6, n-3), which are synthesised from linoleic and α-linolenic acid. These long-chain PUFAs accumulate in the brain during the third trimester and immediate post-delivery period, when the brain grows at its maximum rate. A deficiency of such fatty acids during the formative period cannot be to the brain's advantage. If either n-3 or n-6 is deficient then there is an increase in the fatty acid family that is present in larger amounts, with unknown consequences on the function of the brain.

FAT STORES

Fat is stored in the adipose organ, which has two distinct tissues, white adipose tissue and brown adipose tissue (BAT). The organ is a single structure storing saved nutritional energy in the form of fat. The two tissues, white and brown, are interconvertible, but morphologically and functionally dissimilar. Brown fat has a rich vascular and noradrenergic innervation. Adipose tissue structure is different in hot and cold climates, fasting and obesity, and responds differently to leptin and uncoupling protein-1, which are genetically expressed differently in the white and brown tissue. Brown adipose fat is rich in mitochondria, in contrast to white adipose fat in which mitochondria are much less prolific.

Fat is stored inside the abdomen in amphibians and reptiles. In mammals and many birds the fat is distributed around the body in discrete compartments in close contact with other tissues. The deposition, size and site of individual fat deposits continue to be a topic for conjecture. Intermuscular depots of fat are the most metabolically active. Fat cell volume may be important in a particular site. Activity is peculiar to any one site and inferences from studies on that site may not necessarily be extrapolated to the entire fat component of the body. Fat distribution differs from species to species and from individual to individual. Appetite and exercise may be important in dictating the relative lipid masses. In humans there are important gender differences in the distribution and abundance of fat tissue.

An inverse relationship between the total number of fat cells in the body and the age of onset of obesity was demonstrated in the early 1970s. The result was a belief that there is an inevitable progression to an adult body habitus. 'Cells for storing fat in the body develop primarily in the first year of life. They persist throughout life, so a fat baby becomes a fat adult who is unable to control weight.' Later work showed the need for caution in the interpretation of fat cell counts. It is possible that the number of such fat cells reflects the degree of obesity rather than the age of onset of obesity. The fat cell pool contains mature fat cells, mature fat cells that are reverting to precursor cells, fat cell precursors and replicating fat cells: an actively changing system. The cellular development that accompanies fat tissue growth involves both cellular hyperplasia and hypertrophy at all stages of life.

White adipose tissue

White adipose tissue is primarily a long-term reserve of energy which can be drawn upon as fatty acids during periods of deprivation. It is widely distributed throughout the body, largely subcutaneously, and has insulating and protective functions. The fat is held in adipocytes, large single lipid globules surrounded by a ring of cytoplasm. These cells are unusual in being able to expand, and can absorb fat from circulating lipoproteins. Such a process requires hydrolytic breakdown of the triacylglycerols, through release of fatty acids by lipoprotein lipase. The fatty acids are transported into the cell before being incorporated into triacylglycerols.

An important organ of fat storage is the breast, where the duration of lactation is important for the newborn. Milk consists of globules composed of triacylglycerols, small amounts of cholesterol, fat-soluble vitamins and hydrophobic complex lipids. The milk fat globule is surrounded by protein phospholipid and cholesterol, and has an average diameter of 1–2 μm. During milk production, fat globules and droplets are formed in the mammary cells within the endoplasmic reticulum membrane and migrate to the apical regions of the mammary secretory cell, to be enveloped in the plasma membrane. The neck of membrane is pinched off and the resulting vesicle is expelled into the lumen as a milk fat globule.

The tissue is formed from different cell types, fat cells, adipocytes, fibroblasts and macrophages. Released stored cholesterol is important in steroid hormone synthesis in other tissues. The tissue is an insulating structure, has mechanical structure and has a role in defining some of the features of the young human female figure. The amount of lipid stored within the adipose tissue is dictated by the number of adipocytes and their volume. Adipocyte number is defined over time by multiplication and differentiation of adipocyte precursor cells, and genetic and environmental factors. The number of morphologically identified lipid-filled fat cells can increase even in adult humans. Dietary fish oil PUFAs limit the hypertrophy of the fat depots compared with animal-fat diets. There are regional site specific, differences in the limiting effect of n-3 polyunsaturates on adipose tissue growth and accumulation.

Women have larger femoral–gluteal fat cells than men, while abdominal fat cell size is similar in men and women. Most of the differences in the size of subcutaneous fat depots between men and women at specific sites are due to differences in the number of fat cells. These gender-related differences disappear in the obese. Women are able to tolerate about 30 kg more body weight than men before experiencing comparable degrees of metabolic compromise.

The fat cells can act as macrophages and fat tissue has a role in glucose homoeostasis. A further role for white adipose tissue is as an endocrine organ with the release of leptin, which has a cytokine-like action.

Lipid metabolism is interlinked with protein and carbohydrate metabolism. Adipose tissue takes up glucose and releases alanine, glycerol, glutamine and lactate substrates for gluconeogenesis.

The accumulation of fat in white adipose tissue results from two processes:

- the uptake of circulating triacylglycerol under the control of lipoprotein lipase
- *de novo* synthesis of fatty acids from glucose (lipogenesis).

Fat is deposited in fat tissue by two routes:

- uptake of preformed fatty acids
- uptake of other substrates that can be converted into triacylglycerol.

Fatty acid release follows the induction of lipolysis, the breakdown of triacylglycerols, which is under the control of the adrenergic nervous system.

The molecular events that control fat tissue growth are complex. There is an interplay between the peroxisome proliferator-activated receptor, a nuclear receptor/retinoid X receptor (PPARγ/RXR) and two other transcription factors, CCAATT enhancer binding protein and ADD-1SREBP-1; these act synergistically in response to hormones, e.g. insulin and glucocorticoids. PPARγ activation induces the expression of adipocyte-specific genes involved in lipid storage and control of metabolism. Leptin and tumour necrosis factor are also involved in this regulation of the fat tissue organ. Twin and family studies show that 80% of variation in body fat mass is genetically determined.

After a meal, triacyl-rich chylomicrons circulate, and when passing through the adipose tissue the triacylglycerols are hydrolysed by lipoprotein lipase, which is controlled by plasma insulin concentrations. Post-prandially, the insulin concentration rises, and so does the activity of the fatty tissue lipoprotein lipase. When the chylomicrons pass through the fat tissue, the free fatty acids liberated by lipoprotein lipase activity pass into the adipocytes under the direction of acylation-stimulating protein. The insulin also inhibits the lipolysis of triacyl glycerols within the adipocytes and the influx of glucose for glycerol formation. Glycerol-3-phosphate is conjugated to the free fatty acids to form triacylglycerol. Once the meal response has settled, there is increased hydrolysis of triacylglycerol under the enzymatic effect of lipase. Consequently, there is release of free fatty acids and glycerol-3-phosphate. The free fatty acids are either taken up by muscle and oxidised, or taken up by the liver.

Lipoprotein lipase
Lipoprotein lipase determines the disposal of triacylglycerols in the body and is expressed in a number of tissues. Its regulation is tissue specific. Post-prandially, lipoprotein lipase is activated in white adipose tissue and down-regulated in skeletal muscle and heart, thereby directing the fats to storage rather than active tissue. During fasting the reverse happens. The mammary gland during lactation is a very avid receptacle for triacylglycerols.

Lipoprotein lipase

Lipoprotein lipase is synthesised within the adipocyte and held in an inactive and glycosylated form. The enzyme is exported to and released from adipose tissue capillary walls, and released into the bloodstream in the presence of heparin, sulfonated dextran and other highly charged compounds. Lipoprotein lipase is specific for 1- and 3-linkages in triacylglycerols. The fatty acid at the 2-monoacylglycerol position isomerises to 1(3)-monoacylglycerol before hydrolysis. Adipocytes contain a very active monoacylglycerol lipase. Removal of the first fatty acid of the triacylglycerol is a rate-limiting step. Lipase also removes the second fatty acid and monoacylglycerol lipase removes the third. The result is non-esterified fatty acids and glycerol. The glycerol appears to be transported elsewhere, whereas the fatty acids are available for re-esterification.

Fatty acids are delivered to fat tissue as chylomicron-triacylglycerol (TAG) or VLDL-TAG. Circulating triacylglycerol is hydrolysed by lipoprotein lipase in the capillary lumen. The enzyme is synthesised within adipocytes, modified intracellularly and transferred to the capillary endothelium.

Chylomicrons are a preferred substrate to VLDL for lipase. The whole of this process is initiated by insulin over a period of hours. Some of the released fatty acids pass to the fatty tissue, and are esterified and stored. A highly regulated proportion of the fatty acids spills over post-prandially into the plasma and is exported, bound to albumin.

Lipoprotein lipase activity is low at birth and increases during the first 10 days of life. This is during the active phase of adipocyte proliferation and decreases to very low levels before further increasing after weaning. In humans there is little evidence, during normal life, for *de novo* lipogenesis as a mode of fat deposition.

Hormone-sensitive lipase
The amount of fat in the fat cell is an equilibrium between the rate of lipolysis and the rate of lipid synthesis. Lipolysis is catalysed by lipase, which catalyses the hydrolysis of triacylglycerol to 1,2-diacylglycerol and then to 2-monoacylglycerol. The

Adrenaline, glucagon, adrenocorticotropic hormone (ACTH) and noradrenaline stimulate adenylate cyclase A-kinase signal transduction. Each of the peptide hormones has a receptor on the plasma membrane and noradrenaline reacts with the β-adrenergic receptor, which activates guanosine triphosphate (GTP)-binding protein, G_s. This initiates an enzyme cascade whereby adenylate cyclase is stimulated to produce cAMP, which activates A-kinase, which phosphorylates and activates the hormone-sensitive lipase. The enzyme cascade is modulated by noradrenaline and adrenaline, which act through prostaglandins (E_1 and E_2).

enzyme is activated by phosphorylation by cAMP-dependent kinase under the control of the sympathetic nervous system and insulin. This promotes the activation of cAMP-dependent protein kinase, which phosphorylates hormone-sensitive lipase (HSL). The control by the sympathetic system is very complex and involves a balance between α_2- and β-adrenoreceptors. Insulin also controls HSL activity through cAMP levels.

These are linked to a second GTP-binding protein, G_l. Catecholamines can both stimulate and inhibit lipolysis, depending upon the number of β- and α2-adrenergic receptors of the fat cell.

Insulin influences lipolysis, for example by controlling the phosphatase that dephosphorylates and inactivates hormone-sensitive lipase. A second kinase phosphorylates HSL on a serine next but one to that phosphorylated by A-kinase. Phosphorylation on one serine prevents phosphorylation on the other. Increased concentrations of palmitoyl-CoA activate the AMP-stimulated kinase.

An accumulation of unesterified fatty acids may inhibit lipolysis. Within the fat cell there is a filamentous structure that surrounds the lipid droplet. Access of the lipase to the droplet is controlled by proteins which, in turn, are under the control of A-kinase. HSL is a hydrophobic protein that regulates the mobilisation of intracellular triacylglycerol. This enzyme is activated by phosphorylation and on the stimulation of adrenaline, and suppressed by removal of the phosphorous under the control of insulin.

Lipoprotein lipase and lipase control the flow of fatty acids in and out of the adipocyte. The acylation stimulating protein is important in the uptake and esterification of fatty acids in adipocytes and responds to the arrival of chylomicrons postprandially.

There is metabolic exchange across the membrane of the adipocyte: triacylglycerol, glucose, oxygen, acetoacetate and 3-hydroxybutyrate are extracted from plasma, and non-esterified fatty acids, glycerol, lactate and carbon dioxide are released. The tissue also takes up glutamate and releases alanine and glutamine.

Adipose tissue is an important source of energy in the post-absorptive state. Net nutrient uptake into adipose tissue after a carbohydrate load requires suppression of fat release. Ethanol appears to act on adipose tissue metabolism by unknown but distinct mechanisms.

Leptin

Leptin is a hormone with a molecular weight of 18 kDa, secreted by white and brown adipose tissue and to a lesser extent a number of other tissues. Leptin is a similar type of protein to the long-chain helical cytokine family. The amount secreted by adipose tissue is influenced by the site of the adipose tissue and the ambient temperature, nutritional status, catecholamines and other hormones (Table 34.1). The sympathetic nervous system through the generous innervation of fatty tissue is the major physiological controller of leptin production. Plasma concentrations of leptin parallel total fat mass, percentage body mass and body mass

Table 34.1 Influences on plasma leptin concentration

Increasing	Decreasing
Positive energy balance	Negative energy balance
Plentiful food intake	Starvation
High fat or carbohydrate intake	Cold environment
Insulin, glucocorticoids	
Puberty	
Luteal phase of menstrual cycle	Follicular phase of menstrual cycle
Fertile women	Post-menopausal women
Pregnancy	Falling to normal 24 h post delivery
Foetus	
Placenta	
Bone formation	Reduced bone formation

index (BMI), and it is a sensing hormone relating adipose tissue mass to the hypothalamus and the control of satiety. As fat increases so does the plasma leptin concentration. Low leptin concentrations are important in conserving energy reserves and dampening fertility during starvation. Leptin receptors belong to the cytokine receptor family in several alternatively spliced forms. Kinases (Janus kinases) have a regulatory function on the receptors and they, in turn, are associated with the receptor domain, which is controlled through phosphorylation on ligand binding. Receptors are found in tissues involved in appetite control (hypothalamus, a centre for control of energy balance), energy storage, metabolism and digestion, and the reproductive organs. Leptin influences energy expenditure, a signal to the reproductive system, and metabolic processes, particularly glucose and insulin metabolism. The underlying function of leptin may be as a starvation signal or to deposit fatty acids into fatty tissue so that triacylglycerols are placed in fatty tissue rather than in other tissues. Other hormones secreted by white adipose tissue include angiotensinogen, plasminogen activator inhibitor-1, tissue factor, cytokines and growth factors.

Diet can influence lipolysis by:

- alteration of the serum concentration of acutely acting hormones
- alteration of sympathetic nervous activity
- increased concentrations of hormones.

Brown adipose tissue

A cold environment increases blood flow to the brown fat tissue, which also increases heat transfer. In animals born in a cold environment with no protective coat, an ability to alter metabolic rate in response to changes in ambient temperature (cold-induced non-shivering thermogenesis) is important. Brown fat is a tissue involved in promoting such a protective flexibility in metabolism, in part as a result of increased conversion of thyroxine to triiodothyronine. Sympathetic nervous activity is also important, acting through a receptor increasing cAMP activity, stimulation of lipolysis and fatty acid oxidation. Adrenaline reacts with receptors on the cell surface and activates a series of metabolic pathways metabolising endogenous

triacylglycerol, exogenous triacylglycerol and glucose. BAT grows when stimulated by continued intense activation of the sympathetic supply. Thyroid hormone is responsible for the thermogenic response of BAT to noradrenaline. Glucocorticoids, insulin, glucagon, pituitary hormones, sex hormones and melatonin may be involved in BAT suppression and modulation.

BAT may be regarded as an arrested embryonic form of white adipose tissue. White adipose tissue is a storage organ and BAT a thermogenic organ. There is probably a continuum between the two types of cell. BAT is regarded as a factor in the development of obesity, and its defective functioning may lead to reduced thermoregulatory energy requirements.

Brown adipose fat cells are multilocular and contain several droplets of stored triacylglycerol and characteristically large mitochondria. When the cells are inactive they are filled with lipids and resemble white adipose tissue cells. BAT cells are innervated by sympathetic nerves and also contain mast cells. BAT deposits are found in interscapular, subscapular, axillary and intercostal regions, and along major blood vessels of the abdomen and thorax.

Energy expended for thermogenesis in BAT may be important in total energy expenditure. Thermogenesis may be a response not only to cold but also to eating. BAT thermogenesis may not occur normally in the obese and is a component of facultative thermogenesis. This process may be switched on depending on need, under central and peripheral neural sympathetic control. In contrast, obligatory thermogenesis occurs in all organs of the body as an essential mechanism to maintain life at a temperature above that of the surroundings. Obligatory thermogenesis is controlled to a significant extent by the thyroid hormones.

Thermogenin

Thermogenin, or uncoupling protein 1, molecular weight 32 kDa, binds purine nucleotides on the outer surface of the inner mitochondrial membrane.

BAT contains an uncoupling protein in the inner mitochondrial membrane that allows the flow of protons to the mitochondrial matrix and uncouples oxidative phosphorylation to oxidise endogenous and exogenous substrates, thereby bypassing ATP synthesis. The process is controlled by the intracellular concentration of fatty acids as a result of the breakdown of endogenous triacylglycerol. BAT thermogenesis is conducted through a specific membrane protein (molecular weight 32 kDa), the uncoupling protein; the amount of this is related to the thermogenic capacity of the tissue. The gene coding for the uncoupling protein, specific for BAT, is under transcriptional control and is stimulated by noradrenaline, retinoic acid and the RAR/RXR heterodimer. Transcription of the uncoupling protein gene is stimulated by cAMP which, in turn, is stimulated by thyroxine and fatty acids. The action of thyroxine appears to be due to changes in the leakage of protons across membranes and uncoupling of respiration.

Uncoupling proteins (UCP) and source

- UCP1 (thermogenin): brown adipose tissue
- UCP2: widely distributed
- UCP3: skeletal muscle
- UCP4 and 5: brain.

Foetal development
In the developing foetus the thermogenic capacity of BAT remains at a low level of activity and increases before delivery. There are three phases of growth and development of BAT in the foetus:

- tissue growth as a result of hyperplasia and hypertrophy
- differentiation and ability to generate triiodothyronine
- expression of thermogenin during late pregnancy and birth.

BAT multilocular cells appear at midgestation. During the last month *in utero* the BAT becomes innervated with sympathetic nerves, and there is an increase in 5′-monodeiodinase activity, which converts thyroxine to triiodothyronine, and the expression of genes for thermogenin and lipoprotein lipase.

There appears to be a slow increase in BAT activity over the first few days of neonatal life. The diet and nourishment of the infant thereafter may determine the rate of loss of BAT lipid.

At birth, BAT provides 1–2% of birth weight and is found in the axillary and perirenal regions. Over subsequent months, it is replaced by white adipose tissue. Following this, shivering rather than nonshivering thermogenesis is the mechanism of body temperature control.

Measurement of thermogenesis and the quantity of BAT are neither easy nor practical in humans. It has been suggested that defective thermogenesis may contribute to obesity.

WEIGHT, MORBIDITY AND LIFE EXPECTATION

The deposition, size and site of individual fat deposits are variable in humans. Intermuscular depots of fat are the most metabolically active. Fat cell volume and activity are peculiar to any one site. Gender, appetite and exercise are important in dictating the distribution and abundance of fat tissue.

Excessive fat is stored in the white adipose tissue when energy intake persistently exceeds energy output. It is reasonable to define obesity as a BMI (weight/height^2) greater than 30. It is not known why people become fat. Biological inheritance accounts for only 5% of the chances of having a particular BMI and amount of subcutaneous fat, but for 20% of the propensity for the manner in which the fat is distributed. There is very little evidence to suggest a genetic basis for human obesity. The condition has a strong cultural and social background. In most obese patients high leptin concentrations have been found, interpreted as a reduced sensitivity to leptin's physiological effects of this hormone.

The type of obesity is important, i.e. whether the fat is distributed around the waist, which is dangerous, or the gluteofemoral region, which is not. Visceral adipose tissue is drained by the portal vein, directly into the liver. The release of free fatty acids from the waist, i.e. portal vein drained fat, can be rapid and is a consequence of regional differences in the activity of lipolysis-regulating hormones, catecholamines and insulin. Central obesity is associated with increased glucocorticoid production, and the number of glucocorticoid receptors is greater in the visceral than in subcutaneous fat depots, whereas leptin gene expression is greatest in the subcutaneous tissue.

Little is known about the effect of weight change on longevity. In the adult who changes weight there are often concomitant changes in smoking habits and exercise levels. In a long-term study of weight changes and longevity in Harvard graduates, the lowest all-cause mortality was in individuals who maintained a stable body weight over 15 years. If there was an increase or decrease in weight of over 5 kg during that period then there was an increase in mortality. This was primarily due to an increase in coronary heart disease rather than to deaths from cancer. These changes in mortality were not influenced by smoking habits or exercise levels.

A long-term study between 1922 and 1935 followed up adolescents aged 13–18 years who were overweight (BMI greater than 75th percentile). Mortality rates were compared with lean contemporary subjects with a BMI between the 25th and 75th percentiles. In middle age (analysed in 1968) the only health risk from adolescent obesity was diabetes mellitus. When the group became elderly, there was an increased mortality among those males who had been fat in adolescence. There was an increase in death from all causes, including coronary heart disease, stroke and colorectal cancer. The morbidity associated with early obesity in women included an increased incidence of coronary heart disease, atherosclerosis and arthritis.

Weight loss is a complex dietary management problem. A high-fat and consequently high-energy diet can be delicious and difficult to resist. Red pepper, chilli and mustard increase the thermogenic properties of a meal. The capsaicinoids in red peppers also increase the lipid oxidation properties of a meal in women; this may be related to their sympathoadrenal system effects.

Thermogenic natural chemicals in foods

- caffeine in coffee, tea and cola drinks
- catechin-polyphenols in green tea
- medium-chain triglycerols in coconut oil
- capsaicinoids in red peppers.

KEY POINTS

1. Liver and adipose tissue are the most important tissues for fatty acid biosynthesis. Most naturally occurring fatty acids have even numbers of carbon atoms. The first step in fatty acid synthesis is the carboxylation of acetyl-CoA to malonate, catalysed by acetyl-CoA carboxylase. Acetyl-CoA is formed within the mitochondria. Because fatty acid synthesis occurs in the cytosol, acetyl-CoA is transported across the membrane as citric acid.

2. Fatty acid synthesis from malonyl-CoA is a series of condensation additions, catalysed by fatty acid synthase, with the endproduct usually palmitic acid. Fatty acids are converted into metabolically active thiol esters before further metabolism.

3. Fatty acids are lengthened in the endoplasmic reticulum, catalysed by type III synthases or elongases, by adding malonyl-CoA, to preformed acyl chains requiring NADPH. Dietary essential fatty acids are lengthened to the higher polyunsaturated fatty acids, n-3 and n-6 series.

4. Fat synthesis decreases during starvation or by eating a high proportion of dietary fat, especially polyunsaturated fatty acids. Sucrose ingestion increases liver lipogenesis.

5. Fatty acid synthesis is controlled by acetyl-CoA carboxylase with a hydroxy tricarboxylic acid, e.g. citrate or isocitrate, as substrate. Regulation of acetyl-CoA carboxylase depends on nutritional status, hormonal developmental and genetic status.

6. Unsaturated fatty acids are important for physical properties of lipoproteins and membranes, regulation of metabolism in cells and as precursors for physiologically active compounds, e.g. eicosanoids.

7. The biosynthesis of unsaturated fatty acids is an oxidative step in which a double bond is introduced directly into a saturated long-chain fatty acid, a double bond at the C9 position (Δ^9 desaturase), and C4, C5 and C6, but not beyond C9. Unsaturated fatty acids beyond C9 have to be met from the diet and are essential, i.e. linoleic acid 18:2 $\Delta^{9,12}$ and α-linolenic acid 18:3 $\Delta^{9,12,15}$.

8. Fatty acid breakdown involves oxidation at defined bonds in the acyl chain or oxidation at defined double bonds in particular unsaturated fatty acids. The main forms of oxidation are termed α, β and ω, depending on the position of the carbon of the acyl chain that is oxidised. The endproduct is acetyl-CoA, which passes into the TCA cycle.

9. The glycerol phosphate pathway for triacylglycerol formation is the progressive esterification of glycerol 3-sn phosphate and 1-acylglycerol 3-sn phosphate with long-chain acyl-CoA fatty acids using phosphatidic acid in both phospholipid and triacylglycerol biosynthesis.

10. Triacylglycerols are resynthesised in the enterocyte from monoacylglycerols absorbed following small intestinal hydrolysis, are converted into lipoproteins and circulate in the blood. Fatty acids are released from the acylglycerols, enter the cells and are then re-esterified into acylglycerols.

11. Lipases are important in the splitting of the fatty acid ester at positions 1 and 3 from the primary hydroxyl groups of glycerol.

12. Triacylglycerols in humans are a source of fatty acids when energy demands exceed immediate requirements and hence act as a metabolic fuel. When there is a preponderance of fat in the diet, fat synthesis from carbohydrate in the tissues is depressed.

13. Glycerol-3-phosphate is regulated by similar factors to glycolysis and gluconeogenesis. Starvation reduces glycerol-3-phosphate cell concentrations, which are restored by feeding.

14. The biosynthesis of phospholipids takes precedence over triacylglycerols, as membrane turnover and biosecretion are biologically more significant.

15. The ratio of circulating insulin to glucagon influences the fate of fatty acids entering the liver; high ratios favour esterification of fatty acids into acylglycerols and a low rate of β-oxidation.

16. The synthesis of lipid by adipocytes is determined by high concentrations of insulin, glucose, free fatty acids and triglycerides as lipoproteins. The activation of lipase is controlled by phosphorylation–dephosphorylation. This is regulated by protein kinase A through adenylate cyclase-generated cAMP and insulin-activated protein phosphatase.

17. Breast milk is an important organ of fat storage; the duration of lactation is important for the newborn animal.

18. The general principle of energy balance is that Energy consumed = Energy expended + Change in body energy stores. Amino acid oxidation adjusts to dietary protein intake. Glycogen reserves are maintained at a balanced amount that prevents hypoglycaemia, and excess carbohydrates are channelled into lipid stores. Fat balance, oxidation and metabolism are not dependent on the fat content of the meals; fatty meals lead to fat accumulation and obesity.

19. The accumulation of fat in white adipose tissue results from: (i) the uptake of circulating triacylglycerol under the control of lipoprotein lipase; and (ii) de novo synthesis of fatty acids from glucose (lipogenesis). Fat is deposited in fat tissue by two routes: (i) uptake of preformed fatty acids; and (ii) uptake of other substrates that can be converted into triacylglycerol.

20. Brown adipose tissue thermogenesis is conducted through a specific membrane protein, the uncoupling protein. The amount of this enzyme in the brown adipose tissue is related to the tissue's thermogenic capacity.

21. Leptin is a hormone that responds to body stores of fat. Leptin acts on the hypothalamus as an appetite suppressant and also has actions in sexual development, reproduction and bone formation.

22. Obesity is a body mass index (weight/height^2) greater than 30. Appetite and exercise may be important in dictating the relative lipid masses. In humans there are important gender differences in the distribution and abundance of fat tissue.

23. Young, fat males have an increased incidence of vascular disease in old age compared with those who were not obese in youth.

THINKING POINTS

1. Lipids are a separate entity in biology through their poor solubility in water, which creates and acts as a separate phase.

2. This has enormous biological importance, particularly in the large lipid organs, e.g. brain and nervous tissues are central to the role of humans as intelligent beings.

NEED TO UNDERSTAND

1. The diverse ways in which fat is absorbed, synthesised and degraded.
2. The ways fats are synthesised and elongated and the different oxidation pathways.
3. The anatomy and metabolic characteristics of adipose tissue.
4. This is a multifaceted topic, but there is a relationship between energy intake, leptin response and the fat structure.

FURTHER READING

Ahima. R.S. and Flier, J.S. (2000) Leptin. *Annual Review of Physiology*, **62**, 413–38.

Arner, P. (1998) Not all fat is alike. *Lancet*, **351**, 1301–2.

Baile, C.A., Della-Fera, M.A. and Martin, R.J. (2000) Regulation of metabolism and body fat mass by leptin. *Annual Review of Nutrition*, **20**, 105–27.

Belury, M.A. (2002) Dietary conjugated linolese acid in health. *Annual Review of Nutrition*, **22**, 505–31.

British Nutrition Foundation Task Force Report (1992) *Saturated Fatty Acids; Nutritional and Physiological Significance*. Chapman & Hall, London.

Cinti, S. (2000) The adipose organ: morphological perspectives of adipose tissues. *Proceedings of the Nutrition Society*, **60**, 319–28.

Dulloo, A.G. (1998) Spicing fat for combustion. *British Journal of Nutrition*, **80**, 493–4.

Feilding, B.A. and Frayn, K.N. (1998) Lipoprotein lipase and the disposition of dietary fatty acids. *British Journal of Nutrition*, **80**, 495–502.

Frayn, K.N., Coppack, S.W. and Potts, J.L. (1992) Effect of diet on human adipose tissue metabolism. *Proceedings of the Nutrition Society*, **57**, 409–18.

Freake, H.C. (1998) Uncoupling proteins: beyond brown adipose fat. *Nutrition Reviews*, **56**, 185–9.

Fruhbeck, G. (2001) A heliocentric view of leptin. *Proceedings of the Nutrition Society*, **60**, 301–18.

Gurr, M.I. (1996) Dietary fatty acids with transunsaturation. *Nutrition Research Reviews*, **9**, 259–79.

Gurr, M.I. and Harrow, J.L. (1991) *Lipids*. Chapman & Hall, London.

Hajri, T. and Abumrad, N.A. (2002) Fatty acid transport across membranes. *Annual Review of Nutrition*, **22**, 383–415.

Halliwell, B. (1993) Renaissance of peroxisomes. *Lancet*, **341**, 92.

Harris, R.B.S. (2000) Leptin–much more than a satiety signal. *Annual Review of Nutrition*, **20**, 45–75.

Jensen, M.D. (1997) Lipolysis: contribution from regional fat. *Annual Review of Nutrition*, **17**, 127–40.

Kelley, D.E., Goodpaster, B.H. and Storlein, L. (2002) Muscle triglyceride and insulin resistance. *Annual Review of Nutrition*, **22**, 325–46.

Must, A., Jacques, P.F., Dallal, G.E. *et al*. (1992) Long-term morbidity and mortality of overweight adolescents: a follow up of the Harvard Growth Study of 1922 to 1935. *New England Journal of Medicine*, **327**, 1350–5.

Pollack, O.J. and Kritchevsky, D. (1981) *Sitosterol*. Karger, Basel.

Pond, C.M. (1992) An evolutionary and functional view of mammalian adipose tissue. *Proceedings of the Nutrition Society*, **51**, 367–77.

Raclot, T. and Oudart, H. (1999) Selectivity of fatty acids on lipid metabolism and gene expression. *Proceedings of the Nutrition Society*, **58**, 633–46.

Rangwala, S.M. and Lazar, M.A. (2000) Transcriptional control of adipogenesis. *Annual Review of Nutrition*, **20**, 535–60.

Rasmussen, B.B. and Wolfe, R.R. (1999) Regulation of fatty acid oxidation in skeletal muscle *Annual Review of Nutrition*, **19**, 463–84.

Rocchi, S. and Auwerx, J. (2000) Peroxisome proliferator-activated receptor γ, the ultimate liaison between fat and transcription. *British Journal of Nutrition*, **84**, (Suppl. 2), S223–7.

Samra, J.S. (2000) Regulation of lipid metabolism in adipose tissue. *Proceedings of the Nutrition Society*, **59**, 441–6.

Symposium on 'Lipid absorption and metabolism: physiological and molecular aspects' (1996) *Proceedings of the Nutrition Society*, **55**, 1–154.

Symposium on 'New perspectives on adipose tissue function' (2001) *Proceedings of the Nutrition Society*. **60**, 319–80.

Trayhurn, P. and Beattie, J.H. (2001) Physiological role of adipose tissue: white adipose tissue as an endocrine and secretory organ. *Proceedings of the Nutrition Society*, **60**, 329–39.

Wainwright, P. (2000) Nutrition and behaviour: the role of n-3 fatty acids in cognitive function. *British Journal of Nutrition*, **83**, 337–9.

Wolf, G. (1995) A regulatory pathway of thermogenesis in brown fat through retinoic acid. *Nutrition Reviews*, **53**, 230–1.

Vergroesen, A.J. and Crawford, M. (1989) *The Role of Fats in Human Nutrition*, 2nd edn. Academic Press, London.

Vernon, R.G. (1992) Effects of diet on lipolysis and its regulation. *Proceedings of the Nutrition Society*, **57**, 397–408.

35

Eicosanoids

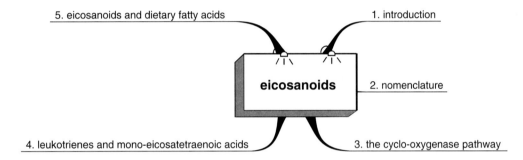

Fig. 35.1 Chapter outline.

INTRODUCTION

The eicosanoids are a family of hormones that are specific oxidation products of C20 polyunsaturated fatty acids (PUFAs), derived from arachidonic acid. They are very potent biologically; they are important local hormones generated *in situ*, rapidly metabolised and briefly active in the immediate vicinity to where they are synthesised.

NOMENCLATURE

The different eicosanoids all consist of a cyclopentane substituted ring, the structure of which dictates their biological differences. The names are usually abbreviated: for prostaglandins to PG, followed by the letter E, F, G, H or I; and for thromboxanes to TX, followed by the letter A or B.

The subscript 1, 2 or 3 indicates the number of double bonds in the side-chain structure in all series:

- 1 is *trans* $\Delta 13$
- 2 is *trans* $\Delta 13$, *cis* 5
- 3 is *trans* 13, *cis* 5, *cis* 17.

There are two major families, determined by the synthetic pathway:

- the cyclo-oxygenase-dependent pathway for prostanoids: prostaglandins (PG), prostacyclins (PG_1) and thromboxanes (TX). Five main naturally occurring prostanoids exist (prostaglandin PGD_2, PGE_2, $PGF_{2\alpha}$, prostacyclin PGI_2 and thromboxane TXA_2)
- the lipoxygenase-dependent pathway for leukotrienes (LT).

Within the cell the concentration of arachidonic acid is low. The immediate source of arachidonic acid is from cell membrane phospholipids, phosphatidylcholine and phosphatidylinositol. Cellular membrane phospholipids act not only as structural chemicals but also as sources of secondary messengers produced by intracellular and extracellular phospholipidases. The release of arachidonic acid is catalysed by phospholipase A_2 (PLA_2) and C hydrolysing the ester link of arachidonic acid at C2 of the glycerol. There are two forms of PLA_2, an intracellular form of which produces eicosanoids and the extracellular form which produces lysoglycerophosphoryl-choline, the precursor platelet activating factor. The arachidonic acid may also be re-esterified to membrane phospholipid (Figure 35.2).

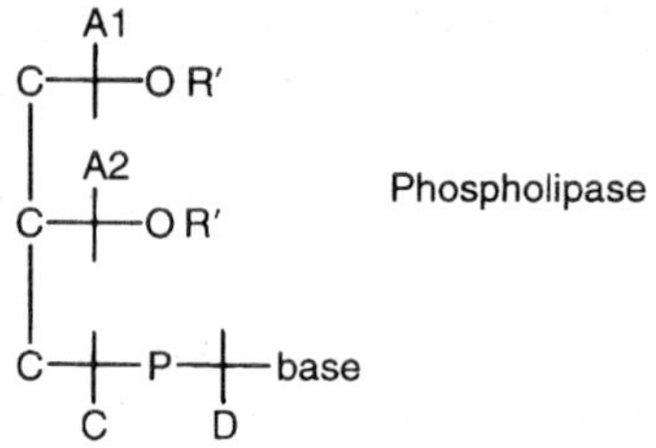

Fig. 35.2 Classification of phospholipases based on the bond in the phospholipid that is hydrolysed: A_1, A_2, C, D. Phospholipase B hydrolyses lysophospholipids, releasing a fatty acid.

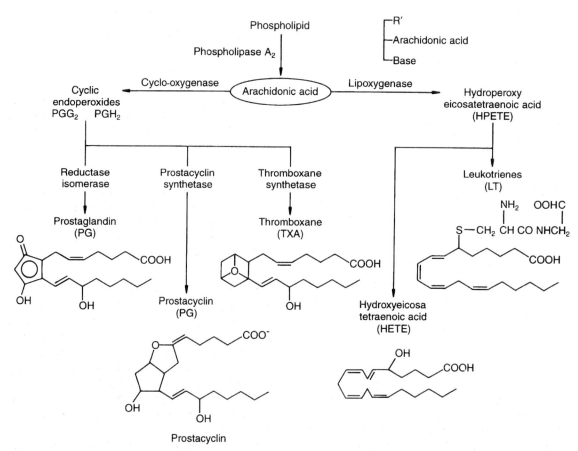

Fig. 35.3 Arachidonic acid metabolism to eicosanoids. The eicosanoids are products of the cyclo-oxygenase or lipoxygenase pathways.

THE CYCLO-OXYGENASE PATHWAY

The biosynthesis of prostanoids involves the following sequence.

1. Stimulated hydrolysis of arachidonate from glycerophospholipids involving PLA_2.
2. Oxygenation of arachidonate to produce prostaglandin endoperoxide H_2 by prostaglandin endoperoxide H synthases 1 and 2 (generic name COX-1 and COX-2).

   The two isoforms of COX are almost identical in structure, but have important differences in substrates and inhibitor sensitivity. Both will accept arachidonic acid and dihomo-γ-linolenate as substrates, but COX-2 will accept other fatty acids. COX-2 is inducible. COX-1-derived prostaglandins maintain the integrity of the stomach, intestine and kidneys. COX-2-derived prostaglandins are associated with inflammation.
3. Conversion to biologically active products, the five primary prostanoids, PGE_2, $PGF_{2\alpha}$, PGI_2, TXA_2 and PGD_2.

   The synthesis of prostaglandins, prostacyclins and thromboxanes occurs by the oxidation of arachidonic acid followed by cyclisation to form a cyclopentane ring, C8 to C12. Substitutions to the cyclopentane ring R_1 and R_2 determine biological activity (Figure 35.3).

   The fatty acid prostaglandin endoperoxide H synthase (a cyclo-oxygenase) is a microsomal enzyme (Figure 35.4), which:

   - adds molecular oxygen as a peroxide across C9 and C11 of the arachidonic acid
   - adds a hydroperoxide (–OOH) at C15 to form the cyclic endoperoxide PGG_2. The next transformation is catalysed by the peroxidase to the 15-hydroxy PGH_2, which is the starting point for subsequent metabolism.

4. Each prostanoid is synthesised in specific compartments within the body. They act through specific G-protein-coupled receptors (GPCRs), of which there are eight: EP(1–4) are the PGE_2 receptors, and FP, DP, IP and TP are receptors for $PGF_{2\alpha}$, PGD_2, PGI_2 and TXA_2, respectively. There are many subtypes of prostanoids and receptors.

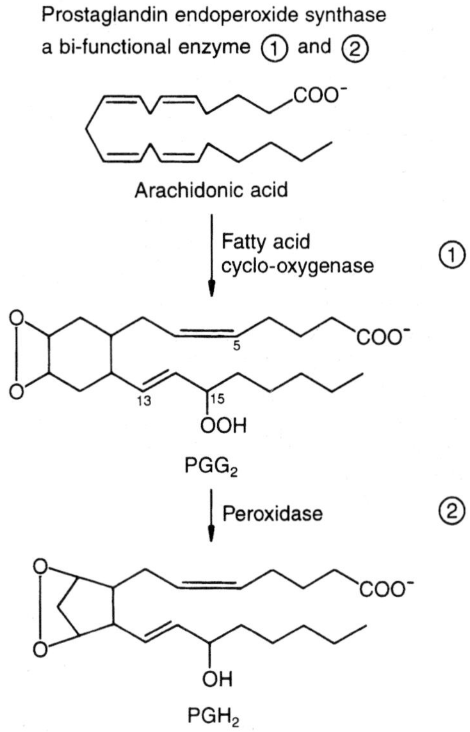

Fig. 35.4 Cyclo-oxygenase pathway from arachidonic acid with 15 PGH_2 as the starting point for subsequent metabolism (enzymes: fatty acid cyclo-oxygenase and peroxidase).

While most cells can produce all three types of metabolite there is a bias within platelets and macrophages to produce thromboxane, and for endothelial cells to produce prostacyclin. Mast cells predominantly produce PGD_2 and microvessels PGE_2.

The *nomenclature* of these compounds is based on prostanoic acid, an acid that does not exist in nature (Figure 35.6). They contain 20 carbon atoms, including a five- or six-carbon cyclic structure. Prostaglandins and prostacyclins have a cyclic ring of five carbons and thromboxanes a ring of six carbons. The C8 to C12 positions are closed to form a five-membered ring, prostanoic acid, in prostanoids. Most of the prostaglandins have an OH group at the C15 position.

Prostaglandins have a wide range of activities. PGD_2, found in mast cells and the nervous system, inhibits platelet aggregation. PGE_2, produced in

Cyclo-oxygenase activity and non-steroidal anti-inflammatory drugs

Non-steroidal anti-inflammatory drugs (NSAIDs), e.g. aspirin or indomethacin, inactivate fatty acid cyclo-oxygenase COX-1 but not COX-2, which will oxidise arachidonic acid to 15-hydroperoxy eicosatetraenoic acid (15-HETE). NSAIDs, e.g. ibuprofen, compete with the fatty acid substrate for the prostaglandin endoperoxide synthase active site. Aspirin acetylates a serine hydroxyl at or near the active site, which permanently inactivates the COX-1 enzyme. The acetylenic fatty acids such as eicosa-5,8,11,14-tetraenoic acid have the same effect (Figure 35.5).

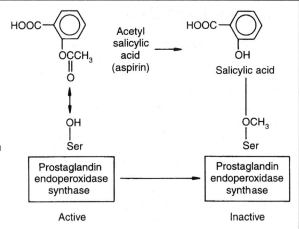

Fig. 35.5 Prostaglandins and aspirin. Inhibition of prostaglandin endoperoxidase synthetase by acetylation by acetyl salicylic acid.

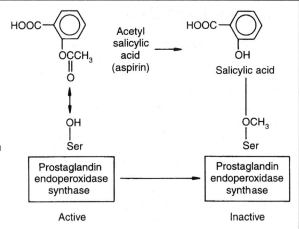

Numbering of eicosanoids based on prostanoic acid, a hypothetical compound

Fig. 35.6 Prostanoic acid, a theoretical acid. This structure is used to number the carbons of the eicosanoids.

The difference between the E and F prostaglandin series lies in the keto or hydroxyl group at position 9. The E-type PGs are 11,15-dihydroxy-9-keto compounds and the F-type 9,11,15-trihydroxy structures. The suffix α or β indicates the stereochemistry of the hydroxyl at C9. The suffix 1, 2 or 3 refers to how many double bonds are contained in the prostaglandin structure. There are two side-chains, one of which (R_1) is attached to C8, and carries a carboxyl group, the other (R_2) is attached to C12 and has a hydroxyl group at C15.

most cells, increases cAMP concentrations and stimulates bone resorption. PGI_2 is important in smooth-muscle contraction throughout the body and has a vasodilatory effect, whereas thromboxane is a vasoconstrictor and stimulates platelet aggregation. Prostaglandins are involved in inhibition of platelet release reactions, lysosomal enzyme release from neutrophils, and inhibition of mast cell and basophil histamine release. The prostanoids have a short (less than 5 min) half-life in tissues and are excreted in urine.

Prostacyclins are synthesised largely in the vascular and gastric tissues. They also have antiaggregator and pulmonary vasodilator functions.

LEUKOTRIENES AND MONO-EICOSATETRAENOIC ACIDS

The leukotrienes have a role in smooth-muscle contraction, mononuclear leucocytes and tumour cells. A lipoxygenase catalyses the formation of 5-hydroperoxy-6,8,11,14-eicosatetraenoic acid (5-HPETE) from arachidonic acid, which is then enzymatically dehydrated to form LTA_4. Two series of products are then produced according to needs.

Leukotriene metabolism

- **Enzymatic hydrolysis to LTB$_4$**: this causes chemoattraction in neutrophils and subsequent aggregation. The role is to recruit circulating cells at inflammatory sites.

- **Peptidoleukotriene formation**: the addition of glutathione at C6 forms LTC$_4$. (Figure 35.7). Loss of glutamine (enzyme, γ-glutamyltransferase) forms LTD$_4$ and glycine residues (enzyme, dipeptidase) form LTE$_4$ in sequence from these reactions. These leukotrienes participate in a number of inflammatory processes and in anaphylaxis. The peptidoleukotrienes have profound effects on the tone in arteries and microvascular vessels. They also have a role in microvascular leakage.

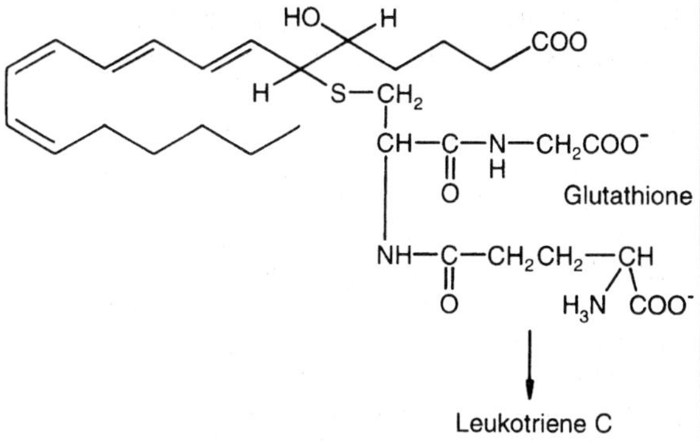

Fig. 35.7   Leukotrienes and glutathione substitutions.

EICOSANOIDS AND DIETARY FATTY ACIDS

It has been suggested that only those fatty acids capable of being converted into the $\Delta^{5,8,11,14}$-tetraenoic fatty acids of chain length C19, C20 and C22 are essential, because these give rise to physiologically active eicosanoids. Eicosanoids are metabolised very rapidly and are excreted in urine or bile. The dietary intake (10 g) of essential fatty acids thought necessary contrasts with the 1 mg of prostaglandin metabolites formed in 24 h by humans. A deficiency of substrates for prostaglandin synthesis is unlikely to occur.

The n-6 unsaturated fatty acids, linoleic and arachidonic acid, are synthesised to the 3-series and 4-series leukotrienes respectively, whereas the α-linolenic acid n-3 of fish oil origin is synthesised to the 5-series leukotrienes. Linoleic acid and arachidonic acid are synthesised to the 1- and 2-series prostaglandins, respectively, whereas α-linolenic acid is synthesised to the 3-series. The relative contribution of n-3 and n-6 fatty acids in the diet will therefore dictate the spectrum of types and biological potencies of the prostanoids and leukotrienes. Other than this dietary control, the production of eicosanoid formation is dependent on PLA$_2$ activity. This function is activated and inhibited by a number of messengers in a similar manner to the inositol cyclase system.

KEY POINTS

1. The eicosanoids are a family of important, potent, locally acting hormones and are specific oxidation products of C20 polyunsaturated fatty acids, derived from arachidonic acid.

2. The different eicosanoids consist of a cyclopentane substituted ring; biological differences are dictated by the structure of the substituted ring.

3. There are four main groups of such cyclic compounds and other biologically active products of lipoxygenase and mono-oxygenase activity on arachidonic acid.

4. The immediate source of arachidonic acid is from cell membrane phospholipids, phosphatidylcholine and phosphatidylinositol. The release of the arachidonic acid is catalysed by phospholipase A$_2$ and C hydrolysing the ester link of arachidonic acid to C2 of the glycerol.

5. There are two major families dependent on two synthetic pathways: the cyclo-oxygenase-dependent COX pathway (prostaglandins, prostacyclins and thromboxanes) and the lipoxygenase-dependent pathway (leukotrienes).

6. The two isoforms of COX are almost identical in structure, but have important differences in substrates and inhibitor sensitivity. COX-2 is inducible. COX-1-derived prostaglandins maintain the integrity of the stomach, intestine and

kidneys. COX-2-derived prostaglandins are associated with a response to inflammation.

7. The first step in the synthesis of prostaglandins, prostacyclins and thromboxanes is the oxidation of arachidonic acid, followed by cyclisation to form a cyclopentane ring, C8 to C12. Substitutions to the cyclopentane ring R_1 and R_2 determine biological activity. The fatty acid cyclo-oxygenase is a microsomal enzyme.

8. Non-steroidal anti-inflammatory drugs, e.g. aspirin and indomethacin, compete with the fatty acid substrate for the prostaglandin endoperoxide synthase active site. Aspirin also acetylates a serine hydroxyl at or near the active site, which permanently inactivates the COX-1 enzyme. COX-2 will only synthesise 15-HETE.

9. It has been suggested that only those fatty acids capable of being converted into the $\Delta^{5,8,11,14}$-tetraenoic fatty acids of chain length C19, C20 and C22 are essential, because these give rise to physiologically active eicosanoids.

THINKING POINTS

1. Eicosanoids are an example of a vital hormone system that is directly dependent on an adequate dietary intake of an essential nutrient.

2. It is of interest that a plant secondary metabolite, aspirin, has such an effect on eicosanoid activity.

NEED TO UNDERSTAND

The metabolic pathways from arachidonic acid to the eicosanoids.

FURTHER READING

Balsinde, J., Balboa, M.A., Insel, P.A. and Dennis, E.A. (1999) Regulation and inhibition of phospholipase A_2. *Annual Review of Pharmacology and Toxicology*, **39**, 175–89.

Breyer, R.M., Bagdassarian, C.K., Myers, S.A. and Breyer, M.D. (2001) Prostanoid receptors: subtypes and signalling. *Annual Review of Pharmacology and Toxicology*, **41**, 661–90.

Smith, W.L., DeWitt, D.L. and Garavito, R.M. (2000) Cyclooxygenase: structural, cellular and molecular biology. *Annual Review of Biochemistry*, **69**, 145–82.

Vane, J.R., Bakhle, Y.S. and Botting, R.M. (1998) Cyclooxygenase 1 and 2. *Annual Review of Pharmacology and Toxicology*, **38**, 97–120.

36

Cholesterol and lipoproteins

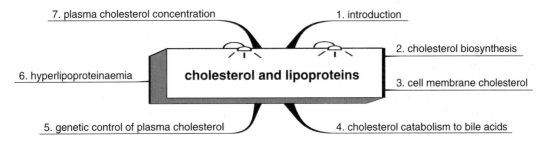

Fig. 36.1 Chapter outline.

INTRODUCTION

The synthesis of sterols is closely related to growth, development and differentiation of all cells. All cholesterol is synthesised from acetate or ingested in the diet.

CHOLESTEROL BIOSYNTHESIS

In the synthesis of cholesterol (Figures 36.2 and 36.3) three acetates condense to form 3-hydroxy-3-methylglutaryl-coenzyme A (HMG-CoA), which is then catalysed by the enzyme HMG-CoA reductase to form mevalonic acid.

Mevalonate is converted by two kinase reactions to 5-diphosphomevalonate, losing a carbon atom *en route*. The enzyme has a requirement for Mg^{2+} and uses adenosine triphosphate (ATP) as a substrate. Two isomers are formed, isopentenyl diphosphate and 3,3-dimethylallyl diphosphate, which condense to form geranyl diphosphate.

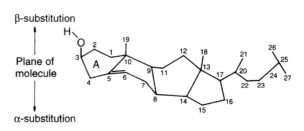

Fig. 36.2 Structure of cholesterol, including the three-dimensional structure. Substitutions above the plane of the molecule are β; substitutions below the plane of the molecule are α.

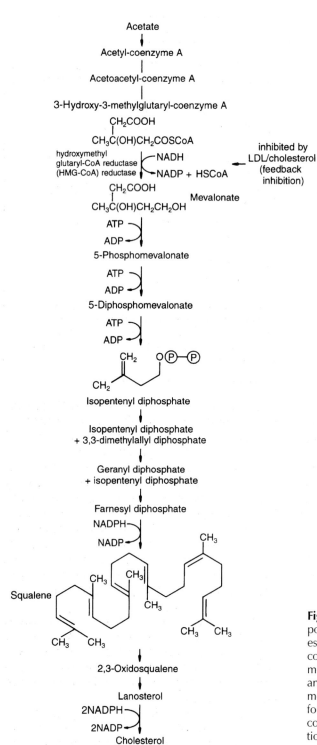

Fig. 36.3 Cholesterol synthesis. The starting compound is acetate, which in the synthetic process passes through five isoprenoid intermediates. The conversion of 3-hydroxy-3-methyl-glutaryl-CoA to mevalonate is the rate-limiting step. This is irreversible and is catalysed by HMG-CoA reductase. Three molecules of isopentenyl diphosphate condense to form farnesyl diphosphate, two molecules of which condense to form squalene. There is further cyclisation to form cholesterol.

HMG-CoA reductase

This is an irreversible reaction, a rate-limiting step, requiring two molecules of reduced nicotinamide adenine dinucleotide (NADH). Coenzyme A is released. HMG-CoA reductase is controlled by an elaborate phosphorylation system (Figure 36.4). The enzyme is inactive when phosphorylated by HMG-CoA reductase kinase. The phosphorylation is reversed by HMG-CoA reductase phosphatase. The HMG-CoA reductase kinase is active in the phosphorylated form, this being catalysed by HMG-CoA reductase kinase. Many factors regulate cholesterol biosynthesis and many of these are involved in the activity of HMG-CoA reductase.

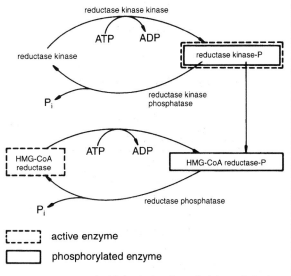

Fig. 36.4 Control of β-hydroxy- β-methylglutaryl-CoA reductase. The enzyme is activated by phosphorylation. This phosphorylated state is controlled by HMG-CoA reductase kinase, which in itself is active in the phosphorylated form.

There follows a series of condensation reactions with the eventual formation of squalene, followed by lanosterol and finally a series of oxidation steps to form cholesterol.

There appears to be a diurnal pattern to cholesterol synthesis. This is largely due to changes in the circadian rhythm with the activity of HMG-CoA reductase, cholesterol 7-α-hydroxylase, which is involved in bile acid synthesis, and lysosomal acid cholesteryl ester hydrolase, which hydrolyses cholesteryl esters derived from lipoproteins. The sterol carrier protein, which is a major regulatory protein of lipid metabolism and transport, has a diurnal cycle.

The input of cholesterol to the liver is provided by two sources:

• uptake of circulating lipoprotein cholesterol
• direct *de novo* synthesis of cholesterol.

The balance between input and output determines the concentration of cholesterol inside the liver cell. Excess cholesterol that is not readily disposed of can be converted to the fatty acyl ester by the action of the liver enzyme acyl-CoA:cholesterol acyltransferase (ACAT). HMG-CoA reductase

activity and low-density lipoprotein (LDL) receptor expression can be regulated by the concentration of free cholesterol. The pool of cholesterol forms part of a self-regulatory system.

There are wide species variations in the rate of synthesis of cholesterol, but 10 mg/day/kg body weight is typical in humans. Endogenous synthesis in humans is important in the adjustment of the cholesterol body pool. Ingestion of cholesterol increases plasma cholesterol concentration, dependent on the dietary unsaturated/saturated fatty acid content. There are wide variations in the ability to absorb dietary cholesterol; humans can absorb 2–4 mg/day/kg body weight.

Cholesterol feeding markedly inhibits hepatic cholesterogenesis, varying with species. In rats and dogs, inhibition is almost complete; in humans, it is 40%. Cellular cholesterol concentration is a balance between synthesis or uptake of preformed cholesterol and degradation.

Most of the cholesterol-rich lipoprotein is removed by the liver. Remnants of chylomicrons generated by the action of the lipoprotein lipase are cleared by the liver by a saturable receptor-mediated process. Only a fraction, corresponding to 50–60% of very low-density lipoprotein (VLDL) remnants, is directly removed by the liver in humans. The major cholesterol-carrying lipoprotein is LDL, up to 85% of these particles being taken up by the liver at apolipoprotein (apoB) receptors and to a lesser extent by non-specific processes.

VLDL is the major lipoprotein secreted by the liver. Its metabolism in the blood leads to the production of intermediate-density lipoproteins (IDLs) and LDL (apoB-100-containing lipoproteins). The liver is the major organ that clears these modified plasma lipoproteins through receptors for apoB-100 or apoE. Ingestion of significant amounts of dietary cholesterol and saturated fatty acids can raise the concentration of plasma lipoprotein cholesterol.

There is a general stimulatory effect of dietary lipids on cholesterogenesis. However, the effect of fats on HMG-CoA reductase activity may be related to the chemistry of the lipid. The microscopic fluidity of high-density lipoproteins (HDLs), which are responsible for cholesterol efflux from the cell, is increased following dietary intake of unsaturated fats. This increased fluidity may allow more cholesterol to be taken into solution by the HDL molecules. This allows greater cellular efflux of cholesterol and reduces endproduct inhibition effects on HMG-CoA reductase.

The synthesis of HMG-CoA reductase is inhibited by LDL. Cholesterol enters the hepatic cell as cholesterol esters and cholesterol, transported on LDL, and influences sterol synthesis through feedback regulation on the concentration of LDL membrane receptors and on the concentration of HMG-CoA reductase. There are lipoprotein receptors on the surface membranes of liver, fibroblasts, smooth muscles and lymphocytes. LDLs bind to the receptor and then enter the cell through endocytosis. The LDL protein is degraded to amino acids and the cholesterol esters are hydrolysed. The free cholesterol is then transported into the cytosolic compartment, on a sterol carrier protein. Cholesterol from LDL reduces HMG-CoA reductase enzyme activity by accelerating degradation and reducing synthesis. This may be through a reduction in the amount of messenger RNA (mRNA) responsible for the reductase or through phosphorylation of the enzyme. The

increased degradation may be through localisation of cholesterol in the membrane domain of the reductase gene.

Inhibition of HMG-CoA reductase

The active inhibitor of transcription of the reductase may be the oxysterol derivative of cholesterol. The 25-hydroxylated cholesterol may attach to a protein which interacts with the genetic machinery, at either the transcriptional or translational level.

Cytosolic protein factors belong to a family that can influence the effect of lipids on the activity of HMG-CoA reductase; these include sterol carrier proteins, fatty acid binding protein and z protein. These may influence the binding of the hydroxysterol metabolites of cholesterol or may bind lipid inhibitors.

CELL MEMBRANE CHOLESTEROL

The mechanisms that control the amount of cholesterol and fatty acids in the cell wall are very sensitive to the lipid content in the cell wall. A feedback system relates gene transcription for LDL receptor and the enzymes involved in lipid biosynthesis to the cellular cholesterol. Sterol regulatory element binding proteins (SREBPs) are membrane-embedded proteins that are regulated by the sterol content of the cell.

CHOLESTEROL CATABOLISM TO BILE ACIDS

In the degradation of cholesterol to bile acids, the first step, 7-α-hydroxylation, a microsomal enzyme reaction, is rate limiting, Cytochrome P450 NADPH and molecular oxygen are required. There is then hydroxylation at C12 for the precursor of cholic acid, following which, in sequence, the C4/C5 bond is saturated and the carbonyl group at

C3 reduced. There is a series of oxidative steps in the C20 to C27 side-chain in the mitochondria. This leads to oxidation to a carboxyl of the alcohol group at C26.

In this manner, cholic acid, 3,7,12-α-trihydroxy-cholanoic acid and chenodeoxycholic, 3,7-α-dihydroxycholanoic acid are formed. Bile acids are amphiphilic molecules (one side is hydrophobic and the other hydrophilic) as a result of hydroxyl groups They are conjugated with taurine or glycine, become more water soluble and are excreted in bile to the enterohepatic circulation.

Bile acids are a major product of the hepatic degradation of cholesterol and may exert a regulatory role on the overall hepatic sterol metabolism. Depletion of the enterohepatic circulation, as with ileal bypass or as a result of cholestyramine bile acid binding therapy, depletes the bile acid pool and alters hepatic metabolism of cholesterol. Bile acid synthesis increases, and this causes an increased rate of cholesterol synthesis and increased LDL receptor activity. This may act through a decrease in the hepatocyte regulatory pool of cholesterol. Not only the size but also the composition of the bile acid pool may contribute to the regulation of hepatic sterol metabolism. This may relate to the physicochemical characteristics of the constituents of the bile acid pool. The hydrophobic–hydrophilic balance of the pool seems to dictate most of the effects of bile acids on hepatic cholesterol metabolism.

The bile acid pool of humans consists of cholic acid and chenodeoxycholic acid in approximately equal amounts (40% of the total pool), and the bacterial degraded bile acids deoxycholic acid (15–20%) and trace amounts of lithocholic acid and ursodeoxycholic acid.

Lithocholic acid is the most hydrophobic bile acid, followed by deoxycholic, chenodeoxycholic and cholic acids. Hydrophobic bile acids such as deoxycholic and chenodeoxycholic acid inhibit HMG-CoA reductase, whereas cholic acid does not appear to have this effect. The more hydrophobic the bile acid that predominates, the greater the inhibitory effect on endogenous bile acid synthesis.

GENETIC CONTROL OF PLASMA CHOLESTEROL

ApoA-I, C-I, A-IV gene cluster

The risk of developing coronary artery disease (CAD) is inversely correlated with plasma HDL cholesterol and apoA-I concentrations. There are at least 12 variants of apoA-I, but in general such variants are rare, occurring in less than 0.1% of the population. As the genes for apoA-I, C-III and A-IV are clustered, polymorphism of one may also affect the others.

Apolipoprotein genes

Chromosomal location
The genes for apoA-I, apoC-II and apoA-IV are clustered on the long arm of chromosome 11. The apoC-III gene is approximately 2.6 kb downstream from the apoA-I gene, but in the opposite transcriptional orientation. The apoA-IV gene is 7.5 kb downstream from the apoC-III gene. The genes for apoE, apoC-I and apoC-II are found on

---

The genes for apoA-I, A-II, A-IV, C-I, C-II, C-III and E belong to a multigene family with a common ancestral gene. ApoB is not thought to be part of this family since its exon–intron organisation is so different to that of the other apolipoprotein genes. From protein and DNA sequences a common structural element is suggested. In general, there are four exons and three introns. The diversion results probably from a series of duplication events.

Genetic polymorphism of apoE is derived from three alleles, e2, e3 and e4, at a single autosomal gene locus. These give rise to six phenotypes, E2/2, E3/2, E3/3, E4/4, E4/2 and E4/3.

- E4/4 homozygous subjects have raised LDL concentrations compared with E3/3 subjects.
- E4/4 subjects have an increased plasma cholesterol on an enhanced cholesterol-containing diet compared with E3/3.
- E4/4 subjects are characterised by IDL particles being more readily taken up by α_2-macrophages in the liver than other types.

chromosome 19. The genes for apoB and apoA-II are on the short arm of chromosome 2 and the long arm of chromosome 1, respectively. The gene for apoD is on the long arm of chromosome 3. The lipoprotein lipase gene is on the short arm of chromosome 8. The gene for cholesteryl ester transfer protein is on chromosome 16, next to the lecithin:cholesterol acyltransferase (LCAT) gene (16q21).

> The concentration of plasma LDL is dependent on VLDL secretion rate, conversion to LDL and its removal. The rate of VLDL to LDL conversion depends on the allelic difference in the apoE phenotype as well as VLDL particle size. ApoE binds with high affinity to the apoB receptor, and hence the rate of removal of LDL may be affected by competition. The apoB receptor regulates the rate of removal of LDL as well as its synthesis from VLDL.

ApoA-I and apoB, the major lipoproteins of HDL and LDL, respectively, are markers of CAD. The genes that influence HDL-cholesterol concentration are encoded for apoAI–CIII, lipoprotein lipase and LCAT. The cholesterol efflux regulatory protein is encoded by the adenosine triphosphate (ATP)-binding cassette (ABC1) transporter gene, a member of the ABC superfamily whose gene members encode a number of transmembrane proteins that transport diverse substances across membranes.

In measuring such lipoproteins, cholesterol-lowering diets and β-blocker drugs have effects on cholesterol concentrations that may distort the results, e.g. propranolol has a profound influence on lipid concentrations, and β-blocker drugs may increase triglyceride concentrations, lower HDL cholesterol and apoA-I and reduce LDL cholesterol, with little effect on apoB concentrations. This results in the formation of more dense LDL particles associated with hypertriglyceridaemia. ApoB is less directly related to the risk of CAD than LDL-cholesterol and even total cholesterol concentrations. For these reasons an expert panel, the National Cholesterol Education Program of the United States, suggests that total cholesterol in HDL-cholesterol is useful for screening in the non-fasting state. In the fasting state, total cholesterol,

triglyceride and HDL-cholesterol can be measured, so that LDL-cholesterol can be calculated.

Hepatic receptors to apoB and apoE are important in regulating cholesterol concentrations.

The binding capacity of apoB is determined genetically. However, hormonal factors such as corticosteroids and oestrogens increase, and dietary factors including cholesterol decrease the number of active LDL receptors. LDL concentrations in humans are influenced more by rates of LDL synthesis than by removal, as LDL receptor activity is low in humans. Linoleic acid replacing saturated acids may reduce LDL synthesis rates. The lipid composition of lipoprotein particles may affect their physical properties and hence their interactions with receptors.

HYPERLIPOPROTEINAEMIA

Classification

The World Health Organisation (WHO) classification of hyperlipoproteinaemia is simple, and allows meaningful recording and treatment regimes to be instituted. However, the more subtle features of the genetic basis are not identified by this classification, and more narrow lipid bands are discernible (Table 36.1).

Familial hypercholesterolaemia is due to defective hepatic receptors to apoB and premature development of atherosclerosis. Increased concentrations of cholesterol result from increased conversion of VLDL to LDL and a slow rate of removal of LDL from blood. This defect does not respond to diet, so drug treatment is more appropriate. The common polygenic hypercholesterolaemia leads to mild increases in LDL; individuals with the apoE4/4 phenotype respond better to such treatment than those with apoE3/3. Type III hyperlipoproteinaemia is often found in patients who are homozygous for apoE2/2 phenotype. This is characterised by increased IDL and reduced LDL concentrations. The high IDL concentrations are possibly due to poor binding of the defective apoE to the hepatic B/E receptor. This condition is associated with atherosclerosis in the peripheral vessels and responds well to a reduced fat intake.

Table 36.1 Classification of hyperlipoproteinaemia

Type	Frequency	Plasma cholesterol	Plasma triglyceride	Lipoprotein increases	Cause (deficiency)
I	Rare	Normal	Markedly increased	Chylomicron	Lipoprotein lipase (apoC-II)
IIa	Common	Increased	Normal	LDL	(LDL receptor) defect
IIb	Common	Increased	Increased	LDL, VLDL	Overproduction of VLDL
III	Rare	Markedly increased	Markedly increased	IDL, chylomicrons	(apoE-2 defect), delayed VLDL remnant clearance
IV	Common	Slightly increased	Markedly increased	VLDL	Overproduction of VLDL (defective lipoprotein lipase)
V	Rare	Slightly increased	Markedly increased	VLDL, chylomicrons	Genetic or diabetes, alcohol or obesity (lipoprotein lipase VLDL triglyceride)

Major genetic hyperlipidaemias

WHO type	Frequency	Plasma cholesterol	Plasma triglyceride	Lipoprotein increase	Cause (deficiency)
Familial hypercholesterol-aemia IIa, IIb	Uncommon	Markedly increased	Normal	LDL	(LDL receptor activity)
Polygenic hyper cholesterolaemia IIa	Common	Increased	Normal	LDL	LDL overproduction, reduced catabolism
Familial combined hyperlipidaemia IIa, IIb, IV	Common	Increased	Increased	LDL, VLDL	Overproduction of VLDL apoB-100, impaired metabolism
Familial hyper-triglyceridaemia IV, V	Uncommon	Increased	Markedly increased	Chylomicrons, VLDL	Impaired VLDL, triglyceride and apoB-100 metabolism

Major secondary hyperlipidaemias

	Plasma cholesterol	Plasma triglyceride
Hypothyroidism	Increased	Normal
Nephrotic syndrome	Increased	Increased
Diabetes mellitus	Normal	Increased
Alcohol excess	Normal	Increased
Anorexia nervosa	Increased	Normal

Such classifications of the population indicate that an overall or relative excess of a particular item of diet will test the enzyme constitution of an individual. Such a constitution will be determined genetically.

The beneficial effect on plasma lipids of n-3 unsaturated fatty acids in hyperlipidaemic patients is very much dependent on the nature of the hyperlipidaemia and genetic makeup. In contrast, the effect on plasma lipids of n-6 unsaturated fatty acids in hyperlipidaemic patients is minimal.

Atherosclerosis

The process of the development of atherosclerosis is increased in the presence of:

- high plasma concentrations of cholesterol, more particularly the transporting lipoproteins, e.g. VLDL, IDL, LDL, apoB and lipoprotein(a) [Lp(a)]
- reduced concentrations of HDL, especially HDL$_2$ and apoA-I.

High concentrations of plasma cholesterol are associated with increased concentrations of LDL, VLDL or IDL. Increased plasma triacylglycerol concentrations are associated with increased VLDL or IDL or chylomicron remnants.

Hyperlipoproteinaemias IIa, IIb, III and IV, lipoprotein apoB, LDL and VLDL and low concentrations of HDL are associated with an increased incidence of atherosclerosis.

Dietary linoleic acid and dietary intervention, e.g. reduced fat intake and increased dietary fibre, may result in atherosclerotic regression.

The atherogenic process
If the protein fractions and lipid components of VLDL, LDL, IDL and chylomicron remnants are modified by oxidation, acetylation or glycosylation, these can be ingested by monocytes that have become tissue macrophages. Glycosylation can occur in high glucose concentrations. Polyunsaturated fatty acids (PUFAs) are particularly sensitive to oxidation. Linoleic-rich LDL particles are more readily oxidised than oleic acid-enriched particles. The lipid peroxides and breakdown products form oxidation products with cholesterol and the result is a modified apoB structure that no longer enters the normal LDL receptor but is scavenged. Antioxidants such as vitamin E and ascorbic acid prevent oxidation occurring. Lp(a) may be particularly taken up by the scavenger pathway, rather than the normal apoB receptor pathway. Lp(a) inhibits tissue plasminogen activity and inhibits the breakdown of mural thrombi.

When modified lipoproteins are engorged with cholesterol they are taken up by macrophages to form foam cells. When native LDL is attached to a normal cell receptor the result is not atherogenic. Foam cells are trapped in the vascular intimal lining and become the fatty streak of the arterial intima. Platelet activation occurs and as a result of an interaction with the vascular wall and the production of growth factors, hyperplasia of smooth muscle occurs with resultant intimal thickening. A relaxing factor derived from the epithelium (possibly nitric oxide) is inhibited by foam cell formation and the smooth muscle of the vessels is less relaxed. The shape and form of the lipoproteins affect how they are taken up by the cell receptors. This can be modified and altered by genetic and dietary influences.

Vegetable oils (n-6 enriched) are associated with less atherosclerosis than saturated acid-rich diets.

Eicosapentaenoic acid (EPA; 20:5, n-3) and docosahexaenoic acid (DHA; 22:6, n-3) decrease the concentrations of VLDL, IDL and chylomicron fractions, but increase LDL in some people. These effects may well be independent of the receptor system. Intimal thickening due to proliferation and migration of proliferated smooth muscle cells from deep layers is reduced by EPA and DHA.

Dietary proteins influence cholesterol metabolism. Animal protein, e.g. casein, is more cholesterolaemic and atherogenic than protein of plant origin, e.g. soya protein. The mechanism may include the absorption and turnover of cholesterol. There may be effects on essential fatty acid turnover.

PLASMA CHOLESTEROL CONCENTRATION

In heart disease, which is multifactorial in origin, environmental factors, diet, exercise, stress and genetic influences act on a variety of lipoproteins, apolipoproteins, enzyme and tissue-specific events involved in lipoprotein metabolism. All of these are highly regulated and potentially causally related to vascular disease. Other host factors such as vascular wall biology and platelet function are important. Age, blood pressure, tobacco smoking, increased LDL-cholesterol, decreased HDL-cholesterol and diabetes are significant independent factors. Serum fibrinogen is also an independent risk factor.

There is therefore considerable interest in plasma cholesterol screening and subsequent intervention, although the advice is not always consistent. Individual variation in serum total cholesterol has strong genetic origins, but HDL-cholesterol is affected by lifestyle. The total cholesterol concentration gradually increases from youth to middle age, with associated increases in LDL and declining HDL concentrations. Smoking interferes with HDL metabolism and is associated with an accumulation of atherogenic remnants of triglyceride-rich particles in the arterial wall. Exercise in excess of 20 km a week is favourable to HDL concentrations. Similarly, moderate alcohol intake in sedentary individuals is associated with increased HDL concentrations. Diets containing a ratio of polyunsaturated to saturated fats of 0.45 or more are recommended. There is a seasonal rhythm of plasma cholesterol; in the same individuals the concentration between November and January is lower than between February and April. The timing of the trough varies, but persists in both women and men. There are similar changes in lipoprotein and apolipoprotein concentrations.

Saturated fats differ in their effects on serum cholesterol. Palmitic (C16), myristic (C14) and lauric acid (C12) raise the serum cholesterol. Lauric acid and palmitic acid raise the total and LDL lipoprotein concentration, which is in contrast to the stable triglycerides and HDL-cholesterol. Oleic acid has no effect on cholesterol concentrations. Low-fat diets lower plasma LDL but also HDL-cholesterol concentrations. Individuals eating dietary carbohydrate with a low glycaemic index (beans, apples and other fruit) have increased plasma HDL-cholesterol concentrations. Alcohol has the same effect. Dietary plant sterols and stanols reduce the absorption of cholesterol, with average reductions in the serum concentrations of 0.33–0.55 mmol/l, dependent on and increasing with age.

The dietary intake of saturated fatty acids is the principal environmental determinant of plasma concentrations of total cholesterol and LDL. If there is a change from a highly saturated diet to one with more PUFAs, the response is variable. Genes involved in such variability include those encoding for apolipoproteins, lipid metabolism enzymes and lipoprotein particle receptors. The variability includes:

- genetic variation affecting the level of a plasma lipid trait in an individual, e.g. apoC-III and apoB
- genetic variation affecting the ability to respond to environmental change, e.g. LDL gene.

The apoA-I protein is important in HDL and lipid metabolism. A common variant is adenine to guanine transition (G/A), and individuals with the A allele have higher HDL concentrations than those with the more common G allele. Individuals with the A allele respond more to dietary changes involving PUFAs.

ApoA-IV exists in several isoforms, of which the most common is apoA-IV*1. ApoA-IV*2 is associated with a modest response to lipid diet thera-

py and more pronounced adverse response to smoking and saturated fat intake compared with other isoforms. This may be a result of delayed hepatic clearance of chylomicron remnants.

ApoE is part of chylomicrons, VLDL and HDL, is a ligand for the LDL receptor and LDL receptor-related protein, and is important in the clearing of these proteins. There are three alleles of importance, E*4, E*3 and E*2, with the plasma total cholesterol, LDL-cholesterol and apoB being highest in the apoE4 group and lowest in the apoE2 isoform. The response to diet follows the same pattern. There are also significant gene × gender interaction and gene × diet interactions.

Plasma apoC-III is a contributor to chylomicrons, VLDL and HDL, and the apo3 gene locus is involved in LDL-cholesterol response to dietary fat.

ApoB is the main component of LDL; the Xbal restriction fragment length polymorphism (RFLP) mutation is associated with variations in plasma lipid concentrations. Individuals with the X+X+ or X+X– genotype plasma lipids respond more to a low-fat diet than individuals with the X–X– genotype.

Lipoprotein lipase gene has a number of alleles. The HindIII RFLP is associated with variability in response to lipid dietary changes.

Cholesteryl ester transfer protein facilitates the transfer of neutral lipid core constituents (cholesteryl ester in triacylglycerol) between plasma lipoproteins. Individuals with the B2 allele have lower lipid transfer activity and raised HDL-cholesterol concentration. There is significant interaction between smoking and the B2 allele.

Key's equation

This describes a change in plasma cholesterol that occurred in volunteers when alterations were made in the dietary intake of saturated and polyunsaturated fats (all *cis*-linoleic and α-linoleic acids):

Change in plasma cholesterol (mg/100 ml) = $1.3 (2\Delta S - \Delta P)$

where ΔS = difference in percentage energy derived from saturated fat, and ΔP = difference in percentage energy derived from polyunsaturated fat.

A low-lipid, high-carbohydrate diet can result in raised triacylglycerol concentrations and reduced HDL concentrations. The reduced fat content of the diet may also alter the distribution of the LDL fraction to the more atherogenic LDL pattern B.

Plasma cholesterol concentrations should be under 6.5 mmol/l; between 6.5 and 7.8 mmol/l is regarded as moderately increased, and above this figure is severely increased.

The Sheffield risk and treatment table gives clear indications for cholesterol lowering for the primary prevention of coronary heart disease.

Low serum cholesterol

A low serum cholesterol concentration is not necessarily beneficial.

Cholesterol and behaviour

Depression is associated with cholesterol concentrations under 4.14 mmol/l. This is age dependent, especially in men. Depression may be associated with a reduction in dietary intake, weight loss and hence reduced serum cholesterol. That is, the reduction in serum cholesterol may have antedated the study or be an effect rather than a cause of the depression.

There is an increased suicide rate in trials where the serum cholesterol has been reduced by either diet or drugs. Engelberg suggested that changes in the central nervous neurotransmitter serotonin may be important in this association. A low cholesterol concentration in the brain reduces the number of serotonin receptors. The blood cholesterol is in equilibrium with the membrane cholesterol and therefore changes in one will affect the other.

A curious anomaly is that there is an enhanced rate of coronary heart disease in smokers, in whom the tissue adipose linoleic content is reduced, yet there is an association between smoking and suicide.

KEY POINTS

1. The synthesis of sterols is closely related to growth, development and differentiation of all cells.

2. All cholesterol is synthesised from acetate. The irreversible, rate-limiting reaction in cholesterol synthesis is catalysed by HMG-CoA reductase. This enzyme is inactive when phosphorylated by HMG-CoA reductase kinase. Many of the factors that regulate cholesterol biosynthesis are involved in HMG-CoA reductase activity.

3. Plasma cholesterol enters the hepatic cell as cholesterol esters and cholesterol, transported on low-density lipoproteins (LDL), and influences sterol synthesis through feedback regulation on the concentration of LDL membrane receptors and of HMG-CoA reductase.

4. There appear to be diurnal and seasonal cycles in cholesterol synthesis, due largely to changes in the activities of HMG-CoA reductase and cholesterol 7-α-hydroxylase, which is involved in bile acid synthesis, and lysosomal acid cholesteryl ester hydrolase.

5. Excess cholesterol is esterified to fatty acids by the liver enzyme acyl-CoA: cholesterol acyltransferase (ACAT).

6. The first step in the degradation of cholesterol to bile acids is a rate-limiting, 7-α-hydroxylation, a microsomal enzyme reaction. Cytochrome P450, NADPH and molecular oxygen are required. There is then hydroxylation at C12 for the precursor of cholic acid. Cholic acid, 3,7,12-α-trihydroxycholanoic acid and chenodeoxycholic-α-3,7-dihydroxycholanoic acid are formed and conjugated with taurine or glycine and excreted in bile to the enterohepatic circulation.

7. Bile acids have a major regulatory role in overall hepatic sterol metabolism. Not only the size but also the composition of the bile acid pool may contribute to the regulation of hepatic sterol metabolism.

8. The risk of developing coronary artery disease is inversely correlated with plasma HDL-cholesterol and apoA-I concentrations. As the genes for apoA-I, C-III and A-IV are clustered, polymorphism of one of these genes may also affect the others.

9. The hyperlipoproteinaemias are classified by the changes in chylomicron, HDL, LDL and VLDL concentration. The type of abnormality determines outcome and treatment.

10. A low-fat diet is important in reducing serum

cholesterol. The response to this diet and the type of fatty acids eaten have a variable effect on the serum cholesterol and HDL and LDL concentrations. This variation in response to dietary treatment is in part decided by the individual's genetic makeup, and smoking, weight, exercise and health.

THINKING POINTS

1. The pattern of serum cholesterol and the lipoproteins is very dependent on genetic makeup and environmental factors.
2. The response to diet is a balance between age, smoking, weight, diabetic problems and the genetic makeup.

NEED TO UNDERSTAND

The environmental and genetic strands that determine a serum lipid concentration and pattern.

FURTHER READING

Brown, M.S. and Goldstein, J.L. (1998) Sterol regulatory binding proteins (SREBPs): controllers of lipid synthesis and cellular uptake. *Nutrition Review*, **56**, S1–3.

Carulli, N., Loria, P., Bertolotti, M. *et al.* (1990) The effects of bile acid pool composition on hepatic metabolism of cholesterol in man. *Italian Journal of Gastroenterology*, **22**, 88–96.

Edwards, P.A. and Ericsson, J. (1999) Sterols and isoprenoids: signalling molecules derived from the cholesterol biosynthesis pathway. *Annual Review of Biochemistry*, **68**, 157–86.

Engelberg, H. (1992) Low serum cholesterol and suicide. *Lancet*, **339**, 727–9.

Fisher, E.A., Coates, P.M. and Cortner, J.A. (1989) Gene polymorphisms and variability of human apolipoproteins. *Annual Review of Nutrition*, **9**, 139–60.

Haq, I.U., Jackson, P.R., Yeo, W.W. and Ramsay, L.E. (1995) Sheffield risk and treatment table for cholesterol lowering for primary prevention of coronary heart disease. *Lancet*, **346**, 1467–71.

Hayes, K.C. (2000) Dietary fatty acids, cholesterol and the lipoprotein profile. *British Journal of Nutrition*, **84**, 397–9.

Humphries, S.E., Talmud, P.J., Cox, C. *et al.* (1996) Genetic factors affecting the consistency and magnitude of changes in plasma cholesterol in response to dietary change. *Quarterly Journal of Medicine*, **89**, 671–80.

Krauss, R.M. (2001) Dietary and genetic effects of low-density lipoprotein heterogeneity. *Annual Review of Nutrition*, **21**, 283–96.

Kritchevsky, D. (1992) Variation in plasma cholesterol levels. *Nutrition Today*, **27**, 21–3.

Kritchevsky, D. (1995) Dietary protein, cholesterol and atherosclerosis: a review of the early history. *Journal of Nutrition*, **125** (Suppl.), 589–93S.

Law, M. (2000) Plant sterol and stanol margarines and health. *British Medical Journal*, **320**, 861–4.

Ordovas, J. (1999) The genetics of serum lipid responsiveness to dietary interventions. *Proceedings of the Nutrition Society*, **58**, 171–87.

Ostlund, R.E. Jr (2002) Phytosterols in human nutrition. *Annual Review of Nutrition*, **22**, 533–49.

Owen, J.S. (1999) Role of *ABC1* gene in cholesterol efflux and atheroprotection. *Lancet*, **354**, 1402–3.

Roche, H.M. (1999) Dietary carbohydrates and triacylglycerol metabolism. *Proceedings of the Nutrition Society*, **58**, 201–7.

Unwin, N., Thomson, R., O'Byrne, A.M., *et al.* (1998) Implications of applying widely accepted cholesterol screening and management guidelines to a British adult population: cross sectional study of cardiovascular disease and risk factors. *British Medical Journal*, **317**, 1125–30.

37

Amino acid metabolism

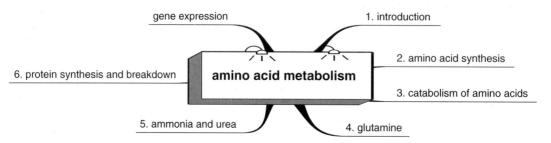

Fig. 37.1 Chapter outline.

INTRODUCTION

Amino acids can be classified as essential or non-essential. An essential amino acid is one that has to be supplied in the diet to maintain a positive nitrogen balance. Fewer than half of the protein amino acids can be synthesised by *de novo* pathways. The remainder must be supplied by nutrients.

The liver is important in protein synthesis. The non-essential amino acids (alanine, glycine, glutamic acid and glutamine) are normally present in many times greater amounts in the liver than in the plasma, whereas the concentrations of the essential amino acids are the same in liver and plasma.

AMINO ACID SYNTHESIS

Amino acid synthesis arises from a few key intermediates from the glycolytic pathway, pentose phosphate pathway or the tricarboxylic acid (TCA) cycle.

Amino acids found in adult humans

Essential	*Non-essential*
Isoleucine	Alanine
Leucine	Arginine
Lysine	Asparagine
Methionine	Aspartate
Phenylalanine	Cysteine
Threonine	Glutamate
Tryptophan	Glutamine
Valine	Glycine
	Histidine
	Proline
	Serine
	Tyrosine

The synthesis of amino acids, with the exception of cysteine and tyrosine, is linked to the glycolytic TCA cycle by transamination or ammonia fixation. The α-amino group is central to all amino acid synthesis and is derived from ammonia from the amino groups of L-glutamate. From this glutamine, proline and arginine are synthesised.

Glutamic dehydrogenase facilitates a reversible reaction between glutamic acid and oxaloacetic acid. Glutamic acid is the key source of amino groups for transamination. This reaction of transamination is important in generating amino acids and deaminating amino acids.

Glutamate + oxaloacetate

$$\xleftrightarrow{\text{aspartate amino transferase}}$$

α-Ketoglutarate + aspartate

CATABOLISM OF AMINO ACIDS

Amino acids that are catabolised come from three different sources:

- dietary proteins
- storage proteins
- metabolic turnover of endogenous proteins.

All cells turn over their protein-containing structures and the constituent amino acids are recycled into other proteins or other metabolic pathways. This depends on local or total body needs.

Protein catabolism begins with the hydrolysis of the covalent peptide bonds linking amino acid residues in a polypeptide chain. This proteolytic process, by the action of peptidase, yields free amino acids and peptides. Endopeptidases hydrolyse peptide bonds remote from the ends of the molecule, whereas exopeptidases remove amino acids from the end of the molecule. Such peptidases are either aminopeptidases or carboxypeptidases according to the end of the peptide at which digestion takes place. The degradation of amino acids requires the removal of the α-amino nitrogen through two forms of deamination, i.e. transamination or oxidative deamination.

Transamination occurs when an amino acid gives its amino group to α-ketoglutarate producing α-keto acid and glutamate. Most transaminases contain pyridoxal-5′-phosphate as a coenzyme. So that α-ketoglutarate is regenerated for further transamination, oxidative deamination is necessary, using nicotinamide adenine dinucleotide (NAD)-linked glutamate dehydrogenase. This allows the net conversion of amino acid groups to ammonia.

An interesting phenomenon is the highly active and widely distributed D-amino acid oxidase.

The malate shuttle

This allows the transfer of reducing equivalents from the cytoplasm to the mitochondria. Mitochondrial oxaloacetate cannot cross the inner mitochondrial membrane, so is converted into aspartate, which crosses the mitochondrial membrane on a specific carrier to the cytosplasm and is deaminated, yielding oxaloacetate. This reacts with cytoplasmic NADH catalysed by malate dehydrogenase to form malate, which is then transported back across to the mitochondria. Inside the mitochondrial inner membrane space, malate is reoxidised to oxaloacetate by a mitochondrial isoenzyme of malate dehydrogenase. Both isoenzymes are NAD linked, so this allows the movement of electrons from cytoplasmic NADH to mitochondrial NADH.

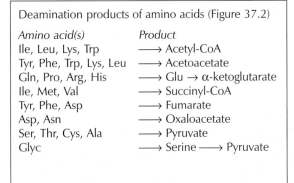

Deamination products of amino acids (Figure 37.2)

Amino acid(s)	Product
Ile, Leu, Lys, Trp	⟶ Acetyl-CoA
Tyr, Phe, Trp, Lys, Leu	⟶ Acetoacetate
Gln, Pro, Arg, His	⟶ Glu → α-ketoglutarate
Ile, Met, Val	⟶ Succinyl-CoA
Tyr, Phe, Asp	⟶ Fumarate
Asp, Asn	⟶ Oxaloacetate
Ser, Thr, Cys, Ala	⟶ Pyruvate
Glyc	⟶ Serine ⟶ Pyruvate

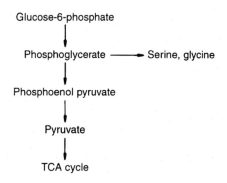

Fig. 37.2 Contribution of glycolysis to amino acids.

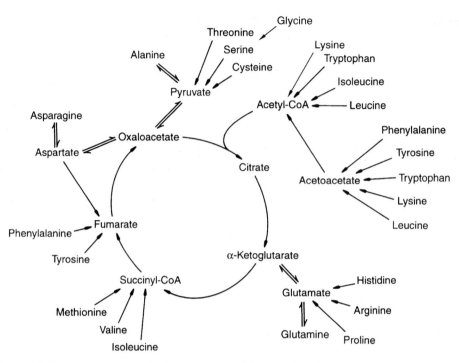

Fig. 37.3 Relationship between amino acids, deamination and the tricarboxylic acid (TCA) cycle.

D-Amino acids are seldom encountered in animals, except as breakdown products of bacterial cell walls. It is possible that this enzyme is protective against bacterial amino acids.

Central to the catabolism of amino acids is the formation of a dicarboxylic acid intermediate of pyruvate or acetyl-coenzyme A (CoA) in the TCA cycle. The four-carbon dicarboxylic acids can stimulate TCA function. They leave the cycle either by:

- the conversion by gluconeogenesis of oxaloacetate to phosphoenolpyruvate; such amino acids are called *glycogenic*
- the formation of pyruvate, which may be converted to acetyl-CoA and completely oxidised to carbon dioxide and water.

There is a close relationship between the products of deamination of amino acids and the TCA cycle (Figure 37.3). Acids having deamination products that are directly metabolised to acetyl-CoA or acetoacetate are ketogenic; leucine and lysine are directly ketogenic. Amino acids having deamination products that directly enter the citric acid cycle as pyruvate or citric acid are glucogenic and produce a net synthesis of glucose. Eighteen of the amino acids yield glucose and therefore are important as energy sources as well as having structural importance. This is of significance during starvation or when the diet is reduced in carbohydrate content. Phenylalanine, tyrosine, isoleucine and tryptophan are both ketogenic or glucogenic.

The transaminase *aspartate aminotransferase*, as well as catalysing the synthesis of aspartate, is important in the transport of reducing equivalents between mitochondria and cytoplasmin in the malate shuttle.

The *malate shuttle* (Figure 37.4) is important in reoxidising NAD to NADH, which is generated in abundance during glycolysis in the cytoplasm. NADH cannot cross the mitochondrial membrane. Reactions that require NADH may produce reaction products which, after oxidising NADH in the cytoplasm, cross into the mitochondria, are reoxidised and then return to the cytoplasm.

The transaminase *alanine aminotransferase* catalyses the reaction:

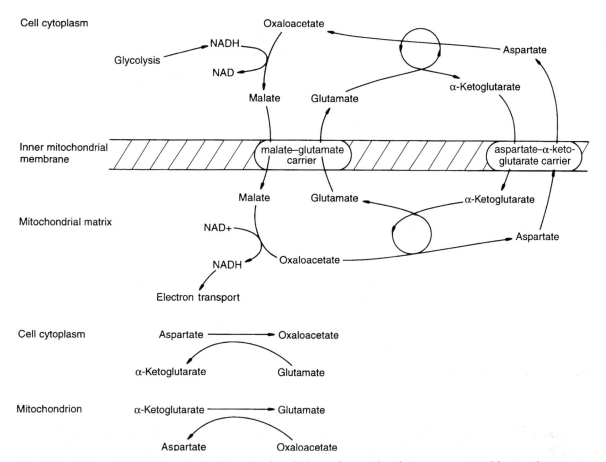

Fig. 37.4 Because NADH cannot cross the mitochondrial membrane, the electrons are carried by a malate–aspartate shuttle.

Pyruvate + Glutamate $\longleftrightarrow$ Alanine + α-Ketoglutarate

in the alanine cycle, which transports nitrogen and carbon from muscle to liver. During starvation, when muscle protein is a major source of gluconeogenesis, the carbon substrate is carried from the muscle as alanine. In the liver this is converted to pyruvate. Nitrogen is present in the liver as glutamic acid.

Another mode of transporting nitrogen around the body is by glutamine:

Glumate + NH$_3$ + ATP $\longleftrightarrow$ Glutamine + ADP + P$_i$

(NH$_3$: ammonia; ATP: adenosine triphosphate; ADP: adenosine diphosphate; P$_i$: inorganic phosphate).

In this manner glutamine can deliver ammonia to the liver for urea production, or to the kidney for excretion as the NH$^+$ cation. The ammonia derived from metabolised amino acids is disposed of as urea in humans. Urea is non-toxic but metabolically expensive, requiring four high-energy bonds for its synthesis.

Serine and glycine are interconvertible (Figure 37.5). Serine undergoes a transhydroxymethylation reaction, being synthesised from 3-phosphoglyceric acid. Glycine is degraded by two routes. The route to pyruvate involves the conversion of glycine to serine and the addition of hydroxymethyl through 5,10-methylenetetrahydrofolate. The serine is then converted to pyruvate by serine dehydratase. Most glycine, however, is oxidised to CO$_2$, NH$_4^+$ and methylene (–CH$_2$–), which is accepted by tetrahydrofolate in a reversible reaction.

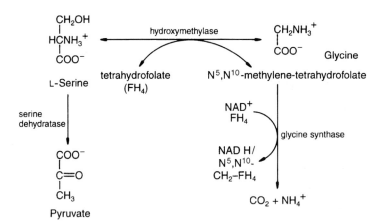

Fig. 37.5 Serine and glycine inter-relationship and catabolism. This transmethylation reaction involves tetrahydrofolate and N^5, N^{10}-methylene tetrahydrofolate.

Alanine is involved in a reversible transaminase reaction to pyruvate as part of the glucose alanine cycle.

Tyrosine catabolism is catalysed by tyrosine–glutamate transaminase. Tyrosine can also be the starting point of the synthesis of the skin colour pigment melanin. The enzyme involved, tyrosinase, is found solely in melanosomes, which are specialised pigment-producing cells in the skin and other tissues. Dopa (3,4-dihydroxyphenylalanine) is synthesised from tyrosine by tyrosine hydroxylase and is a precursor of noradrenaline and adrenaline synthesis in the adrenal glands.

Phenylalanine degradation occurs through the intermediary tyrosine by the action of phenylalanine-4-mono-oxygenase (Figure 37.6). This requires tetrahydrobiopterin as a cosubstrate. This biopterin remains in the reduced form through the action of NADPH. Tyrosine is not an essential amino acid unless phenylalanine dietary intake is reduced; when there is an absence or deficiency of the hydroxylation to tyrosine, high concentrations of phenylalanine are found in the blood. This is known as phenylketonuria.

The major pathway for *tryptophan* catabolism in the liver is through kynurenine, which is metabolised in the liver through α-ketoadipate (also an intermediate in lysine degradation) (Figure 37.7). Kynurenine is also involved in the synthesis of the coenzyme nicotinamide.

Arginine, histidine, proline, glutamic acid and *glutamine* are readily converted to α-ketoglutarate (Figure 37.8). Arginine is not transaminated but is a precursor of various essential polyamines and is important in the urea cycle.

Methionine, isoleucine and *valine* are degraded to succinyl-CoA. The three keto-acids produced by deamination of valine, isoleucine and leucine are decarboxylated by the same enzyme complex. This enzyme also acts on pyruvate and α-ketobutyrate, which are products of both threonine and methionine metabolism.

The turnover of methionine exceeds the dietary intake; therefore, recycling through homocysteine is important, with the vitamin B_{12}-dependent methionine synthase.

Aspartate and *asparagine* are deaminated to oxaloacetate, and then to the metabolic pathway into the TCA pool.

Regulation of amino acid catabolism

Amino acid catabolic enzymes are under hormonal control, although the activity of some is influenced by diet (Figure 37.9).

The degradation of arginine (and its precursor ornithine), serine and tryptophan is affected by the protein content of the diet. High-protein diets stimulate the enzymes involved, whether they be ornithine-glutamate transaminase, urea cycle enzymes or deaminases. Threonine deaminase is also stimulated by a high-protein diet. In contrast, tryptophan oxygenase and tyrosine-glutamate transaminase are stimulated by glucocorticoids.

These catabolic enzymes may vary in activity dependent on age. Tryptophan oxygenase activity is low in the newborn rat, but increases after 12 days, an increase associated with a rise in adrenal activity. Glucocorticoids induce the formation of

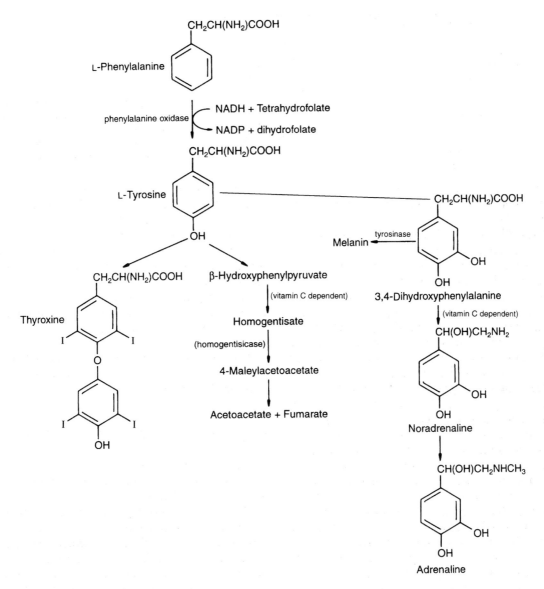

Fig. 37.6 Aromatic amino acids. Phenylalanine, an essential amino acid, is an important source of tyrosine, which may be catabolised to fumarate and acetoacetate or to 3,4-dihydroxyphenylalanine and then to melanin, which is a pigmented cutaneous polymer catalysed by tyrosinase. 3,4-Dihydroxyphenylalanine may also be synthesised to noradrenaline and adrenaline. L-Tyrosine may also be iodinated to thyroxine or degraded to acetoacetate and fumarate. (Note that tyrosine is not an essential amino acid unless phenylalanine is deficient.)

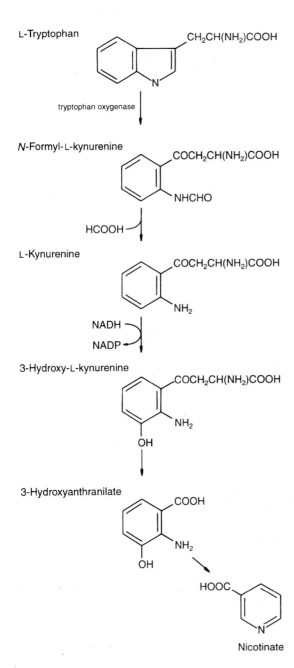

Fig. 37.7 Tryptophan is the only amino acid with an indole ring and is an essential amino acid. It can be catabolised to kynurenine and synthesised to the coenzyme NAD.

the enzyme in young rats and stimulate enzyme production in adults. Ornithine transcarbamoylase and the other urea-forming enzymes are synthesised after birth and are induced by a high-protein diet.

Many amino acids are transported into cells by sodium ion-dependent transport systems (Figure 37.10), which convert the energy of the electrochemical sodium gradient across the plasma membrane into osmotically active amino acid gradients with intracellular/extracellular concentration ratios of up to 30. Such gradients allow water to move into the cell and lead to cell swelling. Liver cells swell by as much as 12% within 2 min with the influx of glutamine, and this increased cellular hydration is maintained as long as the amino acid is present. Hormones also change cellular hydration, i.e. cell volume, by modulating the activity of the ion transport system in the plasma membrane. Insulin increases cellular hydration by causing Na^+, K^+ and Cl^- to accumulate within the cell through activation of the Na^+/H^+ antiporter, Na–K–2 Cl cotransport and the Na+/K^+-ATPase. Glucagon, in contrast, induces cell shrinkage.

Cellular hydration status is an important determinant of protein catabolism in health and disease.

In the liver, *cell swelling* inhibits the breakdown of glycogen, glucose, RNA and protein, and at the same time stimulates synthesis of glycogen, RNA, DNA and protein. The opposite metabolic pathway is triggered by cell shrinkage. Cell swelling is a proliferative anabolic signal, whereas cell shrinkage is antiproliferative and catabolic, i.e. concentration dependent. Hormone-induced changes in cellular hydration are second messengers of hormone action. It is possible that the antiproteolytic effects of some amino acids and insulin and the proteolytic action of glucagon may be explained by the influences of these on cellular hydration.

GLUTAMINE

Glutamine is a non-essential amino acid and is the most abundant free amino acid in the body. It has the highest plasma concentration of any amino acid and provides approximately 5% of the whole body

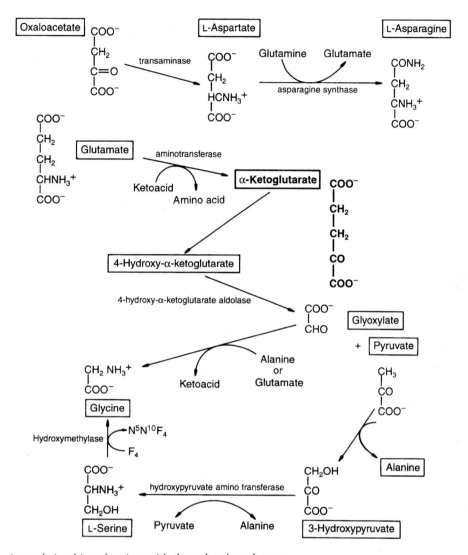

Fig. 37.8 Interrelationships of amino acids through α-ketoglutarate.

free amino acid pool, 25% of the plasma amino acids and 60% of the muscle free amino acids. Glutamine is an obligatory fuel for intestinal cells and other rapidly dividing cells, e.g. the cells of the immune system, and in the regulation of acid–base balance in renal ammoniagenesis. Glutamine provides precursors for nucleic acid biosynthesis and their regulation, purine, pyrimidine and nucleotide synthesis, and protein synthesis and its regulation. Glutamine has a C5 chain and two nitrogen atoms, which makes it a powerful donor of C and N. Glutamine is important in the synthesis of proline, citrulline, arginine and glutathione.

Sites of glutamine metabolism

Intestines
Intestines contain high glutaminase activity and very little glutamine synthetase activity. The intestines therefore break down glutamine, which provides an important energy source in addition to glucose, short-chain fatty acids and ketone bodies.

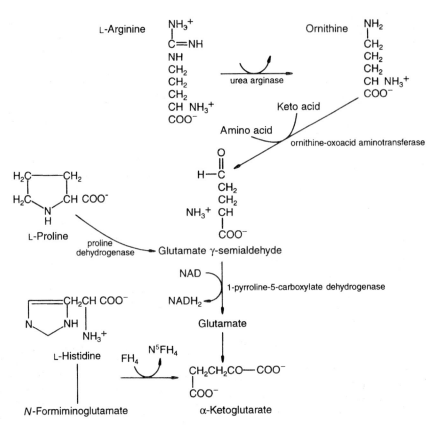

Fig. 37.9 Regulation of diet and amino acid catabolism. Arginine, ornithine, serine and tryptophan degradation is increased by a high protein content of the diet.

The glutamine is derived from either the blood-stream or the intestinal lumen. Most of the gluta-mine is used by the intestinal mucosa. The large bowel uses much less glutamine than the small intestine.

Intestinal glutamine uptake and metabolism account for approximately 60% of the ammonia from the viscera drained by the portal vein. Glut-amine is converted to ammonia and glutamate, which is then transaminated to alanine and to a lesser extent to other amino acids and organic acids. Colonic bacteria in the gut lumen produce ammonia by splitting urea, creating another source of ammonia. Glutamine breakdown and urea splitting make the intestines a major ammo-nia-producing organ. Ammonia and amino acids are carried in the portal vein to the liver and then to the urea cycle. The alanine carbon skeleton is used in hepatic gluconeogenesis.

Muscle
Glutamine synthetase activity in skeletal muscle is low. However, because muscle occurs in such sub-stantial quantities, it is one of the principal gluta-mine-synthesising organs. In addition, skeletal muscle is an organ of net glutamine release in the physiological situation through glutaminase activ-ity. Skeletal muscle contains 70–80% of the total body free amino acid pool and glutamine forms 60% of the muscle pool. Glutamine release from skeletal muscle increases with muscle protein turnover or release from the free glutamine pool. Glutamine forms approximately 30% of the amino acid released from skeletal muscle, but con-stitutes only 5% of muscle protein amino acids. Glutamine is a carbon and nitrogen carrier from skeletal muscle to splanchnic organs.

The cellular tissue concentration of glutamine falls during severe illness. Glutamine is considered

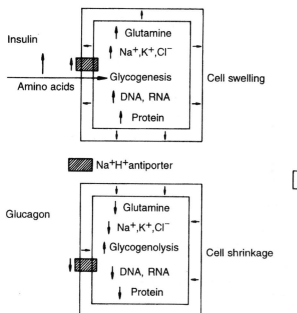

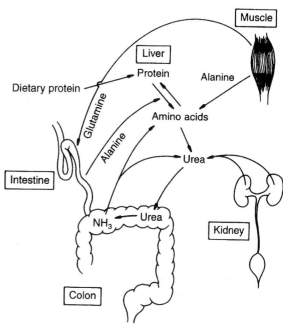

Fig. 37.10 The entrance of amino acids into the cell through the sodium-dependent transport system increases the osmotic active pressure within the cell, which swells. Insulin increases the activity of the Na^+/H^+ antiporter, increasing glycogenesis and DNA, RNA and protein synthesis. Glucagon has the opposite effect.

Fig. 37.11 Urea is produced in the liver from dietary and endogenous protein amino acids. Some 70% of the urea is excreted in the urine, with 30% being retained in the body. Most tissues release nitrogen as alanine or glutamine. Alanine results from the transamination of glutamate to pyruvate. Glutamine utilises ammonia (enzyme, glutamine synthase).

to be an essential fuel for small intestinal function. This leads some clinicians to regard glutamine as being conditionally indispensable in critical illness.

AMMONIA AND UREA

Ammonia is converted to urea (Figure 37.11), a soluble endproduct that is readily excreted in urine at approximately 30 g/day. Ammonia is a toxic substance, whereas urea is relatively harmless to tissue function and well-being. All of the nitrogen in urea is derived from two precursors, the ammonium ion and aspartate. Ammonia, mainly coming from the gut, enters the cycle as NH_3, not NH_4^+, a pH-dependent equilibrium that may be a control on urea synthesis. The ammonia is absorbed from the colon, transported to the liver in the portal vein and added to the amino-N pool by transamination. These new amino acids are non-essential amino

acids, this has the potential to alter the ratio of essential to non-essential amino acids, but in practice this is not a problem.

Glutamine dehydrogenase and ammonia

Glutamine is an abundant amino acid and is readily transaminated by other amino acids. Glutamate is derived from alanine, aspartate and other transaminating amino acids. In a reversible reaction,

The transfer of nitrogen from an amino group is to a keto acid; using aspartate aminotransferase:

L-Glutamate + Oxaloacetate $\longrightarrow$ α-Ketoglutarate + L-aspartate

The aminotransferase contains pyridoxal phosphate.

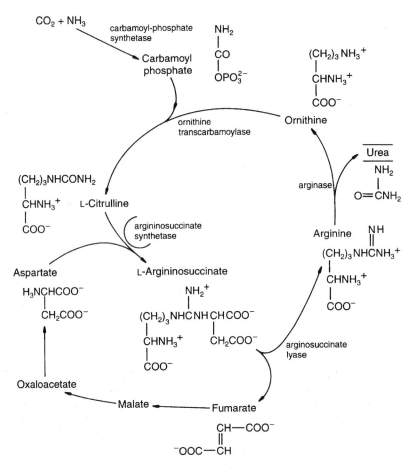

Fig. 37.12 The urea cycle. Ammonia reacts with carbon dioxide and ATP to produce carbamoylphosphate within the mitochondria. The urea cycle produces urea, which diffuses into the blood, is carried to the kidney and excreted.

glutamate is oxidatively deaminated to α-ketoglutarate and ammonia by the mitochondrial enzyme glutamate dehydrogenase.

Glutamine synthetase

Glutamate is the prime amino acid precursor of NH_3.

Ammonia can be carried to the liver as glutamine, formed in a reaction catalysed by glutamine synthetase, in which NH_3 is added to glutamate to form glutamine. Once the glutamine reaches the liver or small intestine the enzyme glutaminase releases the ammonia.

Skeletal muscle transports NH_3 to the liver in the

form of alanine. This is derived from a transamination reaction between pyruvate and glutamate. In the liver alanine reacts with α-ketoglutarate to form pyruvate and glutamate, a reaction catalysed by alanine transaminase. If the blood glucose concentration is low, then pyruvate is converted to glucose via gluconeogenesis. This glucose can be returned to the skeletal muscle for energy purposes. This is known as the glucose alanine cycle and is important in the muscular activity of the organism.

Urea cycle

Urea is derived from the hydrolysis of arginine

The urea cycle

Five enzymes are involved:

- Carbamoyl phosphate synthetase I (carbamoyl phosphate synthetase):

$$\text{Carbon dioxide} + \text{Ammonia} \longrightarrow \text{Carbamoyl phosphate}$$

- Ornithine transcarbamylase (L-ornithine carbamoyltransferase):

$$\text{Carbomyl phosphate} + \text{Ornithine} \longrightarrow \text{Citrulline}$$

Citrulline is transported from the mitochondria.

- Argininosuccinate synthetase (L-citrulline L-aspartate ligase):

$$\text{Citrulline} + \text{Aspartate} + \text{ATP} \longrightarrow \text{Arginosuccinate} + \text{AMP}$$

- Argininosuccinate lyase (L-argininosuccinate arginine-lyase):

$$\text{Arginosuccinate} \longrightarrow \text{Arginine} + \text{Fumarate}$$

- Arginase (L-arginine ureohydrolase):

$$\text{Arginine} \longrightarrow \text{Ornithine} + \text{Urea}$$

Fumarate is in equilibrium with malate. In this way urea production is tied into other metabolic pathways. Malate is converted to pyruvate in fatty acid synthesis or gluconeogenesis as required.

catalysed by arginase, leaving L-ornithine, which is recycled, enabling a continuous production of urea.

The urea cycle (Figure 37.12), which is confined to the liver, is a metabolic pathway for the disposal of ammonia. In the liver the urea cycle enzymes are found predominantly in the periportal hepatocytes. In each cycle, two nitrogens are eliminated; one from the oxidative deamination of glutamate and the other from the α-amino group of aspartate. Urea is excreted into the bloodstream and removed by the kidneys in the urine.

In addition to the removal of ammonia, the urea cycle is important in pH homoeostasis by regulating bicarbonate concentrations. Some of the enzymes of the urea cycle are found in the small intestine and liver, forming an independent arginine biosynthetic pathway.

Each enzyme is a single polypeptide chain encoded by a single-copy nuclear gene. The first two enzymes of the urea cycle are located within the mitochondrial matrix and the other three are cytosolic (Figure 37.13). The first enzyme, carbamoyl phosphate synthetase I, is not reversible and controls the flow through the cycle. This enzyme has an absolute requirement for cofactor N-acetylglutamate. The substrates move sequentially from one enzyme to another by channelling.

These enzymes are highly inducable by diet and hormones. Urea production in the adult human varies with the dietary protein intake. The metabolic regulation of urea cycle enzymatic activity is very much species specific, perhaps depending on the type of diet to which an animal is normally adapted. With increasing dietary protein the activity of all of the enzymes increases two- to threefold. Reducing the dietary protein has the opposite effect. Following starvation, urea output and enzyme activity, except for arginase, doubles. These changes occur within 8 h and appear to be the result of increased amounts of protein rather than an allosteric effect. The amino acid composition of the proteins has little or no effect on enzyme activity. Diet-dependent changes in urea cycle activity are the consequence of changes in enzyme mass and altered enzyme synthesis rates. Therefore, dietary regulation of enzyme level is acting at a pretranslational step. There is a co-ordination in the regulation of the five messenger RNAs (mRNAs) involved. Urea production is constant over the day and night, but urea excretion increases during the day and falls at night. Corticosteroids, glucagon and cyclic adenosine monophosphate (cAMP) are inducers, and insulin and glucose are suppressers of activity.

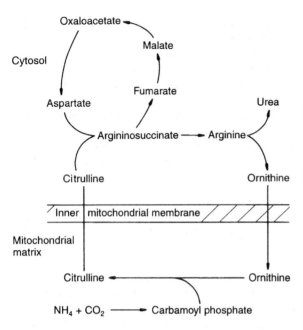

Fig. 37.13 Urea cycle compartmentalism. Part of the urea cycle takes place within the mitochondria. Ornithine must cross the mitochondrial membrane to be available for the formation of citrulline. The transport of ornithine into the mitochondria uses the same transporter system that carries citrulline out of the organelles.

Sepsis, trauma, uraemia and cancer alter urea synthesis and levels of urea cycle enzymes.

Arginine biosynthesis
The importance of endogenous arginine synthesis is highly dependent on age, physiological state and species of animal. Young animals require dietary arginine for optimal growth, whereas endogenous arginine synthesis meets the arginine requirements of most adult omnivores.

The small intestine is the principal source of citrulline in adult mammals, the synthesis being catalysed by carbamyl phosphate synthetase I and ornithine transcarbamylase in mucosal epithelial cells. The kidney has a significant capacity for converting citrulline to arginine, by argininosuccinate synthetase and argininosuccinate lyase, the third and fourth enzymes of the urea cycle in the proximal tubules of the kidney. The kidney is a major site of arginine biosynthesis and renal production of arginine is limited by the availability of citrulline. Renal argininosuccinate synthetase and argini-

nosuccinate lyase activities and the responsible mRNA increase proportionally with dietary protein intake.

> Regulation of carbamyl phosphate synthetase I (CPS-I) is dependent on the concentration of its essential cofactor, *N*-acetylglutamate. Arginase is a rate-limiting enzyme at a junction point in the pathway wherein arginine may be used for ureagenesis, protein synthesis or polyamine synthesis.

Free ammonia formed by oxidation and the deamination of glutamine is converted into carbamoyl phosphate. The carbamoyl group is transferred to the terminal amino group of ornithine to form L-citrulline, which enters the urea cycle.

PROTEIN SYNTHESIS AND BREAKDOWN

Whole body protein turns over at about 3% a day, i.e. approximately 300 g.

The manner in which different tissues behave will vary. With increased protein intake, synthesis increases by up to 20% and breakdown decreases. Oxidation increases with higher intake. Synthesis takes priority and progresses at a steady rate, and excess amino acids not required for synthesis are removed by oxidation. High protein intakes amplify the diurnal swings in synthesis and breakdown. Insulin is the hormone that affects protein synthesis in the short term, an effect that runs in parallel with the availability of amino acids. When the dietary amino acid supply is sufficient more than to compensate for the inhibition of normal tissue breakdown, tissue amino acid levels are sufficiently increased to stimulate protein synthesis.

GENE EXPRESSION

Reduction in the amino acids arginine, cystine and all of the essential amino acids results in increased expression of insulin-like growth factor-binding protein-1 and CCAAT/enhancer binding protein (C/EBP) homologous protein (CHOP) mRNA and protein CCAA.

KEY POINTS

1. Dietary amino acids are either essential or non-essential. Non-essential amino acids can be synthesised from key intermediates in the glycolytic pathway, pentose phosphate pathway or TCA cycle. Some amino acids may become essential under stress, e.g. glutamine, or due to the lack of a precursor e.g. tyrosine.
2. The synthesis of amino acids involves transamination or ammonia fixation. The α-amino group is generally derived from the amino groups of L-glutamate.
3. The catabolism of dietary proteins yields amino acids for recycling. Other sources of amino acids for catabolism include storage proteins and the metabolic turnover of endogenous proteins.
4. Protein catabolism involves the hydrolysis of covalent peptide linkages. The degradation of amino acids requires the removal of the α-amino nitrogen through deamination in the form of transamination or oxidative deamination. Transamination is the donation of the amino group to α-ketoglutarate, which is then regenerated by oxidative deamination.
5. There is a close link between the deamination products of amino acids and the TCA cycle. Amino acids directly converted to acetyl-CoA are ketogenic, but deamination products directly entering the TCA cycle are glucogenic.
6. The malate shuttle is important in maintaining a required balance between NAD and NADH across the mitochondrial membrane. This involves NAD-linked enzymes and the movement of aspartate and malate across the mitochondrial membrane, producing oxaloacetate on either side; the process is then repeated.
7. The transaminase alanine aminotransferase reaction allows the transportation of nitrogen from muscle to liver in the form of alanine.
8. Amino acid catabolic enzymes are under hormonal and dietary control.
9. Glutamine, while being a non-essential amino acid, is important as the most abundant free amino acid. It is an obligatory fuel for intestinal and immune cells, has a role in acid–base balance, provides α-amino groupings for renal ammoniagenesis, and is a precursor in nucleic acid biosynthesis.
10. The endproducts of nitrogen catabolism are ammonia and urea. Ammonia is toxic and is carried to the liver as glutamine. Muscle transports ammonia to the liver in the form of alanine.
11. In the urea cycle, urea is produced by the sequential removal of nitrogen atoms. Urea production varies as a function of dietary protein intake, being reduced in starvation.

THINKING POINT

It is interesting that while amino acid and protein metabolism is central to the knowledge of nutrition, comparatively little is known of the molecular biological background behind interactions between genes and amino acids/proteins.

NEED TO UNDERSTAND

1. The interrelationships between the amino acids and their recycling, conservation and losses.
2. The role of essential and non-essential amino acids.
3. The role of glutamine and urea.

FURTHER READING

Bruhart, A., Jousse, C. and Fafournoux, P. (1999) Amino acid limitation regulates gene expression. *Proceedings of the Nutrition Society*, **58**, 625–32.

Crim, M.M. and Munro, H.N. (1994) Protein and amino acids. In *Modern Nutrition in Health and Disease*, 8th edn. (M.E. Shils, J.A. Olson and M. Shike) Lea and Febiger, Philadelphia, PA, pp. 3–36.

Fuller, M.F. and Garlick, P.J. (1994) Human amino acid requirements. *Annual Review of Nutrition*, **14**, 217–42.

Griffiths, R.D. (2001) The evidence for glutamine use in the critically ill. *Proceedings of the Nutrition Society*, **60**, 403–10.

Kilberg, M.S., Stevens, B.R. and Novak, D.A. (1993)

Recent advances in mammalian amino acid transport. *Annual Review of Nutrition*, **13**, 137–65.

Lacey, J.M. and Wilmore, D.W. (1990) Is glutamine a conditionally essential amino acid? *Nutrition Reviews*, **48**, 297–309.

Morris, S.M., Jr (2002) Regulation of enzymes of urea cycle and arginine metabolism. *Annual Review of Nutrition*, **22**, 87–105.

Souba, W.W. (1991) Glutamine: a key substrate for the splanchnic bed. *Annual Review of Nutrition*, **11**, 285–308.

Waterlow, J.C. (1995) Whole body protein turnover in humans – past, present and future. *Annual Review of Nutrition*, **15**, 57–92.

Waterlow, J.C. (1999) The mysteries of nitrogen balance. *Nutrition Research Review*, **12**, 25–54.

Windmueller, H.G. (1982) Glutamine utilization by the small intestine. *Advances in Enzymology*, **53**, 201–37.

38

Amino acid neurotransmitters

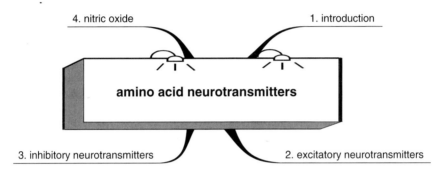

Fig. 38.1   Chapter outline.

INTRODUCTION

Nerve cells are the basic units of the nervous system, which incorporates the brain, spinal cord and nerves. Nerves in the periphery may be motor or sensory, that is, stimulating or transmitting information to organs or tissues. A nerve cell receives, conducts and transmits signals over large distances. Although nerve cells are present in a wide variety of forms, the form of the signal is always the same: changes in the electrical potential across the nerve cells' plasma membranes.

Stimuli are received in a variety of ways, including directly onto the nerve cell surface. Neuronal cells transmit from one to another via synapses (Figure 38.2). The small chemical neurotransmitters are very varied and pass from one synapse to the next at great speed. The important property of the nerve cell is its excitability. Whatever the signal, voltage-gated cation channels generate the action potentials.

An action potential is set off by a depolarisation of the plasma membrane, to a less negative value. The proteins of these channels are very similar in their amino acid structure among a wide range of species, in accordance with the evolution of these systems from quite primitive to complex organisms.

There are also guanosine triphosphate (GTP)-binding protein (G protein)-linked receptors that respond to signals evoked by neuropeptides. These are more complex and longer acting. Unlike the G protein-coupled receptors, the ligand-gated channels do not require second messenger systems for signal transduction.

Metabolically driven pumps are effective in establishing concentration differences across neuronal and glial cell membranes. Membrane gates or channels can be classified into two types, controlled by chemical molecules or ligands on transmembrane voltage. Opening and closing the gates allows ions to flow across the membrane in the direction required, creating the electrical neuronal activity.

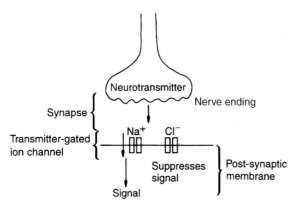

Fig. 38.2 Signals pass from one nerve ending to another at specialised sites called synapses. A presynaptic cell is separated from the post-synaptic cell. The neurotransmitter crosses the synaptic space and binds to a transmitter-gated ion channel. Opening the channel gate provokes an electrical change and a neurological signal is transmitted.

Both excitatory and inhibitory transmitters are known. Nitric oxide (NO), an important biogenic messenger with potent actions and a modulator of transmission, is less readily classified and is dealt with separately, indicating that sometimes these classifications are not clear-cut.

EXCITATORY NEUROTRANSMITTERS

The most studied is the nicotinic acetylcholine receptor. The brain also contains important excitatory amino acids, glutamate and aspartate. These are widely distributed through the spinal cord and brain and are active at concentrations of 10^{-15} M. They induce rapid membrane depolarisation, in a manner resembling nicotinic acetylcholine receptor activity.

Once aspartate and glutamate have been released into the synapse they are rapidly taken up by a high-affinity transport system in the nerve endings.

Glutamate is transformed to glutamine in the glial cells and, once in contact with the glutaminergic nerve endings, is deaminated to glutamate. A similar transport system applies to aspartate.

INHIBITORY NEUROTRANSMITTERS

These include γ-aminobutyric acid (GABA$_A$), an inhibitory transmitter in the brain, and glycine, which is effective in the spinal cord and brainstem. They operate by controlling a channel specific to small anions. The inhibitory action of GABA$_A$ is potentiated by the psychoactive drugs benzodiazepines and barbiturates. The glycine-activated channels are found on post-synaptic membranes in the brainstem and spinal cord of mammals. They are very selective for small anions, e.g. chloride, and show marked affinity for strychnine.

Most neurotransmitters use two types of receptors and neurotransmitters; GABA$_A$ and nicotinic acetylcholine act by directly opening ion channels. GABA$_A$, 5-hydroxytryptamine-1 (5-HT$_1$), 5-HT$_2$, muscarinic acetylcholine and glutamate are linked by G proteins to a variety of effector molecules, including ion channels and enzymes, that generate diffusible second messengers. Glutamate is the major excitatory neurotransmitter in the brain. In the spinal cord and brainstem glycine is the dominant inhibitory neurotransmitter, whereas in higher brain regions GABA is the dominant inhibitor.

Glutamate receptors, important in neuronal activity, exist as a diverse family of five distinct subgroups, comprising three subtypes. The GABA$_A$ receptor is the major molecular site of the inhibitory activities of the brain. The GABA$_A$ brain synapse receptor is the site of action for:

Excitatory

These open the cation channel, and an influx of Na$^+$ depolarises the post-synaptic membrane to fire an action potential:

- acetylcholine
- glutamate
- serotonin.

Inhibitory

These open the Cl$^-$ channel, keep the post-synaptic membrane polarised:

- GABA
- glycine.

Action potentials

In nerves, action potentials are produced by voltage-gated sodium channels that allow Na^+ to enter the cell along an electrochemical gradient. Another system is the Ca^{2+} channel. The membrane has an automatic inactivating system. A voltage-gated K^+ reverses the charge by an efflux of K^+, which reverses the polarity. These channels may be present in one of three forms, which reflect the energy state:

- membrane at rest: highly polarised gates closed
- membrane energy low: depolarised gate open
- membrane inactivated: inactivated.

GABA$_A$ receptors

The receptor is a heterotetrameric protein with an array of sites that span the channel. There appear to be two subunit types, α (Molecular weight 53 kDa) and β (57 kDa). The GABA sites are multimeric with α, β, γ and ρ subunits. The receptor contains a proline moiety that may give the receptors flexibility, with a bend of 20–25°, and a helix that is hydroxy rich on one side and has aliphatic side-chains on the other. The latter may interact with lipid hydrocarbon chains. Clusters of arginine and lysine molecules at the channel mouth act in both GABA$_A$ and glycine receptors as an anion-concentrating device and to increase the driving force for anion flow upon opening the channel.

- GABA agonist/antagonist
- benzodiazepine
- picrotoxin
- depressants, including the barbiturates.

NITRIC OXIDE

NO is a neurotransmitter, produced enzymatically in post-synaptic structures in response to activation of amino acid receptors. NO is derived from arginine by enzymatic removal of one of the terminal guanidino nitrogens of the amino acid L-arginine by nitrogen oxide synthase, which is found in six isoforms including endothelial, neuronal and inducible. NO synthase is found in all tissues of the brain, the highest in the cerebellum and the lowest in the medulla. The granule cell in the neurone appears to be particularly active in NO synthesis. Haemoglobin is an important antagonist of NO activity. Arginine metabolism in the brain is associated with urea metabolism. Some citrulline is formed during NO synthase activity. The brain urea cycle resynthesises arginine from the coproduct ornithine. Synthesis of NO from L-arginine can be blocked by N^G-monomethyl-L-arginine and asymmetrical dimethylarginine.

NO diffuses to act on other cellular pre-synaptic nerve endings and astrocyte receptors. The major action of NO is to activate soluble guanylate cyclase and to increase cyclic guanosine monophosphate (cGMP) levels in target cells. NO is highly reactive and an unstable free radical species, with a half-life of 4 s.

A major role of NO is to stimulate cGMP synthesis, which directly regulates cation channels and inhibits inositol phospholipid hydrolysis. Arachidonic acid and its metabolites mimic or oppose NO at the guanylate cyclase level. NO binds to the iron–sulfur centres of enzymes, e.g. those involved in the mitochondrial electron transport chain, citric cycle and DNA synthesis.

NO acts as a neurotransmitter in the brain and peripheral nervous tissues, and may be the neurotransmitter in the non-adrenergic, non-cholinergic neurotransmission system, e.g. the gastrointestinal tract. There is a possible role for NO in angiotensin and oxytocin release. In the peripheral nervous system NO regulates pain perception.

NO regulates blood flow by acting on the endothelial cells lining the vessels, binding to iron in a haem moiety attached to guanylyl cyclase, and activating the enzyme to form cGMP. This causes smooth muscle to relax. Through the action of cGMP, NO inhibits platelet aggregation and may function as an endogenous, antithrombotic agent in endothelial cells.

The delivery of NO at tissues may be by diffusion, but this seems to be a somewhat random system. It is possible that NO is transported in haemoglobin on Fe^{2+}, a conserved thiol group in haemoglobin producing S-nitroso-haemoglobin. The NO is released by passing to the plasma membrane of the red cell, to be attached to anion-exchange protein AE-1, allowing release from the red cell, usually in oxygen-deprived tissues where the NO allows vasodilatation.

KEY POINTS

1. Nerve cells, regardless of anatomy or function, signal to each other from one synapse to another using chemical neurotransmitters, thus inducing an action potential.
2. The signals are received at voltage-gated channel receptors.
3. There are both excitatory and inhibitory neurotransmitters, which include amino acids.
4. Nitric oxide, which is widely distributed throughout the body and has many functions, is a rapidly acting neurotransmitter derived enzymatically from arginine.

THINKING POINTS

1. Amino acids and peptides are important in message transmission.
2. What are the implications for nutrition of the availability of these in the diet and their effect on the mind?

NEED TO UNDERSTAND

Amino acids and their metabolites are powerful signalling agents.

FURTHER READING

Boger, R.H. and Bode-Boger, S.M. (2001) The clinical pharmacology of L-arginine. *Annual Review of Pharmacology and Toxicology*, **41**, 79–100.

Conn, P.J. and Pin, J.-P. (1997) Pharmacology and functions of metabotropic glutamate receptors. *Annual Review of Pharmacology and Toxicology*, **37**, 205–38.

Corringer, P.-J., Le Novere, N. and Changeux, J.-P. (2000) Nicotinic receptors at the amino acid level. *Annual Review of Pharmacology and Toxicology*, **40**, 431–58.

Davis, K.L., Martin, E., Turko, I.V. and Murad, F. (2001). Novel effects of nitric oxide. *Annual Review of Pharmacology and Toxicology*, **41**, 203–36.

Edmunds, B., Gibb, A.J. and Colquhon, D. (1995) Mechanisms of activation of glutamate receptors. *Annual Review of Physiology*, **57**, 495–519.

Furchgott, R.F. (ed.) Nitric oxide: special topic (1995) *Annual Review Physiology*. **57**, 659–790.

Garthwaite, J. (1991) Glutamate, nitric oxide and cell–cell signalling in the nervous system. *Trends in Neurological Sciences*, **14**, 60–7.

Gross, S.S. (2001) Vascular biology. Targetted delivery of nitric oxide. *Nature*, **409**, 577-8.

Liebman, S.W. (2001) Prions. The shape of a species barrier. *Nature*, **410**, 161–2.

Myers, S.J., Dingledine, R. and Borges, K. (1999) Genetic regulation of glutamate receptor ion channels. *Annual Review of Pharmacology and Toxicology*, **39**, 221–42.

Stuehr, D.J. (1997) Structure function aspects in the nitric oxide synthases. *Annual Review of Pharmacology and Toxicology*, **37**, 339–60.

Vallance, P. (2001) Importance of asymmetrical dimethylarginine in cardiovascular risk. *Lancet*, **358**, 2096–7.

Wu, G. and Neininger, C.J. (2002) Regulation of nitric oxide synthesis by dietary factors. *Annual Review of Nutrition* **22,** 61–86.

39

Organ metabolic fuel selection

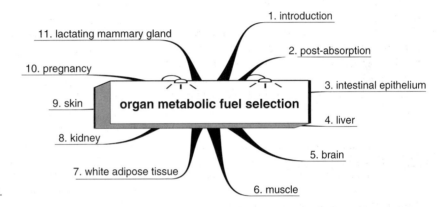

1. introduction
11. lactating mammary gland
2. post-absorption
10. pregnancy
3. intestinal epithelium
9. skin
organ metabolic fuel selection
4. liver
8. kidney
5. brain
7. white adipose tissue
6. muscle

Fig. 39.1 Chapter outline.

Table 39.1 Pathways involved in organ fuel selection

Tricarboxylic acid cycle (page 495)

Catabolism	**Anabolism**
Carbohydrates	
Glycogenolysis (page 500)	Gluconeogenesis (page 502)
Glycolysis (page 492)	Glucose alanine cycle (page 558)
Pentose phosphate shunt (page 499)	
Glycogen synthesis (page 500)	

Amino acids, proteins and nucleotides

Amino acid degradation	Protein synthesis (page 93) (page 555)
Urea cycle (page 564)	DNA and RNA synthesis (page 281)
Nucleotide synthesis (page 281)	
Hormone and neurotranmitter synthesis (page 569)	

Lipids and sterols

Fatty acid β-oxidation. (page 519)	Fatty acid synthesis (page 511)
Ketone body oxidation (page 504)	Triacyl glycerol synthesis (page 522)
Cholesterol metabolism (page 547)	Cholesterol synthesis (page 543)
	Phospholipid synthesis (page 189)

INTRODUCTION

There are differences in substrate metabolism between organs in the body, in the fasting, resting and exercising phases, all of which affect nutrient requirements. The important fuels in humans are carbohydrates (glucose, glycogen, lactate, pyruvate), the amino acid alanine, and lipids (free fatty acids, triacylglycerols) (see Tables 39.1 and 39.2). Glucose is essential for cells that are obligatory anaerobes and also for the brain.

POST-ABSORPTION

After a meal there are two responses, rapid and delayed. The rapid responses are mediated by nerve networks or hormones and the slower ones by metabolic feedback. An important determinant of nutrient delivery, absorption and release to and from a tissue is the blood supply. Various factors

Table 39.2   Total fuel use (%) in humans

	Postprandial	Overnight fast	40 days' starvation
Carbohydrate	50	12	0
Fat	33	70	95
Protein	17	18	5

From Randle in Organ Fuel Selection (1995).
Post-prandially, the brain uses half of the ingested carbohydrate, after an overnight fast 80%, and after a prolonged fast 100% of protein and carbohydrate is used by the brain.

may affect blood flow which may increase many fold post-prandially.

Another factor is solubility and hence transport in blood. A readily water-soluble nutrient, e.g. glucose, is easily transported, but transport of insoluble lipids is limited by the availability of carriers, e.g. fatty acids by albumin.

Following a meal, glucose concentrations increase three-fold; alanine, lactate and triacylglycerol ten-fold; free fatty acids, 15-fold and ketone bodies 100-fold.

INTESTINAL EPITHELIUM

Nutrients present in the intestinal lumen are selectively absorbed by the intestinal epithelium. This is associated with variable feeding patterns (time, frequency, content) and physiological conditions.

The fasting gastrointestinal tract uses some 20–25% of the body's oxygen uptake. This increases after a meal, largely through increased blood flow. This high oxygen usage is due to high protein synthesis rates and turnover of epithelial cells. Glutamine, glucose and ketones are taken up by intestinal tissues, with glutamine (35%) and ketone bodies (50%) being important oxidative substrates. In humans following a protein meal 80% of the total oxygen uptake of the jejunum is to oxidise glutamine. Glucose is not an important source of energy to the intestine.

In the colon short-chain fatty acids, especially butyric acid, are important sources of fuel. The expression of nutrient transporters controls the metabolic fuel selection by the intestinal epithelium. This will respond to intracellular messengers, e.g. cyclic adenosine monophosphate (cAMP), hormones and nutrients. Dietary fructose can increase GLUT2 expression.

LIVER

The liver is one of the largest organs in the body, weighing 1200–1500 g, about 2% of the total weight of an adult. In the infant it is proportionately larger and contributes to the baby's characteristic rotund abdomen. The liver is important in the metabolism and storage of nutrients, particularly because it is the first organ to which nutrients are exposed after absorption from the intestine.

Anatomy and blood supply

The liver has two blood supplies: the hepatic artery supplies the liver with arterial blood and the portal vein carries venous blood from the intestines and spleen. These vessels enter the liver through the lower surface of the right lobe of the liver. The hepatic artery and portal vein divide to perfuse both the right and left lobes of the liver, and are joined by the right and left hepatic bile ducts, together forming the common hepatic duct. The venous drainage from the liver is into the right and left hepatic vein and then into the inferior vena cava. Lymphatic vessels drain into glands around the coeliac axis.

The liver cells (hepatocytes) form 60% of the liver. They occupy a significant position between blood and bile, with distinct sinusoidal and canalicular membranes. They are polygonal in shape and approximately 30 μm in diameter. The hepatocyte has three surfaces, one facing the sinusoid and the space of Disse, the second facing the canaliculus, and the third facing neighbouring hepatocytes. The space of Disse is a tissue space between the hepatocytes and sinusoidal lining cells. Tight junctions between hepatocytes maintain the

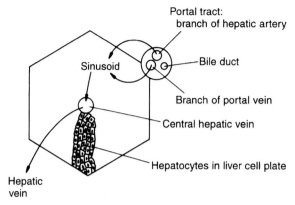

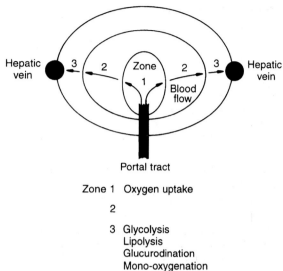

Zone 1 Oxygen uptake

 2

 3 Glycolysis
    Lipolysis
    Glucurodination
    Mono-oxygenation

Fig. 39.2 Diagrammatic representation of a hepatic lobule with a central vein and portal tracts on its periphery, separated by radially arranged hepatocyte plates and sinusoids.

Fig. 39.3 The hepatic acinus divided into zones, with the portal tract at the centre and the hepatic vein peripherally. The predominant metabolic processes in periportal and perivenous regions of the liver acinus are shown.

polarity and prevent the mixing of canalicular and sinusoidal contents.

The liver was described in terms of hepatic lobules by Kiernan in 1833. Pyramidal lobules consist of a central hepatic vein and at the periphery a portal triad containing the bile duct, portal vein radicle and hepatic artery branch (Figure 39.2). Columns of hepatocytes and blood vessels containing sinusoids separate these two systems. Hepatocytes radiate from a central vein and are interlaced by sinusoids. Liver cellular tissue is permeated by portal tracts and hepatic central canals. These run perpendicularly, are never in contact and are separated by about 0.5 mm. The sinusoids are irregularly placed, normally perpendicular to the plane of the central veins. The terminal branches of the portal vein carry blood into the sinusoids and the direction of flow is a function of the higher pressure in the portal vein than in the hepatic vein. The central hepatic canals contain branches of the hepatic veins and are surrounded by a limiting plate of liver cells, which is the interface between the portal tract and hepatic parenchyma. This is perforated by blood and lymphatic vessels and biliary radicles.

The acinus, first described by Rappaport, is the basis of a functional description of the liver, distinct from the anatomical concept of the central hepatic vein and surrounding liver cells. The liver acinus is a mass of hepatic parenchyma, dependent on blood from hepatic arterial and portal venous

branches which flows into sinusoids and drains to several veins supplying the intervening hepatic parenchyma. There is an oxygen gradient across the zone. Each acinus is centred on the portal triad (Figure 39.3). The zone next to this is zone 1, which is well oxygenated. The hepatic venules are peripheral. The periphery of the acinus adjacent to terminal hepatic veins (zone 3) has a reduced oxygen supply and, as such, is more vulnerable to injury, whether viral, toxic or anoxic.

Each efferent vein drains blood from several acini. Cells in zone 1 are nearest the portal tract and those in zone 3 farthest from the tract. Complex acini are formed from three or more simple acini, supplied by a common large portal tract, the vessels of which divide to enter the terminal portal tracts of each simple acinus.

Metabolism in the liver

The liver accounts for 20–25% of the resting energy expenditure, that is a high organ metabolic rate, some 840 kJ/kg liver/day, which contrasts with 54 kJ/kg for muscle.

The liver is the major source of protein synthesis, albumin, coagulation factors, complement factors, protein mineral carriers, e.g. caeruloplasmin and transferrin, and protease inhibitors. The liver is also a storage organ for minerals, iron, copper and vitamins, e.g. A, D and B_{12}.

The liver is involved with the dietary and endogenous sources of energy interacting with the organs that use energy. The liver is an aerobic organ, using some 2–10 µmol/g liver/min oxygen, largely for mitochondrial metabolism. In the fasting state, free fatty acids, pyruvate and amino acids are the preferred fuels for hepatic energy metabolism, which includes the synthesis of urea, gluconeogenesis, protein synthesis, Na^+/K^+-ATPase, secretion of biliary excretion products and ketogenesis. Post-prandially, amino acids and pyruvate assume importance as fuels, and carbohydrates are stored as glycogen. There is little hepatic oxidation of exogenous glucose or hepatic lipogenesis. A meal causes spanchnic vasodilatation and an increase in splanchnic blood flow.

Substrates passing from the liver act as prompters to other tissues, e.g. muscle, to activate or inhibit metabolic paths that reflect back on hepatic metabolic function. That is an interactive system throughout the body. Oxygen tension, substrate supply (free fatty acids, glucose), blood flow, hormones (insulin, glucagon, growth hormone, thyroid hormone, cortisol), autonomic factors and cytokines are determinants of liver metabolic activity.

The liver is the site of nutrient processing and distribution:

- amino acid metabolism
- citric acid cycle
- carbohydrate metabolism
- carbohydrate anabolism
- fat metabolism
- fat anabolism
- nucleotide metabolism
- oxidative phosphorylation
- protein synthesis
- detoxification mechanism and biliary excretion
- synthesis and release of prohormones and mediators
- inactivation of hormones and mediators
- storage.

Key enzymes and location in liver zones

Periportal	Perivenous
Carbohydrate metabolism	
Phosphoenolpyruvate carboxykinase	
Fructose-1,6-bisphosphate	Fructose-1,6-bisphosphate
	Glucokinase
	Pyruvate kinase
Amino acid metabolism	
Tyrosine aminotransferase	
Serine dehydrate	
Glutaminase	Glutamine synthase
Lipid metabolism	
HMG-CoA reductase	
Xenobiotic metabolism	
Cytochrome P450	

In the liver the mitochondrial enzymes in the periportal zone predominantly catalyse glucose production, oxidative energy metabolism, amino acid utilisation, urea formation, bile acid and haem metabolism.

The pericentral zone is important in glucose uptake and glutamine metabolism. This metabolic difference produces decreasing or increasing periportal to pericentral concentration gradients of glucose, amino acids, fatty acids, glycerol, ketone bodies and other nutrients. The magnitude and direction of gradients vary with the diurnal rhythm and during absorption and post-absorptive phases. The rate of enzyme synthesis, oxygen tension, and the effect of insulin and glucagon will also affect mitochondrial function. The nature of the diet, high carbohydrate, protein or fat, can alter these gradients.

The periportal zone produces ammonia which, in addition to the ammonia from the portal-drained visceral-derived blood, affects hepatic urea synthesis. Any ammonia escaping detoxification in the urea cycle is trapped in the perivenous glutamine synthetase-containing cells. Urea that comes into contact with the perivenous glutamine synthetase system is detoxified by glutamine synthesis. The liver synthesises and degrades glutamine.

The distribution of enzyme activity within the liver suggests that the periportal cells are important in oxidative respiration, with a high activity of cytochrome oxidase. The hepatocytes in the periportal area may be more active in gluconeogenesis, while those in the perivenous area may be more active in glycogenolysis. Perivenous hepatocytes contain more of the smooth endoplasmic reticulum and cytochrome P450 system, which is important in drug metabolism. Under physiological conditions hepatocytes in the periportal region are involved in bile acid transport from the sinusoids to the biliary canaliculi.

Perivenous hepatocytes may be more involved in the synthesis of bile acids. In general, the metabolic potential of many hepatocytes is not fully activated. Their activity will depend on blood flow, oxygen supply, and hormone and nutrient substrates in the blood.

This means that there is traffic across the liver of substances in varying degrees of metabolism. This may be of importance for plant chemicals, drugs and other noxious substances.

Biliary system

The excretory system of the liver is the bile canaliculi. These radicles converge to form bile ducts of increasing sized. The bile ducts amalgamate to form the common bile duct, which drains into the duodenum through the sphincter of Oddi. Bile is stored in the gallbladder so that a concentrate of bile can be mixed with the ingested meal to facilitate lipid absorption and digestion in the duodenum. Contraction of the gallbladder is subject to the control of the vagus nerve and hormones, of which cholecystokinin is probably the most important. Through this system are eliminated chemicals with a molecular weight in excess of 300–400 Da, dependent on the species. The primary or canalicular bile is modified by a mixing of ductular bile and the reabsorption of water and electrolytes passing through the biliary tree. Canalicular flow can be measured using inert markers, e.g. erythritol or mannitol, which pass unchanged through the biliary tree. In humans, canalicular flow is in the order of 450 ml/24 h. Canalicular secretion is dependent on concentration gradients derived from osmotic forces. There is active secretion and a local osmotic

pressure gradient. There are two secretion systems, each contributing half of the secretory drive:

- bile acid-dependent
- bile acid-independent, but sodium-dependent.

There is a linear relationship between biliary secretion of bile acids and bile flow, called the choleretic effect. In humans the two prime bile acids, directly derived from cholesterol, are chenodeoxycholic acid ($3\alpha,7\alpha$-di-hydroxycholanoic acid) and cholic acid ($3\alpha,7\alpha,12\alpha$-tri-hydroxycholanoic acid), which are conjugated to either taurine or glycine. Whether conjugation is principally to taurine or glycine depends on whether the diet is predominantly vegetarian (glycine) or meat (taurine) containing. The bile acids in the newborn child fed on milk are predominantly taurine conjugated. The bile acids are excreted in the bile and involved in lipid absorption through a series of steps:

- adherence to the fat emulsion
- activation of the lipase enzyme
- solubilisation of the lipids through the formation of micelles.

Following absorption of the lipid hydrolysate, the bile acids pass to the ileum to be absorbed. This is an enterohepatic circulation. Some bile acids, however, are not absorbed and pass into the colon, where they lose their amino acid conjugate and the 7-α-hydroxyl grouping, producing lithocholic acid (3-α-hydroxycholanoic acid) and deoxycholic acid (3,12-α-dihydroxy acid). These are in general excreted in the faeces, although there is some colonic absorption.

Bilirubin, the final degradation product of haemoglobin catabolism, is excreted in bile as the bilirubin glucuronide, the conjugation being catalysed by the enzyme bilirubin glucuronyltransferase. The activity of this enzyme is modest at birth, but can be a cause of perinatal jaundice. Bilirubin and other organic anions are extracted from the sinusoidal blood by binding to a protein ligand. This binding is affected by thyroxine, ethinyloestradiol and corticosteroids.

The biliary system also acts as an organ of excretion. Cholesterol is removed from the body, solubilised by bile acids. Other lipid-soluble compounds with a molecular weight of over 300 Da are excreted by this route. These include hormones such as the steroid hormones, thyroxine, xenobiotics such as antibiotics, and other drugs and dietary contaminants, e.g. dichorodiphenyltrichloroethane (DDT). These compounds may initially be oxidised, reduced or hydrolysed. They may then be made more soluble in bile through the addition of hydroxyl, carboxyl or amino groups, followed by conjugation with sulfate, glucuronic acid, or acetylation or methylation. The electrophilic, more water-soluble metabolites of lipophilic compounds, e.g. epoxides of polycyclic hydrocarbons, products of lipid peroxidation, and alkyl and aryl halides, are excreted into bile.

- Uridine diphospho-glucuronyltransferase (UDPGT) catalyses the conjugation of glucuronic acid with aglycones (phenols, alcohols, carboxylic acids, thiols and amines).
- UDPGT enzymes are microsomal membrane-bound.
- Sulfation of endogenous (including steroids and catecholamines) and foreign substances (including alcohols and hydroxylated compounds) is by substrate-specific cytosolic sulfotransferase.
- A substance may undergo both glucuronidation and sulfation, so the process is co-operative.
- Most hepatic glutathione-S-transferases are cytosolic. These catalyse the first step in mercapturic acid formation.
- Amines and hydrazines undergo acetylation, and catecholamines, amines and thiols undergo methylation.

These compounds are excreted and pass along the small intestine to the colon without being absorbed. In the colon they are exposed to the colonic bacteria. A wide range of metabolic processes takes place. Some of the metabolites are absorbed from the colon and reappear in bile. This constitutes the enterohepatic circulation, where substances may remain for a prolonged period. The non-absorbed fraction of the chemical is excreted in the faeces.

Kupffer cells and endothelial cells are in contact with the lumen of the sinusoids. These are mobile macrophages that take up particles such as old cells, tumour cells, bacteria, yeasts, viruses and parasites by endocytosis or phagocytosis.

Protein synthesis

The liver is the main site of synthesis of plasma proteins, including albumin, fibrinogen, prothrombin, other clotting factors and caeruloplasmin. The normal liver produces approximately 10 g of albumin/day, the half-life of albumin being approximately 22 days. Prothrombin has a much shorter half-life.

In healthy humans, only 15–30% of hepatocytes in the liver contain albumin, although all hepatocytes are capable of its synthesis.

BRAIN

The brain uses glucose almost exclusively for its metabolism; over half of the body's glucose utilisation is by the brain. The principal metabolism (90%) of glucose by the brain is to carbon dioxide and water, the remainder passing through the pentose phosphate pathways or undergoing glycolysis to lactate and pyruvate. There is virtually no storage of glucose in the brain, although the brain has a full capacity for metabolising the other fundamental nutrients. Of great importance is the glucose transporter system from blood across the endothelial cells of the blood–brain barrier and across the plasma membrane. The two primary glucose transporters are GLUT1 and GLUT3. GLUT1 functions in the blood–brain barrier, choroid plexus, ependyma and glia, and GLUT3 in the neuronal transport system. These must be able to function at reduced plasma glucose concentrations to keep the brain operating. Ketones and lactate may be used by the brain under severe glucose deprivation.

MUSCLE

Muscle consists of a variety of fibre types. Striated muscle can be classified as type I and type II A and B. Muscle activity depends on the utilisation and resynthesis of adenosine triphosphate (ATP) using three principal groups of substrates: phosphocreatine, muscle glycogen and blood glucose, ketones and unesterified fatty acids.

Muscle characteristics

ATP utilisation and resynthesis are crucial to muscle activity.

Type I are slow-twitch, fatigue-resistant, red fibres. They have:

- low ATPase, creatine kinase and glycolytic enzyme activity, and a phosphorylase system activation dependent on the availability of phosphorous and AMP
- high oxidative capacity, mitochondrial density, myoglobin content and capillary density
- high capacity for ATP resynthesis.

Type II are short twitch contractor fibres:

- type IIA have high oxidative capacity
- type IIB have low oxidative capacity.

Types I and II both have high myosin ATPase, high creatine kinase and anaerobic glycolysis activity as well as phosphocreatine degradation. The glycogen phosphorylase system is fully activated.

Different muscle fibres are used during different activities. In light exercise the slow twitch type I and fast twitch type IIA are used. These are highly oxidative, have a substantial mitochondrial mass and capillary bed, and use glycogen and fat as substrate. Type I fibres are depleted of glycogen first.

The active muscle mass relies on both stored fuels (glycogen and triacylglycerols) and blood-borne fuels (glucose and free fatty acids). Muscle proteins are not sources of energy. At rest only a small percentage of muscle fuel is carbohydrate, the principal fuel being non-esterified fatty acids, which continue to be important as exercise continues. With moderate exercise, plasma glucose utilisation increases to 10–30%. During sustained exercise the dependence on carbohydrates increases according to the amount of carbohydrate in the diet before the exercise and the fitness of the person. The time interval after the last meal and the amount of glycogen stored in the muscles will dictate the relative uptake from exogenous and endogenous sources of fuel. Muscle-stored glycogen can account for 60–80% of fuel in the early period of sustained activity. Fatigue and depletion of muscle glycogen are associated, and are dependent on the previous dietary content.

Intense exercise markedly reduces ATP degradation and also increases the myosin, Ca^{2+} and Na^+/K^+-ATPases. The maximum rate of ATP production for carbohydrate oxidation is twice that for fat. The time to reach maximal synthesis rate is 3 min for carbohydrates and 30 min for fat, as the release from triacylglycerols takes some time to be activated by insulin and the sympathetic nervous system. There is suppression of the muscle metabolism of carbohydrate and usage of free fatty acids and ketones if these substrates are available. This is due to:

- inhibition of the pyruvate dehydrogenase complex activity consequent on an increase in acetyl-coenzyme A (CoA) activity
- suppressed phosphofructokinase activity and glycolysis, due to accumulated citrate following lipid oxidation.

Glucose is transported into the muscle cells principally by the GLUT4 insulin-regulated transporter, where insulin-like growth factor-1 control is important. GLUT1 glucose transport is important during rest and inactivity. Even a single episode of exercise can increase the number of transporters.

Training increases the reliance of the muscle on fat rather than carbohydrates. During exercise there is increased plasma and muscle lipolysis of triacylglycerols. Physical activity in the muscle increases sensitivity to insulin action. If an untrained person undertakes a prolonged exercise schedule 20% of the muscle activity is fuelled by glucose. After 3 months of training this has fallen to 15%. Nevertheless, glucose transporters increase with training, as does the muscle mitochondrial mass and capacity to resynthesise ATP. The reliance on and rate of storage of muscle glycogen also increase. The rate of glycogenolysis and the glycogen phosphorylase system are different in the two muscle fibre types.

While protein metabolism is not a significant contributor to muscle energy expenditure and synthesis stops during exercise, amino metabolism is important and contributes to both hepatic gluconeogenesis and the citric acid cycle. Branched-chain amino acids are partially metabolised by muscle during exercise and then transported to the liver. After a meal, muscle is the major source of amino acids in the body.

WHITE ADIPOSE TISSUE

The oxygen consumption of white adipose tissue is modest, at 0.3 ml/min/kg body weight (compared with 44 for the liver and 90 for the heart). The principal energy source for white adipose tissue is glucose, using the GLUT1 transporter for basic transport and GLUT4 transporter for insulin-regulated transport.

The function of adipose tissue is to regulate the flow of energy, providing or storing fatty acid substrates as an energy source or a storage depot. The predominance of one over the other will vary post-prandially or during exercise.

Deposition of fat occurs post-prandially with increased activity of lipoprotein lipase; this catalyses the release of free fatty acids transported by chylomicrons, which are then synthesised into tri-acylglycerol, through the phosphatidic acid pathway, whereby glycerol-3-phosphate is conjugated to three fatty acids, a process stimulated by insulin. Triacylglycerol is also synthesised from lipoprotein particles, glucose and ketone bodies, and stored in adipose tissue.

When a source of energy is needed, as during fasting or starvation, the triacylglycerol is hydrolysed to glycerol and fatty acids through the activation of the hormone-effected lipase enzyme.

KIDNEY

The kidney is a small gland; it is less than 0.5% of body weight and yet receives 20–25% of the cardiac output and uses 10% of oxygen consumption. This high activity is to replenish ATP used during renal excretion. The most common substrates are glucose and lactate, although other substrates, ketone bodies, free fatty acids, citrate, glutamine and glycerol are used in significant amounts. The predominant nutritional fuel is dependent on the location in the nephron segment.

SKIN

The human skin is one of the largest organs in the body, having an average area of $1.8\,m^2$, with a pre-

dominance of keratinocytes and melanocytes in the epidermis, the outer layer. These are active cells turning over every 10 days and using all the essential nutrients that pass from the basal membrane by diffusion or active transport.

PREGNANCY

During the growth of the newly fertilised ovum, up to the time of birth there is a series of metabolic changes and reliance on varying fuel sources.

The newly fertilised ovum is a small, intensely active cell mass using pyruvate, glutamine and lactate as fuel, glucose being a minor contributor. Once cellular differentiation starts, glucose increases in importance, to become essential as a fuel. The early dependence on the pentose phosphate shunt means that glucose-6-phosphate dehydrogenase, the rate-limiting enzyme, becomes especially relevant. This is because this enzyme is encoded on the X chromosome and therefore is doubly represented in the female. There are differences in fuel consumption between the male and female embryo.

The diverse interspecies differences in energy consumption during pregnancy are in part the result of maternal size, length of gestation, size of the offspring at birth and the amount of energy stored in the offspring. In humans the enthalpy of combustion is 8–9 MJ/kg birth weight, double that of the rat. There is a considerable energy expenditure in the development of the baby from conception, which has been estimated at 132 kJ/kg birth weight/day. This is not a uniform rate of consumption of energy during pregnancy, but increases substantially at the end of pregnancy. The distribution of energy consumption between the placenta and foetus varies during pregnancy. The uteroplacental tissues are significant metabolic organs, even as their role declines towards the time of birth. The growth of the placenta is important in determining birth weight, so smoking, which retards placental growth, also retards the baby's growth.

LACTATING MAMMARY GLAND

The mammary gland is not only a secretory gland

with a high metabolic rate but also, by virtue of that secretory activity, a prime exporter of energy from the mother and thus a drain on maternal energy and metabolism. During lactation food intake, intestinal, liver and mammary gland weight all increase. The important substrates for the mammary gland are amino acids, glucose and triacylglycerol. Insulin stimulates lipid synthesis from glucose, lipoprotein lipase activity and the uptake of plasma triacylglycerols. ATP is required in substantial amounts, largely for protein and lactose synthesis and the uptake of plasma triacylglycerol.

KEY POINTS

1. The fuel requirements of the organs of the body vary with the demands on the organ, e.g. metabolism, exercise, excretion or thinking.

2. The intestine is very active metabolically and activity increases after a meal. The resulting increased blood flow uses some 20–25% of the body's oxygen uptake. This high oxygen usage is accompanied by high protein synthesis rates and turnover of epithelial cells. Glutamine, glucose and ketones are taken up by intestinal tissues as important oxidative substrates. In the colon, short-chain fatty acids, especially butyric acid, are important sources of fuel.

3. The liver is important in the metabolism and storage of nutrients, and is the first organ after the intestine to which absorbed nutrients are exposed.

4. The acinus is the anatomical unit of the liver; it depends on blood from the hepatic arterial and portal venous branches, drains into the hepatic vein and secretes into the lymph and bile duct. There is an oxygen gradient from zone 1 next to the portal triad to the periphery of the acinus next to terminal hepatic veins (zone 3); this has a reduced oxygen supply and consequently is more vulnerable to injury, whether viral, toxic or anoxic.

5. The liver contains a multitude of enzymes, sited within the liver structure in a manner that reflects metabolic needs. The periportal zone mitochondrial enzymes predominantly catalyse glucose production, oxidative energy metabolism, amino acid utilisation, urea formation, bile acid and haem metabolism. The pericentral zone is important in glucose uptake and glutamine metabolism. The excretory system of the liver for chemicals, e.g. bile acids, cholesterol, bilirubin, glucuronide, hormones and drugs, is the bile canaliculi. Bile is also an important contributor to the digestion of fat in the duodenum. The liver is the main site of synthesis of plasma proteins, including albumin, fibrinogen, prothrombin, other clotting factors and caeruloplasmin.

6. The brain uses glucose almost exclusively for its metabolism; over half of the body's glucose utilisation is by the brain. The principal metabolism (90%) of glucose by the brain is to carbon dioxide and water, the remainder passing through the pentose phosphate pathways or undergoing glycolysis to lactate and pyruvate.

7. Muscle consists of a variety of fibre types, type I and type II A and B. ATP utilisation and resynthesis are crucial to muscle activity. The principal substrates for this action are phosphocreatine, muscle glycogen and blood glucose, ketones and unesterified fatty acids.

8. At rest the principal fuel is non-esterified fatty acids, which continue to be important during exercise. With moderate exercise plasma glucose utilisation increases to 10–30%. During sustained exercise the dependence on carbohydrates increases according to the amount of carbohydrate in the diet before the exercise and the fitness of the person. The time interval after the last meal and the amount of glycogen stored in the muscles will dictate the relative uptake from exogenous and endogenous sources of fuel.

9. The kidney is less than 0.5% of body weight, receives 20–25% of the cardiac output and uses 10% of oxygen consumption. This high activity is to replenish ATP used during renal excretory activity. The most common substrates are glucose and lactate, although other substrates, ketone bodies, free fatty acids, citrate, glutamine and glycerol, are used in significant amounts.

10. The highly active skin tissue has no critical energy source.

11. During pregnancy the ovum grows into the foetus and the size of the supportive placenta is

very important. The energy requirements alter with the stage of development of the foetus.

12. During lactation the mammary gland is very active, converting glucose triacylglycerols and amino acids into milk constituents for export from the mother.

THINKING POINTS

1. An ingested meal is subject to a series of stripping-down and allocation processes.
2. The metabolism of nutrients is very much dictated by the organ to which the nutrient is directed.

NEED TO UNDERSTAND

1. When a meal is eaten the disposition of the different nutrients is dictated by the individual needs of different organs.

2. Liver function will alter across the acinus.
3. The fuel needs of the other organs will differ with the activity of the organ, whether this be lactation, exercise, illness or thought.

FURTHER READING

Jungermann, K. and Kietzmann, T. (1996) Zonation of parenchymal and nonparenchymal metabolism in the liver. *Annual Review of Nutrition*, **16**, 179–204.

McGee, J. O'D. (1992) Normal liver: structure and function. In *Oxford Textbook of Pathology* (eds J.O'D. McGee, P.G. Issaacson and N.A. Wright). Oxford University Press, Oxford, pp. 1287–426.

Sherlock, S. and Dooley, J. (2001) *Diseases of the Liver and Biliary System*, 11th edn. Blackwell Scientific Publications, Oxford.

Symposium on Organ Fuel Selection (1995) *Proceedings of the Nutrition Society*, **54**, 125-327.

40

Growth

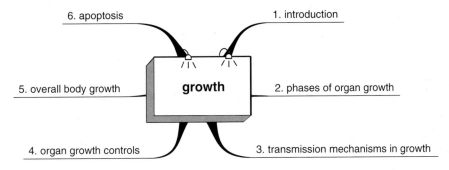

Fig. 40.1 Chapter outline.

INTRODUCTION

The science of nutrition aims to define the overall quantity of nutrients and individual nutrients required by the human population.

Humans deal uniformly badly with deficiency, whether this be in the very short term (oxygen), the short term (water) or longer term (food). Survival times depend on body stores at the onset of deprivation. The consequence of a deficiency of single or several nutrients from the diet may be lethal over a period of time.

Modern Western populations are faced with an excess of food. This may lead to an overgenerous intake of nutrients. The manner in which each individual deals with this is in part dependent on their genetic and isoenzymic constitution. The basal metabolic rate and level of physical activity are also important. The excess intake may be in all nutrients or be confined to a few specific nutrients. The stage of life and health status are also important.

Growth is frequently used as a non-specific term to describe the changes associated with the development of form and function. Growth may readily be measured as length, weight and chemical composition. By such measurements, normal and abnormal growth can be identified.

Growth requires nutrients to be directed towards energy storage, cell multiplication and skeletal utilisation. These metabolic fuels are co-ordinated in their role in growth by systemic and local regulatory factors. Growth includes:

- whole body growth
- individual organ growth
- cellular growth and replication
- tissue turnover and repair
- cell death (apoptosis).

These overlap and are all involved in the achievement of functional maturity. The amount of dietary energy and protein necessary for growth varies between species, and is influenced by the time taken for the growth phase. Differences between species and the genetically determined rate of proliferation influence cell number and body mass.

Hypertrophy is the reversible increase in the size of a cell through the accumulation of more structural components. *Hyperplasia* is an increase in the number of cells in a tissue or organ, and an increase in organ size.

Maternal nutrient supply to the foetus in the latter part of gestation affects the rate of growth and the composition of the infant. Hypertrophy becomes more significant in the more mature foetus, as does the differential growth of different cells, tissue and body protein mass and organs.

The increase in weight from birth to adult maturity is determined by the proportion of the lifespan spent in maturation and growth. The development of reproductive maturity usually means the end of growth. Humans are somewhat different from other mammals in that body weight increases 15-fold from the birth weight. Protein deposition continues for a quarter of the time between birth and death.

Example of the phases of organ growth

In the development of skeletal muscle, which is derived from a population of myoblasts, the formation of cells involves transcriptional activation. Two genes, *myd* (myogenic determination gene) and *MyoD*$_\lambda$ (myoblast determination gene number 1), are activated sequentially at the beginning of muscle growth.

Skeletal muscle differentiation
Cell differentiation continues after the withdrawal of the myoblast nuclei from the cell cycle. The cells differentiate into multinucleated myotubes. Protein products of the differential genes are important in such change, along with promotor-enhancer regions of other genes, e.g. muscle type creatine kinase and α-actin. In the foetus, interactions between fibroblasts, myotubes and growing skeleton lead to the formation of tendon attachments. At birth the skeletal muscles are close to completing the primary stages of differentiation. The muscle then develops into three myosin fibre types. The maturing motor sensory system innervates the muscle to produce externally regulated contractions.

PHASES OF ORGAN GROWTH

There are three phases of organ growth.

1. Formation of the endodermal, ectodermal and mesodermal layers; these cell lines are then committed to a specific lineage of cell specialisation and structure.
2. Differentiation of cell lines into primary differential states.
3. Maturation to full physiological and metabolic function.

TRANSMISSION MECHANISMS IN GROWTH

Communications between cells are important for co-ordinated behaviour in multicellular organisms. There are numerous signalling molecules. Some regulators, e.g. steroids, retinoids and thyroid hormones, circulate in the blood and act on distant targets. They pass through the plasma membrane and interact with cytoplasmic receptor molecules. The vast majority of extracellular signals, e.g. neurotransmitters, nucleotides, leukotrienes, peptides and prostaglandins, act in a localised manner. These molecules act by combining with specific cell-surface receptors.

Insulin-like growth factor (IGF) resembles insulin in hormone structure, receptor structure and action. There are two IGFs, named 1 and 2. The concentration of IGF-1 is low in infants and increases in adults. The gene for IGF-1 is located on chromosome 12, while that for IGF-2 is on chromosome 11. Both are a single chain of amino acids with interchain disulfide bridges connected by a C-peptide and a terminal D extension. Both IGFs stimulate the multiplication of a wide variety of cells, and promote processes related to energy storage. These include amino acid and protein synthesis in muscle, and fatty acid synthesis in the liver. They stimulate processes that are important in skeletal elongation, including synthesis of RNA, DNA, protein and proteoglycan in chondrocytes and cartilage. IGF-2 is important in foetal life, whereas circulating and tissue concentrations are low in the adult except in the brain. IGF-2 may act as a neurotransmitter.

Binding of IGF-1 to its receptor activates a whole cascade of cellular events, including phosphoinositide-derived messenger molecules. This affects glucose transport and the phosphorylation of substrate proteins that mediate slower processes, e.g. the activation and inactivation of genes. IGF-1 may also activate phospholipase C, which hydrolyses cellular membrane phosphoinositides that are important in phosphate energy metabolism. IGF-1 may, through phosphorylation, be involved in the activation of transcription. This acts in the formation of messenger RNA (mRNA), movement of mRNA to the cytosol, ribosomal translation of mRNA, synthesis of protein and intracellular processing of protein, including glycosylation.

Synthesis of IGF-1 in the liver is a switch mechanism that results in the utilisation of nutrients for growth. IGF-1 may amplify the action of endocrine hormones. The level of dietary protein is important in sustaining circulating IGF-1. There is also local production of IGF-1 by many tissues.

Peptide regulatory factor (PRF) has a low molecular weight (< 80 kDa) and a short or intermediate range of action, is very specific and has a high affinity for cell-surface receptors. The peptide also has the ability to affect cellular differentiation and proliferation. Peptide regulatory factor acts locally on adjacent cells or on the secreting cell. The PRF is often glycosylated, and the glycosylated form has an equivalent action to the free form, e.g. granulocyte macrophage colony-stimulating factor. Free forms of erythopoietin do not act equally with the glycosylated form. The free form of follicle-stimulating hormone acts as an antagonist or antihormone to the glycosylated form. PRF is now identified as a group of multifunctional molecules with a range of biological effects.

Transforming growth factor (TGF) was originally described as being capable of inducing phenotypic transformation of untransformed cell lines. TGF-α is now known to be expressed during embryonic development and in adult pituitary cells, epithelial cells and macrophages.

PRF binds to specific high-affinity cell-surface receptors, with the following effects.

- A post-receptor signalling mechanism alters the pattern of gene expression.

- Ligand–receptor complexes are internalised and increase activity or affect down-regulation that may act as a negative feedback loop.

The effect of a particular PRF on a single cell type is not necessarily the same on all occasions. The effect depends on the background set by other signalling molecules, which communicate by a signalling language read by the cell.

Some PRFs may down-regulate other unrelated receptors; this is called *transmodulation*. A cascade of PRF may amplify the original stimulus or lead to a feedback inhibition of the primary mediator. The mechanism is partially understood for muscle contraction and glycogen metabolism. The main regulatory mechanism is through the phosphorylation and dephosphorylation of proteins. The initial transmembrane signalling process is transmitted to long-term patterns of gene expression. This regulation leads to cell proliferation and differentiation.

Phosphorylation of tyrosine residues on proteins is less frequently the control mechanism on the protein than the phosphorylation of serine or threonine. This means that in the regulation of enzymes, phosphorylation of only a limited fraction of the total molecule may significantly change the catalytic activity and so initiate a regulatory cascade.

One signalling pathway in the regulation of cell growth is hydrolysis of the membrane lipid phosphatidylinositol-4,5-bisphosphate, a lipid kinase that phosphorylates phosphatidylinositol.

Serine kinase is a cell cycle regulator and is essential at stage G_1, at the start of the cell cycle and/or the entry of cells into mitosis. Phosphorylation of the tyrosine residues of the enzyme results in increased protein kinase activity, reaching a maximum as cells progress from S phase towards mitosis.

Some receptors transmit their signals through guasonine triphosphate (GTP)-dependent coupling,

Hormonal activation of cyclic adenosine monophosphate (cAMP) formation involves the sequential action of three proteins:

- a receptor
- a guanine nucleotide-dependent coupling protein: G protein, α, β and γ
- adenylate cyclase.

e.g. control of cyclic guanosine monophosphate (GMP) phosphodiesterase, phospholipase A_2 and membrane channels.

The receptor is a transmembrane glycoprotein in which a conformational change takes place when it is bound to hormone. This is transmitted through the receptor protein to the signalling domain. This system can transmit a large amount of information to the cell during regulation. Each stimulus has its own receptor, but the receptors respond to each other. All receptors that interact with G proteins have a common amino acid pattern. Each domain represents one transit of the folded polypeptide chain through the plasma membrane.

ORGAN GROWTH CONTROLS

Increased physiological activity leads to organ enlargement, while disuse leads to atrophy. Trophic hormones are secreted when physiological demand is increased. These stimulate target organs to greater functional activity, and trigger cell hypertrophy and hyperplasia. Some organs react to the physiological demands to which they are committed. The parathyroid hormone responds directly to serum calcium, islets of Langerhans to plasma glucose, and zona glomerulosa of the adrenal cortex to sodium. Skeletal muscle and bone similarly respond to need. Other organs, e.g. the liver, are very complex in the regulatory mechanisms of growth.

Differences in growth control

There are differences in growth control between somatic and visceral organs and tissues. Somatic tissues, muscle, heart, blood vessels, bone, skin and connective tissue, undertake the mechanical functions of the body. Their growth is controlled locally. Visceral organ growth is regulated by other systemic hormonal and nutritional influences.

OVERALL BODY GROWTH

Growth is only possible if energy intake exceeds energy expenditure. Waterlow (1961) showed that the rate of weight gain depends more on the intake of calories than on that of protein (within a range of 100–200 kcal/kg/day and protein intake of 2–7 g/kg/day; in children, 150 kcal/kg/day and a protein intake of 3–4 g/kg/day is adequate). The requirement for weight gain is less in adults. Weight gain of lean tissue is quite different to weight gain of adipose tissue.

Body and tissue chemical composition

As the organ and body mass increase during development, so the hydration of the body decreases. The distribution of water through the tissues alters, with more being found in intracellular compartments. The nitrogen:weight ratio is a measure of relative chemical maturity. As maturity approaches, the protein deposition slows and fat storage increases in importance. Fat stores require little accompanying deposition of water.

Height

There are many important factors affecting height, which include ethnic, genetic, dietary and environmental aspects. The male, on average, is taller than the female (Table 40.1). What is not known is whether the achievement of maximal height is healthy. Do maximum height and maximum growth make for longevity? Do such realisation of potential affect the propensity to obesity, hypertension, diabetes, coronary artery disease and diet-related cancers? It has been shown that energy restriction of as little as 10% subsequently reduces tumour incidence in rodents. Short stature due to malnutrition or illness is undesirable, but this does not mean that feeding children for maximum growth and physical development is advantageous to health and longevity.

Table 40.1 Average height and weight of early and modern humans

	Height (cm)		Weight (kg)	
	Male	Female	Male	Female
Homo sapiens	175	135	65	54
Neanderthal	165	155	84	80
Homo erectus	178	135	63	53
Homo habilis	163	117	37	32

Source: National Geographical Society, 1997.

- Aspects of biology vary with size.
- Larger animals grow more slowly, have slower heart rates, live at a slower pace and live longer.
- An animal's metabolic rate is proportional to body mass$^{3/4}$.

Growth and function

Throughout life, organs respond to the needs of the body in relation to environment and workload. Both hyperplasia and hypertrophy are stimulated. The heart and liver are relatively large in relation to total body protein cell mass at birth than at later stages of development. The intestine and skeletal muscle grow more after birth than *in utero*. The long bones appear to reach a genetically determined length irrespective of growth in other organs.

Growth regulation is divided between genetic–temporal and functional aspects. During foetal life, protein disposition is less sensitive to maternal nutritional deprivation than after birth and lactation. At weaning, when the change to an adult gene expression is virtually complete, organ growth, e.g. muscle, is very sensitive to undernutrition.

From ancient times it has been believed that the span of the arms and the height of a normal man are equal. Vitruvius, the Roman architect, claimed that the perfect proportion of a man was for his span and height to fit within a square or a circle. Such human proportions were central to the artistic and architectural traditions of classical art. Height is greater than span before the age of 4 years, they are equal at 4 years, and the span is greater than height thereafter. This is the case in two-thirds of Caucasian adults. Another example of functional value is the belief that the child is ready to go to school when able to touch the left ear by placing the right arm over the head.

The child who is not growing to expected potential is identified from the use of percentiles with a height measurement at school entry or height and weight charts over a defined period of months or years. The 90th percentile of the distribution for a population, e.g. height, intelligence quotient (IQ) or weight, is the value that 90% of individuals fall short of and only 10% exceed. The 10th percentile is the opposite. The rate of growth is a very useful measurement. In France it is a public health obligation and in some communities the children are measured annually against the wall. Reduced growth can occur for social and economic reasons, or due to familial trends, malnutrition, chronic inflammatory disease, renal insufficiency, cardiac causes and endocrine insufficiency. Pituitary-induced growth hormone deficiency can be treated by recombinant DNA-produced hormone.

Catch-up growth

This is accelerated weight gain. During recovery from an illness inhibiting growth, the child may to some extent catch up the deficient growth, depending on their age and the length of the illness. The earlier in life and the shorter the illness the better. The rate of weight gain may reach 20 times the uncomplicated growth of children of similar age, and starts some 1–3 months after beginning treatment for the underlying problem. In this catch-up period, the diet must be complete, as nutritional deficiencies, single or multiple, will impose a restriction on growth.

Catch-up growth is primarily seen in three groups:

- preterm infants, in whom the aim is to achieve rates of growth similar to those that would normally have occurred *in utero*
- children recovering from severe undernutrition and illness
- adults recovering from the stress of trauma, infection or surgery.

The diet for catch-up growth varies with the needs of the depleted tissue. There is relative preservation of visceral tissue at the expense of muscle and adipose tissue.

Immature animals seek to obtain and use nutrients to enable a rate of protein deposition to achieve maximum growth. After birth the rate of protein development will depend on the quantity and biological quality of dietary essential amino acids and proteins. These enable the genetic programme to be performed.

There is a series of genetically and developmentally regulated priorities for growth. Nutrition is important in the achievement of the genetic potential of the body as a whole and for individual organs. Nutritional deprivation depletes the body

Hormones and growth

Farm animals can be made to grow faster and with more lean meat content with the use of oestrogenic hormones, oestradiol benzoate and progesterone or testosterone. These increase growth rate by 8–15% and feed conversion by 5–10%. Hormonal implants include testosterone analogues and oestrogenic-like substances. The animals have to be adequately fed to achieve the full benefits of the treatment. Such stimulant effects of hormones have also achieved publicity when used by sportsmen and women.

initially of fat, and then of protein. These differences are reflected in changes in the intracellular and extracellular water spaces.

Total body water is used to measure lean tissue mass. During the early phase of rapid weight gain there is a disproportionate increase in body hydration, which returns to normal once recovery is established.

Some amino acids, are claimed to increase growth hormone secretion, e.g. oral ornithine which is believed to be twice as effective as oral arginine.

APOPTOSIS

Apoptosis is a co-ordinated, programmed, genetically regulated form of cell death. A multicellular organism must sustain equal rates of cell generation and cell death to maintain a constant size. Senescent, damaged or abnormal cells that could interfere with organ function must be removed. Physiological cell death is not a random process. Apoptosis is important in organ atrophy and during disease with a decrease in cell numbers. Apoptosis is a rapid process that is directed towards scattered individual cells rather than all the cells in a particular area. It occurs during embryogenesis in the process of tissue turnover and after withdrawal of a trophic hormone from its target tissue. Apoptosis is a mechanism whereby organs and digits in the hand and foot are sculptured out in the evolving foetus.

In the adult some 10 billion cells die each day to balance new production. An example of apoptosis in the adult is a shedding of intestinal cells. Apoptosis may be important in autoimmune disease, degenerative diseases and ageing. The decline in body cell mass with age is probably controlled genetically, as it is related to lifespan.

Early in apoptosis the distinct morphological features include compaction of chromatin against the nuclear membrane, cell shrinkage and preservation of organelles, detachment from surrounding cells, and nuclear and cytoplasmic budding to form membrane-bound fragments (apoptotic bodies). These are rapidly removed by adjacent parenchymal cells or macrophages.

There are three phases to apoptosis.

1. **Initiation**: this can be by noxious agents, e.g. drugs or irradiation, or reduced exposure to interleukin-1 and other cytokines.
2. **Gene expression**: the gene families studied include the *bcl-2* family of 20 or more proapoptotic and antiapoptotic genes. Another antiapoptotic gene is the tumour suppressor gene *p53* (see Colonic cancer section, Chapter 47).
3. **Enzyme phase**: central to the process of apoptosis is the protein-cleaving enzyme family, the caspases (CED-3/ICE family). These are normally inactive until they become active under stimulus, and begin to cleave a cascade of enzymes in the cell.

The initiation of the process of cleaving proteins leads to active enzymes that kill the cell quickly and effectively, attacking the nuclear membrane, the cell DNA and the cell skeleton. Early in the process, a negatively charged phospholipid phosphatidyl serine moves from the inner surface of the cell to the outside, announcing the imminent death of the cell.

Apoptosis is induced through various routes, but they originate from two different signalling routes. One is external on the cell membrane. The other, of internal origin on the mitochondrial surface, follows the release of cytochrome *c* and the cell death pathway continues with an adapter molecule, Apaf-1. Once started, the caspase cascade sets off, with cell death the outcome. The external stimulants to this process may well be varied and tissue dependent. For example, the gastric bacterium *Helicobacter pylori* may affect apoptosis in the gastric mucosa, whereas butyrate, the short-chain fatty acid resulting from colonic bacterial breakdown may influence colonic mucosal cell apoptosis.

The overriding of the controls and initiators of apoptosis has profound consequences for our understanding of the malignant cell process.

KEY POINTS

1. Growth is an increase in weight, height, and composition of body organs, cells and tissue repair. It requires appropriate nutrient intake of energy and protein.
2. Hypertrophy is a reversible increase in cell size. Hyperplasia is an increase in the number of cells. Organ growth is in three phases: the development of cell lines, differentiation and maturation to mature function.
3. Growth at the cellular and organ level is a co-ordinated process, controlled by various specific signalling molecules, many of which are hormones. The growth process at maturity is in response to need. Disuse leads to atrophy.
4. Growth is only possible if energy intake exceeds expenditure. Height is dependent on gender and ethnic, genetic, dietary and environmental factors.
5. Catch-up growth requires sufficient nutritional intake, including high-quality protein and energy content. This growth spurt is seen in children who, following failure to achieve their age growth norms, are subsequently well.
6. A multicellular organism must balance cell generation and cell death to maintain a constant size. Senescent, damaged or abnormal cells are removed. Physiological cell death, apoptosis, is directed towards scattered individual cells rather than all the cells in a particular area.

THINKING POINT

Growth, where the balance between the genetic, environmental and dietary intake is ideal, is unlimited, but is controlled in part by apoptosis.

NEED TO UNDERSTAND

1. The relationship between cell, tissue and organ growth to make the coherent form of the individual, and the important role of nutrition in that process.
2. Hormones and apoptosis keep growth under control.

FURTHER READING

Ashworth, A. and Millward, D.J. (1986) Catch up growth in children. *Nutrition Reviews*, **44**, 157–63.

Burns, H.J. (1990) Growth promotors in humans. *Proceedings of the Nutrition Society*, **49**, 467–72.

Carson, D.A. and Ribeiro, J.N. (1993) Apoptosis and disease. *Lancet*, **341**, 1251–4.

Carter-Su, C., Schwarz, J. and Smit, L.S. (1996) Molecular mechanism of growth hormone action. *Annual Review of Physiology*, **58**, 187–208.

Cole, T.J. (2000) Secular trends in growth. *Proceedings of the Nutrition Society*, **59**, 317–24.

Cryer, A., Williams, S.E. and Cryer, J. (1992) Dietary and other factors involved in the proliferation, determination and differentiation of adipocyte precursor cells. *Proceedings of the Nutrition Society*, **51**, 379–85.

Dauncey, M.J., White, P., Burton, K.A. and Katsumata, M. (2001) Nutrition–hormone receptor–gene interactions: implications for development and disease. *Proceedings of the Nutrition Society*, **60**. 63–72.

Freeman, M. (2000) Feedback control of intercellular signalling in development *Nature*, **408**, 313–8.

Goss, R.J. (1990) Similarities and differences between mechanisms of organ and tissue growth regulation. *Proceedings of the Nutrition Society*, **49**, 437–42.

Jackson, A.A. (1990) Protein requirements for catch-up growth. *Proceedings of the Nutrition Society*, **49**, 507–16.

Koletzko, B., Aggett, P.J., Bindels, J.G. *et al.* (1998) Growth, development and differentiation: a functional food science approach. *British Journal of Nutrition*, **80**, (Suppl. 1), S5–45.

Loveridge, N., Farquharson, C. and Scheven, B.A.A. (1990) Endogenous mediators of growth. *Proceedings of the Nutrition Society*, **49**, 443–50.

Mathers, J.C. (1998) Nutrient regulation of intestinal proliferation and apoptosis. *Proceedings of the Nutrition Society*, **57**, 219–23.

National Geographic Society (1997) Poste: Seeking our origins. Washington, DC.

Nicholson, D.W. (2001) Baiting death inhibitors. *Nature*, **410**, 33–4.

Phillips, L.S., Harp, J.B., Goldstein, S. *et al.* (1990) Regulation and action of insulin-like growth factors at the cellular level. *Proceedings of the Nutrition Society*, **49**, 451–8.

Reeds, P.J. and Fiorotto, M.L. (1990) Growth in perspective. *Proceedings of the Nutrition Society*, **49**, 411–20.

Renehan, A.G., Booth, C. and Potten, C.S. (2001) What is apoptosis, and why is it important? *British Medical Journal*, **322**, 1536–8.

Schott, G.D. (1992) The extent of man from Vitruvius to Marfan. *Lancet*, **340**, 1518–20.

Shirin, H. and Moss, S.F. (1998) *Helicobacter pylori* induced apoptosis. *Gut*, **43**, 592–4.

Strasser, A., O'Connor, L. and Dixit, V.M. (2000) Apoptosis signalling. *Annual Review of Biochemistry*, **69**, 217–45.

Thompson, E.B. (ed.) (1998) Apoptosis. *Annual Review of Physiology*, **60**, 525–666.

Walker, A.R.P, Walker, B.F, Glatthaar, I.I. and Vorster, H.H. (1994) Maximum genetic potential for adult stature that is aimed as desirable. *Nutrition Review*, **52**, 208–15.

Waterlow, J.C. (1961) The rate of recovery of malnourished infants in relation to the protein and calorie levels of the diet. *Journal of Tropical Pediatrics*, **7**, 16–22.

Watson, W.H., Cai, J. and Jones, D.P. (2000) Diet and apoptosis. *Annual Review of Nutrition*, **20**, 342–4.

Whitfield, J. (2001) All creatures great and small. *Nature*, **413**, 342–4.

41

Bone

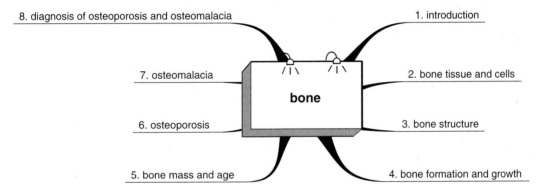

8. diagnosis of osteoporosis and osteomalacia

7. osteomalacia

6. osteoporosis

5. bone mass and age

bone

1. introduction

2. bone tissue and cells

3. bone structure

4. bone formation and growth

Fig. 41.1 Chapter outline.

INTRODUCTION

The skeleton provides scaffolding which enables a mobile terrestrial life. The skeleton consists of bones, joints, tendon sheaths and fascia. The bony skeleton forms the firm attachment for tendons on which muscles pull for movement. Bones consist of 35% mineral salts (largely calcium and phosphorus), 20% organic matter (mostly collagen) and 45% water; 99% of the body calcium and two-thirds of the body magnesium is found in bone.

- The vertebrae support the whole body.
- The long bones of the limbs, humerus, radius, ulna, tibia, fibula and femur, support muscles of movement and give height to the individual; their shape is designed for an upright stance.

Every bone will have some role in each of these functions, but some will be more conspicuous in a particular function than others.

Almost all bones have joints. In the long bones these are at either end. The bones of the wrist and ankle are small and are largely articular surfaces. Some bones, e.g. the scapula, have only one articular surface. The protective function of the bones is best illustrated by the pelvis, skull, vertebrae, sternum and ribs. The pelvic bones protect the ovaries, uterus, bladder and rectosigmoid region of the colon. The skull and vertebrae protect the brain and spinal column, and the sternum and ribs protect the heart and lungs. Each bone has a blood supply, which has a nutrient role A long bone (Figure 41.2) consists of:

- a shaft or **diaphysis**
- an **epiphysis**: the end of the bone, including the articular surface
- a **metaphysis**: a functional zone between the diaphysis and the epiphysis
- an **epiphyseal plate**: cartilage between the epiphysis and the metaphysis; which is important in growing bone.

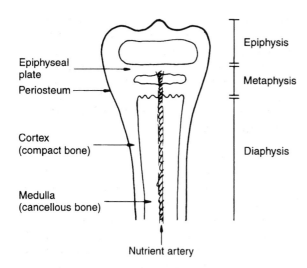

Fig. 41.2 Cross-section through the head of a long bone. The structure is cartilage early in life, which is later replaced by bone. Osteoclasts erode cartilage and bone matrix; osteoblasts secrete bone matrix.

BONE TISSUE AND CELLS

Bone consists of three layers (Figure 41.2):

- **periosteum**: a fibrous membrane covering the bone
- **cortex**: the hard sheath of compact bone
- **medulla**: contains the marrow and spongy (cancellous) bone.

Microscopic structure of bone

Mature bone
In both compact and cancellous bone the structure is formed of lamellar bone plates. Type I collagen fibres are arranged in parallel sheets (lamellae). In cortical bone the lamellae are wrapped around the blood vessels in a concentric manner. These cylinders (Haversian systems or osteons) lie in the long axis of the bone. Between each osteon are interstitial lamellae. Cancellous bone is made of lamellar bone separated by cement lines.

In immature bone, growing bone, repaired fracture and pathological conditions, woven or immature bone is found. There is random packing of the collagen and the matrix is rich in ground substance.

This woven bone is not strong and is replaced by lamellar bone.

Bone cells
There are three types of bone cell.

- **Osteoblasts** line the external surface of the bony trabeculae, the inner aspect of the periosteum and the surface of bone lining the osteons. They produce collagen and proteins forming the organic bone matrix, and deposit and remove calcium.
- **Osteocytes** are osteoblasts trapped in mature bone, which cannot synthesise protein but have a role in mature bone maintenance and are the sensors for changes in mechanical demand.
- **Osteoclasts** are responsible for bone resorption.

BONE STRUCTURE

Bone is an inorganic–bioorganic composite material made of collagen proteins and hydroxy apatite, $(Ca_{10}(PO_4)_6(OH_2))$, which is a crystalline form of calcium phosphate, and a ground substance of glycoproteins and proteoglycans, in the form of lamellae and a mineral matrix of calcium hydroxyapatites deposited on the protein collagen matrix, which give bone its rigidity. The organic lamellae are 90% collagen (largely type I) produced by the osteoblasts. The synthesis of collagen is under the control of several genes. Collagen undergoes a series of post-translational modifications before being deposited in the growing bone, and there is calcification between the collagen molecules. Bone contains other proteins, phosphoproteins and lipids. Many of the trace elements (zinc, manganese and copper) are required for the growth, development and maintenance of healthy bone. Lead and cadmium have a toxic effect on bone. Fluoride increases bone density in advanced osteoporosis. Fluorine readily substitutes for the hydroxyl ion in bone hydroxyapatite, creating a less acid-soluble, more stable crystal. Fluorine does not diffuse into bone, but may be incorporated during growth. Hydroxyapatite crystals run parallel to collagen fibres in bone, whereas fluoroapatite crystals run perpendicularly to the fibres. Fluoride increases osteoblast number and bone formation.

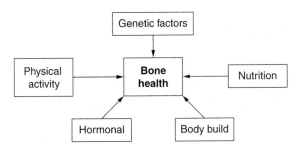

Fig. 41.3 Modifiable and non-modifiable factors influencing bone health. (With kind permission of Dr Susan New and the Nutrition Society.)

Cortical compact bone, which is thick, dense, calcified (80%) tissue, comprises the outer layer of bone. Trabecular (cancellous) bone is spongy and is a lattice of thin, calcified (15–25%) trabeculae. The spaces in trabecular bone are filled with haemopoietic bone marrow.

BONE FORMATION AND GROWTH

Bone is a dynamic tissue in a continuous process of formation and resorption, activities accomplished by osteoblasts and osteoclasts. Bone mass increase or loss is the result of differences in the balance between these two states. Diet, hormones, including oestrogens, and physical exercise can influence this balance (Figure 41.3).

Collagen spontaneously forms fibrils of aligned protein helices on which hydroxyapatite crystals (10–50 nm in length) can grow. The size and the orientation of the crystals are dictated by the collagen template. The relationship between the collagen and hydroxyapatite is critical to the strength of the bone.

Bone formation

Foetal bone
Connective tissue is ossified, i.e. calcified by intramembranous or endochondrial ossification. The resultant woven bone is remodelled by osteoclasts to form the mature skeleton. In flat, bony structures, e.g. the skull and scapula, the centres of ossification are not on articular surfaces but

expand to form a continuous mass of woven bone.

Endochondrial ossification occurs in the epiphyseal growth plate, which is how long bones, vertebrae and the pelvis grow. Cartilage is laid down and then calcified. This growth process stops at maturity and the epiphysis closes. Completion of calcification occurs in different bones at different intrauterine ages.

Bone ossification after birth
The baby must be flaccid to pass through the birth canal without harm to the baby or the mother. At birth, the baby's skeletal calcium content is approximately 25 g. Different parts of the bone complete ossification at different ages, which enables measurement of a person's bone age compared with their chronological age, in nutritional assessment.

For bones with an epiphysis at either end, the first epiphysis to appear is the last to close. Growth continues for longest at the shoulder, knee and wrist.

Ossification is determined by X-ray examination. Full details of the expected age of ossification can be found in atlases of bone ossification, available in radiology departments.

Bone remodelling is a continuous process during adult life. There is a 25% turnover of cancellous bone and 2–3% turnover of cortical bone each year. The rate varies with age and the particular bone. Bones exposed to stress, e.g. weight bearing and exercise, remodel at a different rate to bones exposed to less pressure.

Bone growth

Skeletal growth and metabolism are dependent on a number of factors:

Ossification of the ulna and radius

Age of ossification in sections of bones

Primary centre in shaft	7 weeks
Secondary centre	
Lower end	year 2
Upper end closure	year 5
Upper epiphysis closure	year 18
Lower epiphysis	year 20

Bone remodelling

This begins with the retraction of the lining cells, derived from osteoblasts that cover bone surfaces. Mononucleated osteoclast precursors fuse on the denuded surface to form differentiated osteoclasts. Once activation has started, a volume of bone is replaced over a 2–3 week period. Then the osteoclasts are replaced by mononucleated cells preparatory to new bone formation on lacunar surfaces and the summoning of osteoblast precursors to the resorption lacunae. This is a phase of reversal, converting to formation, controlled by poorly understood systems. Osteoblasts fill the cavity with new organic matrix or osteoid which, after an interval of 25–35 days, becomes mineralised. This cycle takes several months and results in a new area of cancellous bone and a new Haversian system in cortical bone.

- **calcium control**: parathyroid hormone, calcitonin and 1,25-dihydroxycholecalciferol
- **skeletal growth control**: growth hormone, insulin-like growth factor-1 (IGF-1), thyroid hormone, adrenal corticosteroids, androgens, oestrogens, vitamin C, vitamin A
- **other control mechanisms** (the overall rate of remodelling): parathyroid hormone activity, 1,25-dihydroxyvitamin D, calcitonin.

Long bone
At birth, in the long bone, the columnar structure of the epiphyseal growth plate is incomplete. Longitudinal growth at the ends of the bone results from the increased production of cells (hypertrophic chondrocytes) originating in the germinal layer which then form the proliferative layer of the bone. These cells produce the cartilaginous matrix, which then becomes calcified, resorbed and replaced by osteoblast-mediated bone formation. Bone longitudinal growth is dependent on the increased production of cells and their subsequent expansion. After birth, bone growth is activated by growth hormone. Growth in width results from intermembranous ossification and bone-forming periosteal surface activity. The growth in width of bone continues slowly throughout life.

The important hormones involved are the growth hormone–IGF axis, the gonadal axis, the pituitary–thyroid axis and, to a lesser extent, insulin. The growth hormone–IGFs are either free or bound to protein in the circulation. There are two binding proteins (> 100 kDa and 80–85 kDa). The 80–85 kDa protein is responsible for 80–90% of the growth hormone binding. The concentrations of these two proteins vary from subject to subject and in sickness and in health. The concentrations are low in neonates, but increase at 1 year. The biological significance of these proteins is not known, but they may have a protective role and may also prolong the half-life of the hormones.

Vitamin D influences the availability of calcium, with effects on bone metabolism. The degree of mechanical loading also affects bone modelling. Vitamin C is essential for the synthesis of connective tissue, through the hydroxylation of proline and lysine. Vitamin A stimulates osteoclast bone resorption. Vitamin K has effects on bone through osteocalcin, a small protein that accounts for up to 15% of non-collagenous bone. Its role is yet to be defined.

Osteoclast maturation and gene function require and are regulated by the transcription factor c-Fos and the surface proteins RANK and RANKL (ligand). Osteoprotegerin is a soluble receptor of the tumour necrosis factor receptor superfamily. Osteoprotegerin ligand binds RANKL, promotes osteoclast function and bone resorption, and is regulated by anti-inflammatory cytokines and hormones. Osteoprotegerin production declines with age, but increases with oestrogen therapy. Osteopontin is involved in the regulation of mineralisation of bone, and is expressed in both osteoblasts and osteoclasts. Osteopontin may be involved in bone resorption and be controlled in part by parathyroid hormone. Osteoclasts also have feedback systems governing their activity.

Exercise, especially of the high-impact type, affects bone mass. The exact mechanism is not clear, but physical activity, physical fitness, muscle strength and bone mass are related. However, in the young woman with an eating disorder and associated amenorrhoea, and who exercises to excess, there is a decline in bone mass.

BONE MASS AND AGE

The variations in bone mass over the life cycle are shown in Figure 41.4.

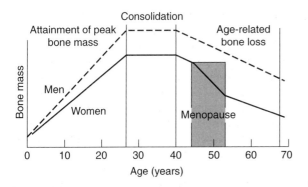

Fig. 41.4 Alterations in skeletal mass throughout the life cycle. (With kind permission of Dr Susan New and the Nutrition Society.)

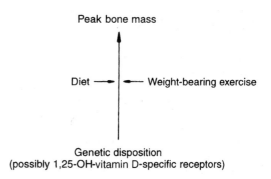

Fig. 41.5 Peak bone mass is dependent on diet and weight-bearing exercise, but most of all on genetic disposition, possibly mediated through the 1,25-dihydroxy-vitamin D-specific receptors.

Foetal bone mineralisation is affected by season of birth, birth weight and diabetes in the mother. Maternal vitamin D status is an important influence on the foetal bone.

Bone mass increases rapidly during the first year of life and during the rapid growth at the time of puberty (40% of bone mass). Pubertal growth is greater in the male than the female. The most critical needs during the growth phase are dietary proteins and, to a lesser extent, vitamin D and calcium. During growth, bone mineral mass increases through bone size rather than bone density. During childhood the main hormones involved in bone structure are the growth hormone–IGFs and thyroid hormones.

The pubertal spurt occurs for 2 years after the menarche in girls, with a maximum velocity at 12.5 years, and for 2 years in the male, with a maximum at 14 years. During this period calcium accumulates in the bone of girls at about half the rate of boys. By the age of 16–18 years calcium retention decreases. At puberty the growth plate becomes fully calcified and fused, and bone growth stops. Dietary supplementation of calcium, vitamin D supplements and physical exercise during the pubertal spurt in children result in significant increases in bone mass, which may be of lifelong value. Sex hormones are important in the pubertal spurt and during other phases when sex hormones are secreted. If there is a calcium deficiency, catch-up is feasible, provided calcium supplementation is maintained.

Peak bone mass, i.e. the amount of bone at the completion of linear growth, is under genetic control, as well as being affected by the dietary provision of calcium during growth and mechanical stress (Figure 41.5). There does not appear to be a genetic component to the rate of bone loss. Bone loss is greater in females than in males of the same age.

Peak bone mass is, on average, achieved at the ages 35–44 years for cortical bone and somewhat earlier for trabecular bone. White males have a 5–30% greater peak bone mass than females, and African–Asians 10% greater than Caucasians. Age-related bone loss results from gradual thinning of trabeculae through declining osteoblastic function.

Bone strength and the menopause

Rapid post-menopausal bone loss is due to increased activity of osteoclasts, as oestrogen activity declines. Once osteoclastic resorption has breached the trabecular plate, new bone formation is not possible and tissue is rapidly lost. Trabeculae are separated and intertrabecular connective tissue is reduced. The rapid disruption of trabecular microarchitecture after the menopause seriously reduces bone strength.

Each year, 0.3% cortical bone loss occurs in males and females up to the menopause, when there is a decrease in oestrogen production and an accelerated loss in females. The periosteal circumference increases slowly, but there is also an expansion of the medullary cavity. Osteoclasts are important in this process. The post-menopausal bone loss may be independent of calcium intake, but this is a somewhat controversial area.

Bone loss begins in the fourth or fifth decade of life and varies from bone to bone. The mass of the skeleton shrinks and in advanced old age will have fallen to approximately 70% of the bone mass of youth. This is reflected in a deterioration of the ratio of the cortical bone area to the total bone area in bones such as the metacarpal bone.

During confinement to bed and during space travel (see Chapter 45) there is a negative calcium balance. The relationship between bone density and dietary calcium intake is not immediate or direct. Calcium supplementation in the mature individual only benefits those with a particularly pronounced lifelong deficiency in dietary calcium.

Exercise, especially of the weight-bearing type, is important in maintaining bone density. Smoking, alcohol and poor diet are predisposing factors in reducing bone density. The incidence of vertebral fractures is up to six times more common in women than in men. Men are protected for several reasons. Age for age, their bone density is higher, in part because the bones are larger and in part because androgens have a direct effect on the growth plate chondrocytes and on osteoblasts. The anabolic effect of androgens on muscles increases the stress on muscles during exercise and increases bone calcium deposition. Testosterone and oestradiol circulation continues well into old age in the male. Men die on average 5 years earlier than women, which reduces the chance of developing an age-related condition. Predisposing illnesses include treatment with steroids and malabsorption, e.g. following gastric surgery. Heavy tobacco smoking, excessive drinking, a low-calcium diet and a slothful lifestyle are other factors. Curiously enough, obesity is protective in men. Steroids inhibit bone formation and osteoclastic activity continues. Hypogonadism leads to trabecular perforation rather than thinning.

With age, the control of calcium intake and output is less efficient, and intestinal calcium absorption and the renal ability to hydroxylate 25-hydroxyvitamin D decline. Less time may be spent in the sun. The ability to synthesise vitamin D in the skin and the response of intestinal absorption to parathyroid hormone is reduced. Secondary hyperparathyroidism may then occur. This may stimulate bone remodelling through activation of osteoclast activity and, as there is reduced available calcium, the bones thin. In contrast, in the post-menopausal state the rate of bone loss may be accelerated (by 1–2%/year for cortical and 2–3%/year for trabecular bone) by several factors, such as smoking and loss of oestrogen production. Oestrogen depletion results in increased bone turnover, with osteoclast activity exceeding osteoblastic formation and reduced bone mass. Urinary calcium excretion increases after the menopause, again in part attributable to oestrogen depletion. Low bone density will also coincide with ageing and frailty, especially in the female, who has an increased risk of bone fractures. The low bone density, in addition to increasing the risk of fracture, is likely to be a marker of other variables, including diet, which influence mortality. Old women with low bone density are also at risk of dying of non-traumatic causes, e.g. stroke. Deteriorating bone structure is more pronounced in osteoporosis, where there is a reduction in bone density. Supplementation of the diet with vitamin D_3 and calcium (cholecalciferol) in elderly women reduces the risk of hip and other fractures. Furthermore, dietary protein supplementation is of value in the care of the elderly recovering from fractures.

Genetics and bone structure

The inherited component of stature is between 50–80%, unless the environment changes from that in which the parents and family grew up. The variability in the regulation of bone formation comes in part from the serum bone specific alkaline phosphatase and osteocalcin activity, which reflect osteoblast activity. Other genes include the vitamin D receptor, collagen-1-α-1, and the hormones involved. Some 70–80% of variation in bone mineral mass is accounted for by genetic factors.

OSTEOPOROSIS

Clinical osteoporosis is a thinning of the bone despite normal mineralisation. For a fracture to occur, the trauma must be greater than the strength of the bone. In osteoporosis, fractures occur with minimal trauma. Factors that increase the chance of fracture include reduced bone mass, loss of trabeculae in cancellous bone and skeletal fragility, trauma and the type of fall. Protective muscle mass, which declines in the elderly, can cushion and protect from the effects of trauma.

Ovarian function (menopause, surgical removal of ovaries, athletic pursuits, stress-related amenorrhoea, anorexia nervosa) are associated with loss of bone structure and negative bone homoeostasis.

Osteoporosis occurs in patients on long-term treatment with corticosteroids. Osteoporosis in Crohn's disease, ulcerative colitis and autoimmune chronic hepatitis may be due to inhibition of osteoblast activity and a decrease in intestinal calcium absorption. Osteoporosis is a common finding in individuals with vertebral fractures and in people with kidney, heart and liver transplants.

In hip fracture there is a 2.6-fold increase in risk for each standard deviation reduction in bone density. A woman whose femoral neck bone density is at the 10th percentile would have a 25% lifetime risk of hip fracture, compared with an 8% risk for a woman at the 90th percentile. The decline in bone density and the increased incidence of falls account for the increasing risk of hip fracture with age. Although there is a doubling of the risk of fracture with age, falls directly increase the risk. It has been suggested that present-day women have a reduced bone density compared with previous generations.

The elderly with osteoporosis and its attendant complications have increased chances of breaking a bone, are less able to perform daily tasks,

Proximal femur bone density in 100–200-year-old human skeletal material of known age at death

Restoration of a church in London required the temporary removal from a crypt of bodies buried between 1729 and 1852. Dual-energy X-ray absorptiometry showed the bone density to be greater in that generation than in the present population, in both pre-menopausal and post-menopausal women. The physical activity and lifestyle of the eighteenth and nineteenth century women were hard, with many working as weavers.

suffer loss of independence, pain and reduced social activities, and may be confined to a nursing home.

Treatment with fluoride (therapeutic range 30–50 mg NaF/day) does not reduce the fracture rate. Fluoride therapy in osteoporosis increases unmineralised osteoid tissue and delays mineralisation. New bone formation occurs in the axial skeleton, which is mostly trabecular bone. The new bone matrix has a woven rather than lamellar appearance. The treated bone looks similar to that in osteomalacia and is not altered by calcium and vitamin D supplements.

A 5% increase in peak bone mass would lead to a 40–50% reduction in fracture rate.

OSTEOMALACIA

Osteomalacia is a failure of bone mineralisation and in the adult results in thin bony cortex and incomplete pathological fractures (Looser's zones). These fractures do not heal and unite until the nutritional problem is resolved. An important feature is osteoid mineralisation failure. Other complicating bony changes may take place as there may be multiple associated deficiencies.

Osteomalacia and osteoporosis may be complications of chronic gastrointestinal and liver diseases, e.g. coeliac disease, Crohn's disease, partial gastrectomy and pancreatic insufficiency. Primary biliary cirrhosis and other chronic conditions of bile insufficiency, e.g. biliary atresia and hypoplasia, are important causes of osteomalacia and bone demineralisation. Insufficient calcium phosphate and vitamin D absorption occur in these conditions. The symptoms and signs of osteomalacia include bone pain, muscle weakness, hypophosphataemia, increased serum alkaline phosphatase and parathyroid hormone concentrations.

DIAGNOSIS OF OSTEOPOROSIS AND OSTEOMALACIA

A 'rough and ready' screening test for the development of osteoporosis is reduction in height. Women's height peaks at 27 years and men's at

21 years. Men of predominantly northern European stock will be 2.6 cm shorter at 60 years and 6 cm shorter at 80 years of age; women will be 2.6 cm shorter at 60 years and 6.7 cm shorter at 80 years. Assessments of bone include bone mineral density, total lumbar spine (dual-energy X-ray absorption), plasma alkaline phosphatase, plasma osteocalcin and serum parathyroid hormone.

The only method to distinguish between osteomalacia and osteoporosis is with a full-thickness iliac crest bone biopsy. Early bone demineralisation can be detected by radiogrammetry, photonabsorptiometry and tomography. Radiometry provides magnified views of bone, particularly metacarpal bones, and indicates the thickness of cortical bone. However, it does not indicate total skeletal mass. Iodine-125 photon absorptiometry is used for measurements on the radius of the non-dominant arm. This precise and accurate method correlates with total skeletal mass, but not trabecular bone in the iliac crest or vertebral bodies. It does not distinguish between osteoporosis and osteomalacia. A complicating factor is that peripheral bones, arm and leg bones, axial bones, and the pelvis and vertebrae may react differently to deficiencies. Radiogrammetry and ^{125}Iphoton absorptiometry may be insensitive in the early detection of osteoporosis, where the axial skeleton may be more involved.

KEY POINTS

1. The skeleton consists of bones, joints, tendon sheaths and fascia. The bony skeleton forms the attachment for tendons, allowing muscles to contract. Bones consist of 35% mineral salts (largely calcium and phosphorus), 20% organic matter (mostly collagen) and 45% water; 99% of the body calcium is found in bone.
2. Each bone has a blood supply, which provides nutrients. A long bone consists of a shaft or diaphysis, an epiphysis with an articular surface, a metaphysis, a functional zone and an epiphyseal plate; cartilage between the epiphysis and the metaphysis is important in growing bone.
3. Bone is formed in three layers: periosteum, cortex and medulla. Periosteum is a fibrous membrane covering the bone. The cortex is the hard sheath of compact bone. The medulla contains the marrow and spongy (cancellous) bone.
4. There are three types of bone cell. Osteoblasts line the external surface of the bone trabeculae, the inner aspect of the periosteum and the surface of bone lining the osteons; they produce collagen and proteins forming the organic bone matrix, and deposit and remove calcium. Osteocytes are osteoblasts trapped in mature bone; they have a role in mature bone maintenance and are the sensors for the changes in response to mechanical demand. Osteoclasts are responsible for bone resorption.
5. Bone consists of lamellae and a mineral matrix of calcium hydroxyapatites deposited on a protein collagen matrix, which gives bone rigidity. The organic lamella is 90% collagen (largely type I) produced by the osteoblast, and calcification occurs between the collagen molecules. Bone contains other proteins, phosphoproteins and lipids.
6. Bone is continuously remodelled throughout life. The rate varies with age. Bones exposed to stress, e.g. weight bearing and exercise, will remodel at a different rate from less pressured bones.
7. With age, bone develops osteoporotic changes wherein bone structure and density decline with a continued calcium content.
8. Bone calcium content declines in osteomalacia.

THINKING POINTS

1. Bone is a support and reservoir for minerals.
2. Bone is also a tissue that reflects the ageing process.
3. Nutrition and exercise are important ways to ameliorate the ageing process on bone.

NEED TO UNDERSTAND

The greatly different controls of bone homoeostasis over the years of life and the vital role that nutrition plays in this process.

FURTHER READING

Alliston, T. and Derynck, R. (2002) Interfering with bone remodelling. *Nature*, **416**, 686–7.

Anderson, D.C. (1992) Osteoporosis in men. *British Medical Journal*, **305**, 489–90.

Anderson, J.J. (1992) The role of nutrition in the functioning of skeletal tissue. *Nutrition Review*, **50**, 388–94.

Branca, F., Robins, S.P., Ferro-Luzzi, A. and Golden, M.H. (1992) Bone turnover in malnourished children. *Lancet*, **340**, 1493–6.

Browner, W.S., Seeley, D.G., Vogt, T.M. and Cummings, S.R. (1991) Non-trauma mortality in elderly women with low bone density. *Lancet*, **338**, 355–8.

Cullen, K. (1992) Motivating people to attend screening for osteoporosis. *British Medical Journal*, **305**, 521–2.

Cummings, S.R. and Melton, L.J. III (2002) Epidemiology and outcome of osteoporotic fractures. *Lancet*, **359**, 1761–7.

Cummings, S.R., Black, D.M., Nevitt, M.C. *et al.* (1993) Bone density at various sites for prediction of hip fractures. *Lancet*, **341**, 72–5.

Dawson-Hughes, B., Harris, S.S., Krall, E.A. and Dallal, G.E. (1997) Effect of calcium and vitamin D supplementation on bone density in men and women 65 years of age or older. *New England Journal of Medicine*, **337**, 670–6.

Delmas, P.D. (2001) Osteoporosis in patients with organ transplants: a neglected problem. *Lancet*, **357**, 325–6.

Dempster, D.W and Lindsay, R. (1993) Pathogenesis of osteoporosis. *Lancet*, **341**, 797–801.

Greenfield, E.M. and Goldberg, V.M. (1997) Genetic determination of bone density. *Lancet*, **350**, 1264–5

Johnston, C.C. and Slemenda, C.W. (1992) Changes in skeletal tissue during the ageing process. *Nutrition Reviews*, **50**, 385–7.

Keay, N. (2000) The modifiable factors affecting bone mineral accumulation in girls: the paradoxical effect of exercise on bone. *British Nutrition Foundation, Nutrition Bulletin*, **25**, 219–22.

Kun, Z., Greenfield, H., Xueqin, D. and Fraser, D.R. (2001) Improvement of bone health in childhood and adolescence. *Nutrition Research Review*. **14**, 119–51.

Leader (1992) Maximizing peak bone mass: calcium supplementation increases bone mineral density in children. *Nutrition Reviews*, **50**, 335–7.

Lees, B., Molleson, T., Arnett, R.A. and Stevenson, J.C. (1993) Differences in proximal femur bone density over two centuries. *Lancet*, **341**, 673–5.

Loveridge, N., Farquharson, C. and Scheven, B.A. (1990) Endogenous mediators of growth. *Proceedings of the Nutrition Society*, **49**, 443–50.

Namgung, R. and Tsang, R.C. (2000) Factors affecting newborn bone mineral content: *in utero* effects on newborn bone mineralisation. *Proceedings of the Nutrition Society*, **59**, 55–63.

New, S.A. (2001) Exercise, bone and nutrition. *Proceedings of the Nutrition Society*, **60**, 265–74.

Prentice, A. (2001) The relative contribution of diet and genotype to bone development. *Proceedings of the Nutrition Society*, **60**, 45–52.

Ralston, S.H. (1997) The genetics of osteoporosis. *Q. J. Med.*, **90**, 247–51.

Reeve, J., Green, J.R., Hesp, R. *et al.* (1990) Determinants of axial bone loss in the early post menopause: the Harrow postmenopausal bone loss study. In *Osteoporosis 1990* (eds C. Christiansen and K. Overgaard). Osteopress, Copenhagen, pp. 101–3.

Schneider, V.S., LeBlanc, A. and Rambaut, P.C. (1989) Bone and mineral metabolism. In *Space Physiology and Medicine* (eds A.E. Nicogossian, C.L. Huntoon and S.L. Pool). Lea & Febiger, Philadelphia, PA, pp. 214–21.

Seeman, E. (2002) Pathogenesis of bone fragility in women and men. *Lancet*, **359**, 1841–50.

Symposium on Nutritional Aspects of Bone (1997) *Proceedings Nutrition Society*, **56**, 903–87.

Warrell, D.A., Cox, T.M., Firth, T.D. and Benz, E.J. Jr (eds) (2003) *Oxford Textbook of Medicine*, 4th edn. Oxford University Press, Oxford.

Weaver, C.M. (2000) The growing years and prevention of osteoporosis in later life. *Proceedings of the Nutrition Society*, **59**, 303–6.

Wosje, K.S. and Specker, B.L. (2000) Role of calcium in bone health during childhood. *Nutrition Reviews*, **58**, 253–68.

Part VII

Special nutritional requirements and conditions

- Pregnancy, lactation and weaning
- Childhood and youth; middle age and old age
- Sport
- Nutrition in outer space
- Dietary deficiency
- Nutrition in the aetiology of disease

42

Pregnancy, lactation and weaning

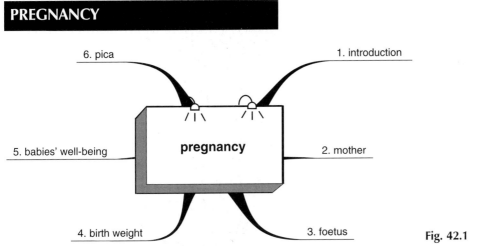

6. pica

1. introduction

5. babies' well-being

pregnancy

2. mother

4. birth weight

3. foetus

Fig. 42.1 Section outline.

INTRODUCTION

Pregnancy is a normal physiological process. The diet and well-being of the mother are important to maximise the prospects for the baby's future life.

MOTHER

Ideally, an expectant mother needs a good mixed diet, both before and during pregnancy, adequate in total number of calories, protein, vitamins and minerals. Folic acid supplementation before and in early pregnancy is important. Nutrition well before pregnancy is most important as this will establish the long-term prospects for the baby, as a child and into middle and even old age. During pregnancy, weight and diet should be monitored. Iron, calcium and folic acid supplements (as milk) are important. Nausea and vomiting in early pregnancy affect 50–90% of pregnant women. The effect on the outcome of the pregnancy is not, however, unfavourable to birth weight or length of pregnancy.

The total amount of fatty acids (of all types) in the plasma phospholipids and vitamin E concentration increase by 50% over the period from 10 to 40 weeks of pregnancy.

If a woman has previously been undernourished, particularly if there was rickets during childhood and adolescence, stunted growth with a resulting small pelvis can result. The passage of the baby

A woman should maintain weight during the first two trimesters and thereafter gain 0.5 kg/week until term. Weight and fat gain during pregnancy is some 11 kg and 5 kg, respectively, put on primarily from 14 to 24 weeks. The increase in weight is made up of 4.8 kg foetus, placenta and liquor, 1.3 kg uterus and breasts, 1.25 kg blood and 1.2 kg extracellular water. When the expectant mother is obese, hypertension is a dangerous complication. Women who are underweight at the beginning of pregnancy should gain weight at a greater rate than normal-weight women, i.e. 0.58 kg/week. Adolescent mothers should also put on weight at a rate similar to the underweight group to allow for normal growth of the mother.

Increased maternal weight [body mass index (BMI) > 25] before pregnancy increases the risk of late foetal death, independent of the presence of hypertension or diabetes.

Many women associate the onset of the development of obesity with one or more of their pregnancies. Those who become obese develop central obesity.

through this distorted pelvis may lead to a difficult and prolonged labour. This is now a rarity in Western obstetric practice. The chance of conception is reduced if there is a reduction in energy intake to less than 6.3 MJ/day. Such restriction, as in anorexia nervosa, inhibits ovulation. Maternal blood pressure may be an important factor in the baby's birth weight and a contributor to the relationship between low birth weight and subsequent hypertension.

Mortality during pregnancy is considerable in many developing countries, where 20–45% of deaths among women of child-bearing age are related to pregnancy. This compares with less than 1% in the UK. World-wide, 500 000 women die of pregnancy-related causes annually, 99% in the developing countries. Bangladesh, Bhutan, India, Nepal, Pakistan and Sri Lanka account for 43% of this total. In Nepal, for example, traditional maternal practice was for no one, even members of family, to touch a woman during and for several weeks after delivery. The woman was confined to a cow-byre, to look after all the details of birth, including cutting the umbilical cord. In many countries there are economic, social and cultural barriers to changing practices that are dangerous to a

pregnant woman. In developing countries iron deficiency (450 million women world-wide) and iodine deficiency (5.7 million world-wide) are major hazards in pregnancy. Women in rural Africa have a 1 in 21 chance of dying of pregnancy-related causes, in south Asia 1 in 38, and in Latin America 1 in 73, compared with 1 in 6366 for the USA and 1 in 9850 for northern Europe. The reasons for this difference are poor education, poverty, insanitary conditions and malnutrition, and whether the family budget is controlled by the husband or wife. The development of agricultural co-operatives has had a positive effect on nutrition through improved food production. Refugee camps are associated with malnourishment and increased pregnancy-related mortality. In earlier times in Britain the pregnant woman, in addition to preparing clothes for the baby, would sew her funeral shroud as it was frequently needed.

Single mothers now form a significant proportion of the population. Women in this group may be disadvantaged and have a higher death rate than mothers in a partnership.

FOETUS

The weight of the baby is approximately 3300 g, with an wide range of normal. The weight is influenced by the protein-energy intake of the mother. Protein-calorie malnutrition at this stage may have consequences for later infant development. In the second trimester the mother should be laying down adipose tissue in preparation for later foetal requirements. In the third trimester the mother's weight gain affects the infant's final weight. This underlines the significance of the timing of maternal dietary supplementation, i.e. first, second or third trimester.

In the development of the foetus, if any developmental process is restricted during the period of its fastest rate by any agency, at any time, not only will this delay the process, but the effect can be long-standing, and the ultimate value of that development will be restricted. This applies even when the restricting influence is removed and the fullest rehabilitation obtained. The vulnerable period hypothesis states that when there is stress to the pregnancy, then the older the foetus, the better it can cope with that stress. This is reflected in the potential for development, e.g. the quantity and rate of growth, and the height and number of cells in certain organs. Some developments occur only during one period, others during two separate periods, e.g. increase in height and weight occur both during infancy and at puberty. If a stress occurs at an early stage in the growth phase then catch-up growth is possible.

The foeto-placental growth is substantially dependent on the provision of nutrient from the mother's diet and the blood supply. A reduction in placental bed blood flow or nutrient supply results in the placental release of growth-suppressive peptides, which slows foetal growth. When blood flow and nutrient supply improve, this secretion decreases and growth accelerates. Regular exercise during pregnancy increases placental growth and function, and results in smaller babies with a reduced fat content. There is a direct relationship between maternal blood glucose concentrations and the size of the baby at birth.

The effects of malnutrition at the time of birth are long-standing. In rural Gambia the season of the birth predicts mortality. Individuals born in the annual hungry period are ten times more likely to die prematurely in young adulthood. The hungry period is the wet season (July to October) when the staple foods from the previous harvest are exhausted.

Equal numbers of adult males and females are the ideal. In practice, 5% more boys are born in communities where girl babies are welcomed as much as boys. In some cultures there is manipulation of this ratio by aborting female foetuses or neglecting baby girls, and the female to male ratio is 0.9 to 0.95. There are fewer males born to insulin-dependent diabetic mothers. Male foetuses are more vulnerable and are more frequently lost from the pregnancy, especially at the early stages of gestation. Severe placental dysfunction is more common in a pregnancy with a male than a female foetus. Parental preconception smoking (more than 20 cigarettes/day in both parents), environmental toxins, e.g. dioxin and methylmercury, and stress reduce the male to female ratio. The number of male births is said to increase after wars.

Mouth movements *in utero* may have little value, but it is essential for the infant to suck, to gain nourishment and survive. Such movements

Foetal brain development

The development of the baby's brain and neurological system, both *in utero* and during the early stages of extrauterine life, is at risk during the vulnerable periods. The brain undergoes neuroblast development during the first trimester and nerve glial development occurs during the third trimester, continuing into the first year of life. Nutritional deficiency can lead to psychomotor retardation. The later period of gestation has been likened to a culture medium. Excess or deficient availability of nutritional growth factors may have long-term consequences that extend even into middle life. Premature babies may require specialised feeding so that normal growth and development may be achieved. The provision of the long-chain fatty acids docosahexaenoic acid and arachidonic acid is important for brain development *in utero* and during the first months of life.

appear early in gestation and are more advanced in female than in male foetuses.

BIRTH WEIGHT

The birth weights of infants of well-fed mothers are on average higher than those of poorly fed women. The baby is particularly at risk when the mother is 12–14 years old, and has not completed her full growth and development before pregnancy. The reduced weight of the baby may be due to prematurity, retarded intrauterine growth or multiple pregnancies. A multiple birth in a primiparous woman over the age over 30 years carries a risk of infant mortality approaching 27%. The average twinning rate is 1.12 % of births, but the number varies for populations (range 0.6–3.4%).

If the mother's weight is less than 40 kg, the baby is particularly at risk of low birth weight. When a baby's weight is less than 2500 g the chances of survival are reduced. Preterm babies are very vulnerable. Babies born before 22 weeks of gestation rarely survive, and 27% of preterm babies born from 23 to 28 weeks of gestation suffer severe disability. Careful feeding regimens are important in the care of these and older preterm babies. If such children are tested for cognitive performance at the of age 7½–8 years (when cognitive scores predict adult scores), then their nutrition is shown to be important in determining adult cognitive levels. The brain in the third trimester foetus and early life is undergoing rapid and defining growth. Babies of lower birth weight born full term do not show deficiencies in cognitive performance when measured in adult life.

Other causes of low birth weight in babies are social status, smoking and excess alcohol consumption; these factors also influence the infant's mental development. The birth weight of babies born to mothers smoking up to ten cigarettes a day was approximately 100 g less than that of babies born to non-smokers, and babies born to mother smoking more than 10 cigarettes a day weighed approximately 200 g less than the babies born to non-smokers. At 6 months these differences were not apparent. Caffeine intake increases this reduction in birth weight in smokers.

Epidemiological studies have linked poor foetal nutrition with health problems in adult life. The findings in studies on foetal nutrition are inconsistent and flawed by incomplete and incorrect statistical interpretation and unforeseen selection biases.

Consequences of poor foetal nutrition

- Mothers who themselves weighed < 2000 g at birth have a enhanced risk of losing a baby.
- Subsequent pregnancies in which the baby is of low birth weight dependent on social status.
- Other outcomes include:
  adult hypertension
  ischaemic heart disease
  non-insulin-dependent diabetes
  suicide.

BABIES' WELL-BEING

The children of mothers who smoke tend to wheeze, cough and cry more than those of mothers who do not smoke. Colic is also more frequent. Since the thalidomide disaster, when the babies of mothers prescribed this drug failed to develop normal limbs, there has been misgivings about the prescription of any drugs to pregnant women. A useful treatment should not be stopped for pregnancy, but many women stop treatment without discussion with their doctor.

PICA

Pica is an unusual craving for normal food constituents or for substances not commonly regarded as food by the local culture. The name 'pica' is derived from a mediaeval Latin word meaning 'magpie'. The magpie was known to pick up a range of objects to satisfy hunger or curiosity. The diagnosis of pica depends on cultural attitudes, as well as the amounts ingested and degrees of craving.

Pica has been described since the time of Ancient Greece and sometimes can have quite devastating effects. On the plantations of the USA and the Caribbean, slaves sometimes showed a craving for clay. When pica is superimposed on a diet that is conducive to pellagra, i.e. a diet of salt pork, corn bread and molasses, a condition known as cachexia africane develops, with weakness, pallor, oedema, enlargement of the liver, spleen and lymph nodes, anorexia, tachycardia, ulceration of the skin and death.

Conditions in which pica occurs

The craving for particular food substances during pregnancy is a widely recognised phenomenon. In a survey of pregnant women, cravings for fruit and other sweet, sour or sharp-tasting foods were not uncommon. Pregnant women may eat clay and starch, soil and refrigerator frost. It is debatable whether chewing tobacco is a form of pica. Pica is prevalent among children, particularly psychotic, children with learning disabilities.

Causes of pica

Pica has been suggested to be a craving produced by nutrient or mineral deficiency. The salt lick of wild animals is widely considered a response to a deficiency. Alternatively, pica has been suggested to be due to deeply ingrained cultural customs within societies. However, pica may not be limited to any age, gender or racial grouping.

Consequences of pica

These depend on what is being eaten, e.g. lead toxicity may occur if there is lead in the material being eaten. Nutritional status may be affected by pica; the consumption of excessive amounts of a single substance may reduce the intake of normal dietary constituents. For example, excessive ingestion of laundry starch may depress intakes of required food. If the amylophagia does not interfere with appetite then obesity may result. Pica may reduce the bioavailability of minerals. Alternatively, pica may be of no adverse significance.

KEY POINTS

1. The expectant mother needs a good, mixed diet before and during the pregnancy. Breast feeding and anorexia nervosa reduce the chances of conception.
2. The weight of the baby is influenced by the protein-energy intake of the mother. The provision of nutrients for brain development is important. If the mother weighs under 40 kg then the baby is liable to have a reduced birth weight. Young, growing mothers are another group whose babies are vulnerable.
3. Pica is a craving for a normal food constituent or unusual substances. This may be secondary to some explicable or inexplicable nutritional deficiency. Unless the substance is toxic or there is an underlying deficiency, the phenomenon is harmless.

THINKING POINTS

1. Pregnancy is a normal process, requiring normal nutrition.
2. If a women had a tumour the size of the gravid uterus she would be very ill and cachexic, yet a pregnant woman flourishes.

3. Problems arise with socioeconomic and cultural mores, along with illness, obesity, smoking and alcohol intake.

NEED TO UNDERSTAND

1. The deviations from the normal in pregnancy and their impact on the baby.
2. The importance of normality in the mother's diet, mother's weight, birth weight and care after birth.

FURTHER READING

Barker, D.J.P. (1992) Infant origins of common. In *Diseases in Human Nutrition; A Continuing Debate* (eds M.A. Eastwood, C. Edwards and D. Parry). Chapman and Hall, London, pp. 17–30.

Clapp, J.F. (2002) Maternal carbohydrate intake and pregnancy outcome. *Proceedings of the Nutrition Society*, **61**, 45–50.

Cook, D.G., Peacock, J.L., Feyerabend, C. *et al.* (1996) Relationship of caffeine intake and blood caffeine concentrations during pregnancy to fetal growth: prospective population based study. *British Medical Journal*, **313**, 1358–62.

Craft, N. (1997) Life span: conception to adolescence. *British Medical Journal*, **315**, 1227–30.

Danford, D.E. (1982) Pica and nutrition. *Annual Review of Nutrition*, **2**, 303–22.

Edwards, A., Megens, A., Peek, M. and Wallace, E.M. (2000) Sexual origins of placental dysfunction. *Lancet*, **355**, 203–4.

Fukuda, M., Fukuda, K., Shimizu, T. *et al.* (2002) Parental periconceptual smoking and male:female ratio of newborn infants. *Lancet*, **359**, 1407–8.

Godfrey, K, and Robinson, S. (1998) Maternal nutrition, placental growth and fetal programming. *Proceedings of the Nutrition Society*, **57**, 105–11.

Harries, J.N. and Hughes, D.E. (1957) An enumeration of the 'cravings' of some pregnant women. *Proceedings of the Nutrition Society*, **16**, 20–1.

Hepper, P.G., Shannon, E.A. and Dornan, J.C. (1997) Sex differences in fetal mouth movements. *Lancet*, **350**, 1820.

Lucas, A., Morley, R. and Cole, T.J. (1998) Randomised trial of early diet in preterm babies and later intelligence quotient. *British Medical Journal*, **317**, 1481–7.

Lucas, A., Fewtrell, M.S. and Cole, T.J. (1999) Fetal origins of adult disease – the hypothesis revisited. *British Medical Journal*, **319**, 245–9.

Martyn, C., Gale, C.R., Sayer, A.A. and Fall, C. (1996) Growth in utero and cognitive function in adult life: follow up study of people born between 1920 and 1943. *British Medical Journal*, **312**, 1393–6.

Moore, S.E., Cole, T.J., Poskitt, E.M.E. *et al.* (1997) Season of birth predicts mortality in rural Africa. *Nature*, **388**, 434.

Oostenbrug, G.S., Mensink, R.P., Al, M.D.M. *et al*, (1998) Maternal and neonatal plasma antioxidant levels in normal pregnancy, and the relationship with fatty acid unsaturation. *British Journal of Nutrition*, **80**, 67–73.

Rees, J.M., Engelbert-Fenton, K.A. and Gonq, E.J. *et al.* (1992) Weight gain in adolescents during pregnancy: rate related to birth weight outcome. *American Journal of Clinical Nutrition*, **56**, 868–73.

Reproduction and Development Group Symposium (2002) Manipulating early diet. *Proceedings of the Nutrition Society*, **61**, 51–77.

Rjasanowski, I., Kloting, I. and Kovacs, P. (1998) Altered sex ratio in offspring of mothers with insulin-dependent diabetes mellitus. *Lancet*, **351**, 497–8.

Rubin, P. (1998) Drug treatment during pregnancy. *British Medical Journal*, **317**, 1503–6.

Skjaerven, R., Wilcox, A.J., Oyen, N. and Magnus, P. (1997) Mother's birth weight and survival of their offspring: population based study. *British Medical Journal*, **314**, 1376–80.

Soltani, H. and Fraser, R.B. (2000) A longitudinal study of maternal anthropometric changes in normal weight, overweight and obese women during pregnancy and post partum. *British Journal of Nutrition*, **84**, 95–101.

Stein, Z., Sussex, M., Sanger, G. and Marolla, E. (1975) Mental performance after prenatal exposure to famine. In *Famine and Human Development; The Dutch Hunger Winter of 1944–45*. Oxford University Press, New York, pp. 197–214.

Thapa, S. (1996) Challenges to improving maternal health in rural Nepal. *Lancet*, **347**, 1244–6.

Tin, W., Wariyar, U., Hey, E., for the Northern Neonatal Network (1997) Changing prognosis for babies of less than 28 weeks gestation in the north of England between 1983 and 1994. *British Medical Journal*, **314**, 107–11.

Walker, B.R., McConnachie, A., Noon, J.P., *et al.* (1998) Contribution of parental blood pressure to association between low birth weight and adult blood pressure: cross sectional study. *British Medical Journal*, **316**, 834–7.

Wharton, B. (1992) Food and biological clocks. *Proceedings of the Nutrition Society*, **51**, 145–53.

LACTATION

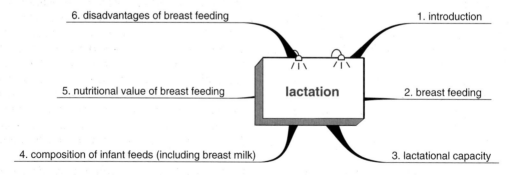

Fig. 42.2 Section outline.

INTRODUCTION

Human breast milk is the best nutrition for human babies. Mothers in developing countries breast feed their babies. Many supplement their milk with water or tea from the first week of life in the belief that it will relieve pain, colic and earache, prevent and treat colds and constipation, soothe fretfulness and quench thirst. Human milk contains approximately 70 kcal gross energy, 1.0 g protein, 4 g fat and 7 g lactose per 100 g. For the first 5 days after birth, milk is rich in colostrum and immunoglobulins. The nitrogen content of human milk decreases rapidly during the early weeks of lactation and slowly thereafter. The nutrient content of human milk at parturition is adequate for growth, except for iron (0.6 mg/l at 2 weeks).

Most mothers prefer to cradle the baby on one side, and most instinctively chose the left. The left cradling preference is present in all cultures and may be due to right handedness in the mother.

BREAST FEEDING

Healthy infants at 2, 4 and 6 months need, respectively, about 800, 900 and 1000 ml of milk daily. Most mothers can produce sufficient milk to meet the needs of their baby at 4 months, but only a minority can at 6 months. Supplementary feeding starts when the baby is aged between 4 and 6 months.

Supplementing breast milk in the first 4 months of life is unnecessary, even in hot climates, and may be harmful. Breast milk has an osmolarity that rarely exceeds 700 mmol/l and in all environments, even in high temperatures and varying degrees of humidity, is within the normal concentrating ability of the child's kidneys. Breast feeding, particularly in developing countries, is important in ensuring a regimen that is sterile during the first 4–6 months of life.

The lactational amenorrhoea method of contraception is based on the belief that a mother who is breast feeding, or almost fully breast feeding, her infant and who remains amenorrhoeic, has a less than 2% chance of pregnancy during the first 6 months after childbirth.

LACTATIONAL CAPACITY

An important influence on the amount and nutrient content of maternal milk production is the maternal lactational capacity. The amount of milk that the child is able to drink will affect the infant's milk nutrient intake and subsequent growth. Maternal physical activity, the thermic effect of food, and maternal or infant illness may also affect the amount and content of milk produced. Maternal dietary intake before and during pregnancy affects maternal adipose tissue and nutrient stores at parturition and lactational capacity. Whether the child is solely fed on the breast or whether there is supplementary feeding will affect the infant's growth. Human milk from mothers of very preterm babies is of a very high quality for the infant's development.

Lactational capacity is probably a function of genetic heritage, age, parity, breast enlargement during pregnancy and nutritional history. It may respond to improved dietary intake and increased infant demand. Lactational capacity is usually measured by milk production, infant milk intake plus residual milk. For well-nourished women lactational capacity is greater than milk production. Milk production requires adequate lactational capacity, adequate nutrition, adequate infant demand and for the baby to have good suckling ability. The relationship between maternal dietary intake, maternal nutritional status, milk production and infant growth will vary during lactation.

Among well-nourished women dietary intake accounts for approximately 13% of the variability in infant milk intake. The size of the mother is not associated with lactational performance during the first 1–4 months post-partum. If there is prolonged lactation, i.e. 3–12 months, there is some relationship between maternal nutritional status and milk composition. In general, however, the mother can maintain milk production, even in poor circumstances, at the expense of her own body needs.

The proportion of ingested nutrients available for milk biosynthesis is influenced by maternal nutrient stores, including adipose tissue stores. For the mother, lactation requires markedly increased food intake. This may deplete some body stores. Fat synthesis is reduced and there is loss of adipose tissue.

Seasonal food shortages and reduced dietary intakes result in a decrease in milk production. In undernourished women given a dietary supplement, infant milk intake increased by 100 ml/day, although there was no effect on the protein content. Infants of the food-supplemented mothers did not gain significantly more weight during the supplemented period, although there was an increase in maternal body fat content.

COMPOSITION OF INFANT FEEDS (INCLUDING BREAST MILK)

Modified infant formulae have been fed to millions of infants with no apparent ill-effects. If modified milks are incorrectly made up in unhygienic conditions, there may be contamination of the milk or a high sodium intake. Another alternative to breast feeding is modified cow's milk, boiled and then cooled for drinking. This should be given only when the baby is approaching 6–12 months of age.

Sodium content of various milks (mmol/150 ml)

Human	0.9
Whey-based	1.0
Infant formula	0.9–2.0
Cow	3.3

Constituents of human milk

Protein: caseins, α-lactalbumin, β-lactalbumin

Non-protein nitrogen: urea, creatine, creatinine, uric acid, glucosamines, α-amino nitrogen, nucleic acids, nucleotides

Immunological factors: secretory IgA, immunoglobulins, lactoferrin, lysozyme

Enzymes: α-amylase, bile salt-stimulated lipase, glutathione peroxidase, γ-glutamyltransferase, lipoprotein lipase, trypsin

Hormones and growth factors: pituitary hormones, brain gut peptides, growth factors, steroids, non-steroid hormones

The disadvantages of supplementary feeding are of inadequate hygiene and consequent infection.

Cow's milk has a high sodium content, between 20 and 25 mmol/l (human milk has 7 mmol/l). Soya-based infant milks contain isoflavones.

The bioavailability of nutrients in human milk is high. Iron concentrations in breast milk decline to 0.3 mg/l at 20 weeks. The absorption efficiency of iron and zinc is high. The infant is born with substantial iron stores.

Milk proteins are very digestible and are a ready source of amino acids to the infant. α-Lactalbumin forms 25–30% of milk protein and is a major nitrogen source. This protein has a role in the synthesis of lactose and also chelates calcium and zinc.

NUTRITIONAL VALUE OF BREAST FEEDING

The newborn baby is helpless, the gastrointestinal tract is underdeveloped and the infant has no teeth. Milk therefore is the ideal food. The constitution of milk is very species dependent, and bioavailability is maximal when the milk and baby belong to the same species. The baby seal drinks a milk rich in fat (490 g/l). The shrew doubles its body weight in 24 h drinking milk with a protein content of 10 g/l. These milks contain double the equivalent nutrient values of human milk.

Milk contains many discrete systems and compartments (aqueous phase; colloid dispersion; caseins); emulsion (fat globules); fat globule membrane (protein, phospholipids, cholesterol, enzymes, minerals) and cells (macrophages, neutrophils, lymphocytes, epithelial cells). Milk provides clean water to the infant. Oligosaccharides are found in relatively large quantities in human milk (6% lactose). Fatty acids are the only constituent of milk that can be significantly affected by the mother's diet. The entry of iron and zinc but not selenium into milk is regulated. The mechanism of transfer of calcium and magnesium to milk is not known.

The newborn receives immunoglobulins, trophic factors, digestive enzymes, physiologically active peptides and oligosaccharides in the milk. Breast milk is rich in secretory immunoglobulin A (sIgA), which resists gastric hydrolysis. Lactoferrin and sIgA provide 30% of the milk protein, giving passive protection at the gastrointestinal epithelium to exclude foreign antigens. Antigens to which the mother has been exposed in her diet are recognised at M cells within Peyer's patches in the maternal small intestine. Primed plasma cells pass to the lymphatic system and to the breasts, where specific sIgA is synthesised and secreted in milk. These factors are present in milk in highest concentrations during the early phase of lactation and help to protect the baby against infections of the gastrointestinal tract and respiratory system.

During the first year of life endocrine function is not fully developed in the infant. Milk-borne hormones are important in supplementing the endogenous secretions of the child. Such hormones are not present in formula feeds. Bile salt-stimulated lipase augments the modest pancreatic function of the infant and ensures good lipid digestion during the period of lactation.

Human milk is particularly suited to ensure human brain development. The linoleic acid, α-linolenic acid, arachidonic acid and docosahexaenoic acid content of milk is particularly important. The fatty acid composition of human milk is very variable, depending on the diet of the mother. A topic of interest is whether vegetarian and omnivorous mothers produce milks of equivalent essential fatty acid content (Table 42.1). Breast milk from vegan mothers is enriched in linoleic acid and reduced in DHA. Breast milk has a role in the adaptation of the gastrointestinal tract of the newborn infant to oral feeding. Milk contains both nutrients and non-nutrient factors that are important in this adaptation. Exclusively breast-fed babies have slightly higher intelligence quotients (IQs), but it is difficult to separate the social environment from the nutritional value of the milk.

Table 42.1 Essential fatty acids in human breast milk by diet

	Omnivores	Vegetarians
Linoleic acid	10.9 ±1.0	22.4 ±1.26
α-Linolenic	0.49 ± 0.06	0.70 ± 0.91
Docosahexaenoic acid (DHA)	0.31 ± 0.07	0.11 ± 0.08

Data are shown as mean ± SEM.

The neonatal infant's gastrointestinal tract becomes adapted to post-natal requirements. The trophic factors secreted in milk include epidermal growth factor (EGF), a small polypeptide with mitogenic, antisecretory and cytoprotective properties. This peptide is also present in amniotic fluid and colostrum. Its role is to activate mucosal function, to reduce gastric hydrolysis of milk macromolecules and to protect the gastrointestinal epithelium. EGF receptors are found on enterocytes from week 19 of gestation, increasing slowly during the first two trimesters and rising steeply thereafter. EGF has a role in inducing intestinal lactase and depresses the activity of sucrase.

The newborn baby has an immediate requirement for fat for energy, insulation, neural tissue and membrane synthesis. As the pancreatic (10% of adult) and hepatobiliary function (50% of adult) are not developed, milk lipase is important. The benefit of such depressed hydrolytic systems is that immunoglobulins and enzymes in milk are not hydrolysed in the gastrointestinal tract. The immature infant's intestine readily absorbs macromolecules and micromolecules. Predominantly breast-fed babies grow more slowly, but have a greater head circumference than formula-fed babies.

DISADVANTAGES OF BREAST FEEDING

The linear growth and weight gain decrease after 4–6 months of breast feeding. The zinc content of the breast milk declines from 40 μmol/l at 1 month to 10–15 μmol/l at 6 months. If children of poorly fed mothers, breast fed over a prolonged period are to maintain growth, then 5 mg of zinc restores weight gain to anticipated average values. Supplementation with iron and ergocalciferol is also important during prolonged breast feeding.

Breast milk from mothers who smoke contains cotinine, a stable metabolite of nicotine (at concentrations ten times those of controls). Cotinine attributed to passive smoking was found in the milk of 10% of mothers who did not smoke. By 1 year there appears to be no measurable effect of maternal smoking on infantile growth.

Other pollutants (e.g. polychlorinated biphenyls) are of concern. Cow's and infant formula milk come from many sources. A mother's milk reflects the positive and negative environmental effects on that mother.

There is concern over the transmission of the human immunodeficiency virus (HIV) from mother to infant during pregnancy, delivery and breast feeding. HIV has been found in human milk, concentrations being highest in milk from recently infected women and those with the advanced disease. The viruses appear to be shed into milk intermittently, so that while a sample may appear to be free from the virus, this may not rule out the possibility of viral excretion in a subsequent sample. Breast-fed babies have a higher chance of contracting HIV than those who have been artificially fed, especially after the loss of maternal antibodies. Where there are adequate supplies of properly prepared infant formula milk, women infected with HIV are advised not to breast feed. In developing countries, however, the benefits of exclusive breast feeding for 6 months, not longer, exceed the potential risk of HIV transmission. So there are problems with advice regarding whether the mother can supply milk that is free from infection or HIV. In many countries the threats of dirty artificial milk make breast feeding preferable. Where clean artificial feeds can be ensured, formula feeding is the better option.

KEY POINTS

1. Breast milk is the best food for the baby and does not require supplementation in the first months of life. The nutritional constituents of milk reduce with time.
2. The maternal lactational capacity is important, and is determined by genetic heritage, age, parity and nutritional history. Seasonal food shortages and dietary intake may reduce milk production.
3. Supplementary feeds introduce the risk of infection and harmful constituents, e.g. excess sodium.
4. The bioavailability of nutrients in human breast milk is high. Human milk protects the baby against infections. Milk-borne hormones

may be of importance to the baby. The human milk content of essential and long-chain fatty acids is of paramount importance in brain development.
5. Viruses can be intermittently transmitted in human milk.

THINKING POINTS

1. Breast feeding is wholesome and best.
2. It is important that breast feeding in public becomes acceptable.

NEED TO UNDERSTAND

Breast feeding provides all of the nutrient and energy requirements for the baby during the first 6 months of life. In developing countries this is especially important as breast milk is also clean. However, the AIDS epidemic has complicated this advice and this is an evolving situation.

FURTHER READING

Ellis, L.A. and Picciano, M.E. (1992) Milk borne hormones: regulators of development in neonates. *Nutrition Today*, **27**, 6–13.

Gale, C.R. and Martyn, C.N. (1996) Breastfeeding, dummy use and adult intelligence. *Lancet*, **347**, 1072–5.

Heining, M.J. and Dewey, K.G. (1997) Health effects of breast feeding for mothers: a critical review. *Nutrition Research Reviews*, **10**, 35–56.

Klein, K.O. (1998) Isoflavones, soy based infant formulas and relevance to endocrine function. *Nutrition Reviews*, **56**, 193–204.

Latham, M.C. and Preble, E.A. (2000) Appropriate feeding methods for infants of HIV infected mothers in sub-Saharan Africa. *British Medical Journal*, **320**, 1656–60.

Lonnerdal, B. (2000) Regulation of mineral and trace elements in human milk: exogenous and endogenous factors. *Nutrition Reviews*, **58**, 223–9.

Maas, Y.G.H., Gerritsen, J.G., Hart, A.A.M. *et al.* (1998) Development of the macronutrient composition of very preterm human milk. *British Journal of Nutrition*, **80**, 35–40.

Martino, M. de, Tovo, P.A., Tozzi, A.E. *et al.* (1992) HIV-1 transmission through breast milk: appraisal of risk according to duration of feeding. *AIDS*, **6**, 991–7.

Rasmussen, K.M. (1992) The influence of maternal nutrition on lactation. *Annual Review of Nutrition*, **12**, 103–19.

Ruff, A.J. (1992) Breast feeding and maternal infant transmission of human immunodeficiency virus type 1. *Journal of Pediatrics*, **121**, 325–9.

Sanders, T.A.B. and Reddy, S. (1992) Infant brains and diet. *British Medical Journal*, **340**, 1093.

Schrezenmeir, J., Korhonen, H., Williams, C.M., *et al.* (2000) Beneficial natural substances in milk and colostrum. *British Journal of Nutrition*, **84**, (Suppl.1), S1–166.

Schulte-Hobein, B., Schwartz-Bickenbach, D., Abt, S. *et al.* (1992) Cigarette smoke exposure and development of infants throughout the first year of life: influence of passive smoking and nursing on cotinine levels in breast milk and infants' urine. *Acta Paediatrica*, **81**, 550–7.

Sieratzki, J.S. and Woll, B. (1996) Why do mothers cradle babies on their left? *Lancet*, **347**, 1746–8.

Smith, M.M. and Kuhn, L. (2000) Exclusive breast feeding: does it have the potential to reduce breast feeding transmission of HIV-1? *Nutrition Reviews*, **58**, 333–40.

Symposium on Meeting the Needs of Lactation. (1997) *Proceedings of the Nutrition Society*. **56**, 149–91.

Vernon, R.G. (1992) The effects of diet on lipolysis and its regulation. *Proceedings of the Nutrition Society*, **51**, 397–408.

Walravens, P.A., Chakar, A., Mokni, R. *et al.* (1992) Zinc supplementation in breast-fed infants. *Lancet*, **340**, 683–5.

Weaver, L.T. (1992) Breast and gut: the relationship between lactating mammary function and neonatal gastrointestinal function. *Proceedings of the Nutrition Society*, **51**, 155–63.

Whitehead, R.G. and Paul, A.A. (2000) Long-term adequacy of exclusive breast feeding: how scientific research has led to revised opinions. *Proceedings of the Nutrition Society*, **59**, 17–23.

WEANING

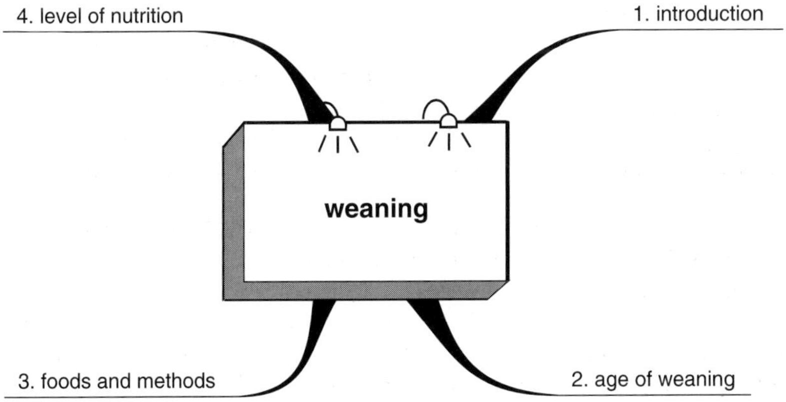

Fig. 42.3 Section outline.

INTRODUCTION

Weaning is the gradual withdrawal of breast milk and introduction of other foods, including suitably prepared adult food and the milk of other animals.

The child is weaned from the breast or formula milk and introduced to semi-solid or solid food, which become the source of energy and nutrient intake. Weaning from maternal milk onto food occurs towards the middle of the first year. An energy gap may develop from that stage.

AGE OF WEANING

The usual practice in Western countries is to wean before 6 months; earlier weaning is practised in some in urban areas. This may be related to the need for women to return to paid employment. In Europe and North America more than 90% of children receive some semi-solid food by the age of 9 months, supplemented by breast milk or a modern infant formula. The age of weaning in developing countries may be different to that in developed countries.

The usual recommendation is that the majority of infants should receive a milk-only diet until 12 weeks. Weaning should be a gradual process thereafter and babies should be offered a mixed diet not later than the age of 6 months. Energy intake per kilogram body weight declines rapidly from birth to the age of 6 months and then rises again, as the baby becomes more active. Babies who are not weaned until 3–6 months of age grow differently to very early weaners.

FOODS AND METHODS

Cereals are the most common first weaning food.

Europe and North America

In the early weaning months breast milk, or a formula, provides a substantial portion of the total energy and nutrient intake. In later infancy and beyond, cow's milk may provide one-quarter of the total energy and one-third of the protein intake. Strained foods are introduced later and are frequently based on full adult meals. Parents are able to apply their knowledge of a reasonable adult mixture of food to their children's diet. It is possible that the occurrence of coeliac disease is a result of premature weaning onto gluten-containing foods, e.g. wheat.

Developing countries

Breast milk is the source of nutrition for the first 6 months of life. In these countries weaning is undertaken by stressed, possibly pregnant, hard-working rural mothers. If the mother is working in the fields, the responsibility may fall upon slightly older sisters.

Traditional weaning foods may be contaminated with enteropathic bacteria. The result is diarrhoea and undernutrition, which may compound the nutritional inadequacies of a child who has been receiving insufficient breast milk. More than half of the developing world's children are undernourished, with retardation of growth and development.

The weaning foods are gruels based on cereal flours, maize, rice, millet, sorghum and wheat, the starch being the important energy source. The boiled starch gelatinises and produces a viscous paste that may contain resistant starch (see chapter 13). The type of cereal is determined by availability. The energy density and fat content is low and the baby has to eat a considerable bulk to meet energy needs. Adding milk increases the protein-energy ratio and overall protein quality. Cereal or milk alone would be inadequate. Water content and hence intake is important, otherwise the gruel becomes very viscous. Germination, malting and roasting reduce viscosity and increase the energy density of cereals. The calorie content may be increased by oils, fat or sugar, and malting may partially digest the starch.

> Cereals are germinated by soaking in the dark for 48–72 h, dried and toasted and, after removal of the sprouting bits, ground and milled to flour. The starches are partially hydrolysed. There may be some solubilisation of proteins, amino acids and vitamins. Their concentrations may increase and trypsin inhibitors and phytic acid content be reduced. The energy content may be doubled by such processes. Fermentation and amylase enrichment may improve both the nutritional content and the hygiene of the feed.

Composition of weaning foods

There are many differences in the approach to weaning in different countries. The recommendations are based on energy and protein content per unit weight or per unit energy. There is often fortification of natural foods.

France has its own detailed recommendations. In Thailand, there is a recommendation for protein of not less than 2.5 g/100 kcal, amino acid score not less than 70% of the FAO/WHO reference pattern, fat 2.6 g/100 kcal and linoleic acid not less than 300 mg/100 kcal. Supplementary food mixtures containing rice and soya bean, groundnuts, sesame or mung beans are also used. This mixes a starch (rice)-containing, relatively low-protein source with a vegetable with a high protein content. This has had profound effects on reducing moderate and severe protein-energy malnutrition.

LEVEL OF NUTRITION

Overnutrition

During the first year of life the deposition of fat increases from approximately 11% of body weight at birth to 25% at 6 months, is steady from 6 to 12 months of age, and slowly decreases to 16% during the toddler years.

Solid foods, particularly those high in protein and electrolytes (added salts), increase the solute loads. The kidney must be able to respond by producing a more concentrated urine. This should result in increased thirst, with the baby drinking more milk or formula to increase weight.

Undernutrition

Weaning may be forced on a mother through insufficient breast milk for the baby's hunger and nutritional requirements. A strong, healthy baby who suckles frequently and well appears to be the most important stimulus to maternal prolactin production and hence milk secretion.

There is a contrast between the health of babies in Europe or North America and the developing world. Babies in Europe or North America who are healthy at 4 weeks old will grow into healthy adults. In the developing world, the early post-natal months and toddler years are very dangerous periods.

The most significant risks of deficiency conditions to the weaning infant and requirements for

supplementation are identified in the chapters on specific nutrients, particularly essential fatty acids and amino acids, calcium and vitamin D, vitamin A, iron and zinc (see Part V).

KEY POINTS

1. Weaning is the process of withdrawal from dependence on breast milk to prepared semi-solid and then solid food. The age of weaning varies with culture, country and economic status.
2. Cereals are the most common first weaning food, with added milk and other protein sources. The weaning food must be adequate in energy, protein, essential dietary constituents and water.
3. The mode of preparation will vary, with the major risk being bacterial contamination of the feed.
4. The correct amount of nutrients given is critical to the baby's future well-being. Depending on the economic environment in which the infant lives there is the potential for under- or overprovision.

THINKING POINTS

1. Infants are vulnerable.
2. Correct weaning is important and rewarding with evidence of satisfactory development.
3. The situation is less enjoyable for the poor, lonely, harassed and unsupported working mother.

NEED TO UNDERSTAND

1. Weaning is the change from a dedicated feeding system, milk, to the wide variety afforded by adult food.
2. The baby is introduced to life-long eating patterns.

FURTHER READING

Barker, D.J.P. (1992) Infant origins of common diseases. In *Human Nutrition; A Continuing Debate* (eds M.A. Eastwood, C. Edwards and D. Parry). Chapman and Hall, London, pp. 17–30.

Brown, K.H. (1997) Complementary feeding in developing countries: factors affecting energy intake. *Proceedings of the Nutrition Society*, **56**, 139-48.

Leader (1991) Solving the weanling's dilemma: power-flour to fuel the gruel. *Lancet*, **338**, 604–5.

Wharton, B. (1997) Weaning in Britain: practice, policy and problems. *Proceedings of the Nutrition Society*, **56**, 105–19.

43

Childhood and youth; middle age and old age

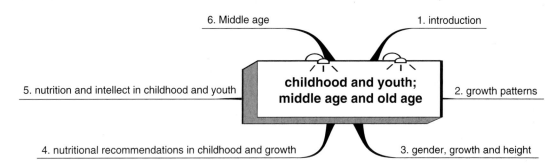

Fig. 43.1 Section outline.

INTRODUCTION

Height is often chosen as an indicator of nutritional status, although the reason for this is not clear, since diet is not the only environmental factor that influences height. Other factors include genetic makeup, childhood illnesses and sleep patterns.

Height velocity is a better measure than height as a single measurement. The short child in the 25th percentile or growing less than 4 cm per year should always be considered for investigation. However, some children grow slowly before achieving their final height. Height is an indicator of past growth rather than present health.

Growth is dependent on a series of factors including the inherited genetic potential, available nutrition to enable the expression of genetic potential and good health.

Normal growth takes place in distinct spurts in a cyclical manner with a periodicity of about 2 years. This cyclical pattern is maintained even during growth lags.

Food that satisfies the energy gap, micronutrient and nitrogen needs is essential for growth and high activity. However, access to effective primary health care is also essential for good growth. The progress of growth can be assessed by regular weight and height measurements and compared with tables for the population. During adolescence there are increased nutritional requirements of adequate protein, vitamins and minerals, and calorie intake.

GROWTH PATTERNS

The pattern of growth is characterised by prolonged infancy, extended childhood and rapid growth during the adolescent growth spurt.

Inadequate food intake in the first 2 years of life is responsible for stunting and poor weight development in millions of children worldwide. Poor breast feeding, weaning and feeding practices are contributory. Intercurrent infections and diarrhoea are also relevant. The way in which the food is provided to the children is relevant. The United Nations Children's Fund (UNICEF) has recommended practices in Early Child Care for Survival, Growth and Development:

- care for women, ensuring adequate prenatal care, safe delivery of the baby and equal access to education
- suitable kitchen facilities: food preparation is a very time-consuming activity. Women cooking over smoky fires in enclosed conditions are liable to develop emphysema
- good hygiene practices
- a healthy home environment, the ready diagnosis of illness, preventive medicine and freedom from pests and accidents.
- good psychosocial care, a loving and caring environment
- feeding, i.e. breast feeding and complementary feeding.

Complementary feeding is the practice of weaning and the child eating in a manner consistent with the culture into which they are born, ensuring adequate intake of nutrition. The child is developing rapidly during these 2 years, when early independence evolves.

By 7 months the gag reflex has moved back to the posterior third of the tongue and allows the swallowing of solids. The child learns how to manage a cup and solid food, and develops the complicated multiple skills in using a spoon. These developments vary with culture and also depend on the time and stamina available to the carer. A working, unsupported, poor, not very intelligent mother with several children is not able to give the same time as an affluent, supported mother with her first child. During this period the child develops behavioural attitudes to feeding that may be life long in their effect.

The head circumference of the child is a physical index of both past nutrition and brain development. It is the most sensitive anthropometric index of prolonged undernutrition during childhood and associated intellectual impairment.

The prepubertal growth spurt is a qualitative as well as a quantitative growth. Body shape and composition also change. Boys enter puberty with one-sixth of the body as fat and end puberty developing muscle, so that the fat content falls to one-tenth. Girls' bodies over the same period change from one-sixth fat to one-quarter fat. Menarche appears to depend on the weight-for-height ratio, and a minimum fat content of 17% is a requirement.

At the pubertal growth spurt, boys grow 20 cm in height and 20 kg in weight, a greater growth than that seen in girls at the same stage.

Stature at the of age 18 years in Austrian men varies by up to 6 mm according to the month of birth. In Denmark there is a 2.2 mm variation in length at birth over the year, being lowest in December and highest in April.

Growth retardation is delayed growth compared with the peer group, and is most common in children aged between 6 and 12 months. The reduced size and function may carry over into later, even adult stages of life, with physiological and economic consequences. Reduced physical development in a country with little mechanisation is detrimental to the individual's work capacity and earning power. Fertility and infant death rate are increased in stunted members of poor communities. Catch-up growth can occur, but in reality only happens if the adverse circumstances change.

Since the 1980s many people in Western countries have developed alternative lifestyles. One such style is the macrobiotic diet, consisting of organically grown cereals, vegetables and pulses, and small amounts of seaweed, fermented foods, nuts and seeds and occasional seafood. There has been anxiety that such a diet may result in health risks. In a study of 4–18-month-old macrobiotic-fed children, a lack of energy-and protein-containing foods led to muscle wasting and intellectual retardation. However, a longer term study found that long-standing mild to moderate malnutrition did not lead to a reduction in mental development. Another dictate of intellectual and emotional

Indian, Japanese and US children have similar growth patterns up to the age of 9 years. Thereafter, a growth gap develops during the remaining years of growth between the first two groups and the US adolescents. It is not clear whether this difference is environmental or genetic. The Indian and Japanese diet is largely cereal derived and there may be dietary deficiency or dietary antinutrients that cause the lack of growth. A survey in 1992 by the Japanese Ministry of Education of 700 000 children aged between 4 and 18 years showed they had grown significantly in height compared with their parents. Boys aged 13–14 years were 9.5 cm taller and 9 kg heavier than their parents at the same age. At 17–18 years they were 5 cm taller in 1992 than Japanese people 30 years previously. Much of this difference was in leg length.

In the Netherlands, there is a tradition of monitoring children's height that goes back to the nineteenth century. During the nineteenth century and the early twentieth century differences of 5–11 cm at various ages were noted between those children whose fathers had a 'low' compared with a 'high' occupational status. This gap has now reduced to differences of 1–3 cm. Similar reduction in height differentials between socially and economically disadvantaged and rich children have been observed in India. A British tradition, unproven except in folklore, is that the child's height at 2 years and 6 months is half that of the final growth achievement.

A curious feature of the development of the stunted child is the anatomy of the deficient height. This may be the sitting height, that is, coccyx to top of head, or standing height, where leg length is important. In stunted Black Americans and Australian Aborigines the sitting height is deficient, in Japanese standing height is deficient, and in Indians the deficit is symmetrical. Possibly some complicating micronutrient is deficient or the timing of the deficiency at some vulnerable period occurs, primarily affecting trunk or leg growth.

development is the social and family environment in which the child is reared. A child that is given attention will make better intellectual and emotional progress than the neglected infant receiving the same nutritional support.

A study of children reared in London on vegan diets showed that such children develop normally, provided that care is taken with vitamin B_{12} replenishment, and that the problems of bulky diets and nutrient dilution are recognised. These children are frequently not immunised and problems can arise in susceptibility to infectious diseases.

The stunted child may be helped by nutritional replenishment, e.g. the child with iron-deficiency anaemia may partially benefit from iron replenishment. However, full restoration of health may depend on other deficient nutrients being replenished. Stunting of growth due to insufficient nutrition may also be aggravated by coincidental infection.

Some teenage girls start smoking in order to lose weight.

GENDER, GROWTH AND HEIGHT

There are 5% more boys born than girls, yet at every stage of life females survive better than males. Girls are more resistant to infection and malnutrition.

In development and normal growth, there is an instinctive feeling that tallness equates with capability. Height may protect against myocardial infarction but not against cancer, and the converse applies to short stature. It has still to be shown that final growth height is advantageous in terms of health.

Height may be a cosmetic attribute useful in certain sporting activities, but it is not necessarily the ultimate measure of nutritional success. In the US presidential elections, the taller of the two candidates has, with one exception, always won. Comparable statistics for other countries are not readily available. Some quite short men, e.g. Napoleon Bonaparte, Alexander the Great, Attila the Hun, Byron, Cervantes, Cromwell, Sir Frances Drake, Louis XIV, Admiral Lord Nelson, Shakespeare, Socrates and St Paul, have been extremely successful. However, tallness in women does not necessarily carry the same prestige in Western society.

NUTRITIONAL RECOMMENDATIONS IN CHILDHOOD AND GROWTH

Several nutrition experts have recommended that all children consume diets containing no more than

30% of calories as fat. It is important to ensure that sufficient calories are provided for growth and energy requirements, and that sufficient polyunsaturated fatty acids (PUFAs) are provided for essential functions.

Children less than 2 years old should not take foods rich in non-starch polysaccharides at the expense of more energy-rich foods that they require for adequate growth. A non-starch polysaccharide intake has not yet been defined for children. Children need energy derived from carbohydrates in all forms. For convenience, their nourishment is facilitated if their simple energy requirements are met at the same time as other needs, e.g. protein and essential nutrients.

Failure to thrive in infancy results from relative undernutrition. In Britain this is less likely to be due to neglect, organic disease or deprivation than to differences in eating behaviour and feeding patterns.

NUTRITION AND INTELLECT IN CHILDHOOD AND YOUTH

There has been considerable debate on whether supplementing the diet with vitamins improves children's performance in intelligence testing. When an improvement is reported, the improvement is in non-verbal rather than in verbal measures. Verbal intelligence reflects educational and other experiences, whereas non-verbal measures basic biological functioning. Improvement may also reflect increased working and attention capacity. A poor diet may be associated with a poorer performance in non-verbal intelligence tests. The response to the trials of supplementation is greater in schools with socially deprived children.

What is not known is the degree of undernutrition that results in reduced intellectual performance. There may be a subgroup of children who are undernourished and whose optimal intellectual development could be ensured by dietary supplements. Such children are found more frequently in developing countries than in the developed world.

Britain has the highest pregnancy rate among 15–19-year-olds in Western Europe. Truancy, low academic achievement and poor sex education are contributory factors. A baby born in these circumstances does not have optimal opportunities.

KEY POINTS

1. Development in growing children is usually measured as height, or preferably the rate of increase in height over a defined period. Height is determined by both genetic background and nutrition.
2. There is a prepubertal growth spurt in which height, body shape and composition change. The characteristic body shapes of males and females are formed at this time. The prepubertal growth pattern varies in different racial and economic groups. Young people on defined diets should ensure that specific nutrient requirements are met, e.g. vitamin B_{12}.
3. The correct dietary intake is critical during childhood and growth.

THINKING POINTS

1. This is the second critical time of the individual's development, following the intrauterine period.
2. Culture, economic environment and availability of the mother are all important to allow the inherent potential to be achieved.
3. In many communities the male is given preference over the female child.

NEED TO UNDERSTAND

1. The importance of the main stages of childhood and adolescent development, the first 2 years and the growth spurt, on build, stamina and emotional well-being.
2. Intrinsically, girls are better equipped to live than boys, which is reversed in some societies by the undue preference shown to boys' needs.

FURTHER READING

Benton, D. (1992) Vitamin–mineral supplements and intelligence. *Proceedings of the Nutrition Society*, **51**, 295–302.

Butler, G.E., McKie, M. and Ratcliffe, S.G. (1990) The cyclical nature of prepubertal growth. *Annals of Human Biology*, **17**, 177–98.

Engle, P.L., Bentley, M. and Pelto, G. (2000) The role of care in nutrition programmes: current research and a research agenda. *Proceedings of the Nutrition Society*, **59**, 25–35.

Evans, D., Hansen, J.L.O., Moodie A.D. *et al.* (1980) Intellectual development and nutrition. *J. Pediatrics*, **97**, 358–63.

Frisch, R.E. (1977) Food intake, fatness and reproductive ability. In *Anorexia Nervosa* (ed. R.A. Vigersky). Raven Press, New York, pp. 149–61.

Geissler, C. (1996) Adolescent nutrition: are we doing enough? *Proceedings of the Nutrition Society*, **55**, 321–67.

Herens, M.C., Dagnelie, P.C., Kleber, R.J. *et al.* (1992) Nutrition and mental development of 4–5 year-old children on macrobiotic diets. *Journal of Human Nutrition and Dietetics*, **5**, 1–9.

Leader (1992) Too tall? *Lancet*, **339**, 339–40.

Mackenbach, J.P. (1991) Narrowing inequalities in children's height (Letter). *Lancet*, **338**, 764.

Nelson, M. (1992) Vitamin and mineral supplementation and academic performance in school children. *Proceedings of the Nutrition Society*, **51**, 303–13.

NNMB (1991) Report of repeat survey (1988–90). *National Institute of Nutrition*, ICMR.

Norgan, N.G. (2000) Long term physiological and economic consequences of growth retardation in children and adolescents. *Proceedings of the Nutrition Society*, **59**, 245–56.

Sanders, T.A. and Manning, J. (1992) The growth and development of vegan children. *Journal of Human Nutrition and Dietetics*, **5**, 11–21.

Wohlfahrt, J., Melbye, M., Christens, P., *et al.* (1998) Secular and seasonal variation of length and weight at birth. *Lancet*, **352**, 1990.

Wright, C., Loughbridge, J. and Moore, G. (2000) Failure to thrive in a population context: two contrasting studies of feeding and nutritional status. *Proceedings of the Nutrition Society*, **59**, 37–45.

MIDDLE AGE

Middle age might be defined as the period between 35 and 59 years of age. Middle age is the established group at the peak of social and pro-fessional achievement. A healthy middle age is dependent on good nutrition in the formative years. Middle age is the time when excess nutrition, especially of fat and alcohol, occurs, with adverse consequences for weight and disease.

The concerns of middle age are:

- the empty nest (children leaving home)
- the mid-life crisis
- change of life, the menopause, etc.
- transition and change before retirement
- the increasing frequency of 'health and illness' problems.

Growth that is of functional value has stopped. During middle age, fat stores usually increase and there is a decline in organ function, especially of pulmonary and renal capacity, which reduce by half between the ages of 30 and 90 years. The decline in organs and systems is gradual, except for the abrupt cessation of ovarian function at the menopause. At the menopause the female is released from the constant threat of iron deficiency through menstruation and pregnancy. The obverse side of this is the loss of the protection afforded by oestrogens against coronary heart disease. This is a period of life when, if there is a sufficiency of food available, food intake, storage and metabolism should be balanced.

In middle age there are increasing numbers of deaths from diseases believed to be associated with an excess of inappropriate foods, too much alcohol and smoking, or all three. Those middle-aged people who die or who suffer from these conditions are disadvantaged by their genetic makeup and consequently by a vulnerability to dietary constituents, alcohol and tobacco. The killers are coronary heart disease, hypertension, stroke, cancer of the lung, colon, prostate and breast, diabetes and chronic pulmonary disease. The individual's weight, especially if male, and the amount of exercise taken are important. An individual should be of acceptable weight [body mass index (BMI) 20–25] and take at least 70 min of exercise a week that results in tachycardia each week.

A broadly based diet is to be commended. It is unclear whether it is too late to alter life expectation by improved diet in middle age. The early years are certainly more important in establishing the individual's constitution. Perhaps the next generation will benefit from improved social and nutritional influences. The health problems that develop in this age group are dependent on a number of factors, only some of which are avoidable:

- vulnerabilities dependent on genetic makeup
- maternal health and nutritional status during uterine life
- nutrition during the first year of life
- exposure to factors including culture, smoking, employment hazards, war and accidents
- exposure to dangerous infections
- excess food challenging the genetic makeup
- overall or individual factors, including amount of food, alcohol, exercise and body weight.

KEY POINTS

1. Middle age is a period of equilibrium in nutrition. There is no further growth except for the laying down of undesirable fat.
2. The decline of body organs begins, and tissue repair becomes increasingly important.
3. Premature death is in part dictated by genetic makeup and early nutritional patterns, but may be reduced by attention to weight, exercise, smoking habits and an adequate diet.

THINKING POINT

Most of the determinants of long life are experienced *in utero* and in childhood: it is necessary to

exercise, not to smoke, to eat a recommended diet and to maintain an appropriate weight if a long life is to be achieved. Why is this incompatible with what many regard as an enjoyable lifestyle?

NEED TO UNDERSTAND

The requirements for a healthy middle age are to enjoy exercise, avoid smoking, follow a recommended diet and maintain an appropriate weight.

FURTHER READING

Abel, T., McQueen, D.V., Backett, K. and Currie, C. (1992) Patterns of unhealthy eating behaviours in a middle aged Scottish population. *Scottish Medical Journal*, **37**, 170–4.

Eastwood, M.A., Edwards, C. and Parry, D. (1992) *Human Nutrition: A Continuing Debate*. Chapman and Hall, London.

Garrow, J.S. (1988) *Obesity and Related Diseases*. Churchill Livingstone, London.

OLD AGE

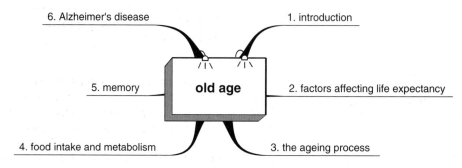

Fig. 43.2   Section outline.

INTRODUCTION

Ageing may be defined as regression of physiological functions accompanied by advancing age. Ageing means increased years, but often also means deterioration. Malnourished populations do not have a long expectation of life. In developed countries, for many people an expectation of life of 85 years or more is being achieved. There is an, as yet undefined, upper limit of life expectancy, and perhaps the quality of overall life should be the objective rather than the extension of life in the frail and disabled.

> There are important differences in the rates at which different individuals age, so there is a distinction between biological and chronological age.

Longevity increased markedly during the twentieth century, with the most marked increase being in Japan (Table 43.1), where the diet has changed during this period (Table 43.2). The Japanese diet is still based on rice with a balance of animal, mostly fish, and vegetable foods.

Table 43.1 Changes in longevity in Japan, 1890–1990

| Year | Life expectancy (years) | |
	Males	Females
1890	36	37
1947	50	50
1990	76	82

1890: New Zealand, Australia and Sweden highest
1947: Sweden and Western Europe highest
1990: Japan highest

Table 43.2 Changes in the Japanese diet, 1910–1989 (daily intake per capita)

Dietary component	1910	1989
Carbohydrate (g)	430	190
Fat (g)	13	59
Animal protein (g)	3	42

Some recommendations for increased life expectancy

Yukaghir of Siberia: 'maintain a few body lice'

Berbers of North Africa: 'always tell the truth'

In the Bible: 'longevity is granted to the righteous'

Avicenna, ninth century physician: 'we should guide the body to its natural span of life'

Ageing through the ages

Palaeolithic (200 000–30 000 BC)	40 years or more
(20 000–6000 BC)	Under 40 years
Neolithic (6000–2000 BC)	25–28 years
Bronze Age (2000–700 BC)	24 years
Minoan and Mycaenian society	35 years
Kings of Judah (if not killed)	24–68 years
Iron Age (700 BC to early AD)	? 40 years
Classical Period (700 BC–AD 400)	66–72 years
Early Middle Ages (AD 400–1000)	36 years
Late Middle Ages (AD 1000–1600)	
English and Scottish kings	48 and 51 years
General population	36 years
Monks	39 years
Seventeenth to nineteenth century	46–58 years
Nineteenth Century (male–female)	40–44 years
Twentieth century (male–female)	72–77 years
British Queen Mother	101 years

These figures are average life expectancies for those who survived infancy and childhood.

Source: MacLennan and Sellars (1999).

FACTORS AFFECTING LIFE EXPECTANCY

The country where the person lives can influence longevity. In Europe and North America longevity is commonplace, but in most of Africa less than 10% of the population are over 60 years old. It is anticipated that in the year 2025, 25% of the US and 31% of the European population will be over 60. Another important element is prosperity and

Factors favouring longevity	Factors militating against longevity
Female gender	Economic inequality
Low cholesterol	Infections
Low blood pressure	Smoking
Non-smoking	Poor nutrition
Physical activity	Hypertension
Healthy diet	High cholesterol
Vegetarianism	Obesity
Early diet and growth	Local homicide rates
Peace	War
Inner peace	Inner turbulence
Relatives who are long lived	Pestilence
Employment status	Famine
Screening for treatable conditions	Poor obstetric care
Social and productive activity	Extremes of weather, cold, and heat
Good available medical care	Pessimism and unhappiness
Optimism	Suicide
Modest alcohol intake	Immodest alcohol intake
Old age	Drugs
Country of domicile	Bereavement
Country of birth	Air pollution
Freedom from diabetes	Immigrant status
Well-stocked refrigerator	
Childhood intelligence quotient (IQ)	

Only the initial factors are in any order of significance, and will vary between countries.

Longevity statistics

Part of the problem in assessing longevity is how and why age is registered in any population. The accuracy of registers of birth is not uniform throughout the world. In some countries it was the practice to take one's father's birth certificate during the late teens to appear older and hence avoid military service.

hence mode of living. When the gross national product exceeds US$7000 per capita, the life expectancy of the inhabitants of the country exceeds 70 years.

Women tend to live longer than men but report more morbidity. Poverty and violence are features of women's life in many communities.

An important factor in longevity is the regard for the elderly by the person, family and community. Although IQ is a favourable factor for longevity, men of high IQ are more likely to be killed in active service during wars.

The nature of the diet through the earlier years, particularly the daily intake of fresh fruit and vegetables and the protein content, will be reflected in a person's life expectation regardless of the country where they live. A protein intake of over 50 g/day is an important divider between short and long life expectations. The contents of the refrigerator reflect the elderly person's way of life: even having a refrigerator, as well as the ability to shop, strength to shop, cognition, money, help, outside interest in their well-being are all predictors of longevity. Night-time (falls, incontinence, confusion, loneliness) and winter (hypothermia, falls on ice, problems with going out for shopping, loneliness) are particular hazards.

THE AGEING PROCESS

It is not known what causes the ageing process, and whether it is at an organ or a cellular level, or is inevitable. Perhaps organs are slowly damaged or compromised by the environment. The brain

Potential contributors to nutritional problems in elderly people

Refusal to eat
Physical factors
Reduced total energy needs
Poor dentition, reduced salivary flow
Declining absorptive and metabolic capacities
Chronic diseases, restrictive diets
Loss of appetite, anorexia
Changes in taste or odour perception
Lack of exercise
Physical disability
Drug–nutrient interactions
Side-effects of drugs (nausea, altered taste)
Alcoholism

Sociopsychological factors
Depression
Loneliness
Social isolation
Bereavement
Loss of interest in food or cooking
Mental disorders
Food faddism
Lack of self-worth
Inadequate diets caused by cultural and religious influences

Socioeconomic factors
Low income
Inadequate cooking or storage facilities
Poor nutrition knowledge
Lack of transportation
Shopping difficulties
Cooking practices resulting in nutrient losses
Inadequate cooking skills

In England and Wales, the mortality rate for immigrants has been high for Scots, Irish and Caribbean men. The increases are due to ischaemic heart disease and lung cancer. The excessive deaths in Irish immigrants takes three generations to reduce to the established population. In Russia, changing social conditions and unemployment have led to increased alcoholism and suicide rates in freezing winters and to a life expectancy for men of 58 years.

shrinks with age, most probably due to cell death. The concentrations of most hormones decline with age, affecting thermoregulatory function and blood glucose concentrations. Imahori (1992) proposed that there are supervising organs, e.g. brain and thymus, which decay before the other organs. The other organs follow an inevitable decline. Alternatively, cells may be genetically programmed to die or wear out. Cell death has been linked to a lethal or senescent gene. Mitochondrial DNA increasingly mutates over the years, the electron transport chain and adenosine triphosphate (ATP) synthase are disrupted, and ATP production is affected. This is followed by cell dysfunction and cell death.

Glycation, the non-enzymatic and irreversible binding of glucose to the N-terminal amino acids of proteins (glycated haemoglobin, and glycated proteins and fructosamine), increases with age.

The only factors that modify the effects of ageing are genetic disposition, nutrition, exercise and blood-pressure control.

Physiology

As the individual ages, physical activity declines and so less dietary energy is required. Energy expenditure in the young and old is very different. Energy expenditure and energy requirements decrease with advancing age, along with a decrease in the basal metabolic rate (BMR). All individuals have to meet the basal needs of both bodily and mental activity; it is the spare energy that varies. The young have abounding energy, well in excess of need. This gives an amplitude of activity that is physical, social and intellectual. As the years accumulate this excess to basal energy requirement reduces. Less free energy is available for physical, social and intellectual activity. The basal energy devoted to basal activity declines less markedly, but assumes a larger proportion of the available energy. This is a source of great frustration to the elderly, as frequently the body declines in strength and stamina in advance of the mind.

Many individuals abandon physical activity after the age of 30 years. The Canada Fitness Survey suggests that the average male over 30 years of age finds walking uphill at 5 km/h (3 miles/h) severe exertion.

As the sedentary way of life becomes more ingrained, the capacity to change decreases and the degree of unfitness increases. When people with a sedentary habit try to exercise, endurance is limited as they draw on reduced available energy stores. Stamina is age related. Some of the deterioration is unavoidable; the remainder is amenable to intervention and is reversible with exercise.

Assessing fitness

Fitness, in general, is measured as $V_{O_2\,max}$ (maximum oxygen intake during exercise).

A more day-to-day assessment of unfitness is the point at which the person is distressed by a degree of exercise and the speed of restoration of well-being is slow.

In the elderly, a small reduction in activity can result in loss of mobility. Physical activity in the elderly is important in maintaining cardiovascular well-being, maintaining muscle mass, reducing falls, osteoblast formation and maintaining bone density. In one study, 1 h of walking twice a week for 8 months increased bone density by 3.5%, compared with a 2.7% decrease in the controls. Flexibility and joint movements also benefit.

Pathology

A distinction has to be made between the fit elderly people living in familiar surroundings and the frail elderly who require care.

Body composition
During adult life there is a slow decrease in lean body mass and total body potassium. By 70 years, 40% of skeletal muscle has been lost compared with young adult life. Women retain their lean body mass up to the age of 50 years, whereas men begin to lose lean body mass from the age of 30. Ageing alters the muscles quantitatively and qualitatively. There is loss of muscle fibres; exercise can affect the fibres that are left but not affect the reduction in numbers. The muscle fibres change shape and grouping, so that in the elderly they change from a regular distribution to clustering in clumps. The fast fibres decay more quickly with age, so that age is associated with increased slow fibres.

There is an increase in body fat, which accumulates throughout life up to the eighth decade. In older people, fat tissue accumulates on the trunk,

in the abdominal region and from subcutaneous tissue to fat surrounding organs.

Total body water decreases with age. This decline begins in middle age in men and in women after the age of 60 years. Bone mass diminishes with age from about the age of 30 years. Bone mineral and matrix disappear more rapidly than deposition of bone tissue. Trabecular bone is lost at an earlier age than cortical bone, which is significant as bone mass is important in bone strength.

Ageing process

Reduction in:
• organ system function
• lean body mass
• total body potassium
• skeletal muscle mass (40% reduced at 70 years)
• muscle protein breakdown
• BMR
• body water
• bone mass.

Increase in:
• body fat, with redistribution to the trunk and around organs.
• urinary creatine clearance (an index of muscle mass).

There are age-related effects on the gastrointestinal tract. The changes observed with age include reductions in gastric acid, mucus, gastric enzymes, pancreatic enzyme excretion, bile and intestinal wall strength. The latter occurs in part because of cross-linkage changes in the collagen of the intestinal wall. Constipation is said to be more common in the frail elderly.

There are increases in blood pressure, and also cardiac enlargement with decreased contractility of the heart muscle and cardiac output. Circulating concentrations of testosterone and oestrogen, parathyroid hormone, triiodothyronine and aldosterone are reduced. There is a reduction in renal function and in kidney size, with the kidney mass being 30% less at the age of 80 than at 30 years. Brain activity changes, with an increase in slow-wave activity, slowing of the α-wave frequency and an increased β-wave activity. The cells of the immune system are affected by age and the T-lymphocytes are reduced. There is a reduction in serum immunoglobulin G (IgG) concentrations and an increase in IgA. While immunocompetence declines with age, such loss is very variable between different individuals. Nutrition is an important determinant of immunocompetence.

Metabolism

The energy requirements of an individual can be described by an energy balance equation:

$$\text{Energy stored} = \text{Energy intake} - \text{Energy expenditure}$$

BMR is affected by familial and genetic influences, and nutritional, metabolic and disease conditions. BMR is reduced in the elderly. This reduction is due to the age-related fall in lean body mass and the loss of the muscle mass. The value is unchanged from younger adults when expressed in relation to lean body, cell or fat-free mass.

The thermic effect of food

This is the energy required for the ingestion, digestion, absorption process and storage of the energy-yielding nutrients. The energy cost of the thermic effect of food varies according to the immediate metabolic fate of these nutrients. There are consequent changes in the metabolic cycle and activation of the sympathetic nervous system, the responsiveness of which declines with age. The size, frequency and composition of meals affect the thermic effect of food. The less food is eaten by the elderly, the less pronounced this effect will be.

The capacity to dissipate excess energy as heat may be different between the elderly and the young adult. However, it is possible that dietary-induced thermogenesis is quantitatively similar in young and elderly subjects in the short term.

Glucose metabolism is altered in elderly people. Insulin deficiency is a contributor to diabetes in the elderly. Total body protein decreases with age as a result of a declining skeletal muscle mass. Whole-body protein synthesis and breakdown and muscle protein breakdown are significantly lower in elderly than in young people. Urinary creatinine excretion, which is an index of muscle mass, is greater in the elderly than in young subjects. It may be that the reduced muscle protein metabolism in the elderly relates to the metabolism of the amino acid gluta-

mine. There is a reduction in the maximal capacity to utilise oxygen during exercise with increasing age.

The total daily energy intake decreases progressively, from approximately 11.3 MJ (2700 kcal) at 30 years to 8.8 MJ (2100 kcal) at 80 years.

FOOD INTAKE AND METABOLISM

Food intake declines with age, as does appetite. The source of energy nutrients in the elderly may be important. There is a deterioration of glucose tolerance with ageing due to impaired peripheral tissue insulin sensitivity, late insulin secretion and altered hepatic glucose output. There are positive connections between fat intake and body composition, suggesting that the composition of the diet is a factor in determining body energy balance and composition. Protein requirements are similar to those in younger adults.

Thirst and water consumption are important to monitor and may be quite varied across the elderly population. Assessment of water intake can be quite difficult in a frail, incontinent person.

Elderly individuals with a fractured neck of the femur do badly if they are underweight. These patients mobilise more readily and without morbidity if they are given supplementary food during the convalescent period.

Once old age has been reached, alteration of the diet, e.g. to reduce obesity, has little effect on longevity, unless the diet is deficient. Osteomalacia and other consequences of long-standing malnutrition may be corrected, without necessarily benefiting the elderly person.

The elderly person is a normal but older, possibly less mobile person, who will consequently enjoy a broadly based diet that fulfils the nutrient needs of an adult.

MEMORY

The brain contains some 100 billion cells (compared with the 100 million in the liver for example) and is made of discrete units rather than a continuum of related cells or syncytium. The cells vary in

Functions predominantly associated with different parts of the brain

Frontal lobe: behaviour, emotions, organisation, personality, planning, problem solving

Parietal lobe: judgement of object's size, shape, weight, sensation of pressure and touch, understanding of language, spoken and written

Occipital lobe: colour and shape recognition

Hippocampus: object recognition, meaning of words and places

Temporal lobe: smell, hearing and sound sensation, short-term memory

Cerebellum: balance, muscle co-ordination, posture

Brain stem: basic body functions, breathing, blood pressure, cardiac function

The collective activity of these regions encompasses the mind.

shape, size and axon lengths. The brain comprises two halves, left and right, joined through the corpus callosum and other axonal bridges.

Memory is a complicated process: visual, spatial, verbal, short-term and long-term memory form mental ability in association with reasoning, attention, psychomotor co-ordination and environmental awareness.

Nutrition plays its role in these processes, as shown by vitamin, iodine and nutrient deficiency in children. Glucose ingestion can benefit short-term memory, rapid information processing, word recall, attention, maze learning and arithmetic ability. This benefit is not achieved by correcting hypoglycaemia, but does coincide with increased blood glucose concentrations. There are cognitive deficits in patients with poor glucose tolerance that are reversible by treatment.

Memory is based on the inner surface of the temporal lobe, in the hippocampus and amygdala. These form part of the limbic system. Also involved is the diencephalon in the midbrain and the limbic system, which are involved in a circuit that creates memory. The actual memory is held in the cortical area where the sensation that created the memory originated. Cells in the cortical neural assembly are changed by feedback from the limbic system and diencephalons, which may take place during sleep. Memory recognition occurs when the neural assembly is reactivated by an appropriate stimulus.

A second, more automatic memory system, is independent of the limbic/diencephalon/cortical system, operates through the striatum in the forebrain.

Short-term memory for simple things is due to the modification of proteins by phosphorylation. Longer term memory may require more permanent change, as in changes in gene expression, e.g. the immediate-early gene (IEG) family. These encode the transcription of proteins that express other genes. Long-term potentiation, i.e. learnt or considered thought, may take place in the hippocampus. The transmitter is glutamate. Sensory experiences are remembered by alterations in the effectiveness of synapses between neurones. The strengths of these increase or decrease and the pattern is a memory. These changes in synaptic strength are due to modifications in phosphorylation or the removal of phosphates in synaptic proteins.

Memory begins to fail as the years progress, and is a major cause of distress in the elderly. The role of nutrition in memory is not clear, although its role in the development of the child's brain and long-chain polyunsaturated fatty acids is recognised. Subclinical deficiencies in vitamins and metabolic disorders, e.g. diabetes, may be important in the elderly.

Women with high blood concentrations of non-protein-bound and bioavailable oestradiol are less liable to develop cognitive impairment than women with low concentrations, as higher concentrations of endogenous oestrogens prevent cognitive decline. The male brain shrinks more rapidly than the female, which may influence cognition and behaviour.

ALZHEIMER'S DISEASE

Dementia occurs primarily with Alzheimer's disease and cerebrovascular disease. Both conditions are very common in old age, and are the cause of much misery to the individual and their partner, family and friends. There is loss of memory, orientation and independence.

Alzheimer's disease may afflict individuals from late middle age, but it is not an inevitable feature of the ageing process. This condition is the cause of 75% of dementias. There is an inherited, autosomal element to Alzheimer's, although head injuries and exposure to aluminium may have a role in the aetiology.

Alzheimer's disease is caused by the loss of nerve cells in parts of the brain including, importantly, the hippocampus and cerebral cortex. The loss of nerve cells is accompanied by a loss of acetylcholine transmitters. Proteins accumulate in the affected brain.

- **Neurofibrillary tangles**: These are made of *tau* protein. Tau protein binds to the protein tubulin, which forms microtubulin structures in the cell. The gene that encodes tau gene is on chromosome 17. Mutations in this gene result in undesirable binding of tau to tubulin.
- **Amyloid protein plaques** with reactive inflammatory cells, (microglia): the amyloid plaques contain β-amyloid pecursor protein. The β-amyloid pecursor protein gene is on chromosome 21. This confirms the inevitable development of Alzheimer's disease in people with Down's syndrome where there is trisomy of chromosome 21. The β-amyloid pecursor protein straddles cell membranes, and the β-amyloid peptide is cleaved from the protein to yield a peptide fraction p3. Alternatively, β-amyloid pecursor protein may be cleaved by β-secretase, yielding C99-βAPP, which in turn is cleaved by γ-secretase to produce the β-amyloid peptide. In general, these are 40 amino acids long, but a form with 42 amino acids exists which is toxic to nerve cells, affecting calcium regulation and damaging mitochondria, with consequent inflammation. The enzymes presenilin-1 and presenelin-2 cleave membrane-bound proteins; the genes for these enzymes are on chromosomes 14 and 1, respectively. Mutations in the genes encoding these enzymes result in a very aggressive form of early-onset Alzheimer's disease. In general, these enzymes overproduce β-amyloid peptide, especially the 42 amino acid version.

Apolipoprotein E (apoE) is a plasma protein involved in cholesterol transport. It is also produced and secreted in the central nervous system by astrocytes. The brain contains large amounts of apoE messenger RNA in amounts second only to the liver. ApoE may be involved in the pathogenesis of late-onset or familial Alzheimer's disease.

This lipoprotein is in three forms, ε_2, ε_3 and ε_4. ApoE-ε_4 is found in 40% of Alzheimer's patients, rather than the usual 6–37%. ApoE-ε_4 successfully competes with β-amyloid peptide removal from the intercellular space by a serum pan-protease inhibitor (A2M), and thus the peptide accumulates.

The apoE-ε_4 allele predisposes to cognitive decline in a general population of elderly men. Oestrogen is not protective in women who have the apoE-ε_4 allele.

There is no indication of an environmental or nutritional cause for these processes, although weight loss is an important complication at all stages of the condition. The weight loss can progress to other complications, infections, skin ulcers, falls and reduced quality of life. Weight loss of more than 5% in a year is a significant predictor of death.

Smoking neither protects or exacerbates the condition. Raised systolic blood pressure and high serum cholesterol increase the risk, from middle age into later life. Individuals with poor linguistic skills in early life are more at risk than those with well-developed skills.

The elderly carers of individuals with Alzheimer's are stressed, preoccupied and suffering. They are at increased risk of infections and their nutritional needs are just as important as all the other support systems that they require.

KEY POINTS

1. The ageing process is a generalised decline in physiological function and stamina, which is a feature of the number of years lived, rather than of a disease process.
2. Longevity is more likely with a good diet and regular exercise, although there is a genetic contribution.
3. There is a slow reduction in body mass, mineral and water with age. Fat may accumulate in the centre of the body. BMR and other measures of metabolism are reduced with age.
4. Alzheimer's disease is a progressive dementia with characteristic clinical and pathological lesions in the brain.

5. In old age the general debility may alter nutritional intake for physical and/or intellectual reasons. However, once old age has been reached, changes in diet have little effect on longevity, unless the diet is deficient.

THINKING POINTS

1. The ageing process is a period of decline, ending in death.
2. Quality of life is all important.
3. By living to old age the nutrition must have been correct for a particular person.
4. The only useful corrections are where deficiencies have developed.

NEED TO UNDERSTAND

1. Fit elderly people are no different from when young or middle aged, in that their way of life must be respected.
2. Frail individuals however, need compassionate care where the declining needs are met, with the knowledge that there are only a few special nutritional requirements, e.g. vitamin D.

FURTHER READING

Andrews, G.R. (2001) Promoting health and function in an ageing population. *British Medical Journal*, **322**, 728–9.

Bales, C.W. and Ritchie, C.S. (2002) Sarcopenia, weight loss and nutritional fraility in the elderly. *Annual Review of Nutrition*, **22**, 309–23.

Bear, M.F. (1997) How do memories leave their marks? *Nature*, **385**, 481–2.

Bellisle, F. (2001) Glucose and mental performance. *British Journal of Nutrition*, **86**, 117–18.

Boumendjel, N, Herman, F., Girod, V. *et al.* (2000) Refrigerator content and hospital admission in old people. *Lancet*, **356**, 563.

Chandra, R.K. (1992) Nutrition and immunity in the elderly. *Nutrition Reviews*, **50**, 367–71.

Craft, N. (1997) Women's health is a global issue. *British Medical Journal*, **315**, 1154–7.

Cronin-Stubbs, D, Beckett, L.A., Scherr, P.A. *et al.* (1997) Weight loss in people with Alzheimer's disease: a prospective population based analysis. *British Medical Journal*, **314**, 178–9.

Doll, R. (1997) One for the heart. *British Medical Journal*, **315**, 1664–8.

Donaldson, G.C., Tchernjavskii, V.E., Ermakov, S.P., *et al.* (1998) Winter mortality and cold stress in Yekaterinburg, Russia: interview survey. *British Medical Journal*, **316**, 514–18.

Fielding, R.A. (1995) Effects of exercise training in the elderly: impact of progressive-resistance training on skeletal muscle and whole body protein metabolism. *Proceedings of the Nutrition Society*, **54**, 665–75.

Fries, J.F. (1980) Aging, natural death and the compression of morbidity. *New England Journal of Medicine*, **303**, 130–5.

Gonzalez-Gross, M., Marcos, A. and Pietrzik, L. (2001) Nutrition and cognitive impairment in the elderly. *British Journal of Nutrition*, **86**, 313–21.

Hitt, R., Young-Xu, Y., Silver, M. and Peris, T. (1999) Centenarians: the older you get, the healthier you have been. *Lancet*, **354**, 652.

Hosoda, S., Bamba, T., Nakago, S. *et al.* (1992) Age-related changes in the gastrointestinal tract. *Nutrition Reviews*, **50**, 374–7.

Huijbregts, P., Feskens, E, Rasanen, L. *et al.* (1997) Dietary pattern and 20 year mortality in elderly men in Finland, Italy, and the Netherlands: longitudinal cohort study. *British Medical Journal*, **315**, 13–17.

Imahori, K. (1992) How I understand aging. *Nutrition Review*, **50**, 351–2.

Ivanovic, D.M., Leiva, B.P., Perez, H.T. *et al.* (2002) Nutritional status, brain development and scholastic achievement of Chilean high school graduates from high and low intellectual quotient and socio-economic status. *British Journal of Nutrition.* **87,** 81–92.

Key, T.J.A., Thorogood, M., Appleby, P.N. and Burr, M.L. (1996) Dietary habits and mortality in 11000 vegetarians and health conscious people: results of a 17 year follow up. *British Medical Journal*, **313**, 775–9.

Khaw, K.-T. (1997) Healthy aging. *British Medical Journal*, **315**, 1090–6.

Khaw, K.-T. (1999) How many, how old, and how soon? *British Medical Journal*, **319**, 1350–2.

Kilpatrick, E.S., Dominiczak, M.H. and Small, M. (1996) The effects of ageing on glycation and the interpretation of glycaemic control in type 2 diabetes. *Quarterly Journal of Medicine*, **89**, 307–12.

MacLennan, W.J. and Sellers, W.I. (1999) Ageing through the ages. *Proceedings of the Royal College Physicians of Edinburgh*, **29**, 71–5.

Marabou Symposium (1992) Nutrition and ageing. *Nutrition Reviews*, **50**, 347–489.

Marcus, E.-L. and Berry, E.M. (1998) Refusal to eat in the elderly. *Nutrition Reviews*, **56**, 163–71.

Masters, C.L. and Beyreuther, K. (1998) Alzheimer's disease. *British Medical Journal*, **316**, 446–8.

Matsuzaki, T. (1992) Longevity, diet and nutrition in Japan: epidemiological studies. *Nutrition Reviews*, **50**, 355–9.

Millward, D.J. and Roberts, S.B. (1996) Protein requirements of older individuals. *Nutrition Research Review*, **9**, 67–87.

Pannemans, D.L.E. and Westerterp, K.R. (1995) Energy expenditure, physical activity and basal metabolic rate of elderly subjects. *British Journal of Nutrition*, **73**, 571–81.

Riviere, S., Gillette-Guyonnet, S., Nourhashemi, F. and Vellas, B. (1999) Nutrition and Alzheimer's disease. *Nutrition Reviews*, **57**, 363–7.

Rolls, B.J. (1994) Appetite and satiety in the elderly. *Nutrition Reviews*, **52**, 59.

Rosenberg, I.H. (ed) (1992) Nutrition in the elderly. *Nutrition Reviews*, **50**, 349–489.

Sayer, A.H. and Cooper, C. (2002) Early diet and growth: impact on ageing. *Proceedings of the Nutrition Society*, **61**, 79–85.

Stephens, T. Craig, C.L. and Ferris, B.F. (1986) Adult physical fitness in Canada: findings from the Canada Fitness Survey. *Canadian Journal of Public Health*, **77**, 285–90.

Terry, R.D., Katzman, R., Bick, K.L. and Sisodia, S.S. (1999) *Alzheimer Disease*, 2nd edn. Philadelphia, PA: Lippincott, Williams and Wilkins.

Trichopoulos, D. and Lagiou, P. (2001) Dietary patterns and mortality. *British Journal of Nutrition*, **85**, 133–4.

Waern, M., Beskow, J., Runeson, B. and Skoog, I. (1999) Suicidal feelings in the last year of life in elderly people who commit suicide. *Lancet*, **354**, 917–18.

Whalley, L.J. and Deary, I.J. (2001) Longitudinal cohort study of childhood IQ and survival up to age 76. *British Medical Journal*, **322**, 819–22.

Wild, S. and McKeigue, P.M. (1997) Cross sectional analysis of mortality by country of birth in England and Wales 1970–92. *British Medical Journal*, **314**, 705–10.

Wilson, M. and Daly, M. (1997) Life expectancy, economic inequality, homicide and reproductive timing in Chicago neighbourhoods. *British Medical Journal*, **314**, 1271–4.

Young, V.R. (1992) Energy requirements for the elderly. *Nutrition Reviews*, **50**, 95–101.

44

Sport

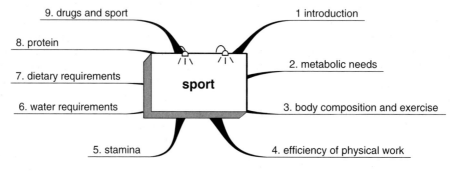

9. drugs and sport   1 introduction

8. protein

7. dietary requirements   **sport**   2. metabolic needs

6. water requirements   3. body composition and exercise

5. stamina   4. efficiency of physical work

Fig. 44.1 Chapter outline.

INTRODUCTION

An appropriate diet for an athlete is dependent on the sport, age of the athlete, fitness and freedom from injury. Modern sport, e.g. football, rugby, athletics, cycling, American football, tennis and hockey, is now so competitive that previously unsuspected demands on physical fitness and strength are expected.

METABOLIC NEEDS

The metabolic needs of endurance athletes (long-distance runners, distance swimmers and cyclists) are different from those for people undertaking intermittent activity (football, hockey, cricket and golf) and sports of short but intense duration, e.g. sprinters and wing three-quarters in rugby. Body-building sportsmen such as weight-lifters have yet different needs (Figure 44.2).

	Endurance sports	Ball games	Strength sports
Requirements	Stamina	Stamina, co-ordination	Strength, co-ordination
Muscle types	1 (slow-twitch)	1 or 2	2 (fast-twitch)
Dietary emphasis	Carbohydrates	Mixed diet	Protein
	Glycogen loading		Muscle mass

Fig. 44.2 General characteristics of requirements in different sports: muscle types and dietary emphasis in endurance sports, ball games and strength sports. All of these dietary emphases are in addition to a balanced diet of carbohydrates, protein, fat, fibre, minerals and vitamins.

To perform well, endurance athletes must establish a store of readily retrievable energy in a frame that is light in weight. The typical long-distance runner or cyclist is a lean individual packed with large stores of glycogen. A first-class football player may run 16 km during a game, yet a goalkeeper may be required to perform intermittently in a gymnastic manner. Sprinters over the range of 100–800 m will rapidly expend energy over short periods of 10 s up to 2 min. Other sports such as cricket, baseball and golf, which are co-ordination sports, require relaxation and concentration. The nutritional needs of a fast bowler at cricket will be different from those of a golfer. It is unlikely that the nutritional needs of this group differ from the prudent advice offered to the population of their age. Players in the strength sports, e.g. weight-lifters, prop-forwards in rugby, heavyweight boxers and American footballers, build massive muscle structure to perform deeds of strength.

There is therefore a range of requirements, including:

- the provision of energy over an extended period from a modest muscle mass, meeting the need to sustain speed for long periods
- the development of a strong physique able to push and pull massive loads and, during the same game, to run considerable distances
- the need for bursts of energy over very brief periods, e.g. sprinters, whether these are athletes or wingers in rugby.

A well-balanced diet should contain 50–60% of the calorie intake as carbohydrate, no more than 35% as fats and approximately 15% as protein. In addition, there should be sufficient amounts of fibre, vitamins and minerals (as suggested for the population in general), but possibly increased in proportion to energy intake. Some sports will require modest increases of a particular nutrient, e.g. carbohydrate for endurance athletes and protein for strength sport. It is important that such diets are sensible and within the overall concept of a balanced diet.

Alcohol is a continuing problem in sport. Athletes are strong, vigorous, young people, sometimes with time on their hands. Victories are to be celebrated. Many athletes have taken an undue amount of alcohol and paid the price.

BODY COMPOSITION AND EXERCISE

Sport has a place for all sizes and shapes of individuals. Overall, with the exception of the massive strength sports, e.g. wrestling, rugby forwards, American football players and even darts players, successful athletes have a lean body mass. Height is very game dependent. Some of the great names in cricket and gymnastics are quite short in stature, whereas tall, fast bowlers are the norm.

In adults, body mass, both lean body mass and fat mass, is regulated at a constant level. Changes are affected by energy intake and expenditure. Successful athletes have a larger lean body mass than their sedentary contemporaries. Body weight influences the response to exercise. If body weight is maintained, then exercise increases the lean body mass. If nutrition is insufficient then lean body mass declines. The body fat content of the individual before exercise influences the extent of the body composition response to exercise. If at the outset the body fat content is small, then the response is the loss or gain of about 0.5 kg of lean body mass for every 1 kg of weight change with exercise. If the initial body fat is larger, then the fat gives a degree of protection, with the energy reserve and lean body mass loss being 0.25 kg/kg change in body weight. Exercise allows weight loss without losing lean body mass. Once a significant weight loss has occurred then body fat content becomes relevant.

If dietary fat is replaced by carbohydrate, then there is an increased post-prandial increase in plasma triacylglycerol concentrations. Daily exercise or a single session, as with a running programme, can prevent this increase. Increased triacylglycerol hydrolysis in skeletal muscle by lipoprotein lipase may be a factor in this reduction. Exercise can have a favourable influence, with increased triacylglycerolaemia, reduced high-density lipoprotein (HDL) cholesterol and hypertension.

A problem for the female athlete is the triad of disordered eating, amenorrhoea and osteoporosis. The most important element in these women is adequate nutrition to sustain normal menstrual and bone function.

However, regular physical activity is good for mood and longevity, and reduces the possibility of type II diabetes, cardiovascular disease and the impact of the ageing process.

EFFICIENCY OF PHYSICAL WORK

Work efficiency may be seen as biochemical or as mechanical efficiency.

- **Biochemical efficiency**: the efficiency of muscle contraction is the product of the coupling efficiency, i.e. the work performed per unit of adenosine triphosphate (ATP) hydrolysed and the efficiency of energy transduction to ATP by oxidation of substrate. Such biochemical efficiency is associated with the availability of substrate, largely provided from glucose.
- **Mechanical efficiency**: is the ratio between mechanical work and the energy expended. To determine the energy cost of the work, energy expenditure at zero load has to be subtracted. This may not be the same as basal metabolic rate (BMR) because of the position and movement of limbs. A further factor is the speed of work, as efficiency is reduced with increasing speed.

While the body mass index (BMI) may range from 20.5 in middle-distance runners to 23.6 in pentathletes, the cost of work in these people (in kJ/kg/m) varies from 3.6 to 3.95, and the mechanical efficiency (as a percentage) from 34.1 to 22.6%, respectively. In contrast, untrained subjects will have a cost of work of 4 kJ/kg/m and a mechanical efficiency of 19–20%. The energy cost in moving 1 kg over 1 m is approximately the same for all athletes.

Training does not produce any change in the metabolic efficiency of the muscles.

The skeletal muscle consists of two filamentary proteins, myosin and actin, which contract. Skeletal muscle is not uniform in type; rather, there are at least two distinct muscle types. *Type I fibres* (slow twitch) are slender and contain an abundance of mitochondria, oxidative enzymes and fat, and are resistant to fatigue. *Type II fibres* (fast twitch) are broader and more coarse than type I, with fewer mitochondria and less fat. The enzymes are for anaerobic metabolism, and fast twitch muscles have

a high glycogen content. Type II muscle fibres subdivide into types IIa and IIx, dependent on their ATPase enzymes and content. The chemistry of the muscles in types I and II is different, as is the neurone supply. The provision and distribution of these types of muscles may well decide the type and excellence of an athlete. There is a positive correlation between the proportion of type I slow-twitch fibres and V_{O_2} at the anaerobic threshold, a measure of maximum working capacity. Slow-twitch fibres are more efficient than fast-twitch fibres in terms of mechanical force development per unit of ATP.

A sprinter will have muscles that are predominantly IIa and IIx, with a few slow type I myosin fibres. A marathon runner will be the opposite, with a lot of slow type I myosin and little fast mysosin.

STAMINA

Endurance athletes

Endurance running can be defined as regular, physically demanding exercise, including frequent sessions of 90 min or more, wherein significant demands are made on body stores of energy.

The limitation of stamina for endurance runners has been shown to include the depletion of glycogen in muscle and hepatic stores, the amount of which is increased by endurance training.

Energy and glycogen

The glycogen content of resting muscle is 1.5 g/100 g wet tissue, which is approximately 300–500 g in 28 kg of muscle. To this should be added 70–100 g of hepatic glycogen. In total, this has the potential of 8.4 MJ (2000 kcal) energy, which may last for 100 min in really vigorous exercise.

The energy expenditure of an individual can be estimated by measuring oxygen uptake, which increases linearly with exercise intensity until a maximum oxygen uptake, $V_{O_2 max}$, is achieved. This is a reflection of the individual's cardiovascular capacity for oxygen transport and an indication of the levels of exercise that an individual might tolerate. The oxygen cost of exercise expressed as a percentage of the maximum oxygen uptake ($\%V_{O_2 \, max}$), gives an indication of the physiological stress on the individual.

During endurance running there is a substantial contribution from carbohydrate for energy metabolism. After 1 h or more, there is a shift towards fat catabolism. The type of exercise is important. Cyclists exercise in a consistent pattern of action on their machines, therefore, they will expend all of the glycogen in a patterned manner. In running, stride length and running pattern change with the undulations of the course and can also be altered consciously by experienced runners. The load is spread over a wider mass of muscles and hence the depletion of glycogen is less profound. As exercise progresses, free fatty acids are mobilised from adipose tissue. This metabolic source does not prevent fatigue as the fatty acid oxidation is associated with a slower rate of resynthesis compared with carbohydrate. Training increases the aerobic capacity of the muscles and allows the more effective use of fatty acids. Increased blood fatty acid concentrations as a result of anxiety at the start of a run may conserve glycogen metabolism for later in the race.

Adequate muscle glycogen stores can be achieved by a diet rich in carbohydrates. In a study of individuals running a 30 km race, glycogen-loading diets did not increase speed but enabled individuals to hold their optimal speed longer. This led to reductions in times of 3.2% in experienced distance runners and 7.6% in active physical education students. The more highly trained individuals utilise glycogen and to some extent lipids more effectively than the average fit individual. A reduction in performance time of 3.2% would improve a personal best marathon time of 2 h 30 min to 2 h 25 min and would justify the regime to some, especially if the profound feeling of exhaustion in the latter part of such a run, known colloquially as 'the wall', is delayed.

The accumulation of glycogen in muscle is dependent on an initial glycogen depletion by exercise and a carbohydrate-rich diet thereafter. The rate of muscle glycogen restoration is faster than liver glycogen repletion, but is dependent on training status. The more glycogen to be restored, the longer duration of feeding necessary, e.g. 1 week for marathon runners. The carbohydrate intake should be in the order of 500 g/day, which is 70% of the calorie intake.

Other distance runners

The energy expenditure for different intensities of exercise for a lightly built woman and man will be different to that for a plump and moderately enthusiastic runner. Ten minutes' mild jogging a day will consume 2.1–2.5 MJ (500–600 kcal) in a week. Such activity will be better for personal feelings of well-being than actual weight loss. Determination is an important factor in extending exercise capability, especially as weight loss and improvements in serum lipid concentrations appear to be dependent on the intensity and duration of the exercise programme. There is a relationship between the amount of exercise performed and the physiological change with exercise. To obtain significant alterations in weight and serum lipids, it is necessary to run at least 15 km and 19 km a week, respectively, for a year. In another study, walking and running for 9–15 miles a week for 8 weeks resulted in weight loss of an average of 1.5 kg, an average increase of maximal oxygen consumption of 0.25 l/min, and an average decrease in serum cholesterol from 5.34 to 5.15 mmol/l, with increases in HDL.

These studies involved middle-aged men and women but the benefits of exercise are not confined to this age group. In another study, elderly men and women (aged on average 63 years) joined in a 12 month endurance programme: 7.4 km of vigorous walking a week for 6 months, followed by 6 months of 100 min of jogging a week. At the end of both periods there were significant improvements in insulin response to a glucose tolerance test and maximal oxygen uptake. Improved serum lipids occurred after the second period. The problem with all of these studies is that there were significant muscular skeletal injuries limiting exercise tolerance.

The majority of runners of all ages have modest ambitions: health, weight control and the occasional marathon, half-marathon or 10 km run. The intense interest in nutrition and exercise comes from long-distance competitive runners. This is an uncompromising pastime with personal best time the omnipresent goal. Improvements in times of a few per cent may make the difference between regional or national representation, a place in the Olympics final or being unplaced in a local race. In the realisation of the marginal differences between success and failure, athletes look to nutritionists for a boost in performance as much as to their inherent natural ability and training programme. Usually the chosen diet has no scientific basis but owes much to the confidence that the athlete has in the trainer or whoever suggests the diet or supplement. An important factor in endurance running is personal resolve, an attribute what no diet or dietary supplement so far has claimed to improve.

WATER REQUIREMENTS

Perhaps the most important single influence on performance over distance is sweating, and the extent to which lost water is replaced during the run. Fluid loss and need for replacement depend very much on the temperature and humidity, varying from 3–4 litres at 38°C and 80–100% humidity to 0.5–1 litres at 15°C or less and less than 40% humidity.

It is well established that a decrease in body weight of more that 2% by exercise-induced sweating places severe demands on the cardiovascular and thermal regulatory systems. Even in a temperate climate the cumulative sweat loss in a marathon is often 3–4 litres, with an associated loss of electrolytes. The problem of fluid loss becomes even more important. The most consistent item of nutrition that is ignored in sport is water intake. Repeatedly in races as diverse as local and Olympic marathon runs, some hero sets out to run the fastest ever marathon and in order to achieve this ignores the watering stations. The great and dramatic failures in marathon history have been caused by dehydration. Acute renal failure has been reported in participants of ultramarathons in South Africa some 24–48 h after completing the run.

During competition in a warm environment, a marathon runner, running at 240 m/min (i.e. a marathon run in 2 h 46 min) will use an estimated 12–14 kcal/min and lose 0.6 l/min, which may mean losses in excess of 6 litres overall. Despite drinking water during the race, the runner may lose 8% of body weight and 13–14% of body water; this is

a hazardous loss, especially in an individual who continues running.

> During a long run, water reserves are maintained by the regular drinking of water and the metabolic water from glycogen metabolism. The water balance of a distance runner is improved if 500 ml of fluid is drunk 15–30 min before the race. Further small draughts of fluid should be drunk at regular intervals during the race. The balance is important. Too much fluid and the runner has to break rhythm to stop and pass urine; too little fluid and dehydration is a prospect. Drinks stations should be sited every 4.8 km in a marathon, with sponges available in between. The drinks should provide electrolytes or just water according to the runners' choice. Runners, especially the inexperienced, should drink at every station. It is also important that the water is absorbed. The osmolality of the drink determines gastric emptying time. It is desirable that gastric emptying time is such to avoid bloating and allow for comfortable running, and so a drink of 250 ml of water or dilute glucose for taste is recommended. The shortest gastric emptying time is achieved with an osmolality of 250 mosmol/l. A suitable drink for endurance athletes contains 25 g/l or less of glucose, 10 mM/l sodium and 5 mM/l potassium. These recommendations apply to any vigorous extended sport in hot conditions, e.g. soccer or rugby played at speed in the heat.

Sometimes after a long run, thirst is insatiable and lots of fluid must be drunk. Urine output is a good guide to need. After demanding runs, the urine may be sparse and concentrated. One rough rule of thumb is that for every 500 g of weight lost, two 250 ml glasses of water should be drunk.

DIETARY REQUIREMENTS

Energy

Energy needs vary with the athlete and the sport. The muscle mass and therefore energy utilisation increase with training. The proportion of energy expenditure as resting metabolic rate is reduced. In the Tour de France cycle run the energy turnover is 3.5–5.5 times BMR, the energy intake being about 35 MJ/day, a huge amount to ingest.

Amenorrhoeic female athletes tend to have a lower calorie intake than menstruating athletes with similar fitness and sporting requirements.

Creatine

Muscle creatine phosphate content is small but very relevant in exercise. The normal daily intake is 1 g, but the exercising requirement may be double this. The limited synthesis is primarily in the kidneys from arginine and glycine. Vegetarians are particularly dependent on endogenous synthesis. Daily intake of 5 g increases creatinine status, but high-performance athletes benefit from four 5 g doses/day for 4-6 days and 1–2 g/day thereafter. Acute supplementation increases body mass.

Protein

The protein needs for endurance athletes (4–18 h/week) are increased above those of the average population at 1.2–1.4 g/kg/day. The athlete will meet all nitrogen needs with a protein intake that is 15% of total energy intake.

Carbohydrates

There are many theories as to the best way to increase the muscle glycogen content before endurance races. Basically, a running workload, that regularly makes demands on the muscle glycogen content is necessary, accompanied by a diet that includes at least 500 g of carbohydrate/day with the fat content correspondingly decreased.

The USA and UK dietary reference value (DRV) for protein is 0.8 g/kg/day. In a large energy intake the additional demands are easily reached. Participants in sports in which lifting strength is important, e.g. body-builders and rugby and American football players, require between 1.2 and 1.7 g/kg/day. The moderately active athlete will have a protein turnover of 1–2% of total protein per day; 75% of this is recycled.

During the 2–3 days before a race, athletes reduce training and replenish their carbohydrate stores with 10 g/kg/day of carbohydrates. The preferred foods are carbohydrates with a high glycaemic index, e.g. bread, potato, pasta, rice or glucose. During long events over several hours, instantly available carbohydrate as glucose is taken to meet immediate needs. Glycogen resynthesis is most rapid in the 4–5 h after prolonged exercise. Maximum rates of resynthesis of glycogen are achieved when the equivalent of 1 g/kg of carbohydrate is eaten every 2 h in the first 5 h after the exercise.

Fat

Stored fat, muscle triglyceride, adipose tissue fat and low-density lipoproteins are important energy sources during moderately intense exercise. Training facilitates the breakdown of fats during exercise, through amounts of tissue lipase, and aids the release of and response to insulin. A diet rich in fat, unlike carbohydrates, is not conducive to better performance. When fat is lost during exercise, it is not known whether it is necessary to replenish tissue fat n-6 and n-3 polyunsaturated fatty acids and vitamin E.

Other nutrients

Despite sometimes strong claims, there is no evidence that any other nutrient, whether mineral, vitamin, protein, fat or whole food, influences performance, although in the growing athlete a balanced, often massive energy input may be necessary. Iron-deficiency anaemia could be a problem in the menstruating female athlete, but iron therapy should be based on biochemical and haematological measurements.

Caffeine mobilises free fatty acids from adipose tissue, increases fat oxidation and spares muscle glycogen, which improves performance in endurance events. There is a wide individual difference in response that may relate to the acetylation rate of the individual for caffeine. Excess caffeine concentrations in the blood (over 12 mg/l) are illegal in sport and cause unpleasant side-effects.

Specific needs

Dancers and gymnasts

These athletes are figure, as well as performance, conscious. Nutrition restriction is a feature of their programmes, with consequent energy and mineral deficiencies; this may be accompanied by eating disorders, endocrine problems and dangers of fractures from thinned bone structure.

Wrestlers

These sports are dominated by theories of nutrition that are ancient in concept and bereft of modern scientific evidence. Bouts last for about 10 min, require muscle power and endurance, and utilise aerobic and anaerobic pathways. The competitors often achieve the weight for a fight by fluid and food deprivation. Wrestlers can lose 2–5 kg in weight during a fight, and fluid and electrolyte replacement is important. A diet of 12% protein, 58% carbohydrates and 30% fat is recommended for their sport.

Hunted deer

The physiological difference between shot and hunted deer is enormous. A hunted deer's blood glucose will initially increase, then fall with exhaustion. The muscle carbohydrate depletion is profound. Plasma cortisol levels are 70 times those of shot animals, and ten-fold increases are seen in plasma haem, creatine kinase and lactate dehydrogenase. Presumably, athletes who compete to exhaustion exhibit a form of this extreme state.

DRUGS AND SPORT

Performance-enhancing substances

The ingenuity of the athletes and their trainers to devise new enhancers of performance is unlimited. It is possible artificially, dangerously and illegally to increase athletic performance with drugs.

Amphetamines

These stimulate the nervous system by bringing about the release of dopamine into the synaptic cleft. Amphetamine also facilitates the release of noradrenaline. Amphetamine is usually taken as a tablet, and as a consequence of increased circulating adrenaline there is an increase in heart rate, breathing and alertness. Such a drug is therefore believed to increase endurance, aggression for competiveness, speed and power, and postpone tiredness and hunger, and is the choice of cyclists. The risk is an increase in heart rate and respiration leading to cardiac failure and death.

Overdosage is also a danger with, in the long term, hypertension, strokes, addiction, delusions, hallucinations and mental illness.

Anabolic steroids

These can be taken as tablets or by injection. The effect is to mimic the male hormone testosterone and increase muscle bulk, body hair and aggression. This is believed to result in increased strength and speed, and these drugs are the choice of some sprinters, weight-lifters and throwers (e.g. shot, discus).

There is an increased risk of liver cancer, hyperlipidaemia and fluid retention in both men and women. Men are at risk of impotence and acne; women of developing male body composition, acne, infertility and increased body hair. Injecting with reused needles carries the usual risk of viral transmission, e.g. hepatitis and acquired immunodeficiency syndrome (AIDS).

Recombinant human erythropoietin

This increases the red cell mass and hence oxygen-carrying potential. Such increased red cell mass can be achieved by living at high altitudes. The use of recombinant human erythropoietin achieves the same at sea level, and is illegal. The problem is to define the normal red cell mass in professional athletes.

Blood doping

A replacement of 1 litre of blood will increase red cell mass and have an effect similar to high-altitude training.

Human growth hormone

This has the effect of increasing muscle mass.

Diuretics

These are use to increase urinary output and aid the loss of illegal drugs from the body.

Narcotics

These are used to relieve the pain of injuries and also help to overcome fatigue.

Other drugs used are the recreational drugs, marijuana, cocaine and alcohol, to relax. β-Blockers are used to steady the hand in target sports, e.g. archery, shooting and snooker.

Drug testing
In championships, and occasionally randomly, athletes are chosen for urine testing. The samples are divided into two containers, which are sealed. One is sent for analysis at an approved laboratory; the other is retained as a back-up sample. If the test is negative then both are destroyed. If the first is positive then the second sample is tested in the presence of the athlete or representative. If the second test is negative then all is well; if positive, then disqualification results.

However, there are hazards in interpreting drug tests. Chemical changes can take place during prolonged storage, provoked by bacterial contamination and changes to natural hormones. Samples are not frozen until they reach the laboratory. Some supplementary foods used by sportsmen and women contain forbidden substances to enhance the apparent natural effect. Urine samples can be tampered with or exchanged. Currently, peptide hormones, e.g. growth hormone and erythopoetin, cannot be detected in blood or urine.

KEY POINTS

1. The diet of athletes must meet their energy requirements and the demands posed by the speed and duration of exercise. Sports requiring co-ordination have no special dietary needs. Increased protein-calorie intake may be required in the body-building sports, whereas a high-carbohydrate diet is required by endurance runners.
2. Sport makes demands on biochemical and mechanical efficiency. Mechanical efficiency declines with the amount of work involved in the sport.
3. Skeletal muscle consists of two types of fibre: type I is for aerobic metabolism and is resistant to fatigue; type II is for anaerobic metabolism.
4. Endurance runners require stores of glycogen to complete their prolonged activity. The glycogen is stored in muscles, the storage capacity being increased by training. Increased carbohydrate intake is required during such training periods.
5. In endurance sports, water is lost and must be replaced during the run, or severe and life-threatening consequences result.
6. Energy requirements vary from sport to sport; the most demanding is the Tour de France cycle race. Protein requirements are modestly and carbohydrate requirements massively increased in endurance sports. Fat has no merit in stamina provision.
7. There is little evidence that other nutrients are required in amounts in excess of the non-exercising population of the same age.
8. It is possible artificially, but both dangerous and illegal, to increase athletic performance with amphetamine- and steroid-type drugs.

THINKING POINTS

1. It is clear that regular exercise is good for health.
2. It is clear that high-grade sports pursuit makes great demands on a participant's body.
3. Where does benefit end and harm begin?

NEED TO UNDERSTAND

1. The different types of sport and their physical, physiological and nutritional requirements.
2. The dangers that can accompany a thoughtless ambition for success.
3. The basis of the benefit of exercise to the average person.

FURTHER READING

Andersen, J.L., Schjerling, P. and Saltin, B. (2000) Muscle, genes and athletic performance. *Scientific American*, Sept. 49–55.

Fentem, P.H. (1985) Exercise and the promotion of health. *Proceedings of the Nutrition Society*, **44**, 297–302.

Forbes, G.B. (1992) Exercise and lean weight: the influence of body weight. *Nutrition Reviews*, **50**, 157–61.

Koutsari, C. and Hardman, A.E. (2001) Exercise prevents the augmentation of postprandial lipaemia attributable to a low fat high carbohydrate diet. *British Journal of Nutrition*, **86**, 197–205.

Mason, G. (1998) The hunted deer. *Nature*, **391**, 22.

Maughan, R. (2002) The athlete's diet: nutritional goals and dietary strategies. *Proceedings of the Nutrition Society*, **61**, 87–96.

Maughan, R.J. (1999) Nutritional ergogenic aids and exercise performance. *Nutrition Research Reviews*, **12**, 255–80.

Milvy, P. (ed.) (1977) *The Marathon: Physiological, Medical, Epidemiological and Psychological Studies*. New York Academy of Sciences, New York.

Nutrition for Sport (1984) Joint publication of the United States National Association for Sport and Physical Education, The Nutrition Foundation, The Swanson Center for Nutrition and the United States Olympic Committee.

Rowe, W.J. (1992) Extraordinary unremitting endurance exercise and permanent injury to the normal heart. *Lancet*, **340**, 712–14.

Saris, W.H., Senden, J.M. and Brouns, F. (1998) What is a normal red-cell mass for professional cyclists? *Lancet*, **352**, 1758.

Shephard, R.J. (1982) *Physiology and Biochemistry of Exercise*. Praeger, New York.

Symposium (1998) Nutritional Aspects of Exercise (1998) *Proceedings of the Nutrition Society*, **57**, 1–103.

Wareham, N.J., Hennings, S.J., Byrne, C.D. *et al.* (1998) A quantitative analysis of the relationship between habitual energy expenditure, fitness and the metabolic cardiovascular syndrome. *British Journal of Nutrition*, **80**, 235–41.

Wasserman, D.H. (1995) Regulation of glucose fluxes during exercise. *Annual Review of Physiology*, **57**, 191–218.

Westerterp, K.R., Donkers, J.H.H.L.M. Fredrix, E.W.H.M. and Boekhoudt, P. (1995) Energy intake, physical activity and body weight: a simulation model. *British Journal of Nutrition*, **73**, 337–47.

Williams, C. and Devlin, J.T. (1992) *Foods, Nutrition and Sports Performance*. E & EN Spon, London.

45

Nutrition in outer space

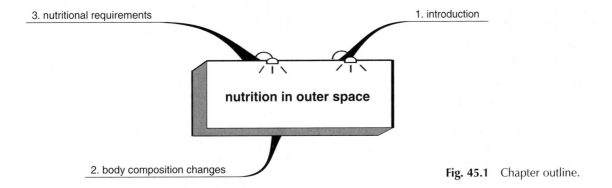

Fig. 45.1 Chapter outline.

INTRODUCTION

The first manned space flight in 1961, by Yuri Gagarin, lasted for 108 min. Since then more than 700 people have spent a total of over 58 person-years in space. Teams of nutritional scientists involved in the care of the American and Russian astronauts have devised meals suitable for space flight. There is no refrigeration in space and food must therefore be storable at ambient temperature. Flights may now extend over 12 months. The available space in the capsules is limited and has precluded studies of metabolic responses. However, it is known that flight can induce persistent negative energy, alter nitrogen and potassium balance, and cause loss of body mass. These probably reflect changes in body composition, energy utilisation and endocrine status.

The conditions and recording in different flights are varied, and many recordings have not been repeated. Sometimes crews exercise or are very busy on assigned tasks, and at other times they are less active, so it is difficult compare like with like.

BODY COMPOSITION CHANGES

Responses to space travel bear on three different tissues: gravity receptors, fluids and weight-bearing structures.

Astronauts have the feeling of being upside down. Motion sickness is a constant problem, with headaches, impaired concentration, loss of appetite and vomiting.

Fluid balance, bone and muscle status are affected at different rates in space. The terrestrial height-related pressure gradient from feet to head is absent and so fluid redistributes. Some of the mass lost is body fluid, in the order of 500–900 ml.

Each leg loses 1 litre of water. Plasma volume decreases by around 6–20% by the end of the flight, with increased plasma concentration.

Anaemia is a feature of even the shortest flight.

The spine is no longer compressed and height increases by 5 cm. There is also bone demineralisation, which is a gradual process dependent on the length of the mission. The lower vertebrae, hips and upper femur lose bone mass at 1%/month. A flight of 184 days resulted in a loss of 20% in bone. Both compact and trabecular bone structure is lost. There is increased excretion of calcium and phosphorus during space flight.

The lungs and other soft tissues exist in a novel gravity-free state, with blood flow differing from that on Earth.

Muscles, particularly of the leg, variably atrophy in space, although the cause may be secondary to inadequate exercise, insufficient food or the effect of altered gravity. As the muscles atrophy, urinary potassium, nitrogen and uric acid increase. The muscle fibrils change, with an increase in faster contractile fibres.

Astronauts are also exposed to radiation levels ten times higher than those on Earth.

NUTRITIONAL REQUIREMENTS

A wide variety of foods prepared for ambient temperature storage is necessary. Freeze-dried fruits, vegetables and meals are available and astronauts have lived for up to 12 months on such fare. Space flight, however, induces persistent negative energy, nitrogen and potassium balances and loss of body mass, despite adequate energy, protein and potassium intake.

Appetite is reduced, possibly owing to the formulation of the food, slower gastrointestinal function, a high carbon dioxide atmosphere (0.3–0.7%) and a warm ambient temperature. It is not usually mentioned that the smell in the capsule from faeces and flatus may be a factor in reducing appetite.

The energy requirements in space are the same as those on Earth, although carbohydrate utilisation may be increased. Mean respiratory quotients may increase from a mean of 0.887 ± 0.09 before flight to 1.041 ± 0.09 during flight, returning to approximately pre-flight figures on return. The total energy requirement for work in space is around 305 kcal/kg/day, depending on body mass, length of flight and activities. The loss of lean body mass is puzzling; however, increasing protein intake may increase the risk of renal stones.

KEY POINTS

1. For space travel, the diet is carefully planned, but is associated with reduced appetite, and negative energy and nitrogen balance.
2. There is redistribution of fluids from the dependent tissues to an equal distribution over the body.
3. Bone readily demineralises.
4. Most of these changes return to normal on return to Earth.

THINKING POINT

The negative balances experienced limit the duration of survival in space that can be achieved for successful return to a terrestrial gravity.

NEED TO KNOW

The changes in space are secondary to pressure redistribution and are similar to those of prolonged bed-rest.

FURTHER READING

Lane, H.W. (1992) Nutrition in space: evidence from the US and the USSR. *Nutrition Reviews*, **50**, 3–6.

Stein, T.P. (2001) Nutrition in the space station era. *Nutrition Research Review*, **14**, 87–117.

46

Dietary deficiency

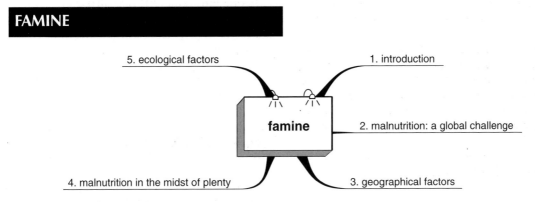

5. ecological factors

1. introduction

famine

2. malnutrition: a global challenge

4. malnutrition in the midst of plenty

3. geographical factors

Fig. 46.1 Section outline.

INTRODUCTION

A definition of health should include the concept of sustainability or the ability of the ecosystem to support life in quantity and quality. Entrapment occurs when a community exceeds the food-carrying capacity of the land, when it lacks the ability to obtain food to sustain its population, or when its people are forced to migrate from a bad to a worse situation. Entrapment leads to dependence on outside aid, forced migration, starvation and possibly civil war. Increased mortality rate, continuing high birth rates, decreased longevity, poor uptake of contraception and precarious food sources raise the question of whether populations are in danger of entrapment.

MALNUTRITION: A GLOBAL CHALLENGE

Malnutrition is the largest and most persistent nutritional problem and dwarfs those problems regarded as being secondary to overeating by the lucky minority. Over a billion people are malnourished, and babies born of low birth weight and children of low weight are counted in millions. The problem of insufficient food has been worsened by civil war, corruption, the acquired immunodeficiency syndrome (AIDS) and drought.

Malthus, in 1798, wrote that the power of population is infinitely greater than the power of the Earth to produce subsistence for man. Population, when unchecked, increases in a geometrical ratio.

Subsistence increases only in an arithmetical ratio. By that law of our nature which makes food necessary to the life of man, the effects of these two unequal powers must be kept equal. This implies a strong and constantly operating check on population from the difficulty of subsistence.

GEOGRAPHICAL FACTORS

There is much starvation throughout the world, but a terrible example of the problem is in southern Africa, where the changing weather patterns, with reduced rainfall have resulted in rivers, wells and water holes drying up. Harvests deteriorate and widespread death from starvation becomes inevitable. A state of famine exists and an inevitable death from starvation is the fate of millions of Africans. Countries such as Zimbabwe, formerly seen as the regional source of food, are now faced with drought and crop failure. Crops are reduced to less than half or even a quarter of past or expected yield. The main problem is lack of rain and all countries have been affected regardless of their political or economic status.

MALNUTRITION IN THE MIDST OF PLENTY

Malnutrition is not uncommonly observable in British hospitals, mainly because of disease. In the community as a whole food poverty still exists. Poor incomes can mean inadequate means of cooking and refrigeration, and hence poor nutrition. Education is an important contributor to cooking skills. The will to combat these problems is an important part of a caring community.

A significant number of people, especially young women, develop eating disorders with serious nutritional outcomes.

ECOLOGICAL FACTORS

Forests are lost when trees are chopped down, for utilitarian but more often financial reasons. This weakens the stability of the soil and allows erosion

to occur. This may be overcome by the planting of fodder trees and grasses. Half of the world's population depends on wood for fuel, used for cooking and keeping warm at night. Trees are a natural sink for carbon dioxide. As trees disappear there is a reduced uptake of carbon dioxide by the trees. They are burned and the result is an increased production of carbon dioxide.

Ozone is an important shield from ultraviolet irradiation and may be lost in the presence of gases such as chlorofluorocarbons (CFCs), which are used in refrigerators.

Nearly three-quarters of the Earth's surface is covered by salt water and unavailable for human needs. Some 1.5% of children in the developing world die of diarrhoea before the age of 5 years, from contaminated water.

Soil is a delicate balance between water, clay, humus and sand. An undue loss of one constituent can lead to a desert of useless soil. Organic waste is needed to replenish the active principles in the soil.

As the Earth warms, the polar ice will thaw and the sea levels will rise. This will particularly affect such countries as Bangladesh, where more than a million of the population live on ground that would be covered by a 1 m rise in the water level. Cyclones are particularly dangerous to such populations and occur when the surface temperature of the sea rises to over 29°C.

War and *civil strife* are important creators of famine. Peace can often only be achieved or continued if both sides feel that aid is reaching them equally. Malnourished people need a balanced diet and the food must be of the correct type. To preserve a population, it is vital that seeds and tools are provided at the correct time for planting. The available crops are largely starch and low in protein content, e.g. derere, a boiled wild okra, and mahewa, a fermented millet. Local maize is more likely to grow than an imported variety. Maize is cheap and plentiful, but beans, oil and fresh fruit and vegetables are also necessary. A clean water supply is critical.

International standards for feeding stations demand high skills, a maximum of 100 inpatients and one carer for every ten patients. In contrast, community-based therapeutic care programmes use the best personnel and local networks in the threatened community, and help the community to believe in its ability to cope. The locally trained women have to be ready to use therapeutic food that can be eaten from the packet, is enjoyed by children and is nutritionally wholesome.

KEY POINTS

1. Famine occurs when a community's food needs exceed its supplies. This a common problem throughout the world. War and pestilence are important contributors to the problem, but the fundamental cause in many areas is lack of rain.
2. The problem is compounded by the felling of trees for fuel and profit, the loss of ozone in the atmosphere, and the consequent effects on the weather, the polar ice mass and sea levels.

THINKING POINTS

1. Is the responsibility for famine relief, local, national or international, with specific aid from the UN, EC and North America?

2. Should such responsibility be to prevent famines or assist when famine occurs.

NEED TO UNDERSTAND

1. The human race has increased in number so much as to endanger its own health and nutrition in many areas of the globe.
2. The terrible plight of malnutrition is worsened by other problems, e.g. war, corruption and infection.

FURTHER READING

Blackburn, G.L. (2001) Pasteur's quadrant and malnutrition. *Nature*, **409**, 397–401.
Smith, R. (1993) Over population and over consumption. *British Medical Journal*, **306**, 1285–6.
Weaver, L.T. and Beckerleg, S. (1993) Is health a sustainable state; a village study in the Gambia? *Lancet*, **341**, 1327–30.

STARVATION AND PROTEIN-ENERGY MALNUTRITION

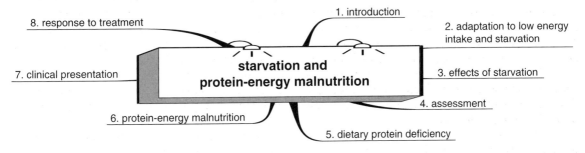

Fig. 46.2   Section outline.

INTRODUCTION

There are many causes of starvation:

• insufficiency of food

• digestive tract malfunction and malabsorption of specific and total nutrients
• impaired appetite due to disease, e.g. cancer, or psychological causes, e.g. anorexia nervosa
• abnormal tissue metabolism, e.g. renal disease, hepatic disease or hyperthyroidism

- severe long-standing infection
- voluntary political hunger strike
- oppression.

> Oppressed groups are found everywhere and in every country. One such group is the begging eunuchs of Bombay, the Hijras or Chakkas, who were sold by poverty-stricken parents, subjected to castration and penectomy without anaesthesia, and thereafter left to beg.

ADAPTATION TO LOW ENERGY INTAKE AND STARVATION

The energy expenditure of subjects engaged in minimum physical activity is 1.4 × basal metabolic rate (BMR). The four major components of energy expenditure are:

- BMR
- physical activity
- growth in children
- pregnancy and lactation.

There are four adaptive processes to starvation:

- weight loss
- reduction in voluntary and conscious activity
- unconscious economy of activity
- true metabolic adaptation.

When starvation is encountered, the body attempts to adapt to the problem. The definition of adaptation to starvation is the process of change of a defined entity, e.g. cell, organ, body or society, in response to a defined cause, e.g. infection and starvation. Alternatively, in an otherwise fit individual successful adaptation is achieved when the body or a function is retained within an acceptable range. Adaptations may be classified as follows.

- **Biological and genetic**: the response that is dictated by the genetic make-up of the individual.
- **Physiological and metabolic**: the body switches metabolic processes from synthetic to conserving, from storage to the organised release of carbohydrates and fats and then proteins, the object being to protect vital organs.

- **Behavioural and social**: in societies where starvation is experienced parents will protect their children. Mothers will give their own food to their offspring. The breadwinner will also be given preference. The level of activity of starving people may decline to match intake. In prolonged starvation these orderly systems break down and individuals become more aware of self-survival rather than the protection of the society and even their family.

There is considerable variation in how much protein and fat is lost during starvation. The initial body fat is a possible determinant of this biological variation and partitioning between fat and protein. It has been proposed that the body compensates for the comparative loss of protein and fat so that:

- during starvation to meet the fuel needs of the individual, the protein and fat both diminish in proportion to ensure that they are proportionately depleted, which ensures maximal survival
- during refeeding, the two energy reserve fractions of protein and fat are restored to the same proportions as before starvation.

> The coefficient of variability of expenditure per square metre of surface area while lying, sitting and standing is about 16%. The coefficient of variability for BMR (adjusted for age, gender and body weight) is 7–10%.
>
> There are great variations between individuals with regard to energy intake, just as there are large differences in recorded intake between similar individuals engaged in similar activities. There are also intraindividual variations, the coefficient of variation in the same individual over 3 weeks perhaps being in the order of 20%. The variability in energy expenditure appears to be less than that in intake. A balance is needed to maintain body weight at a required energy expenditure.
>
> The average amount of protein needed for zero nitrogen balance may have a coefficient of variability of 12.5%. There are substantial interindividual differences in protein turnover. The P ratio is the ratio of protein stored to total energy stored during weight gain. Conversely, the ratio of protein loss to energy loss during weight loss may be characteristic and fixed for each person.

A lower body mass index (BMI) limit compatible with acceptable functional capacity is also an important milestone in a starving population. In many developing countries the average BMI is 18–19, with a range of 15–23. Hard work is possible with a BMI of 15–16 and an estimated body fat content of 6%. It may be that a BMI of 13 in men and 11 in women should be regarded as the absolute lower limit of what is acceptable. Below this survival is unlikely. Such a reduced body mass has little strength, stamina or resistance to illness.

Variations in response to starvation

An individual with substantial lipid stores will cope with starvation better than one who is thin or enfeebled by illness.

The rate of weight loss or BMI status is all important. A rapid loss of weight is very dangerous, whereas a slow loss or failure to achieve acceptable weight may be much more compatible with a healthy life. Death is likely to occur when 40% of body weight has been lost, e.g. a BMI of about 13 in a person whose initial BMI was 22.

Children and starvation

Children are very sensitive to deficient intakes of energy and protein, because of their growth needs, when retardation of growth can be very conspicuous. Diarrhoea is a major cause of short-term growth failure in children in the developing world. Children who have lost weight through diarrhoea have two needs: the diarrhoea must be treated and adequate food must be provided. Many such children in semi-starving situations are severely stunted in height. Stunting of growth in children is an adaptation that demands less food and therefore increases the probability of survival, as survival without an acceptable functional capacity is not a favourable adaptation. It is assumed that everyone has a right to develop their full genetic potential. In terms of food intake this aspiration requires that there is equality of access to a broadly based diet.

EFFECTS OF STARVATION

The main consequences of starvation are due to insufficient macronutrients, carbohydrates, proteins and fats in suitable proportions, compounded by micronutrient insufficiency. There is a reduction in metabolism (adaptation).

There may be a reduction in diet-induced thermogenesis where protein turnover is depressed. Diet-induced thermogenesis uses approximately 10% of the energy value of a meal. Over a whole day this could account for approximately 200 kcal.

Fasting

During fasting, the tissue mass of the body, BMR and energy costs of activities fall until the tissue mass and level of expenditure can be met by the nutrient energy intake. The blood glucose concentrations need to be maintained to ensure cerebral function. Calories are drawn from fat but not protein, in a system controlled by hormonal and metabolic changes.

The sequence of metabolic changes (and the time at which such changes occur) after the onset of starvation is:

1. effects on gastrointestinal absorption (1–6 h)
2. glycogenolysis (1–2 days)
3. gluconeogenesis (12 h to 1 week)
4. ketosis (from 3 days onwards).

The first phase of fasting depends on the carbohydrate concentration of the preceding meal. If the preceding meal is large and predominantly carbohydrate in content, then the liver subsequently removes glucose from the blood in response to increased insulin and decreased glucagon secretion. The glucose is incorporated into glycogen and later metabolised to pyruvate and lactate. The body stores of glycogen are modest (70–100 g in the liver and 300–400 g in muscle) and last for approximately 12–24 h.

After 12–16 h, gluconeogenesis starts, as a result of glucagon excess over insulin, increased hepatic cyclic adenosine monophosphate (cAMP) and an increased concentration of free fatty acids. This leads to increased fat oxidation. Next, the utilisation of ketoacids becomes more efficient. The measurement of the rate at which dependence on glucose or gluconeogenesis occurs is somewhat dependent on the technique used. These differences are quantitative rather than qualitative in their importance.

During prolonged starvation, the body becomes reliant on its own stores. The crucial provision of glucose for the brain and elsewhere depends on liver glycogen, and subsequently on the synthesis of glucose by both the liver and kidneys, initially from muscle protein amino acids. Collagen proteins, which represent 25% of muscle, are preserved. The liver, intestine, skin, brain and adipose tissue, can contribute 1 kg of protein amino acid. Muscle glycogen falls progressively during the first 5 days of starvation and may contribute 140 g of glucose to the brain after hepatic glycogen reserves are exhausted and circulating blood ketones are insufficiently concentrated to supply the brain. Muscle protein catabolism releases predominantly alanine and glutamine. Alanine is the preferred substrate for gluconeogenesis in the liver, and glutamine contributes to gluconeogenesis in the kidneys. In prolonged starvation the flow of alanine from muscle falls and this is reflected in a steady decline in urea synthesis and excretion. After 10 days of fasting, ammonia becomes the main urinary nitrogen product.

There is an increase of ketone bodies from fatty acids in the liver, to be used by most tissues, including the brain. Initially, ketone production is small, but as fasting continues ketones increase progressively to become the dominant substrate. Two main ketone bodies, acetoacetate and 3-hydroxybutyrate, are formed and found in urine, generated from acetyl-coenzyme A in the in liver. Atrophy of tissues is the most characteristic feature of starvation. The wasting and loss of weight are initially rapid, but gradually slow down. The actively metabolising cell mass is reduced and requires less energy to maintain activity. Unnecessary voluntary movements are curtailed.

> A healthy, non-obese subject can lose 25% of weight without endangering life. During starvation, in a 65 kg man, 3 kg of protein, 6.5 kg of fat, 200 kg of carbohydrate, 6 kg of intracellular water and 70% of fat are lost. These represent 300 MJ reserves of nutrition and last for approximately 50 days. The major weight loss in the first week is 1.5 kg of body water, when water-bound glycogen is released and excreted; 1 g of glycogen binds 3–5 g of water

Clinical findings in poor nutrition

Hair: lack of lustre, sparse and thin, straight in Blacks, depigmented

Face: depigmented, nasolabial sebaceous gland dysfunction, 'moon face'

Eyes: Bitot's spots (bilateral, desquamated, thickened conjunctival epithelium), conjunctival and corneal xerosis (dry, thickened, wrinkled, pigmented), keratomalacia (corneal softening)

Lips: angular stomatitis, angular scars, cheilosis

Tongue: smooth or red and swollen, atrophic papillae

Teeth: edentulous, carious, mottled enamel

Gums: spongy, bleeding

Glands: thyroid and/or parotid enlargement

Skin: xerosis, follicular hyperkeratosis (hair follicles plugged with keratin), petechiae (small subcutaneous haemorrhages), pellagrous dermatosis (symmetrical erythema exposed to light and mechanical irritation; dry and scaling), flaky dermatosis, scrotal and vulval dermatitis

Nails: koilynichia

Subcutaneous tissues: oedema of dependent tissues, e.g. legs; sacral oedema, loss of subcutaneous fat

Skeletal system: craniotabes (deformed skull bones), frontal and parietal bone bossing, epiphyseal enlargement, beading of ribs, persistent open anterior fontanelle, deformities of thorax, tender bones, failure to grow to expected height

Muscle/nervous system: muscle wasting, sensory loss, loss of ankle and knee jerks, loss of proprioception (position sense), loss of vibration sense, calf tenderness

Gastrointestinal: enlarged liver, diarrhoea

Haematological: anaemia

Cardiovascular: cardiac enlargement, tachycardia

Infections: tuberculosis, undue sensitivity to infection

Sexual development: correct stages of puberty

Females: affects breast development, onset of menstruation, amenorrhoea, pubic hair development, fertility, size of babies

Males: affects genital (penis) size, pubic hair

Emotional effects: listlessness and apathy; mental confusion

(Modified from Davidson and Passmore (1986).

Protein deficiency in starvation causes a fall in concentration in plasma albumin that also contributes to oedema.

In prolonged starvation there is reduced insulin, insulin-like growth factor-1 (IGF-1) and leptin, which are anabolic, and increased catabolic hormones, glucagon, glucocorticoids, growth hormone and catecholamines and reverse T3.

With insufficient protein intake and hence amino acids the synthesis of critical hormones, insulin, IGF-1 and leptin, is reduced, with metabolic consequences.

Most people with primary undernutrition recover rapidly with access to food. Over 20 MJ/day may be consumed when free food is available.

The effect of weight loss

The effects are variable. There is a rapid initial fall in BMR in response to reduced energy intake, followed by a smaller fall in parallel with loss of weight. Tissues such as muscle and skin with low metabolic rate are preferentially lost, while the visceral tissues and brain with high metabolic rate tend to be preserved. A person with a low body weight has, from a physiological point of view, reduced metabolic rate per unit lean body mass.

BMR appears to be the same for large and small eaters. Indians have a BMR that is lower by approximately 9% than Europeans or North Americans. This may be due to climate, ethnic group, or dietary content or adequacy. The climate may have only a very small effect on BMR. Very underweight Indian labourers have adapted to weight loss, as they are able to continue to be active and fit.

Energy expenditure is related to weight or lean body mass. Total energy expenditure rarely exceeds double the BMR.

> The relationship of BMR (as kcal per person per day) to body weight is not linear. In healthy subjects the BMR/kg rises as body weight falls, and this is independent of height, e.g. a young adult will have an expected BMR of 25 kcal/kg/day, whereas at 55 kg the BMR is 27.6 kcal/kg/day.

In the muscles of malnourished patients there is an increase in the ratio of slow to fast fibres in the muscles. This is a result of a reduction in fast fibres

(type I), the slow fibres (type II) being better preserved. Similar effects on muscle fibres have been shown in hypothyroidism. Hence, it is possible that adaptation is a relative preservation of slow-twitch fibres adapting to a new lifestyle.

ASSESSMENT

The quickest and most effective method of assessment in the community, which is cheap but lacks measurement, is by appearance. Does the person, child or baby look malnourished? Weight and height (length for babies) are precise and allow BMI to be calculated. In adults, mid-upper arm circumference is a good screening test. A value of under 200 mm for men and 190 for women indicates severe malnutrition and a BMI of under 13 indicates a need for supplementary feeding. Under 170 mm for men and 160 for women means a BMI of under 10, where all protein stores have gone and there is a risk of death. Maximum voluntary contraction using a hand grip is a useful field test.

DIETARY PROTEIN DEFICIENCY

Nitrogen balance

Nitrogen balance is obtained from obligatory nitrogen loss and efficiency of restoration of the nitrogen by food protein.

Obligatory losses

In well-nourished young men the average obligatory nitrogen loss is 60 mg/kg/day; 35–40 mg is excreted in urine, 15–20 mg in faeces and 5 mg from the skin. The faecal component depends on the diet and may be increased with a high-fibre diet. Nitrogen lost from the skin as urea is trivial. Urinary nitrogen loss is the most important. Even on minimal protein intake 50% of urinary nitrogen is urea. Ammonia excretion is determined by the need to maintain acid–base balance and is lower on vegetable than an animal protein diets. Uric acid, creatinine and free amino acid losses appear to be consistent.

Efficiency of utilisation

This is obtained from the slope of the line comparing nitrogen balance to intake. Nitrogen intake is required to replace obligatory losses at a constant weight. The protein requirement of different groups is approximately 0.6 g protein/kg/day. These figures are based on short-term studies, and longer term studies may give different results. There are day-to-day variations in urinary nitrogen excretion. Changes from a high to a low protein intake result in the loss of labile protein, the source of which is unknown.

On a normal diet 30% of the urea produced in the liver passes into the colon to be split into ammonia by bacterial urease. This may be recycled to urea and partly taken up as non-essential amino acids. On a low protein intake there is an increase in the proportion of the urea produced and utilised for amino acid synthesis, but no increase in the absolute amount taken up. Urea may be incorporated into amino acids and hence into proteins as a result of transamination of NH_3.

Nitrogen metabolic balances

There are two nitrogen cycles: input/output and *synthesis/breakdown*, which connect through the free amino acid pool. When one is not in balance the other must also be out of balance, since alterations in the size of the free pool are small in relation to flux. The two cycles are not interrelated when they are in balance, but they are related indirectly when there is a reduction in the rate of protein turnover.

If there is a small reduction in energy intake, protein turnover is 15% of the BMR, so a reduction in the rate of protein turnover saves calories. There is less net protein synthesis in response to the ingestion of food and hence there are smaller requirements for essential amino acids. Survival would be possible on a dietary protein mixture of reduced biological value. The increase in protein breakdown in the post-absorptive state is reduced, influx of amino acids into the free pool is reduced and hence there is less loss by oxidation.

Energy balance affects nitrogen intake. Each extra kilocalorie reduces urinary nitrogen loss by about 1.5 mg. Not infrequently, low protein intake and low energy intake go together, so there are small stores of body fat and adaptation to starvation is difficult.

The time-course of reduction in the urea cycle enzymes closely parallels changes in urinary nitrogen output. The rate-limiting enzyme is probably arginosuccinate synthetase. Another adaptation to a reduced protein intake is the rate of input of amino nitrogen to the urea cycle. The enzymes of many amino acid metabolic pathways are modified by dietary protein intake. When urea production is reduced, it may be a result of toxic accumulation of ammonia, which may be removed by recycling to amino acids and hence into protein. However, protein synthesis requires sufficient essential amino acids available in appropriate amounts. The limiting factor is the rate of oxidation of the carbon skeleton of the essential amino acids. It is possible that the important amino acids in this situation are the branched-chain amino acids. These form 20% of the amino acid residues of most proteins, but their concentration in the amino acid pool is relatively low and therefore supply becomes rate limiting. The first step in their catabolism is transamination in muscle, followed by irreversible decarboxylation of the ketoacids by the branched-chain amino acid dehydrogenase complex.

Branched-chain amino acid dehydrogenase is widely distributed in the body. The K_m of the enzyme is close to the concentration of the substrate in the free pool, so activity is concentration dependent. The enzyme exists in an inactive phosphorylated form that is activated by dephosphorylation. There is also an activator protein that reactivates the enzyme without dephosphorylation. These result in a reduction in dehydrogenase activity when dietary protein is restricted.

Adaptation to low protein intakes

Achieving nitrogen balance over a wide range of dietary protein intakes is important. When the capacity to economise on nitrogen metabolism is exhausted there is a reduction in lean body mass. Protein requirement in an individual at a constant height is directly related to lean body mass. In children, there is a reduction in the rate of growth in weight and stunting in height. Pregnancy and lactation are different physiological states, in which the priority is the foetus and its growth is at the expense of the mother's own tissues.

Submaintenance intakes

At submaintenance intakes, rates of turnover of protein are reduced. At the same intake the turnover rate is lower in children with kwashiorkor. Such children are unable to increase their turnover rate in response to an infection and excrete less nitrogen than infected children who are normally nourished. Muscle mass is important in the response of whole-body protein turnover to low protein intakes. The diurnal variation in whole-body protein turnover in response to fasting and feeding runs in parallel with the rate of change of muscle protein synthesis. In children, when the protein intake is reduced there is an immediate fall in the rate of albumin synthesis. Thereafter, there is a fall in the rate of breakdown and a shift of albumin from the extravascular to intravascular compartment. This maintains the intravascular circulating albumin mass.

When amino acid supplies are limited the rate of protein turnover falls in many tissues. Protein turnover is reduced less in the liver and visceral tissues than in muscle. The reduction for the body as a whole is small. The thyroid hormones are important in regulating protein turnover.

The body is very efficient, with a rapid response to variations in amino acid supply, economising when they are in short supply and disposing when in excess. There are, however, limits to this adaptive capacity.

PROTEIN-ENERGY MALNUTRITION

The term protein-energy malnutrition (PEM) is applied to a group of clinical conditions of both adults and children, including kwashiorkor, famine oedema, marasmus and cachexia. Severe undernutrition in adults is found in famine or is secondary to illness, such as anorexia nervosa or cancer.

PEM is the most important social health problem in developing countries and is an important factor in the development, morbidity and mortality of over half the children in such countries who do not survive for more than 5 years.

PEM is not, however, confined to poor countries. This condition may also occur in the families of the poor in the Western world and also as a result of neglectful parenting, ignorance and child abuse. In the affected children there is a failure of growth.

CLINICAL PRESENTATION

Marasmus is caused by a lack of dietary energy and protein, and inadequate amounts of all required dietary components in the growing infant. It occurs in infants under 2 years. The common background is of a family with frequent pregnancies, early and abrupt weaning, and dirty and dilute artificial feeding of the infant. Repeated infections develop and the child may be treated with water, rice water and other non-nutritious foods.

Marasmus also occurs in total starvation. This condition is found in the young baby, leading to severely compromised growth. The baby is cachectic, alert and ravenous.

The term *kwashiorkor* was introduced into modern medicine by Cecily Williams in 1931, and the Ghanaian word means 'the sickness that the second child gets when the next baby is born'. Kwashiorkor occurs due to quantitative and qualitative deficiencies of dietary proteins with an otherwise adequate energy intake. It occurs in the second year of life after a prolonged period of breast feeding. The child is weaned to a traditional diet which, because of poverty, is deficient in protein. There is no supplementation of milk.

There is a range of clinical signs which, at the one extreme can be called marasmus, and at the other, kwashiorkor. All gradations between these two are seen clinically and can occur at all ages. Each of the clinical signs has a biochemical and metabolic basis.

Pitting oedema is always found in kwashiorkor; the oedema is both dependent and periorbital. It is caused by the low serum albumin and the consequent reduced hydrostatic pressure created by the plasma proteins. Because of this there is a failure to bind water by hydrophilic proteins. In addition, there is a leakage of fluid from the vascular compartment into the extracellular tissues, possibly due to increased permeability.

> In kwashiorkor, sodium and water retention in the extracellular fluid may reach 50% in severe cases. There is inappropriate distribution of sodium and water throughout the compartments of the extracellular fluids. The intravascular volume may be depleted. Fluid may accumulate in the peritoneum, pleural cavity or pericardium. In severe cases the entire body and internal organs become oedematous.

The combination of loss of soluble proteins and the excess of sodium and water is responsible for the oedema. There are frequent deficiencies of other intracellular ions, e.g. magnesium, zinc, phosphorus, iron and copper, with consequent effects on metabolism.

Children with PEM fail to grow, are apathetic while resting and cry when nursed. Adults become introspective and apathetic. The higher cerebral functions are most affected, with consequent intellectual impairment.

Not all organs of the body are uniformly affected by PEM, those most affected being the least essential to life. There are reductions in the gastrointestinal tract mucosa, salivary glands, fat stores, muscle mass, heart, liver, pancreas, reproductive organs and thymus. The baby may have a mild normochromic anaemia due to reduced haematopoietic activity. Brain size is unaffected, although it is difficult to know whether the changes in size of an organ result in changes in function. Does a smaller organ function as well as previously? Does a starved brain of constant size function as well as when adequately fed? The marasmic child is more sensitive to bacterial, viral and fungal infections, due in part to a reduced thymus size and circulating T-cell population. The spleen and adrenals may be increased in size. The sufferers readily succumb to infective diarrhoea and hence malabsorption occurs. As a result, kwashiorkor may develop in addition to the marasmus.

Advanced protein malnutrition in adults is associated with progressive weight loss, thirst, craving for food, weakness, lax, pale and dry skin with pigmented patches and loss of turgor; thinned hair and pedal (famine) oedema. There is an increased risk of infections, probably due to reduced serum immunoglobulins. The serum albumin is reduced to under 30 g/l. Skin infections, including tinea versicolor and scabies, are common. This condition has been described in neglected prisoners in overcrowded war camps and civil prisons in developing countries.

RESPONSE TO TREATMENT

Feeding usually results in a restoration of function and growth. Cerebral function may, however, make only a partial recovery, particularly in the infant. It is important not to overload the intestine during the early stages of refeeding. The enzyme systems and body proteins are present in insufficient amounts to cope. The intestinal mucosa may be very thin and unable to tolerate too much food in the lumen. After the liberation of the concentration camps in World War II, some inmates died from intestinal perforation due to the enthusiastic feeding of steaks and other foods for which the intestine was ill-prepared. The important early remedies should include the eradication of infection, the provision of vitamins and trace elements, and then a slow increment of protein and energy intake. A feature of starved people when refed is that the intake of water exceeds the hydrophilic capacity of the body, e.g. proteins. Therefore, in the previously compensated, oedema develops. This will only resolve when protein synthesis is seriously underway. Many adults make a full recovery.

KEY POINTS

1. The causes of starvation are many, but lack of food, especially energy and protein, is a critical factor.
2. During starvation there is adaptation to the new dietary restrictions. The adaptation is both genetically and biologically determined, with physiological, metabolic, behavioural and social changes. There is considerable interindividual variation in adaptation; children are particularly vulnerable.
3. Physiological efficiency is important in determining successful adaptation.

4. The effects of starvation are weight loss, changes in metabolism and increasing dependence on available nutrient stores. The specificity of such release of stores causes some metabolic imbalances, e.g. ketone body production.

5. Adaptations to low energy and low protein intakes are different. Low energy intake leads to weight loss and reduced energy. Dietary protein reduction has a profound effect on protein structure in all forms throughout the body.

6. Protein-energy malnutrition (PEM) is a group of deficiency conditions where all combinations and degrees of energy and protein deficiency are represented.

7. Marasmus is a lack of dietary energy, protein and other nutrients, and is found in total starvation. Kwashiorkor is a deficiency of dietary protein with sufficient calorie intake.

8. In PEM the organs essential for life are conserved if possible, at the cost of the expendable tissues.

9. Feeding can restore growth in the young, but intellectual recovery may not be complete.

THINKING POINTS

1. Malnutrition is a complex problem in which there is the abandonment of all nutritional recommendations.

2. It is a reality, and the timely recognition and correction of the problem is a key resolve of the science and practice of nutrition.

NEED TO UNDERSTAND

The characteristics of the body's response to starvation, and the different effects of starvation for all nutrients and cases where there is a deficiency of protein relative to energy shortage.

FURTHER READING

Allahbadia, G.N. and Shah, N. (1992) India, Begging eunuchs of Bombay. *Lancet*, **339**, 48–9.

American Gastroenterological Association Medical Position Statement (1996) Guidelines for the management of malnutrition and cachexia, chronic diarrhoea and hepatobiliary disease in patients with human immunodeficiency virus infection. *Gastroenterology*, **111**, 1722–52.

Babashola Olubodon, J.O., Jaiyesimi, A.E.A., Fakoya, E.A. and Olasoda, O.A. (1991) Malnutrition in prisoners admitted to a medical ward in a developing country. *British Medical Journal*, **303**, 693–4.

Ben-Tovim, D.I., Walker, K., Gilchrist, P. *et al.* (2001) Outcome in patients with eating disorders: a 5 year study. *Lancet*, **357**, 1254–57.

Black, J.A. (1997) Two hundred years since Malthus. *British Medical Journal*, **315**, 1686–9.

Burges, R.C. (1956) Deficiency disease in prisoners of war at Changi, Singapore. *Lancet*, **ii**, 411–18.

Collins, S. (2001) Changing the way we address severe malnutrition during famine. *Lancet*, **358**, 498–501.

Passmore, R. and Eastwood, M.A. (eds) (1986) *Davidson and Passmore: Human Nutrition and Dietetics* Churchill Livingstone, Edinburgh.

Dulloo, A.G. and Jacquet, J. (1999) The control of partitioning between protein and fat during human starvation: its internal determinants and biological significance. *British Journal of Nutrition*, **82**, 339–56.

Ferro-Luzzi, A. and James, W.P.T. (1996) Adult malnutrition: simple assessment techniques for use in emergencies. *British Journal of Nutrition*, **75**, 3–10.

Henry, C.J.K. (2001) The biology of human starvation: some new insights. *British Nutrition Foundation Nutrition Bulletin*, **26**, 205–11.

Hoare, S., Poppitt, S.D., Prentice, A.M. and Weaver, L.T. (1996) Dietary supplementation and rapid catch up growth after acute diarrhoea in childhood. *British Journal of Nutrition*, **76**, 479–90.

Leader (1992) Insights into fasting. *Lancet*, **339**, 152–3.

Leather, S. (1996) *The Making of Modern Malnutrition.* Caroline Walker Trust, London.

McCarrison, R. (1921) *Studies in Deficiency Disease.* Oxford Medical Publications, Oxford.

McConnell, A.A. and Reid, D.T. (1998) The Irish famine: a century and a half on. *Proceedings of the Royal College of Physicians of Edinburgh*, **28**, 383–94.

Payne, P.R. and Dugdale, A.E. (1977) Model for the prediction of energy, balance and bodyweight. *Annals of Human Biology*, **4**, 425–35.

Smith, D.A. and Woodruff, M.F.A. (1951) *Deficiency Diseases in Japanese Prison Camps.* Special Report No. 274. Medical Research Council, London.

Symposium: Clinical Nutrition in Childhood (2000) *Proceedings of the Nutrition Society*, **59**, 135–62.

Symposium. Nutrition in Clinical Management: Malnutrition in our Midst (1998) *Proceedings of the Nutrition Society*, **55**, 841–62.

Vaz, M, Thangam, S., Prabhu. A. and Shetty, P.S. (1996) Maximum voluntary contraction as a functional indicator of adult chronic under nutrition. *British Journal of Nutrition*, **76**, 9–15.

Waterlow, J.C. (1986) Metabolic adaptation to low intakes of energy and protein. *Annual Review of Nutrition*, **6**, 495–526.

Waterlow, J.C. (1994) Childhood malnutrition in developing nations. *Annual Review of Nutrition*, **14**, 1–20.

Waterlow, J.C. and Stephen, J.M.L. (eds) (1981) *Nitrogen Metabolism in Man*. Applied Science Publishers, London.

Williams, C.D. (1933) A nutritional disease of childhood associated with a maize diet. *Archives of Disease in Childhood*, **8**, 423–33.

World Health Organization (1981) *The Treatment and Management of Severe Protein Energy Malnutrition*, WHO, Geneva.

47

Nutrition in the aetiology of disease

INTRODUCTION

The aetiology of many human diseases includes the consequence of environmental factors. Until recently, infection was the major cause of premature mortality in the developing countries, but this is changing. When the gross national product per capita in a country becomes greater than US$1200 per annum, the proportion of deaths from cardiovascular disease increases sharply and that from cancer increases progressively. The proportion of animal fat in the diet also increases progressively with increasing gross national product.

Diet, smoking and industrial pollution are important factors. Populations living in the Western world constantly seek the various elements in the environment that can be changed to prevent premature death, hence an interest in diet in relation to coronary artery disease, and cancers such as breast and colon. In addition, human immunodeficiency virus (HIV) is causing significant numbers of deaths, particularly in Africa.

The interplay among diet, environment and genetic predisposition is important in most diseases. Two problems, cancer and coronary heart disease, are discussed in this chapter. Diet is a recognised aetiological factor. The individual's genetic predisposition determines an individual response, which is dependent on the isoenzyme constitution.

CANCER

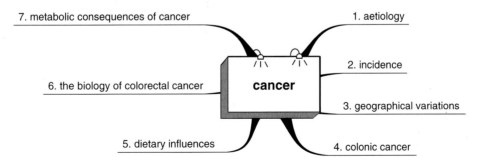

Fig. 47.1   Section outline.

In any malignant neoplasm, a carcinoma is derived from epithelial cells. A carcinoma does not have a clearly defined boundary. Malignancy implies growth, wherein the cells infiltrate the surrounding normal tissues and spread by metastasis to grow at sites distant from the origins of the neoplasm.

AETIOLOGY

Both epidemiological and experimental evidence indicates that cancer results from an accumulation of several distinct molecular events. Cancer is a prime example of the influence of environment and external agencies on the development of disease, e.g. smoking and lung cancer, and certain industrial processes, e.g. tyre manufacture and cancer of the bladder. The individual's genetic makeup predisposes to cancer, an important example being cancer of the colon (Figure 47.2). Cancer of the breast and other cancers may be less well studied but are equally important.

The susceptibility to cancer is determined by individual variation in handling carcinogens. Carcinogen-metabolising enzymes have variable activity (polymorphic), secondary to inherited or environmental influences. Procarcinogens are converted to carcinogens by enzymes that exhibit variable prevalence and penetrance. Dietary ingredients may induce or inhibit these carcinogen-metabolising enzymes, contain electrophilic scavengers or be inducers of DNA repair. The carcinogens may be activated in the liver by P450 enzyme systems, e.g. CYP PIA1, which acts on polycyclic hydrocarbons, or CYP PIA2, which acts on aryl and heterocyclic

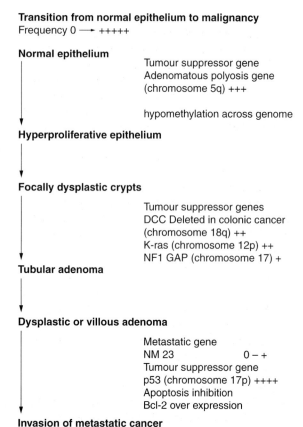

Transition from normal epithelium to malignancy
Frequency 0 ⟶ +++++

Normal epithelium

Tumour suppressor gene
Adenomatous polyosis gene
(chromosome 5q) +++

hypomethylation across genome

Hyperproliferative epithelium

Focally dysplastic crypts

Tumour suppressor genes
DCC Deleted in colonic cancer
(chromosome 18q) ++
K-ras (chromosome 12p) ++
NF1 GAP (chromosome 17) +

Tubular adenoma

Dysplastic or villous adenoma

Metastatic gene
NM 23   0 – +
Tumour suppressor gene
p53 (chromosome 17p) ++++
Apoptosis inhibition
Bcl-2 over expression

Invasion of metastatic cancer

Fig. 47.2 The histological and gene changes in the transition from normal colonic epithelium to a cancer.

amines. The enzymes involved in procarcinogen conversion include acetyl transferase, sulfotransferase, epoxide hydroxylases and cyclo-oxygenases COX1 and COX2. These polymorphic forms may act as slow or fast metabolisers of procarcinogens, respectively creating carcinogens slowly or quickly. Different diets and genes will have different effects on this process.

INCIDENCE

In 1980, there were approximately 6.3 million new cases of cancer throughout the developed and the developing world. The mortality rates for cancer are significantly lower in the developing than in the

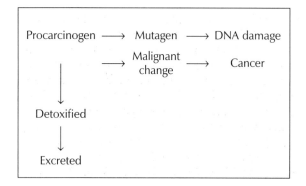

Procarcinogen ⟶ Mutagen ⟶ DNA damage
                    ⟶ Malignant ⟶ Cancer
                       change
Detoxified
Excreted

industrialised countries. In Thailand, cancer mortality rates per 100 000 per annum are 54 for males and 36 for females. The figures for Mexico are 77 and 78, and < 100 per 1000 for most South American countries. In contrast, the cancer mortality rates are > 100 for females and 150 for males per 1000 in most developed countries. Lung cancer accounts for 25–33% of cancer-related mortality in men.

In the USA, one-third of human cancer cases have been attributed to dietary and nutritional factors. These include excess calories in the diet, the type and amount of fat intake, dietary contaminants, e.g. moulds, cooking-related mutagens, naturally occurring toxins, and lack of fruit and vegetables in the diet.

Any diet may contain a number of carcinogenic materials that can be classified into naturally occurring chemicals, synthetic compounds and compounds produced by cooking. The naturally occurring group includes mycotoxins and plant alkaloids, the second group food additives and pesticides, and the third group polycyclic aromatic hydrocarbons and heterocyclic amines.

Some constituents of moulds are carcinogenic. Aflatoxin B_1 is associated with liver cancer. Other suggested carcinogens include hydrazines in some mushroom species, allylisothiocyanate in brown mustard, oestragole in basil leaves and safrole in natural root beer. Biogenetically engineered food constituents are untested in their potential for carcinogenesis.

Cancers in which infective agents have been suggested to be important in the pathogenesis are cancer of the uterine cervix, hepatoma, nasopharyngeal cancer and cancer of the bladder infected with bilharzia. Of the cancers in which cigarette smoking and possibly diet are important, lung, breast and colon are the most common.

Lung cancer rates are increasing at 0.5% per year, while stomach cancer rates are falling by about 2% per year. As cigarette smoking becomes more common in Asia, China and Africa, so lung cancer is beginning to be a problem there. Colorectal cancer is almost twice as common in the industrialised countries as in the developing countries. Cancers of the upper digestive system account for one-third of cancer in the world, and are associated with tobacco chewing, smoking habits and diet.

GEOGRAPHICAL VARIATIONS

Africa and the Middle East

In Africa, the important cancers in men are hepatoma, lymphoma, Kaposi's sarcoma, melanoma, and prostatic, bladder, stomach, oesophageal and penile cancer. Cancer of the lung is rare. In women, cancer of the cervix, followed by breast, liver and stomach are the most common. There are differences in different parts of equatorial Africa in the frequency of these cancers. In Middle Eastern countries bladder cancer caused by endemic schistosomiasis is common.

Asia

The cancer rate and type vary with region and religious groups. In women, cancer of the cervix predominates, particularly in southern India, followed by cancer of the breast, mouth, oesophagus and stomach. In affluent Indians breast cancer is as common as in industrial countries. In men, cancer of the stomach and oesophagus predominate, followed by cancer of the mouth and pharynx. Oral cancer is associated with chewing 'pan' (areca-lime and tobacco wrapped in betel leaves). In Pakistani women breast cancer is more common than cervical cancer. In south-east Asia, liver, lung, oesophageal, stomach and nasopharyngeal cancers are among the most prominent cancers in men. There are differences between different racial groups within the same geographical area.

Latin America

The differences depend on socioeconomic developments. The type and rate vary between the developed countries (e.g. Argentina and Chile) and very poor countries (e.g. Bolivia). The prevalent disease also depends on the relative numbers of migrant European, native Indian or African individuals in the population. There is a high incidence of gallbladder cancer in Bolivia and southern Mexico, oesophageal cancer in southern Brazil, northern Argentina, Paraguay and Uruguay, and gastric cancer in Chile, Columbia and Costa Rica. The highest incidence of cervical cancer in the world is found in Brazil.

COLONIC CANCER

Colonic cancer is a good example of the contributions of genetic predisposition and environment. Colorectal cancer is the fourth most common cancer, with nearly 700 000 new cases a year worldwide. There are two inherited types, familial adenomatous polyposis and hereditary non-polyposis colorectal cancer. The majority of colorectal cancers are sporadic colorectal cancer.

There are community differences in the incidence of colonic cancer, with Scotland having a two- to three-fold higher prevalence than the south of England. A person raised in Scotland who moves south retains the enhanced risk. A move north increases the risk, although the timescale is long.

Most cancers of the colon arise spontaneously, but there is a distinct familial predisposition. Some individuals are very much at risk of cancer of the colon, polyposis coli and rare proliferative adenomatous states. Family history makes their surveillance more defined and necessary. As the number of relatives who have had cancer of the colon increases so does the risk. One relative imposes a trivial increased risk, but if there are two or three affected relatives then surveillance for polyps by regular testing of faeces for occult blood and by flexible sigmoidoscopy is mandatory. If a polyp is found in the left side of the colon or a defined

---

Colonic cancer may develop as a sporadic event in 75% of the population, or be related less commonly to a genetic predisposition, wherein the individual is born with a gene mutation. Such gene mutations may be one of several required for malignant transformation. These at-risk individuals will develop cancer at an earlier age than the overall population and at multiple sites within the gastrointestinal tract. They include familial adenomatous polyposis coli and hereditary non-polyposis coli family syndromes (Lynch types I and II). The same accumulation of molecular events occurs in all types of colonic cancer, but in the sporadic older age group at a later stage.

---

hereditary risk is identified then examination of the entire colon by colonoscopy is required.

The aetiology of colorectal cancer and the adenomatous polyp to carcinoma progression is multifactorial. Colonic cancer is characterised by a well-defined premalignant phase in the adenomatous polyp. The first change may take place in one cell in the crypt. This may occur frequently and there may well be apoptotic processes that respond to such a conversion. Sometimes a changed cell survives, with the prospect of growth, polyp formation and malignancy.

DIETARY INFLUENCES

Dietary factors have an important but complex role, which includes excessive energy intake, and possibly a high consumption of saturated fat and protein and a low consumption of dietary fibre and micronutrients. The rate of occurrence of colorectal cancer in various countries increases with the consumption of red meat and animal fat and with low fibre consumption.

It has been shown that caloric (i.e. energy) restriction will inhibit the growth of spontaneous or experimentally induced tumours. Exercise reduces the risk of chemically induced tumours in rats and vigorous occupational activity has been shown to reduce the risk of colonic cancer.

Epidemiological evidence suggests that the incidence of colonic cancer increases with:

- high dietary fat
- high dietary red meat
- low dietary fibre and resistant starch
- alcohol
- sedentary occupation
- cigarette smoking

and that protective factors are:

- exposure to the sun and raised concentrations of blood vitamin D
- fruit and vegetables
- aspirin consumption
- physical exercise.

There are international differences in the effect of red meat on colon cancer rates. This raises the possibility that there are differences in meat production techniques; an important factor, rarely discussed, is the addition of growth factors, anabolic steroids or antibiotics to the feed of animal stock. Red meat may be a risk factor through N-nitroso compounds, polycyclic aromatic hydrocarbons and heterocyclic amines generated by cooking. Heterocyclic amines are metabolised by acetylation, for which there is genetic polymorphism of the cytochrome P450 enzymes (CYP1A2 and N-acetyltransferase type 2), so slow acetylators may be more at risk of colonic cancer.

In epidemiological studies fruit and vegetable intake has been suggested to be important in prevention. Hence, interest arose in vitamins, antioxidants and dietary fibre. Of the treatments tried, vitamins, e.g. vitamins A, C and E, have proved to be of little use, and vitamin A supplementation was shown to worsen outcome. Vitamin D and to a lesser extent folate have promise in reducing disease incidence and growth rate. It may well be that the secondary metabolites in fruit and vegetables confer the protection. Calcium supplementation has modest benefits.

The protective role of fibre is not yet proven. There is no reduction in the risk of colorectal cancer with 25 g of fibre a day. It may be that 30–35 g of fibre a day is necessary, i.e. at least three times the usual Western intake. Dietary fibre has a complex relationship with the causation of colon carcinoma. There should be differences between fermentable and non-fermentable fibres in their protective potential against colon cancer. Fermentable fibres produce short-chain fatty acids through fermentation, while poorly fermentable fibres dilute intestinal contents. Fibre has complex effects on the colon, altering intestinal microfloral activity, aqueous phase bile acids, mutagenicity of intestinal contents, bacterial enzymes, and responses to hormones and other peptide growth factors, whether these be local or systemic. Dietary fibre affects the enterohepatic circulation of hormones, intestinal transit time and colonic pH, as well as delaying the absorption of dietary energy. It is difficult to separate the value of dietary fibre from that of other chemicals present in fruit and vegetables.

The average stool weight for a range of countries varies from 70 to 470 g/day, and average stool weight in a population appears to be inversely related to colon cancer risk: the lower the stool weight the greater the risk. There is a significant correlation between fibre intake and mean daily stool weight, suggesting that diets providing increased fibre and hence larger faecal output may be protective against the development of cancer.

Non-steroidal anti-inflammatory drugs (NSAIDs) are associated with a reduced risk of colorectal cancer and adenomatous polyps. The activity is possibly but not absolutely through an action on apoptosis and COX-2. COX-2 expression is increased in sporadic colorectal cancer.

THE BIOLOGY OF COLORECTAL CANCER

Despite epidemiological and experimental evidence that cancer requires a number of distinct molecular alterations, there is still hope that a single cause, e.g. the control of cell division, lies behind the genesis of the cancer. The cell cycle is regulated in a similar manner in all higher organisms. There are two major control points in the cycle, one at the G_1/S transition, i.e. where DNA replication starts, and the other at entry to mitosis. These are determined by protein kinases, enzymes regulated by protein cofactors (cyclins), the concentrations of which increase and fall during the cell cycle. Cyclin-dependent kinases (CDKs) and cyclins have many subfractions. The gene involved in cyclin D_1 is located on human chromosomes 11q13 and is involved in a number of tumours, including β-cell lymphoma and parathyroid cancer. Amplification and/or overexpression of cyclin D_1 have been shown to be involved in breast and oesophageal cancers.

The majority of tumours are aneuploid (i.e. the chromosome number is not an exact multiple of the haploid number, e.g. extra single copies of chromosomes as in trisomic Down's syndrome) with a variable chromosome number. This is related to mutations in a gene that controls the formation of the mitotic spindle (hBUBI).

Most tumours are sporadic and associated with mutations in cell growth (oncogenes and tumour suppressor genes) and DNA repair. Different gene pathways may lead to colonic tumour development. There is also differential activation of various enzymes (kinases) and hormones (insulin-like growth factor).

Sporadic colorectal cancer occurs primarily in the older population. For a tumour to develop it is likely that several cell defects must occur, including mutational activation of oncogenes and inactivation of tumour-suppressing genes (Figure 47.2). Some of these changes may be inherited, and though in themselves they are not enough to cause malignant transformation, may reduce the number of stages in the development of a tumour.

Many types of human tumour have abnormal control of the transcription from the G_1 to S phase of the cell cycle. The $P16^{INK4}$ gene encodes a G_1-specific cell cycle inhibitor, which is a tumour suppressor frequently deleted or mutated in tumours. There is a strong relationship between the extent of DNA methylation and hence suppression of the gene, although this varies with tumour type. In the transition from dysplasia to carcinoma there is an increasing frequency of $P16^{INK4}$ hypermethylation.

The *APC* gene is important in the development of carcinoma and has been called the gatekeeper gene. The role of the *APC* gene is in cell-to-cell adhesions, signal transduction, apoptosis, cell differentiation, cell cycle regulation and chromosomal stability. *APC* associates with the catenins. These are a multigene family of cytoplasmic proteins involved in cell adhesion and signalling. Mutation of *DCC* (a gene named from 'deleted in colonic carcinoma'), which encodes a tumour suppressor, (a cell adhesion molecule) and *k-ras* (an oncogene that regulates cell growth and differentiation) causes loss of normal cell adhesion. Loss of *k-ras* is also associated with increased cell proliferation. More than 90% of identified germline mutations are in the DNA mismatch genes *hMSH2* or *hMLH1*.

Peroxisome proliferator activated receptor δ (PPARδ) belongs to the nuclear receptor superfamily (steroid and thyroid hormones and retinoids) and is a ligand-dependent transcription activator. NSAIDs and the gene product of *APC* downregulate the transcription activity of peroxisome proliferator-activated receptor δ.

When the gene mutations in tumours are identified it is possible to compare these cancer markers and the prognosis with that type of tumour.

The potential for colon cancer to metastasise is affect by sialylated carbohydrate structures on mucin apoproteins, and in particular the mucin encoded by the *MUC2* gene.

Tumour recurrence is associated with the expression of *Bcl-2*, a cytoplasmic protein localised to mitochondria, endoplasmic reticulum and the nuclear membrane, which has a role in the inhibition of apoptosis.

Resistance to chemotherapy

Biochemical changes in malignant cells give rise to resistance to chemotherapy, which may be either intrinsic or acquired. Some tumours, such as those of the colon, are inherently resistant to chemotherapy. It has been suggested that the more cells present in a tumour, the greater the risk of resistance. A small mature colonic tumour may go through many divisions but remain small by shedding cells. The following steps occur in the sensitivity of cells to drugs.

1. **Multiple drug resistance** associated with p-glycoprotein 170 found in cancer cells. Drugs against which resistance readily develops have a common origin in that they are all obtained from plants, fungi and bacteria. Resistance appears to be related to the amount of p-glycoprotein 170 in the tumour cell. The function of p-glycoprotein is to pump toxic substances (particularly of plant origin) from the cell. This perhaps accounts for why the oesophagus, stomach and colon are so resistant to chemotherapy. These tissues are exposed to and may provide protection from noxious roots and berries. The multidrug resistance-1 gene associated with p-glycoprotein 170 is amplified in

---

Gene profile and some indicators of prognosis with colorectal cancer

Oncogenes	Ras-mutated	
Tumour suppressor genes	p53 mutations	
Apoptosis pathways	Bcl-2 expression increased	Good prognosis
Metastasis/invasion	Vascular endothelial growth factor: positive staining	

patients receiving drugs of plant or bacterial origin. Placement of this gene into a previously drug-sensitive cell makes that cell resistant to chemotherapy.

2. **Gene amplification** results in an increased enzyme production, e.g. the gene controlling the production of dihydrofolate reductase, which is specifically inhibited by methotrexate. Cells become resistant to methotrexate in various ways. Methotrexate passes through the cell membrane by simple diffusion or an energy-dependent mechanism. On passing through the cell it is polyglutamated and cannot diffuse out. Mutations leading to impaired active transport or a failure of polyglutamation lead to a decreased uptake and hence the cell becomes resistant. The cell may become resistant to methotrexate when the drug, having passed into the cell, meets a variant of the enzyme dihydrofolate reductase. This affects the binding of methotrexate to the enzyme. The most common mechanism of resistance is by amplification of the gene for dihydrofolate reductase.

3. **The presence of topoisomerase II** is important in the action of the chemotherapeutic agents doxorubicin, amsacrine and etoposide. These agents bind to topoisomerase II, preventing the binding of the DNA strands broken as a result of therapy. If topoisomerase II is reduced or absent, the drugs cannot bind to DNA, DNA strand religation occurs and the cells can then divide.

These approaches to the biology of cancer provide encouraging news for the ultimate treatment of cancers, particularly those of the gastrointestinal tract, which are so refractory to chemotherapy and radiotherapy.

METABOLIC CONSEQUENCES OF CANCER

Cachexia

Neoplastic disease is not infrequently complicated by wasting, weakness, anorexia and anaemia. As the tumour increases in size, muscle mass and adipose tissue diminish. It is curious that the liver, kidney, adrenal glands and spleen are spared and may even enlarge. Early in the process, total body protein may be unchanged, although redistributed from muscle to tumour. At a later stage, total body protein declines as anorexia is more pronounced. The mechanism responsible is unknown.

Cachectic cancer patients may not only have protein-calorie undernutrition, but also be deficient in vitamins and minerals. The amount of weight loss varies and may precede clinical presentation of the cancer in a good proportion of patients. The frequency of weight loss varies between 14% with breast cancer, 31% with non-Hodgkin's lymphoma, and 87% with gastric carcinoma. There may also be reduced creatinine:height indices, serum albumin and vitamins A and C. Patients with visceral protein and lean body mass depletion have a worse prognosis than patients in whom weight is retained. However, while there is a general association between protein-calorie malnutrition and survival, a cause-and-effect relationship has not been established. Weight loss may be because of reduced food intake, gastrointestinal malabsorption or endogenous metabolic abnormalities, leading to combinations of impaired protein synthesis, breakdown or hypermetabolism. Mechanical factors, dysphagia, intestinal obstruction and ascites are important reasons for tissue weight loss, as are chemotherapeutic drugs that reduce appetite.

The mechanism by which tumours depress appetite is unknown. Other factors decreasing appetite include pain, drugs for pain relief, radiation enteritis and depression. Intestinal absorption appears to remain intact.

Metabolic abnormalities

There is a variable metabolic response to cancer. There is no consistency between tumour type and increases and decreases in metabolic rate. There is variable production of hormones such as cytokines, which may be due to differing tumour tissue types and degrees of differentiation. The progressive wasting of host tissue contrasts with the vigorous growth of tumour tissue. Tumour cells may divide under conditions where host cells atrophy.

The hexoses taken up by a malignant cell may, in addition to being involved in a glycolytic pathway, be shunted to the pentose phosphate pathway for the synthesis of both DNA and RNA. Hexoses in malignant cells are also used in glycosylation of membrane structures, proteins and lipids. The cancer cell is not infrequently a high consumer of glucose and a producer of lactate. Hexoses used by many malignant cells may support proliferation in ways other than the production of energy, ultimately contributing to the growth advantage of these cells. The ability of tumours to synthesise fatty acid varies widely, although the synthesis rate is inadequate for replication. Consequently, tumour cells may obtain required fatty acids from host tissues.

There may be differences in the uptake of amino acids by malignant cells and normal cells. Malignant cells may use disproportionately large amounts of certain amino acids. There is a marked loss of weight and content of protein and glycogen in the liver. Hepatic protein synthesis is reduced in tumour-containing livers. There are marked changes in the activity of many liver enzymes, with abundant production of foetal isoenzymes. Enzymes important in carbohydrate and amino acid metabolism are altered, such that there is increased glycolysis and disproportionate metabolism of some amino acids.

Skeletal muscle

Skeletal muscle mass declines as the tumour grows. This appears to be due to decreased incorporation of amino acids into muscle protein, which is probably the result of a tumour-specific defect in protein synthesis. Alternatively, these changes may due to starvation. Glucose metabolism is also reduced in the muscles of patients with carcinomatosis. The rate of endogenous glucose production and turnover is increased in undernourished compared with normally nourished cancer patients. Lactate production is increased in patients with metastatic cancer, but the range of production rates is broad. Adipose tissue loss is very marked in patients with cancer.

Tumour cells also produce hormones and hormone-like factors. It is possible that these tumour-secreted, metabolically active products have a deleterious effect on host metabolism. However, all studies comparing tumour growth rates with and without nutritional supplementation show an acceleration in tumour growth rate when nutrient intake is increased.

KEY POINTS

1. Diet, smoking and industrial pollution are important aetiological factors in the disease process in humans. The impact of these on any individual will be determined by exposure, the genetic makeup, gender and geographical location. There is a relationship between socioeconomic status and the prevalence of types of disease.
2. Cancer and coronary heart disease are good examples of this interplay.
3. Some cancers have been attributed to dietary causes, e.g. liver cancer and aflatoxin B_1.
4. Colonic cancer has both genetic and dietary components to its aetiology. Most cancers of the colon arise spontaneously, but there is a distinct familial predisposition.
5. Colonic cancer develops as a polyp which undergoes malignant transformation, with accompanying gene changes. The genes that mutate include oncogenes that induce and maintain cell transformation, and tumour-suppressor genes. There can also be mutation of genes involved in DNA mismatch repair, resulting in a characteristic pattern of DNA damage in some tumours. During the change from polyp to cancer there is an increasing *ras* mutation and loss of specific chromosomal regions containing tumour-suppressor genes (allelic loss).
6. The dietary contributions to this cancer include a deficiency of dietary fibre, particularly fruit and vegetables, and an excess of red meat, protein and fat in the diet. Excessive energy intake may be a factor.
7. Once the malignant transformation has occurred, there are complex metabolic changes which have implications for treatment, including chemotherapy. A damaging change is the very complicated process of cachexia.

THINKING POINTS

1. Cancer is a complex process in which molecular, biological, nutritional and chemical irritations have a role.
2. Not everyone who has the environmental predisposition develops cancer, although it is uncommon for the person with a genetic predisposition to escape this disease.

NEED TO UNDERSTAND

The basic lesion in cancer development is usually dependent on the individual's genome, and brought to its realisation by environmental predispositions.

FURTHER READING

Burns, J., Chapman, P.D., Bishop, D.T. *et al.* (2001) Susceptibility markers in colorectal cancer. In *Biomarkers in Cancer Chemoprevention* (eds A.B. Miller, H. Bartsch, P. Boffetta *et al.*) No 154. IARC Scientific Publications, Lyon.

Chung, D.C. (2000) The genetic basis of colorectal cancer: insights into critical pathways of tumorigenesis. *Gastroenterology*, **119**, 854–65.

Cummings, J.H. and Bingham, S.A. (1998). Diet and the prevention of cancer. *British Medical Journal*, **317**, 1636–40.

Diana, J.N. and Pryor, W.A. (1993) Tobacco smoking and nutrition; the influence of nutrition on tobacco and associated risks. *Annals of the New York Academy of Sciences*, **686**, 1–11.

Doll, R. and Peto, R. (1976) Mortality in relation to smoking: 20 year observations in male British doctors. *British Medical Journal*, **ii**, 1525–36.

Dunlop, M.G. (1997) Colorectal cancer. *British Medical Journal*, **314**, 1882–5.

Forman, D. (1999) Meat and cancer: a relation in search of a mechanism. *Lancet*, **353**, 686–7.

Gottesman, M.M. and Pastan, I. (1993) Biochemistry of multidrug resistance mediated by the multidrug transporter. *Annual Review of Biochemistry*, **62**, 385–427.

Hardman, A.E. (2001) Physical activity and cancer risk. *Proceedings of the Nutrition Society*, **60**, 107–13.

Hayes, J.D. and Wolf, C.R. (1990) Molecular mechanisms of drug resistance. *Biochemical Journal*, **272**, 281–95.

Ilyas, M, Hao, X-P., Wilkinson, K. *et al.* (1998) Loss of Bcl-2 expression correlates with tumour recurrence in colorectal cancer. *Gut*, **43**, 383–7.

Kim, Y.I. (2000) American Gastroenterological Association Medical position statement: Impact of dietary fiber on colon cancer occurrence. *Gastroenterology*, **118**, 1235–57.

Kritchevsky, D. (1993) Colorectal cancer: the role of dietary fat and calorie restriction. *Mutation Research*, **290**, 63–70.

Langman, M. and Boyle, P. (1998) Chemoprevention of colorectal cancer. *Gut*, **43**, 578–85.

Langman, M.J., Cheng, K.K., Gilman, E.A. and Lancashire, R.J. (2000) Effect of anti-inflammatory drugs on overall risk of common cancers: case control study in general practice research data base. *British Medical Journal*, **320**, 1642–6.

Matsuda, Y., Ichida, T., Matsuzawa J. *et al.* (1999) P16^{INK4} is inactivated by extensive CpG methylation in human hepatocellular carcinoma. *Gastroenterology*, **116**, 394–400.

Mcgraff, I. and Lidvike, G. (1993) Cancer in developing countries: opportunities and challenges. *Journal of the National Cancer Institute*, **85**, 862–73.

Midgely, R. and Kerr, D. (1999) Colorectal cancer. *Lancet*, **353**, 391–9.

Midgley, R, and Kerr, D. (2000) Towards a post-genomic investigation of colorectal cancer. *Lancet*, **355**, 669–70.

Orr-Weaver, T.L. and Weinberg, R.A. (1998) A checkpoint on the road to cancer. *Nature*, **392**, 223–4.

Peto, R., Darby, S., Deo, H. *et al.* (2000) Smoking, smoking cessation, and lung cancer in the UK since 1950: combination of national statistics and two case control studies. *British Medical Journal*, **321**, 323–9.

Schatzkin A, Lanza E, Corle, D. *et al.* (2000) Lack of effect of a low fat, high fibre diet on the recurrence of colorectal adenomas. *New England Journal of Medicine*, **342**, 1149–55.

Sidransky, D. (2002) Emerging molecular markets of cancer. *Nature Reviews Cancer*, **2**, 210–19.

Thomas, H.J. (1998) Genetic instability in colorectal cancer. *Gut*, **43**, 450–1.

US Office on Smoking and Health (1979) *Smoking and Health*. A Report of the Surgeon General. US Government Printing Office, Washington, DC.

CORONARY HEART DISEASE AND ATHEROMA

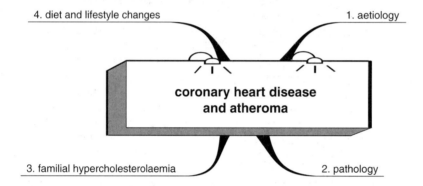

Fig. 47.3   Section outline.

AETIOLOGY

Epidemiological studies have shown that those populations with a high coronary heart disease (CHD) rate have a substantial dietary intake of saturated fat. The consensus, in population studies, is that the higher the average serum cholesterol the greater the risk of CHD. World-wide cross-sectional surveys suggest that low-fat, low-cholesterol diets result in low lipid concentrations and reduced atherosclerotic heart disease. The development of atherosclerosis is influenced by lack of exercise, total calorie intake, obesity, smoking and stress. In an international comparison the French and Japanese have low incidences of CHD (Figure 47.4) and associated mortality rate (Figure 47.5). It is difficult to explain the relative freedom of the French from the CHD problem in the light of their diet and serum cholesterol concentrations. The French cuisine is not based on a low-fat diet. One suggested explanation is that the drinking of red wine provides protection. Possibly a love of good food.

Normal subjects develop increased serum cholesterol concentrations when fed saturated fat compared with concentrated polyunsaturated fat diets. In general, polyunsaturated fats lower plasma cholesterol concentrations. Fatty acids from fatty fish, such as mackerel, salmon and trout contain unsaturated fatty acids of the n-3 type. Vegetable oils contain n-6 fatty acids. Adding fish oils to the diet of normal subjects or hyperlipidaemic subjects results in a decrease in total triglycerides, very low-density and low-density lipoprotein (VLDL and LDL) cholesterol concentrations and prolonged clotting times.

When the percentage of fat in the diet is lowered there will be a matching increase in dietary carbohydrates, preferably as starch, to maintain energy intake. A high carbohydrate diet of sucrose results in increased triglycerides and VLDL triglycerides. Hepatic secretion of VLDL, which contains more triglyceride, increases. There is a fall in high-density lipoprotein (HDL) concentrations.

The recommendation by the UK Committee on Medical Aspects of Food and Nutrition Policy

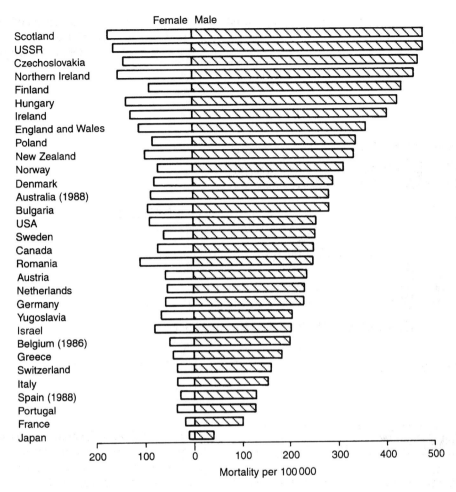

Fig. 47.4 Coronary heart disease world-wide, 1989. Mortality per 100 000, age 40–69 years (WHO data, 1992). (Reproduced from Report of a Working Party to the Chief Medical Officer for Scotland, 1993, with permission of the Scottish Office.) (1996 update, Levy and Kennel 2000.)

(COMA) and other authorities is to decrease the overall intake of fat in the diet to less than 35% of total calorie intake, and that the fat should include polyunsaturated and monounsaturated fats. The energy intake should be maintained by an increase in starch-containing foods, and the daily diet should contain fruit and vegetables.

There are various accounts of the effect of dietary fibre on plasma lipids. The mechanism whereby fibre reduces serum cholesterol has generally been seen to be due to an increase in the faecal excretion of sterols as bile acids. The bile acids are bound to fibre, or lignin within the fibre. However, those fibres that are most successful in reducing the serum cholesterol are fermented in the caecum, e.g. pectin. This suggests that the effect is through some other mechanism that includes the increased activity of bacteria in the colon. The bile acids may be bound to bacteria.

There is a school of thought which does not entirely accept the cholesterol story as the cause of atherosclerosis. The pathological changes in occlusive vascular disease have similarities to those of infections. Great interest has been raised in the possibility that infections with *Chlamydia pneumoniae* and *Helicobacter pylori* are the underlying cause.

People who had a low birth weight or who were thin or short at birth as a result of reduced

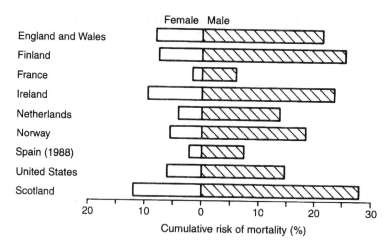

Fig. 47.5 Coronary heart disease, 1989. Cumulative risk of mortality expressed as a percentage of the population aged 35–74 years in a number of countries (WHO data, 1992). (Reproduced from Report of a Working Party to the Chief Medical Officer for Scotland, 1993, with permission of the Scottish Office.)

intrauterine growth have increased rates of CHD and also the predisposing conditions for CHD, i.e. hypertension and type II diabetes. This finding has been confirmed in studies in many countries. Birth weight may be a sensitive indicator of family socioeconomic circumstances *in utero* and during subsequent development. The relationship is restricted to people who have a large body mass index in adulthood. Other risk factors are stressful, overdemanding jobs and cold weather.

PATHOLOGY

There are diffuse thickenings of the musculoelastic intima of the vessels. This abnormal process may start in childhood. Three main lesions are described: the fatty streak, the fibrous plaque and a complicated lesion. The fatty streaks are an accumulation of intimal smooth-muscle cells surrounded by fat. Lipid-laden macrophages are a feature of the early lesion. The lipid in the fatty streak is largely cholesterol oleate in foam cells. The cholesterol deposited in the plaque is from circulating lipoproteins, especially LDL-cholesterol. This uptake is not onto LDL receptors. A modification of the LDL particle may be involved in its uptake by the vascular epithelium, by a scavenger receptor, which is independent of the LDL recep-

tor. The requirements to be taken up include lipid oxidation of the unsaturated fats in the LDL lipid. The size of the LDL particle may determine the oxidation potential.

The fibrous plaque consists of fat-laden smooth-muscle cells and macrophages, the fat being cholesterol linoleate. There are deposits of collagen, elastic fibres and proteoglycan. This lesion undergoes further change, with calcification, cell necrosis, mural thrombosis and haemorrhage. The result is the complicated lesion.

The fibrous plaque and the complicated lesion are associated with vascular occlusion, which is a feature of coronary heart disease (Figure 47.6). The lesions develop at the junction of vessels, more frequently in the arteries of the legs, head and heart, but rarely in the arms. These lesions are more common in the presence of hypertension (cerebrovascular disease) or smoking (peripheral vascular disease).

The occlusion of an artery may result from:

- thrombosis on an atheromatous and stenosed vessel
- haemorrhage into an atherosclerotic plaque
- spasm in a diseased vessel.

Thrombosis is the most common cause of vessel occlusion and occurs as a result of altered blood flow, altered blood constituents or an abnormality of the vessel wall. An abnormal vessel wall can alter

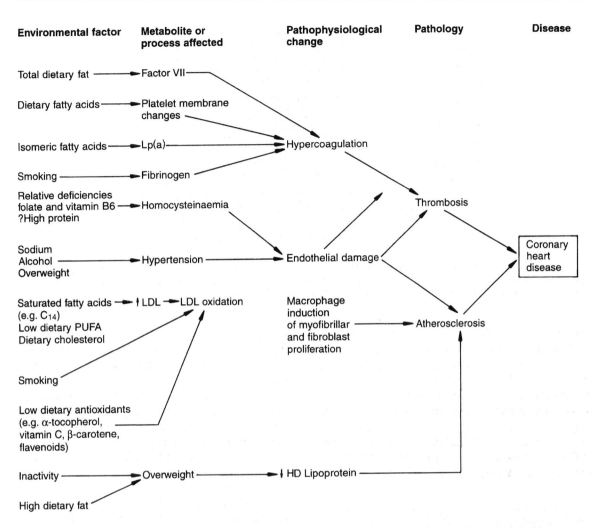

Fig. 47.6 A view of the development of coronary heart disease (CHD). Note: all arrows indicate a stimulatory (i.e. aggravating) effect, except for ↑ LDL: raised LDL; ↓ HD Lipoprotein: lowered HDL. The three well-characterised risk factors are smoking, hypertension and LDL. These are highly interactive but may only explain half of the regional or group variation in CHD. The metabolite response to dietary change shows variation between people; these differences are increasingly recognised as being of genetic origin. Physical activity has many effects apart from increasing HDL concentrations, including physical dilatation of coronary vessels, making them less likely to undergo occlusion. There are also behavioural and metabolic confounders: smokers eat a diet richer in sugar and salt, and with fewer vegetables and fruit. Smoking also accelerates the use of vitamin C which, in this scheme, is shown as a protective factor. Not included in this diagram is the potential programming of one or more metabolic processes in foetal and infant life which may then predispose the adult to CHD; the role of breast feeding is also omitted. (Reproduced from Report of a Working Party to the Chief Medical Officer for Scotland, 1993, with permission of the Scottish Office.)

the binding of platelets, which are negatively charged, to this surface. The vessel wall endothelium is protective against this aggregation process. Metabolic processes in the endothelium reduce the adherence of the platelets.

FAMILIAL HYPERCHOLESTEROLAEMIA

This is characterised clinically by raised plasma LDL concentrations, xanthomas and early CHD due to atherosclerosis. Familial hypercholestero-laemia is an autosomal dominant trait and homozygotes are more severely affected than het-erozygotes. It is a commonly occurring inherited metabolic condition with a population frequency of 1 in 500 for heterozygotes and 1 in 10^6 for homozygotes. There are populations, however, where the frequency is higher, e.g. Lebanese, French Canadians, Afrikaners and Jews of Lithuanian origin. Raised concentrations of plas-ma cholesterol in familial hypercholesterolaemia result from mutations in the LDL receptor gene. Plasma cholesterol and LDL-cholesterol concen-trations may be increased substantially. It is prob-able that differences in lifestyle have no effect on homozygotes with familial hypercholestero-laemia, although there are individual variables in plasma cholesterol concentration. When the homozygotes are subdivided according to LDL receptor gene mutations there is less variability among the groups.

CHD and coronary deaths are more frequent in homozygotes in whom receptor activity is less than 2% of normal than in subjects in whom receptor activity is 20–30% of normal. In homozygotes, mutations that impair rather than abolish receptor function tend to produce lower plasma concentra-tions of cholesterol, and are more responsive to treatment and result in less severe CHD.

There are modifying effects of other genes on cholesterol concentration. Homozygous lipoprotein lipase deficiency in familial hypercholesterolaemia heterozygotes reduces LDL-cholesterol concen-trations to normal. Other genes can a affect the risk of coronary disease.

In liver cells LDL receptor activity is not subject to the normal suppressive effects of cholesterol. This is because of expression of 7-α-hydroxylase in the liver, where this enzyme metabolises hydro-xylated sterols as well as cholesterol to bile acids. Placing the LDL receptor gene into non-hepatic cells causes them to take on the hepatic phenotype of resistance of the LDL receptor to repression by cholesterol. Bile acid sequestrants work by increasing oxysterol flux through this pathway and increasing LDL receptor gene expression.

A diet rich in cholesterol and saturated fats nevertheless has the greatest adverse effect. In a population with a low fat and low cholesterol

intake a genetic propensity to an increased blood cholesterol does not exhibit itself. Nature and nurture both have large roles in familial hypercholesterolaemia.

Homozygosity for the apoE2 allele, which does not bind to the LDL receptor, has severe effects on the familial hypercholesterolaemia phenotype. Inheritance of high concentrations of lipoprotein (a) reduces the risk of coronary disease in subjects with familial hypercholesterolaemia. Transcription of the LDL receptor is negatively regulated by intracellular cholesterol. This process is mediated by hydroxylated cholesterol metabolites.

The E4 allele occurs in 30% of the general population. Heterozygotes with alleles E3/E4 have cholesterol concentrations 10% higher than E3/E3 homozygotes and consequent effects on CHD risk.

Lipoproteins apoB and apoA-I may be better than LDL or HDL-cholesterol as a predictor of coronary artery risk. In the post-absorptive phase, apoB is found not only in LDL but also in VLDL, intermediate-density lipoprotein and lipoprotein (a); apoA-I is found in HDL. Such a measurement allows a measure of total atherogenic particles (apoB) and antiatherogenic particles (apoA-I).

There is a *polymorphism* in the gene for the angiotensin-converting enzyme (ACE). A dele-tion/insertion has been found in intron 16 of the ACE gene. Deletion polymorphism has been found more frequently in patients who have suffered a myocardial infarction. Individuals who are homozygous for the deletion allele have plasma ACE concentrations twice as high as in individuals homozygous for the insertion allele.

Many retrospective studies have shown a positive relationship between moderate *hyperhomocys-teinaemia*, occlusive arterial disease and myocardial infarction. The accumulation of excessive homo-cysteine causes damage to endothelial and smooth-muscle cells, and alters the activity of coagulation factors.

Homocysteine is a sulfur-containing amino acid formed during the metabolism of methionine, which is metabolised by trans-sulfuration to cysteine through cystathionine or by remethylation to methionin, the more important cause of increased plasma homocysteine concentrations. The methyl group may be replaced by a process catalysed by the vitamin B_{12}-dependent methionine synthase, with 5-methyl-tetrahydrofolate as methyl donor, or by betaine-homocysteine methyltransferase, with betaine as the methyl donor. Homocysteinuria is due to a defect in:

- trans-sulfuration.
- or remethylation of homocysteine.

Plasma homocysteine concentrations increase in males with age, in females following the menopause, and with cigarette smoking, coffee drinking and meat consumption.

Hereditary causes of increased plasma homocysteine concentrations include 5,10-methylenetetrahydrofolate reductase and cystathione-β-synthase deficiency.

Hyperhomocysteinaemia is readily corrected by dietary supplementation with folate (400 mg/day) or betaine and is of relevance in clinical improvement in individuals with coronary artery disease problems. Vitamin B_6 supplements of 100–200 mg/day radically reduce the risk of angina and myocardial infarction, and extend the lifespan.

DIET AND LIFESTYLE CHANGES

Many predictors of coronary events are in some way attributable to lifestyle. These include cigarette smoking, weight, serum cholesterol and triglycerides, low HDL-cholesterol, blood pressure, physical activity, alcohol intake, and fruit and vegetable consumption. The most sensitive method of identifying those at risk is to use the total cholesterol concentration of more than 6.5 mmol/l, and more accurately the total cholesterol:HDL-cholesterol ratio and apply these to the Sheffield tables. The Sheffield tables and the New Zealand tables take into account the key variables in coronary artery risk: systolic hypertension, smoking, diabetes, total:HDL-cholesterol ratio, age and gender (Figure 47.7).

- **Smoking**: Coronary deaths occur twice as often in smokers compared with non-smokers. Stopping smoking is possibly the most important step in reducing the risk of CHD. Socio-economic factors acting over the lifetime of the person affect health and the risk of premature death.
- **Obesity** or waist:hip ratio (indicative of central obesity) adversely affects the risk factors by significant amounts. Cardiovascular mortality increases by 40% with a BMI between 24 and 30, and by 100% with a BMI over 30.
- **Cholesterol reduction**: using such a measurement as the serum triglyceride has little predictive value. Every 1% decrease in serum cholesterol is rewarded by a 1.5–2.5 % decrease in risk. This is achieved by diet with a reduced fat intake, by using polyunsaturated fatty acids and reducing weight to the ideal for height. Eating oily fish two or three times a week is helpful. In populations at risk of CHD, there is an individual variation in response to changes in dietary fat. This is not due to variable dietary compliance and may be determined by individual lipid metabolic activities, apolipoprotein concentrations and other polygenic factors.
- **Alcohol**: small amounts are protective, but more than 25 units/week are harmful.
- **Fruit and vegetables** contain many positive additions to a healthy diet and are recommended.
- **Food frequency**: concentrations of cholesterol and low-density lipoproteins are favourably affected by the frequency of eating. Eating six times a day reduces by 5% on average the serum cholesterol and LDLs. Serum cholesterol concentrations fall after the age of 70 years, but without reduction in the rate of CHD.
- **Blood pressure reduction**: this may be helped by weight loss, reducing salt intake, alcohol reduction and exercise, but most of all by hypotensive therapy.
- **Exercise**: helps the general condition and augments lipid-reduction regimens. Maintaining or taking light or moderate exercise reduces mortality and heart attacks in older men with or without diagnosed cardiovascular disease.
- **Educational status** is important; studies have demonstrated that less educated people in India have a higher prevalence of CHD, hypertension and smoking.

Cholesterol concentration (mmol/L) in men

	1	2	3	4	5	6	7	8	9	10	11	12
Hypertension	Yes	Yes	Yes	Yes	Yes	Yes	No	No	Yes	Yes	No	No
Smoking	Yes	Yes	Yes	No	Yes	No	Yes	Yes	No	No	No	No
Diabetes	Yes	No	Yes	Yes	No	No	Yes	No	Yes	No	Yes	No
LVH	Yes	Yes	No	Yes	No	Yes	No	No	No	No	No	No

Age (years)												
70	5.5	5.5	5.7	5.9	6.5	6.8	7.2	8.3	8.4			
69	5.5	5.5	5.9	6.1	6.8	7.0	7.5	8.6	8.8			
68	5.5	5.5	6.3	6.4	7.1	7.3	7.8	9.0	9.1			
67	5.5	5.5	6.4	6.7	7.3	7.6	8.1	9.3				
66	5.5	5.5	6.7	6.9	7.7	8.0	8.5					
65	5.5	5.6	7.0	7.2	8.0	8.3	8.8					
64	5.5	5.8	7.3	7.5	8.3	8.6	9.2					
63	5.5	6.1	7.6	7.9	8.7	9.0						
62	5.5	6.3	7.9	8.2	9.1							
61	5.8	6.6	8.3	8.6								
60	6.0	6.9	8.7	9.0								
59	6.3	7.3	9.1									
58	6.6	7.6										
57	7.0	8.0										
56	7.3	8.4										
55	7.7	8.8										
54	8.1	9.3										
53	8.5											
52	9.0											
<52												

Cholesterol concentration (mmol/L) in women

	1	2	3	4	5	6	7	8	9	10	11	12
Hypertension	Yes	Yes	Yes	No	Yes	Yes	No	Yes	Yes	No	Yes	No
Smoking	Yes	Yes	No	Yes	No	Yes	No	Yes	No	Yes	No	No
Diabetes	Yes	Yes	Yes	Yes	Yes	No	Yes	No	No	No	No	No
LVH	Yes	No	Yes	No	No	Yes	No	No	Yes	No	No	No

Age (years)												
70	5.5	7.1	7.4	9.0								
69	5.5	7.4	7.7	9.4								
68	5.5	7.7	8.0	9.8								
67	5.6	8.0	8.3									
66	5.8	8.4	8.7									
65	6.1	8.7	9.1									
64	6.4	9.1	9.4									
63	6.6	9.5	9.9									
62	6.9	9.9										
61	7.2											
60	7.6											
59	7.9											
58	8.3											
57	8.7											
56	9.2											
55	9.6											
54	10.1											
<54												

Fig. 47.7 The Sheffield risk and treatment table for primary prevention of coronary heart disease. A person whose value falls in the unshaded area has an estimated risk of coronary heart disease of less than 1.5%.

KEY POINTS

1. Coronary heart disease (CHD) is associated with populations who eat a high saturated fat intake and in whom the serum lipids are increased. The CHD in such populations is, to a large extent, concentrated within genetically vulnerable families.
2. Dietary constituents that increase protection from CHD include n-3- and n-6-containing fatty acids and oils, fruit and vegetables, and possibly red wine.
3. The atheromatous plaque formation that is the basis of CHD progresses through stages of a fatty streak, a fibrous plaque and a complicated arterial wall lesion. These are associated with the deposition of cholesterol in the form of lipoproteins, e.g. LDL lipoprotein.
4. Familial hypercholesterolaemia is an autosomal dominant trait with varying frequency in the population. The LDL-receptor gene mutations are well described and the mutation dictates the metabolic response. Hyperhomocysteinaemia is a risk factor correctable with folic acid or betaine supplementation.
5. Other gene mutations, e.g. apoE allele, have considerable effects on blood cholesterol concentrations.
6. There are well-developed risk evaluation tables that take into consideration systolic hypertension, smoking, diabetes, total cholesterol:HDL-cholesterol ratio, age and gender.
7. Many of the risk factors are correctable.

THINKING POINT

The short, overweight, middle-aged man who smokes, enjoys drinking with his friends and takes little exercise is a problem. What approaches should be made to reduce his risk of disease?

NEED TO UNDERSTAND

1. The risk factors of systolic hypertension, smoking, diabetes, total cholesterol:HDL-chole-sterol ratio, age and gender for coronary events.
2. How they may operate and how to treat the risk.
3. Male gender, age and height are significant contributors to these scores that cannot be changed.
4. This means that some risk factors have modest effect on prognosis.

FURTHER READING

Barker, D.J., Winter, P.D., Osmond, C. *et al.* (1989) Weight in infancy and death from ischaemic heart disease. *Lancet*, **ii**, 577–80.

Cook, P.J. and Lip, G.Y. (1996) Infectious agents and atherosclerotic vascular disease. *Quarterly Journal of Medicine*, **89**, 727–35.

Cox, C., Mann, J., Sutherland, W. and Ball, M. (1995) Individual variations in plasma cholesterol response to dietary saturated fat. *British Medical Journal*, **311**, 1260–4.

Day, N.M. and Wilson, D.I. (2001) Genetics and cardiovascular risk. *British Medical Journal*, **323**, 1409–12.

De Lorenzo, F., Sharma, V., Scully, M. and Kakkar, V.V. (1999) Cold adaptation and the seasonal distribution of acute myocardial infarction. *Quarterly Journal of Medicine*. **92**, 747–51.

Frankel, S., Elwood, P., Sweetnam, P. *et al.* (1996) Birth weight, body-mass index in middle age and incident coronary disease. *Lancet*, **348**, 1478–80.

French, C.C. (2001) Apolipoprotein B and A-1 as predictors of risk of coronary artery disease. *Lancet*, **358**, 2012–3.

Goldberg, A.C. and Schonfeld, G. (1985) Effects of diet on lipoprotein metabolism. *Annual Review of Nutrition*, **5**, 195–212.

Gupta, R., Gupta, V.P. and Ahluwalia, N.S. (1994) Educational status, coronary heart disease and coronary risk factor prevalence in a rural population in India. *British Medical Journal*, **309**, 1332–6.

Han, T.S., van Leer, E.M., Seidell, J.C. and Lean, M.E. (1995) Waist circumference action levels in the identification of cardiovascular risk factors: prevalence study in a random sample. *British Medical Journal*, **311**, 1401–5.

Hankey, G.J. and Eikelboom, J.W. (1999) Homocysteine and vascular disease. *Lancet*, **354**, 407–13.

Haq, I.U., Ramsay, L.E., Jackson, P.R. and Wallis, E.J. (1999) Prediction of coronary risk for primary prevention of coronary heart disease: a comparison of methods. *Quarterly Journal of Medicine*, **92**, 379–85.

Levy, D. and Kennel, W. B. (2000) Searching for answers to ethnic disparities in cardiovascular risks. *Lancet*, **356**, 266–7.

McGee, J.O'D., Isaacson, P.G. and Wright, N.A. (1992) *Oxford Textbook of Pathology*. Oxford Medical Publications, Oxford.

Mohan, I.V. and Stansby, G. (1999) Nutritional hyperhomocysteinaemia. *British Medical Journal*, **318**, 1569–70.

Pan, W.-H., Li, L.-A. and Tsai, M.-J. (1995) Temperature extremes and mortality from coronary heart disease and cerebral infarction in elderly Chinese. *Lancet*, **345**, 353–5.

Parthasarathy, S., Steinberg, D. and Witztum, J.L. (1992) The role of oxidized low-density lipoproteins in the pathogenesis of atherosclerosis. *Annual Review of Medicine*, **43**, 219–25.

Ramsay, L.E., Haq, I.U., Wallis, E.J. and Isles, C. (1999) Diet and lifestyle changes in the primary prevention of coronary heart disease. *Proceedings of the Royal College of Physicians of Edinburgh*, **29**, (Suppl. 5), 5–9.

Report of a Working Party too the Chief Medical Officer for Scotland (1993) *Scotland's Health – A Challenge to Us All*. Scottish Office.

Rimm, E.B., Klatsky, A., Grobbe, D. and Stampfer, M.J. (1996) Review of moderate alcohol consumption and reduced risk of coronary heart disease: is the effect due to beer, wine or spirits? *British Medical Journal*, **312**, 731–6.

Schatz, I.J., Masaki, K., Yano, K., *et al.* (2001) Cholesterol and all-cause mortality in elderly people from Honolulu Heart Programme: a cohort study. *Lancet*, **358**, 351–5.

Smith, G.D., Hart, C., Blane, D., *et al.* (1997) Lifetime socioeconomic position and mortality: prospective observational study. *British Medical Journal*, **314**, 547–52.

Symposium on 'Reducing cardiovascular disease risk: today's achievements, tommorrow's opportunities'. (2000) *Proceedings of the Nutrition Society*, **59**, 415–26.

Titan, S.M.O., Bingham, S., Welch, A. *et al.* (2001) Frequency of eating and concentrations of serum cholesterol in the Norfolk population of the European prospective investigation into cancer (EPIC-Norfolk): a cross sectional study. *British Medical Journal*, **323**, 1286–8.

Wannamethee, S.G., Shaper, A.G. and Walker, M. (1998) Changes in physical activity, mortality, and incidence of coronary heart disease in older men. *Lancet*, **351**, 1603–8.

Warrell, D.A., Cox, T.M., Firth, J.D. and Benz, E.J. Jr (eds) (2003) *Oxford Textbook of Medicine*, 4th edn. Oxford Medical Publications, Oxford.

Index